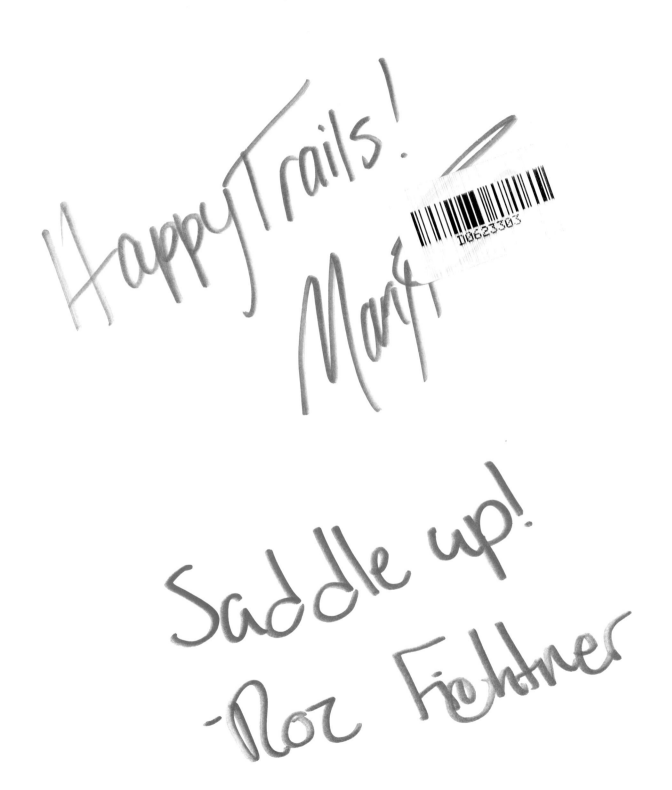

Happy Trails!
Mary

Saddle up!
-Roz Fichtner

This book belongs to

Jace Warren Beck ,

a new friend of Rusty the Ranch Horse

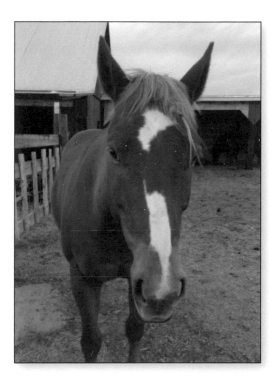

Rusty is honest and true, a dependable work mate and loyal friend. He always does his best and comes to greet visitors, especially if they might have a treat. When you gain his trust he will be a loyal friend for life!

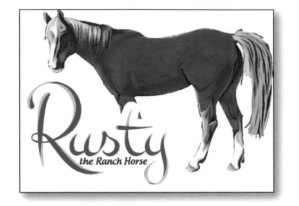

Rusty and His Saddle
A Rusty the Ranch Horse Tale

© 2017 by Mary Fichtner
All rights reserved

Illustrations by Roz Fichtner

Layout and Design by Andy Grachuk
www.JingotheCat.com

Rusty and His Saddle

A Rusty the Ranch Horse Tale

Rusty rose with the sun that matched his bright hue

Leaving orange colored tints on the grass in the dew

Dazzling and smart is how his cowboy saw Rusty

Though once in a while he appeared to be dusty

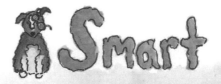 Smart

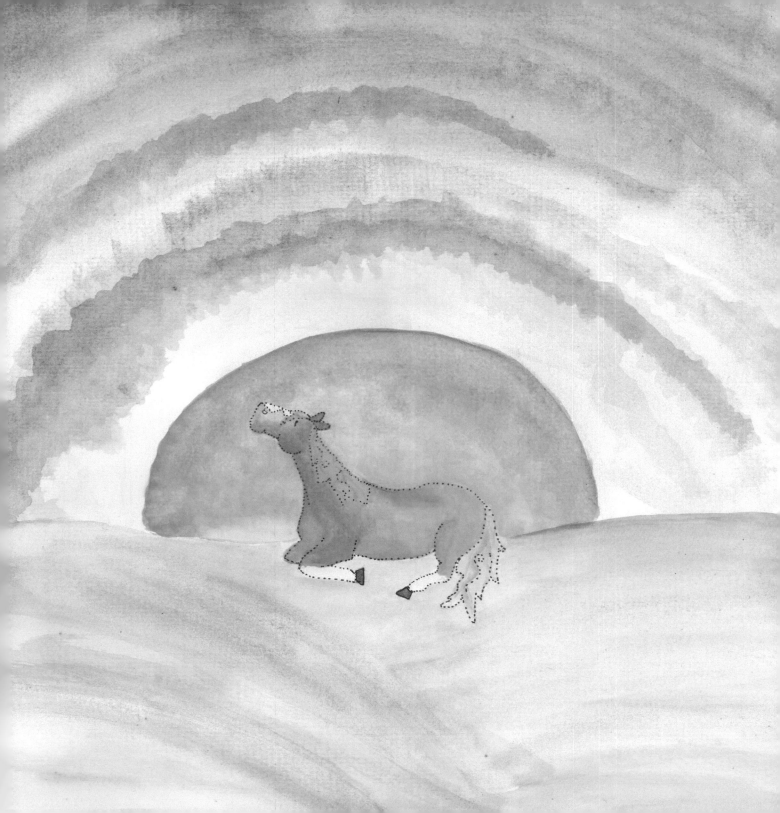

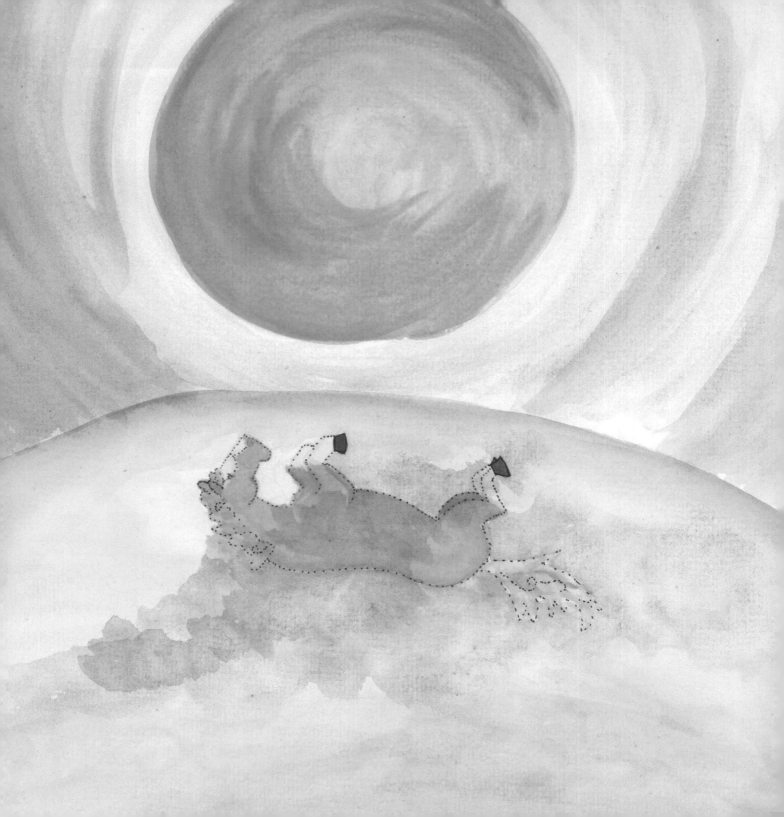

Rusty loved to roll in the soft brown dirt

It seemed there was nothing at all it would hurt

After all a good horse should be comfortable too

There's no need to always look brand spanking new

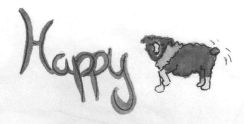

Once in a while his cowboy would ride

Along with some others to work by their side

So he'd brush the fine dirt off Rusty's strong back

And throw on his saddle and other horse tack

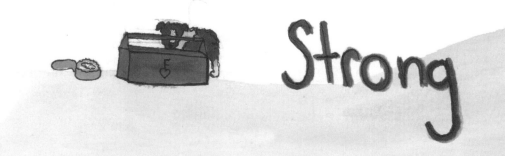

Strong

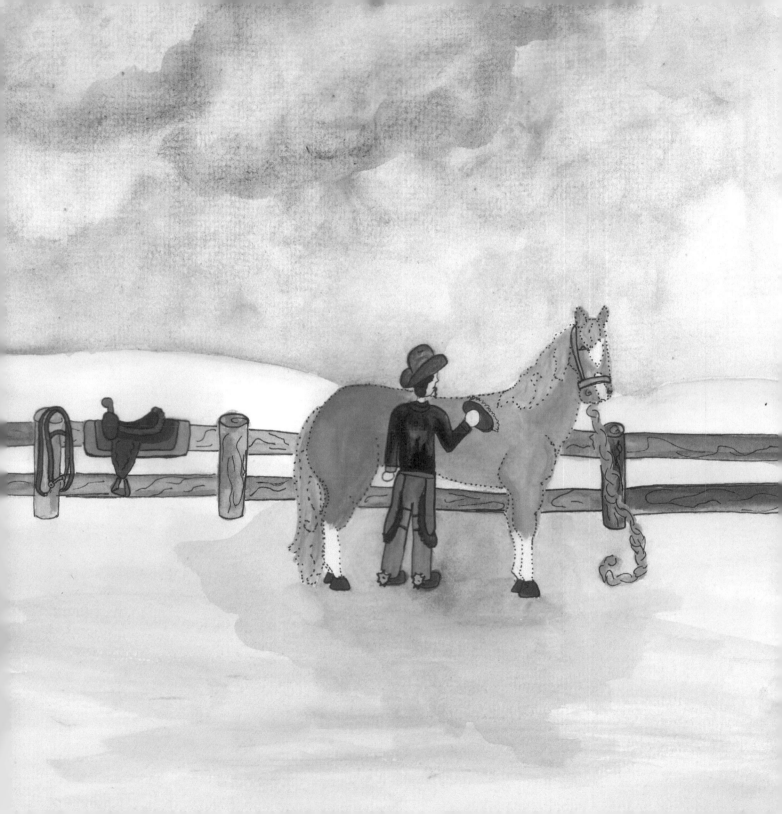

Rusty's saddle was different but he didn't care

Though he noticed the others sometimes would stare

His saddle was scratched and worn and old

While the others had new ones, they'd won them they told

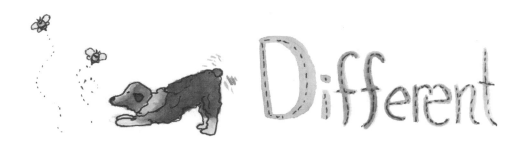

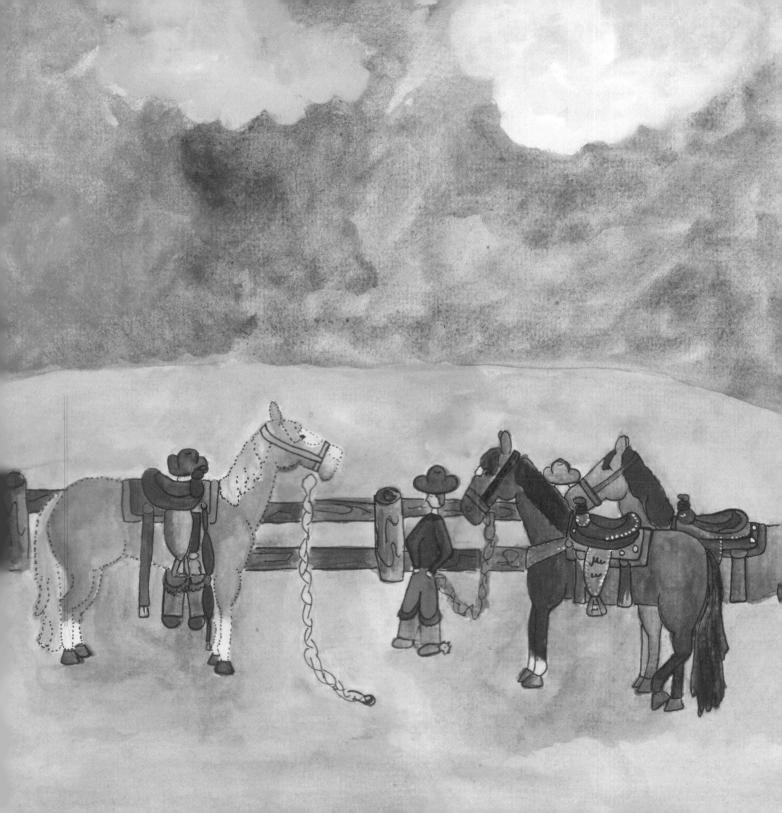

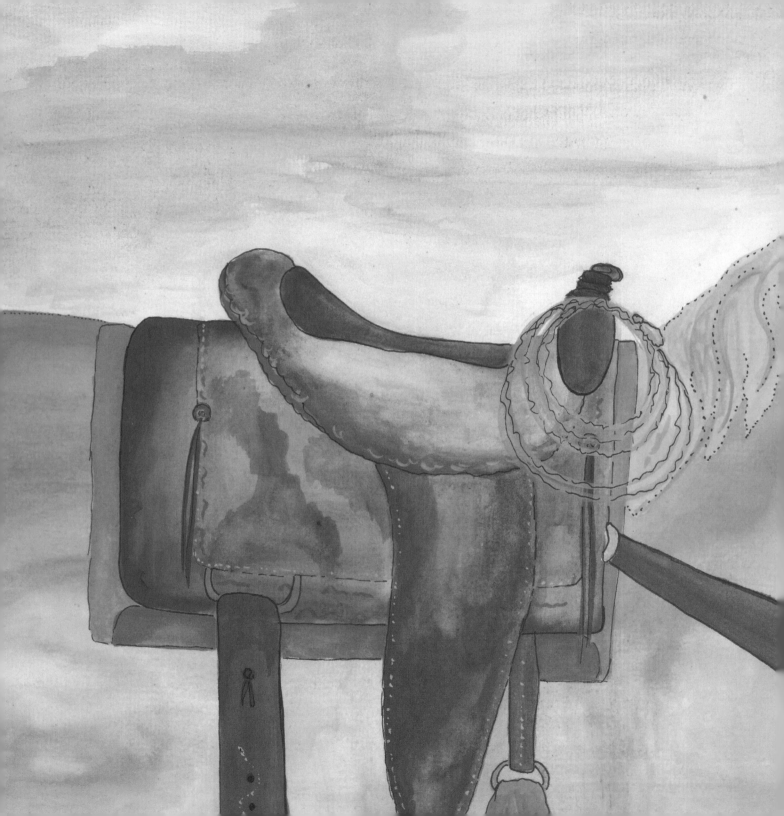

The cowboy loved Rusty's saddle he wore

It fit Rusty just right so he loved it some more

Though it had places on it that needed repair

And spots that could use some mending and care

Love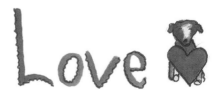

But isn't a saddle's purpose in life

To carry a rider without any strife?

And that's just what it did, you can bet your best hat!

But the others just snickered, snubbing noses at that

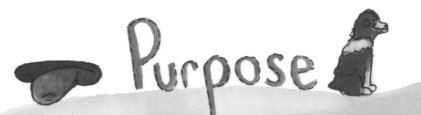

Purpose

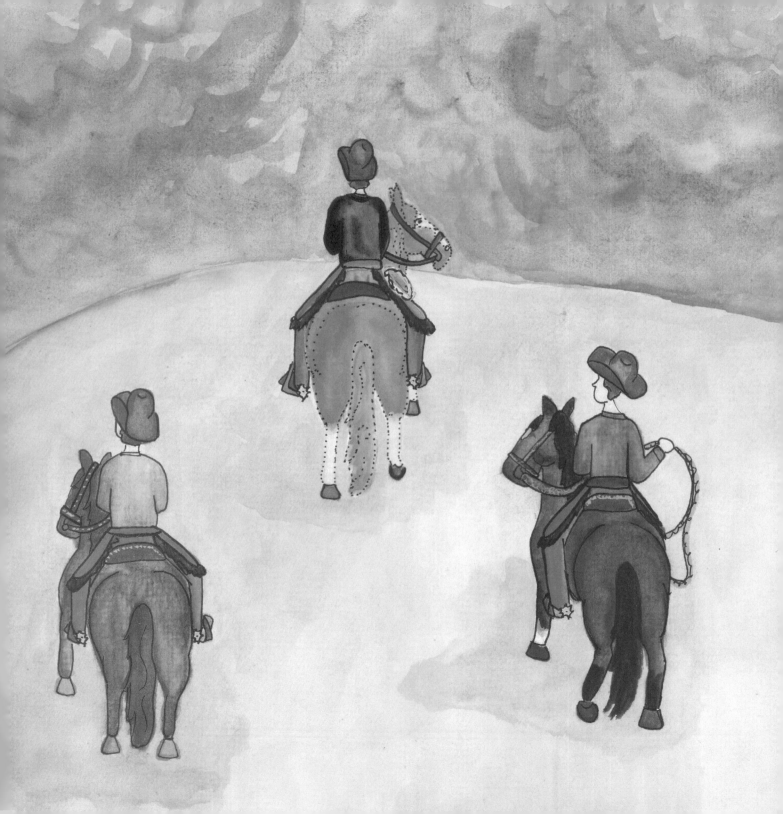

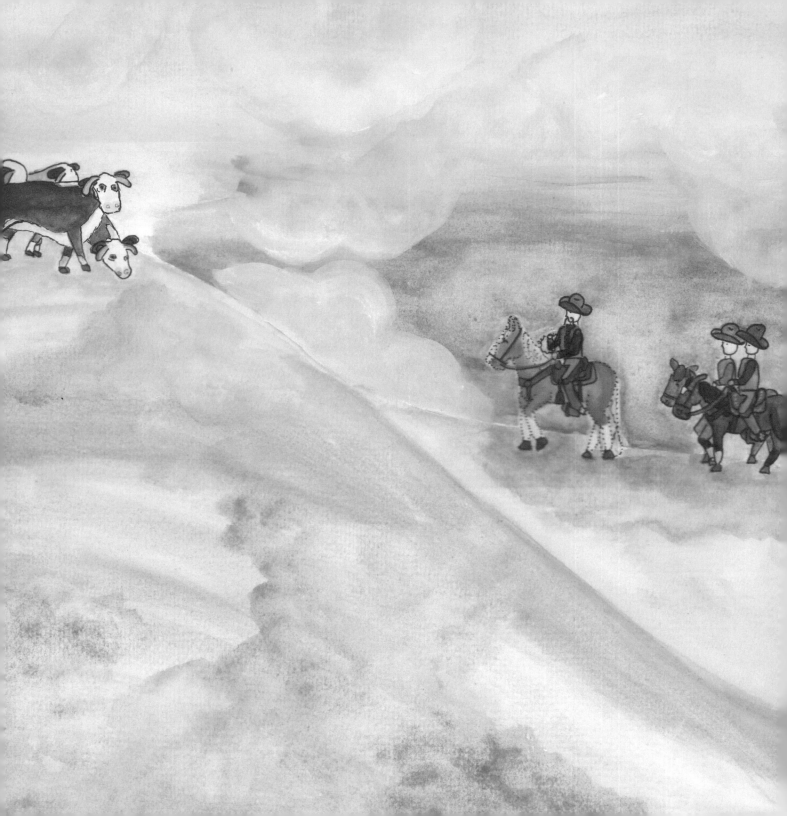

Rusty could see this and it made his heart sad

But at the same time a tad bit of mad

He knew that the outsides don't make someone shine

And maybe they'd notice at just the right time

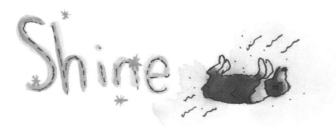

Rusty didn't show off or try to be loud

He just did his work and stood tall and proud

He offered a hoof when help became needed

And jumped at the tasks for which he was deeded

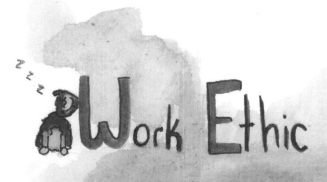

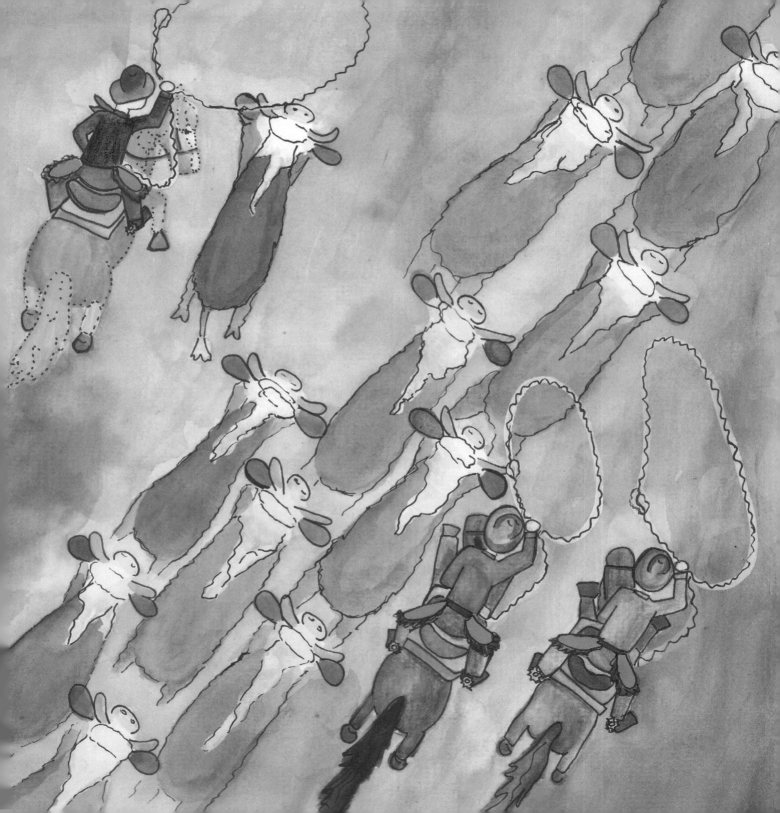

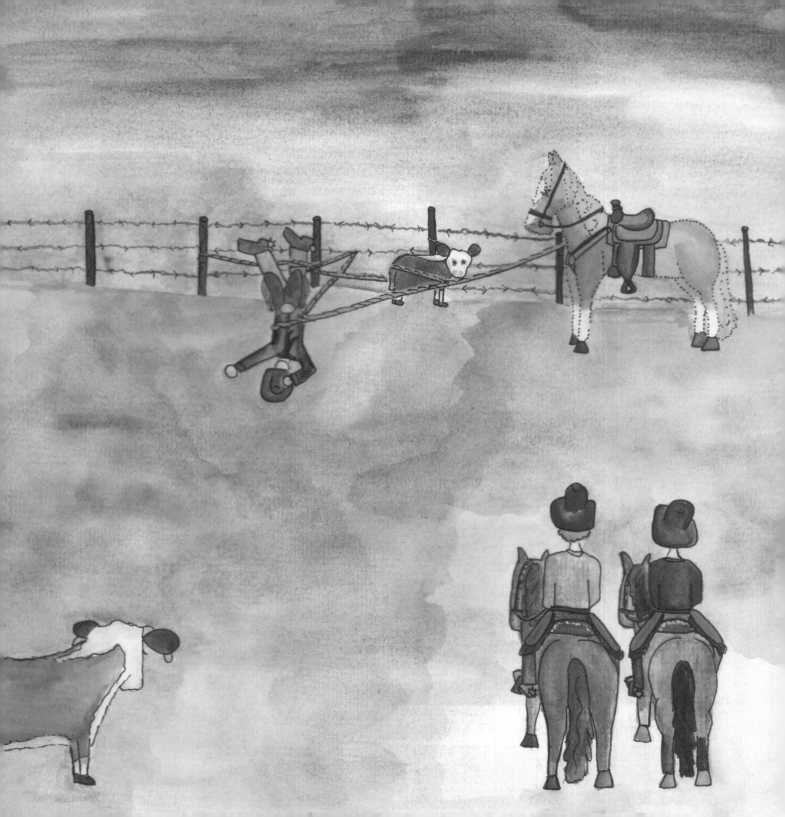

But above all of that when a wreck reared its head

Rusty helped fix it while some others just fled

He never gave up when the going got rough

He proved to himself in his heart he was tough

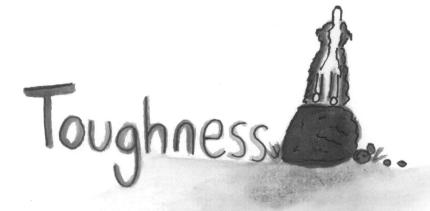

Toughness

After all of this happened time and again

His saddle looked polished because of his grin

It appeared that the others might learn something great

Saddles and outfits don't character make

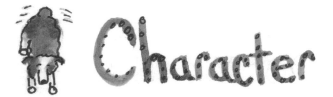 Character

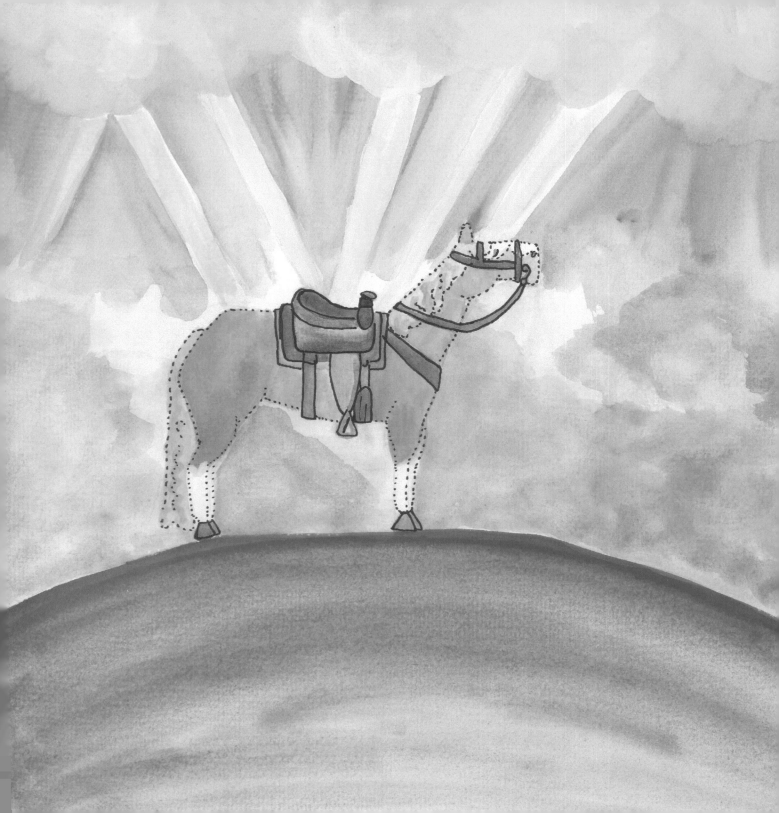

It's what's on the inside that counts most of all

It's where boldness comes from to get up when we fall

For when we are brave on the inside it shines

Through on the outside during hard times

And we can be sure others will know

Our courage inside by the actions we show

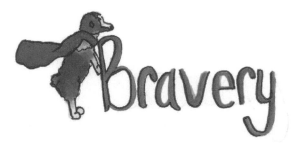

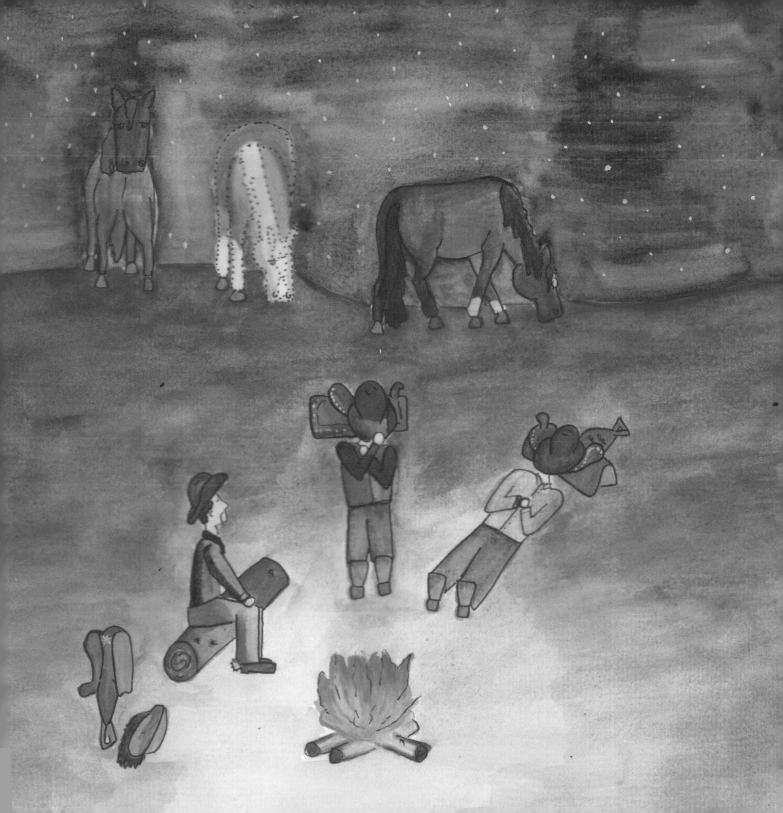

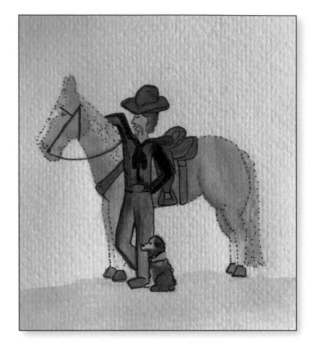

Official Code of Ethics of Wyoming

An Act declaring "The Code of the West" as the official state code of Wyoming was signed into law on March 3rd, 2010. Wyoming is the first state to adopt a code of ethics.

The legislation designates ten ethics derived from the book "Cowboy Ethics" by James P. Owen:

1. Live each day with courage.
2. Take pride in your work.
3. Always finish what you start.
4. Do what has to be done.
5. Be tough, but fair.
6. When you make a promise, keep it.
7. Ride for the brand
8. Talk less, say more.
9. Remember that some things are not for sale.
10. Know where to draw the line.

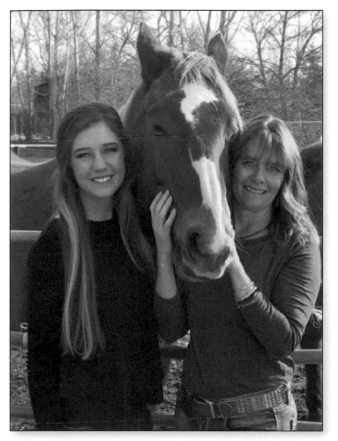

Rozlyn Fichtner, Rusty, Mary Fichtner

"It's the way you ride the trail that counts!"
Dale Evans

A saddle that fits your horse makes for a much happier horse, but ultimately the way you ride matters much more. Choosing to follow the cowboy ethics is a great start. The western lifestyle requires courage and hard work. Mother and daughter, author and illustrator, and horse lovers Mary and Rozlyn hope that as you read about Rusty you will choose to ride your trails in a way that matters and makes the world a better place.

CPSIA information can be obtained at www.ICGtesting.com
Printed in the USA
LVIW01n1900030317
526113LV00003B/3

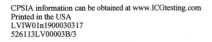

KOREAN
ART

KOREAN ART

FROM

THE BROOKLYN MUSEUM

COLLECTION

ROBERT J. MOES

UNIVERSE BOOKS
New York

Note: Items listed in the catalogue as loans are, without
exception, promised gifts and will all enter the permanent
collection of The Brooklyn Museum within a few years of
this exhibition.

Published in the United States of America in 1987
by Universe Books
381 Park Avenue South, New York, NY 10016

87   88 89 90 91 / 10 9 8 7 6 5 4 3 2 1

Printed in Hong Kong

Library of Congress Cataloging-in-Publication Data
Moes, Robert.
    Korean art.

    Bibliography: p.
    1. Art, Korean—Catalogs.   2. Art—New York (N.Y.)—
Catalogs.   3. Brooklyn Museum—Catalogs.   I. Brooklyn
Museum.   II. Title.
N7362.M64   1987   709′.519′074014723   87-13752
ISBN 0-87663-654-7
ISBN 0-87663-516-8 (pbk.)

Design by John Bellacosa

Cover illustration: **56. Three Jumping Carp**

CONTENTS

Foreword   vii
Preface: The Brooklyn Museum's Korean Collection   ix
Introduction: The Historical Context of Korean Art   1
Prologue: The Uniqueness of Korean Art   19
Catalog   21
   The Chinese Colony at Lo-lang   23
   The Kaya Confederacy   27
   The Silla Period   33
   The United Silla Period   41
   The Koryo Dynasty   47
   The Yi Dynasty   71
   Modern Korea   199
Selected Bibliography   205
Color Plates   207

FOREWORD

The Brooklyn Museum's collection of Korean art is among the most comprehensive in the United States. It includes all periods of Korean cultural history from the Bronze-Iron Age to the mid-20th century and is particularly rich in Korean folk art, seldom seen outside its country of origin.

Although the Museum has for several years maintained the only permanent installation of Korean art in the New York area, limited gallery space has permitted only a fractional portion of the Korean collection to be on display at any one time. A hundred of the finest and most characteristic examples of Korean art from the collection were thus selected for the special exhibition documented by this catalogue. These works represent every important category of Korean art (except architecture), including painting, sculpture, ceramics, lacquer, metalwork, furniture, and embroidery. Few other American museums are capable of mounting such a major Korean art exhibition entirely from their own collections.

Robert Moes, Curator of Oriental Art at the Museum, both selected the objects for the exhibition and wrote this catalogue. In 1985 Mr. Moes was recognized by the government of South Korea for his "valuable contribution to acquainting the American public with Korean culture and promoting friendship between the two countries."

Robert T. Buck
Director, The Brooklyn Museum

PREFACE

THE BROOKLYN MUSEUM'S KOREAN COLLECTION

Stewart Culin (1858–1929) was Curator of Ethnology at The Brooklyn Museum from 1902 to 1928. In those days, The Brooklyn Museum was a museum of science and history as well as of art. Around 1930, the Board of Governors decided to make The Brooklyn Museum an art museum exclusively. Pursuant to that decision, the museum's large collections of stuffed animals, birds, fish, bones, rocks, and plaster casts were transferred to the American Museum of Natural History in Manhattan.

However, a large quantity of anthropological material collected in the field by Stewart Culin was retained at The Brooklyn Museum. By the 1930s this type of material, formerly considered merely ethnographical, had been admitted into the realm of the fine arts as antiquities, or as pre-Columbian, tribal, or folk art. Culin was a remarkably energetic and resourceful man. He made extensive collecting trips to Mexico, Central and South America, Africa, China, Japan, and Korea. Gathering masks and spirit figures from tribal villages in the African bush in the early years of this century was a difficult and sometimes dangerous business, and in Mexico and China, bandits plagued the expeditions.

In 1913 Culin made a collecting trip to Korea. The armor, helmet, and mandarin squares in this exhibition were acquired on that trip. Culin mentioned his Korean trip in a letter dated February 24, 1926 to William H. Fox, The Brooklyn Museum's Director from 1914 to 1933. In that letter Culin complained that the material he had collected was not on display: "The important and beautiful Korean collection I secured in Korea in 1913 is now out of sight in the basement."

When I joined the staff of The Brooklyn Museum in 1973, the situation remained the same; no Korean art was on display, in spite of the fact that many superb Korean works of art had entered Brooklyn's collection during the 1930s, 40s, 50s, and 60s. In order to remedy this, we applied to the National Endowment for the Arts and received a grant to renovate the Japanese Galleries. We sacrificed one-fourth of the Japanese gallery space in favor of Korea. The handsome and functional new Japanese and Korean Galleries opened in 1974 and remain an important part of The Brooklyn Museum's permanent installation.

During the 1970s and the first half of the 1980s, we systematically acquired, through donation and purchase, a wide range of Korean art to fill gaps in the Museum's collection, which is now one of the most comprehensive in the United States. The Brooklyn Museum maintains the only permanent display of Korean art in the New York City area.

Robert Moes
Curator of Oriental Art

ACKNOWLEDGMENTS

The author wishes to express his profound gratitude to Ms. Myung-suk Tae for translating the inscriptions on items in the catalog and to Mrs. Eunwoo Lee for her research on Buddhist paintings and sculpture in the collection.

This catalog and the exhibition, From the Land of Morning Calm: Korean Art at the Brooklyn Museum, were made possible, in part, by support from Republic New York Corporation. The exhibition received generous support from the National Endowment for the Arts, a federal agency.

KOREAN
ART

INTRODUCTION

THE HISTORICAL CONTEXT OF KOREAN ART

The Korean peninsula arches roughly 620 miles southward and slightly eastward from the southeastern corner of Manchuria, which is now part of the People's Republic of China. Its boundary with Korea is formed by two rivers flowing in opposite directions from closely situated sources. The Amnok River (called the Yalu by the Chinese) flows southwest into the Yellow Sea, the body of water separating Korea from the coast of North China. The Tuman River (Tumen in Chinese) flows northeast into the Sea of Japan. Just before reaching the sea, the Tuman River becomes the boundary between Korea and a tip of the USSR near Vladivostok.

The Sea of Japan separates the Siberian coast and Korean peninsula from the Japanese archipelago. The Straits of Tsushima, between the southeastern tip of Korea and the northwest coast of Kyūshū, southernmost of the four main islands of Japan, is only 128 miles wide, easily navigable in good weather even by primitive boats. Since early times, because of its geographic position, the Korean peninsula has functioned as a land bridge through which peoples and cultural developments from mainland Asia have reached Japan.

The area of Korea is about 86,000 square miles. The present population is approximately 53,270,000. The Korean peninsula is rugged and mountainous; hills and mountains occupy about 70 percent of its area and only about one-fifth of the land can be farmed. The great T'aebaek mountain range runs along the east coast, forming the spine of the peninsula and leaving only a narrow strip of land between the mountains and the Sea of Japan. The mighty Nangnim mountain range lies parallel to the Amnok (Yalu) River in northern Korea, forming a barrier between Korea and Manchuria. The T'aebaek chain connects perpendicularly with the Nangnim range.

In early times, the mountains of Korea were densely forested. In recent centuries, forests have survived only in the more remote mountains. All the timber on nearby hills and peaks was cut long ago to burn as firewood against the extreme cold of the winters,

during which a fierce wind from Siberia howls through Korea, penetrating even several layers of clothing. Today an admirable government reforestation program is turning the hills and mountains of South Korea green again.

The most noticeable and characteristic feature of Korean topography is granite: huge, rough masses of exposed granite jut up everywhere among the sparse cover of brush and small trees on the slopes of hills and mountains. In certain areas, such as the famous Diamond Mountains, near the east coast of Korea just above the thirty-eighth parallel, granite boulders have assumed fantastic shapes, like thousands of rock spires.

South of the Nangnim Mountains and west of the T'aebaek range lie numerous river valleys and coastal plains ideal for growing rice and other crops. While the east coast is narrow and almost without harbors, the south and west coasts are broken by countless inlets, bays, and small islands affording excellent harbors. Many varieties of fish abound in the seas surrounding the peninsula and form an important part of the Korean diet.

The Koreans are a hardy people. They are somewhat larger in stature than the Chinese and Japanese. Their personality is direct and rather volatile; they have little patience with pretense and over-refinement. Koreans have a much stronger class consciousness than do the more egalitarian Chinese, and they are less tense and regimented than the Japanese. The ancestors of the Koreans were nomadic peoples of Mongoloid racial stock who came from the forests and grasslands of northern Asia.

The Korean language is related to the Altaic language group, named after the Altai Mountains of Central Asia. Turkish, Manchu, and Mongolian belong to this language group; Finnish and Japanese are related to it. These various languages have dissimilar vocabularies and are mutually unintelligible, but their structures are similar: They are polysyllabic, agglutinative languages, that is, they have words that are often several syllables long, and to many words are added endings indicating their role in the sentence. This is completely different from Chinese, which is monosyllabic and uninflected; a Chinese word's function is indicated entirely by its position in the sentence.

In spite of the total incompatibility of the Korean and Chinese languages, virtually all writing in Korea prior to the mid-15th century was done in Chinese. Lacking a writing system of its own, Korea relied on classical written Chinese, which was introduced into Korea as early as the 3rd century B.C. *Idu*, a hybrid system using Chinese ideograms to represent Korean sounds, was invented in the late 7th century A.D. but never widely used. A simple, nearly perfect system for writing Korean was developed at the command of Sejong, fourth king of the Yi Dynasty, and officially adopted by royal decree in 1446. It was originally called *onmun* (vernacular writing) but is called *han'gul* (Korean letters) today. However, after its introduction, all scholarly and official writing continued to be done in Chinese. *Han'gul* was only used by women and other poorly educated persons. Only since the end of World War II, after the expulsion of the Japanese from Korea, has *han'gul* really come into its own as the standard system for writing the Korean language.

Japan annexed Korea in 1910 and held it until 1945. Its geographic position, with fierce nomadic peoples to the north in Manchuria and Mongolia, the huge and often powerful Chinese empire to the west, and the aggressive Japanese to the east, has unfortunately resulted in frequent incursions, invasions, and conquests by its various neighbors since early times. During the annexation, Japanese was imposed on Korea as the official language. Prior to 1910, the continuous use of classical Chinese as the written language of the educated classes had naturally facilitated wholesale Korean borrowing of Chinese philosophical, political, literary, and artistic forms and ideas. Over and over throughout its history, Korea welcomed overwhelming cultural influence from China. Yet the native cultural substructure remained distinctive and vigorous beneath the official overlay of Chinese civilization. It is in folk art, for example, that the Korean artistic genius expresses itself most vividly, since the art of the court and the scholar bureaucrats usually struggled to be as Chinese as possible.

THE NEOLITHIC PERIOD

In Neolithic times, Korea was occupied by various tribal groups who had pottery and polished stone tools but no agriculture. Primarily of Mongoloid racial stock, these peoples migrated from the forests and steppes of north Asia across the mountainous border into the Korean peninsula by the third millennium B.C. They became the principal ancestors of the Korean people. As noted previously, the Korean language provides evidence for this; it is similar to others associated with the Altai Mountains of northern Central Asia.

Lacking agriculture, the Neolithic inhabitants of Korea were dependent on fishing, hunting, and gathering. The remains of their village sites are often adjacent to shell mounds, indicating that shellfish were a significant part of their diet. These shell mounds, the garbage dumps of antiquity, have yielded pottery shards, as well as implements made of stone, bone, or shell. The pottery is often decorated with combed patterns. A toothed implement was used to scratch designs of short, parallel lines on the surface of the clay before firing. Comb markings are common on Neolithic pottery of Siberia, Manchuria, and Mongolia, but rare on early Chinese ceramics. Neolithic Korean pottery was fired in shallow, open pits; the kiln had not yet been invented.

Some of the Neolithic pottery shards excavated in Korea resemble Japanese earthenware of the Jōmon Period (c. 6000–300 B.C.). From the skeletal evidence of burials near their shell mounds and villages, the Jōmon people were of Caucasoid racial stock. Their ancestors presumably came from Siberia to northern Japan by boat and spread south until they eventually occupied the entire archipelago. The diversity of facial types among modern Koreans, and the fact that some Korean men have relatively profuse facial hair, may indicate a Caucasian strain among their ancestors. Some of the Caucasian tribes in Siberia may have crossed the mountains into the Korean peninsula during the Neolithic Period at the time when others like them were migrating to Japan.

Neolithic Koreans constructed dolmens—huge, table-like stone monuments consisting of two or more upright stones supporting a horizontal stone slab. These dolmens offer further confirmation of the north Asian origin of the early Korean peoples, especially since they are encountered frequently in northern Asia but have not been found in China.

Shamanism, the indigenous religion of Korea, is descended from the animistic beliefs of these early peoples from the forests and grasslands of north-eastern Asia. A sentient spirit dwells in every animal, tree, rock, or mountain, and they must be propitiated by shamans so that they will cooperate rather than work against men.

Tigers and bears were worshiped by Neolithic Koreans, just as they were by many of the early forest peoples of north Asia. The tiger has continued to be a potent Shamanist guardian spirit and frequent subject of Korean folk paintings until recent times (see Cat. 54). A bear and a tiger figure prominently in the story of Tangun, the legendary founder of Korea (traditionally in 2333 B.C.). Comma-shaped stone beads based on the form of a tiger or bear claw were worn by the early inhabitants of Korea. They continued to be used well into historic times, for example as ornaments on the gold crowns and ceremonial belts found in 5th–6th-century Korean tombs of the Silla Period. In the 4th and 5th centuries, Silla warriors invaded Japan and installed one of their clan chieftains as the first emperor, so the *magatama* (curved jewels), which form part of the Japanese imperial regalia, are identical to the comma-shaped beads of early Korea. Shintō, the indigenous religion of Japan, in its orginal form, was very similar to early Korean animism.

THE BRONZE/IRON AGE

During this period, from roughly 350 B.C. until the time of Christ, Korean culture advanced rapidly under the powerful influence of its two prime sources: the northern nomads and the Chinese. While the overlay of Chinese civilization has been more noticeable in historic times, early tribes from Manchuria, Mongolia, and Siberia were the main ancestors of the Korean people and also provided the original and lasting foundation of Korean culture.

Korea, like Japan, had no real Bronze Age, since bronze-casting technology and iron-forging technology were introduced from abroad in well-developed form at about the same time. Early bronze artifacts excavated in Korea have usually been found in conjunction with iron ones. Doubtless, many of the earliest metal implements used in Korea were imported. However, earthenware molds for casting bronze mirrors during this period have been excavated in Korea, indicating that early bronzes were produced locally as well as imported.

Prior to the establishment of a Chinese trading colony on Korean soil in 108 B.C., most of the bronze artifacts in Korea were made in the Scytho-Siberian style rather than the Chinese style. The term "Scytho-Siberian" is used to describe the culture of early nomadic peoples inhabiting the steppes and forests of a vast area stretching from the ancient country of Scythia near the Black and Aral seas all the way to the coast of Siberia. The surviving art of these early nomads consists primarily of small, portable metal artifacts such as weapons, horse fittings, and belt buckles, often taking the form of, or decorated with, figures of animals, and therefore referred to as "the animal style." The nomads raised cattle and sheep for food, hides, and wool. They depended on their sturdy, fast Mongol horses for transportation, hunting, and warfare. They hunted deer, bears, tigers, and other game. Animals were important to them and played significant roles in their spiritual beliefs and folklore as well as in their art.

The migration of northern nomad groups into Korea and the flow of cultural influence across the border from Manchuria, Mongolia, and Siberia continued sporadically until well into historic times. However, this influx of people and ideas was accelerated in the 4th century B.C., when the fierce Hsiung-nu horde from Mongolia menaced other nomadic tribes to its east in Manchuria and Siberia, causing many to flee across the mountains into the Korean peninsula, bringing with them a fully developed bronze and iron technology.

The Hsiung-nu were a federation of Turkish-speaking tribes, the same group known in the West as the Huns—"Hun" being very probably derived from the Chinese "Hsiung-nu." When some of the Hsiung-nu were driven westward around A.D. 200 by the powerful Han Dynasty (206 B.C.–A.D. 220) Chinese armies, they began pillaging eastern and central Europe.

Their fast and deadly mounted archers made the Hsiung-nu a threat not only to other nomad tribes but to the Chinese as well. Like other "Northern Barbarians" before and after them, the Hsiung-nu were constantly raiding towns along the northern frontier of China. It was against such incursions that the Chinese built the Great Wall, but to no avail—the nomads breached it time and again, almost at will. The "Barbarians" sometimes conquered large sections of China, and eventually all of it: the T'o-pa (Northern Wei Dynasty, 386–535) in northwestern China; the Khitan (Liao Dynasty, 947–1125) in north China; the Jurched (Chin Dynasty, 1126–1234) in north China; the Mongols (Yuan Dynasty, 1260–1368) in all of China; the Manchus (Ch'ing Dynasty, 1644–1910) in all of China.

War chariots were the pride of Chinese armies during the Shang Dynasty (c. 1500–1027 B.C.) and the Chou Dynasty (1027–221 B.C.). The much greater speed and maneuverability of nomad cavalry forced the Chinese to abandon the cumbersome chariots and adopt the cavalry techniques of their nomad enemies by the beginning of the Han Dynasty. Uncharacteristically, the normally chauvinistic Chinese also appropriated some of the motifs and treatment of nomad animal-style art for use on their own metalwork at the time.

The nomadic tribes forced into Korea by the troublesome Hsiung-nu were Tungusic-speaking Mongoloid peoples. Tungusic is a subfamily of the Altaic language group. Spoken in Manchuria and eastern Siberia, it includes the Tungus and Manchu languages. The Tungusic arrivals of the 4th and 3rd centuries B.C. introduced important features of the nomadic way of life to Korea: horse and cattle raising and the mounted warrior. The Scytho-Siberian style bronzes they produced included weapons, horse fittings, buckles, mirrors, and bells. Along with independent bells, jingle bells, attached like ornaments to various bronze objects, are characteristic of this style. The cast decoration on Scytho-Siberian style bronzes consists mainly of flat saw-tooth and thin parallel-line patterns. A belt hook in the form of a Mongol horse is one typical nomad bronze artifact subsequently appropriated by the Chinese for their own use (see Cat. 1). In Korean excavations, Scytho-Siberian style bronzes are often found mixed with ones derived from the Chinese.

In the 3rd century B.C., amid the accelerated influx of northern nomads and their culture, Korea received a major infusion of Chinese influence as well. Agriculture, both the wheat farming of North China and the wet-paddy rice cultivation of Central and South China, were introduced to Korea and gradually spread throughout the peninsula. Rice farming prospered best in southwestern Korea, where the land is flatter and the climate is warmer and moister.

By the 3rd century B.C., the state of Yen in northeast China had expanded into southern Manchuria and was in contact with Korea. Choson, the first true Korean state, was founded in the 3rd century B.C. and lasted until 108 B.C. It was located in the northwestern part of the peninsula, nearest the source of Chinese influence. The name "Choson" was later adopted by the Yi Dynasty (1392–1910), and subsequently the Japanese used it as the name for Korea during the annexation of 1910–1945. The establishment of the original state of Choson in the 3rd century B.C. was due in part to the arrival of Chinese refugees fleeing the fighting as nine of the ten Warring States into which China was divided at the time were conquered by the tenth, leading to the unification of China under the first emperor, Ch'in Shih Huang-ti, in 221 B.C. Wiman (Chinese: Wei Man), a Chinese, or possibly a Korean in the service of the Chinese, seized the Choson throne in about 190 B.C. and moved the capital to P'yongyang, today the capital of North Korea. Under Wiman, Choson became a powerful state whose influence was felt throughout the Korean peninsula.

During the Bronze/Iron Age, a new type of pottery appeared in Korea. It consists mainly of globular jars with flaring mouths or well-defined necks and remarkably thin walls. The pots are made of well-washed buff earthenware whose surface has been burnished with a smooth tool prior to firing or sometimes coated with red iron-oxide slip before burnishing. The shapes, techniques, and style of this pottery are very reminiscent of Yayoi pottery in Japan. The Yayoi Period (c. 300 B.C.–A.D. 300) was Japan's Bronze/Iron Age. The Yayoi people are believed to have come to Japan in several waves of migration from the Korean peninsula. Skeletal evidence from burials indicates they were of Mongoloid stock. With their bronze and iron weapons, their better social organization, and their wet-paddy rice farming, they were easily able to dominate Japan's preagricultural, Neolithic Jōmon people. The Yayoi pottery of Japan evolved from Bronze/Iron Age Korean prototypes.

LO-LANG

The increased influence of Chinese culture on Korea due to the presence of Chinese refugees in the state of Choson was further accelerated by the establishment of a Chinese colony on Korean soil in 108 B.C. The colony was named Lo-lang ("Nangnang," according to the Korean pronunciation of the two ideograms pronounced "Lo-lang" in Chinese). The Lo-lang colony played a key role in transmitting Chinese goods, ideas, and institutions to early Korea. Lo-lang survived until A.D. 313, outliving the mighty Han Chinese dynasty (206 B.C.–A.D. 220) that spawned it.

Wu Ti, third emperor of the Han Dynasty, invaded Korea in 109 B.C. Arriving by ship as well as overland, his armies defeated the Korean state of Choson in 108 B.C. His purpose was not so much conquest for its own sake as it was to out-maneuver the Hsiung-nu hordes who were a major threat along China's northern border. Wu Ti was afraid the Hsiung-nu would form an alliance with the Korean state of Choson. Han armies occupied most of central and northern Korea. The Chinese invaders divided the area into four administrative commanderies. However, many of the Korean inhabitants refused to accept Chinese rule. In 82 B.C., the Chinese were forced to pull back to one commandery, Lo-lang, with its capital at Wang-hsien on the Taedong River near P'yongyang.

Lo-lang became a highly profitable trading station, selling Chinese goods to the Korean peninsula as well as to the islands of Japan. It was the custom in China at the time to bury luxury goods in the tombs of deceased dignitaries so they could continue to use them in the spirit world. Tombs of the 1st–2nd-century-A.D. Lo-lang aristocracy near P'yongyang have yielded some of the most splendid Han Dynasty artifacts ever recovered (see Cat. 1), including extremely well-preserved lacquer such as the famous *Painted Basket*, which depicts figures engaged in lively conversation.

All this came to an end when northern nomads overran much of North China at the beginning of the 4th century, cutting off the Lo-lang colony from its source. The Koreans took advantage of the situation and conquered Lo-lang in 313.

During the four centuries when strong Chinese cultural influences were emanating from the Lo-lang colony, the southern half of the Korean peninsula was dominated by a tribal people called the Han. This "Han" is written with a different Chinese ideogram than the one for the Han Dynasty. The name of these early Korean Han people has been chosen as the modern name of South Korea: Han'guk, "The Country of Han."

During the 1st century A.D., agriculture gradually spread throughout southern Korea. The topography and climate of southwestern Korea in particular is ideal for wet-paddy rice farming; this area has continued to be the main rice-producing region of Korea. Large deposits of iron ore in southeastern Korea made it possible for the rulers there to engage in profitable trade with the Chinese at Lo-lang, as well as with Koreans in other parts of the peninsula, and with the Japanese.

THE THREE KINGDOMS PERIOD

This phase of Korean history is named after the Three Kingdoms (Wei, Shu Han, and Wu) into which China was divided for roughly sixty years following the collapse of the Han Dynasty in A.D. 220. The Three Kingdoms Period in Korea began with the conquest of Lo-lang in 313 by the Koguryo Kingdom and ended with the unification of Korea by the Silla Kingdom in 668. Koguryo occupied the northern half of the peninsula, Silla the southeastern quarter, and Paekche the southwest quarter. Each of the three kingdoms traditionally claimed to have been founded in the 1st century B.C. It was not unusual for early Chinese kingdoms, and subsequently Korean and Japanese ones, to claim greater antiquity for the sake of added prestige. Koguryo claimed 37 B.C., Silla 57 B.C., and Paekche 18 B.C.

Koguryo

Koguryo was the first great native Korean kingdom. Whereas the rulers of Choson had been mainly Chinese immigrants, the Koguryo people originally consisted of a group of five tribes among the northern Manchurian nomads known as the Puyo (Chinese: Fu-yu). During the 2nd century B.C., the Koguryo tribes, who were primarily hunters and warriors, migrated south and settled in the rugged mountain forests that separate Korea from Manchuria.

Fierce Koguryo mounted warriors fought against the Chinese troops sent by Han Wu Ti to occupy Korea in 109 B.C. The Chinese invaders were forced to abandon three of their four Korean commanderies and consolidate at Lo-lang in about 75 B.C. The chieftain of one of the five Koguryo tribes then assumed the title of king, which became hereditary. The Koguryo tribes took control of much of northeastern Korea and southeastern Manchuria. The Han Empire dispatched forces to subdue them but was never able to do so.

Koguryo defeated Lo-lang in A.D. 313, taking over its territory and people. Subsequent events followed a pattern that has been repeated many times within China itself: the conquering nomads were quickly Sinicized by their Chinese subjects. Less than sixty years after their victory, the kings of Koguryo set up a complex, Chinese-style bureaucratic government, complete with the necessary system of agricultural taxes to support it. They promulgated a Chinese-style law code and established a university to teach Confucianism and Chinese history. Buddhism was introduced from China in 372. First brought to China by missionaries from India in the 1st–2nd century, Buddhism was adopted as a state religion by the T'o-pa Tartars who conquered northwestern China in the late 4th century. As in 6th-century Japan, Buddhism was given government support in Korea less from belief in its religious teachings than from a desire to obtain the advanced material culture of China that came with it.

In 427, Koguryo moved its capital from Kungnae to P'yongyang, the former capital of Lo-lang and the modern capital of North Korea. Wall paintings in the tombs of the Koguryo nobility near Kungnae and P'yongyang are among the finest known surviving examples of 4th–5th-century Chinese wall painting.

Although Koguryo was invaded by troops from North China in about 342 and forced to pay tribute to various Chinese states, it soon became powerful enough to repulse large Chinese armies. China was divided into a number of smaller kingdoms for most of the time between the fall of the Han Dynasty in 220 and the founding of the Sui Dynasty (581–618). After reunifying China, the Sui emperor decided to conquer Korea. Four times between 598 and 614 he dispatched large expeditionary forces against Koguryo; all four times the Chinese armies were repulsed. These attempts to conquer Korea were so costly that they helped bring about the collapse of the Sui Dynasty.

Five more times between 644 and 659, the first and then the second emperor of the T'ang Dynasty (618–907), one of the mightiest in Chinese history, sent huge armies to conquer Koguryo; each time the Chinese forces were defeated. Obviously, Koguryo could not withstand this kind of punishment indefinitely. T'ang China formed an alliance with the Silla Kingdom in southeastern Korea. Together, the armies of Silla and T'ang destroyed the Kingdom of Koguryo in 668.

Paekche

The Kingdom of Paekche occupied the southwestern quarter of the Korean peninsula. Agriculture, specifically wet-paddy rice farming, spread to this region during the 1st century A.D. While the eastern and southern portions of southwestern Korea are rather mountainous, the northwestern portion consists of wide, flat river valleys. This topography, plus the local climate, warmer and moister than northern Korea, combined to make the area perfect for growing rice. This region has been the main rice-producing area of Korea ever since the 1st century. As a result, it has tended to have a larger population than other parts of the peninsula.

In the days of the Chinese colony at Lo-lang (108 B.C.–A.D. 313) in northwestern Korea, southern Korea was dominated by a tribal people called the Han. The early Paekche kings managed to consolidate the Han tribes of southwestern Korea under their rule in the 3rd–4th century A.D., although they piously claimed a date of 18 B.C. for the founding of their dynasty. The Paekche royal family considered themselves to be descended from the Puyo (Chinese: Fu-yu), nomadic tribes in northern Manchuria, of whom the Koguryo people were originally also a branch.

The Koguryo kingdom maintained direct connections overland with northern China. Paekche was cut off from such contact by the presence of Koguryo in between. Throughout most of their history, Paekche and Koguryo were at war with one another. Paekche, therefore, compensated for its lack of communication with northern China by developing and maintaining relationships with coastal southern China by ship across the Yellow and the East China seas. Paekche also established close maritime connections with Japan: it was from Paekche that Buddhism was introduced to Japan in A.D. 552. Japan welcomed Buddhism primarily because it offered access to the advanced material culture of China; each of the Three Kingdoms in Korea embraced Buddhism for the same reason.

Buddhism was brought to the Kingdom of Paekche by a Chinese monk; the new religion received official recognition and state support from the Paekche court in 384. The first capital of Paekche was at Kwangju, just below the Han River, halfway up the west coast of Korea, not far from the modern city of Seoul. In 475, southward expansion by the powerful Kingdom of Koguryo forced Paekche to move its capital south to Kongju. Continuing Koguryo pressure caused Paekche to move the capital further south to Puyo in 538.

In their struggles against Koguryo and, later, against Silla, their increasingly powerful neighbor to the east, the kings of Paekche requested military assistance from the Japanese. Paekche (pronounced "Kudara" in Japanese) sent some Buddhist monks, nuns, and ritual paraphernalia to Japan with one of its diplomatic missions, offering the new religion as a gift and asking for military aid in return—but to no avail. In 662, T'ang Dynasty Chinese naval forces, with the help of Silla armies, destroyed the Kingdom of Paekche. In 663, Japan finally sent a fleet of warships to rescue Paekche, but the combined T'ang and Silla forces easily defeated the Japanese armada.

Silla

From the 1st century B.C. through the 3rd century A.D., while northwest Korea was under the strong Sinicizing influence of the Chinese colony at Lo-lang, southern Korea was dominated by the Han people. The southwest became Korea's main rice-producing region, while the southeast carried on a profitable iron-ore trade with Lo-lang and other parts of Korea, as well as with Japan. Just as Han tribes in southwest Korea had coalesced to form the Kingdom of Paekche, those in the southeast united during the 4th century to become the Kingdom of Silla. Six of the Han tribes in southeastern Korea formed a confederation and imposed their rule on other tribes in the area. The chieftains of the six ruling tribes met as a council to elect a ruler and decide important issues. Like Koguryo and Paekche, Silla claimed an impossibly early date for the founding of the state: 57 B.C.

The southeast was the quarter of Korea furthest away from Chinese occupation and influence. Sinification came to Silla somewhat later than it did to Koguryo and Paekche. The capital of Silla was near the present town of Kyongju. Tombs of the 5th–6th-century Silla aristocracy in that district have yielded an abundance of impressive luxury goods: pottery (see Cat. 5,6), swords, armor, horse trappings, bronze mirrors, jade jewels, gold crowns, and gold earrings (see Cat. 7). The splendid gold crowns found in the most important Silla tombs have antler-like or treelike superstructures suggesting the animistic beliefs of early peoples from the forests and grasslands of north Asia; these beliefs became the basis for Korean Shamanism.

Silla was frequently at war with Koguryo, Paekche, or the Japanese colony of Kaya (between Paekche and Silla on the south coast of Korea). Koguryo and Paekche had developed efficient, Chinese-style centralized bureaucracies and large, well-organized armies. However, the mounted warriors of Silla were especially fierce fighters. Their vigor and effectiveness resulted from their old tribal loyalties rather than from Chinese-style organization.

As with Koguryo and Paekche, however, Sinification inevitably overtook Silla. In the 5th century, chieftains in the Kim family won the hereditary right to rule the confederation. In 503, they began referring to themselves by the Chinese title of king. During the first half of the 6th century, the Silla kings promulgated a Chinese-style law code and reorganized the government along Chinese bureaucratic lines. Buddhism was made a state religion in 528. As with Koguryo and Paekche, however, the old tribal Shamanism was not rejected. It continued to be practiced along with Buddhism, especially by the common people.

Implementation of Chinese ideas and practices during the first half of the 6th century proved stimulating and beneficial; Silla became increasingly powerful. In 562 Silla formed a military alliance with Paekche and conquered the Kaya confederation that lay between them. Silla armies then advanced up the east coast well into Koguryo territory, turned westward, and fought their way across to the west coast, driving a wedge between Koguryo and Paekche. This move also gave Silla a port on the Yellow Sea and direct maritime access to China. Taking advantage of the situation, Silla subsequently formed a military alliance with the T'ang Dynasty. T'ang warships and Silla warriors combined forces to conquer the Kingdom of Paekche in 662. In 663, they destroyed a Japanese fleet sent to rescue Paekche. Next, they turned their attention to Koguryo. Combined T'ang and Silla armies overwhelmed the Kingdom of Koguryo in 668, making Silla and its Chinese allies masters of the entire Korean peninsula.

The Three Kingdoms Period: Kaya

Kaya is not counted as one of the Three Kingdoms; it is usually treated as a part of Silla, which it did become after its conquest by Silla in 562. However, Kaya was very important in its own right because of its extremely close connections with Japan.

Kaya never coalesced into a unified state as did each of its neighbors, Koguryo, Paekche, and Silla; it remained a confederation of tribal units. Kaya occupied the central third of southern coastal Korea, including much of the lower Naktong River valley. Kaya is sometimes referred to as Karak, the name of the largest principality within it. Karak was traditionally founded in A.D. 42 and had its capital at Kimhae, across the delta of the Naktong River from the modern city of Pusan at the southeastern tip of the peninsula. Kaya was called Mimana by the Japanese, who maintained what amounted to a colony there from the middle of the 4th century until the Silla conquest of 562. The close ties between Kaya and Japan were based on the fact that the dominant Yamato clans in Japan were closely related to the people of Kaya. Tribes of mounted warriors had migrated into Korea from the north and moved gradually through the peninsula to the south coast. Some of them remained there and formed the Kaya confederacy, while others pushed on across the straits of Tsushima to Japan. They arrived in Kyūshū, the large southern island of Japan, in the 4th–5th century. They easily dominated the local Jōmon-Yayoi people, who had never encountered warriors on horseback before. Next, these warriors and their followers moved up through the Inland Sea to what is now the Osaka area, where they installed one of their clan chieftains as the first emperor of Japan. The Shintō myths of the Yamato people, as they called themselves, describe their descent from the plains of High Heaven to the islands of Japan. The archaeological evidence points to the Kaya area of Korea instead. Objects deposited in 5th–6th-century Japanese tombs are virtually identical to those found in Kaya and Silla tombs of the same period.

The material culture of the Kaya confederacy, as evidenced by objects excavated from royal tombs near Kimhae, was substantially the same as that of its neighbor, Silla. However, some of the forms and techniques seem to have been developed in the Kaya area first and then transferred to Silla from there, especially the characteristic dark-gray pottery of the period (see Cat. 2). It typically consists of bowls and jars on tall pedestals with rectangular perforations (see Cat. 3). The nearly identical Sue Ware of the Tumulus Period in Japan derives from it.

THE UNITED SILLA PERIOD

With their conquest of the Koguryo Kingdom in 668, the T'ang Dynasty Chinese expeditionary forces and the Silla armies found themselves in control of the entire Korean peninsula, unified for the first time in history. But the victors inevitably began squabbling among themselves. The Chinese expected to annex Korea to the T'ang Empire. Silla, of course, wanted to rule Korea itself. Fighting broke out between the Chinese occupation forces and the Silla troops. Fortunately for Silla, most of the defeated inhabitants of Paekche and Koguryo decided to join forces with Silla against the Chinese invaders. Still, it took them ten years to drive the Chinese armies out of Korea. It is an indication of the toughness and determination of the Korean people that they were able to humilitate the mighty T'ang Empire and establish their independence. Henceforth, United Silla sent tribute-bearing envoys to the T'ang court on an annual basis; this assured Chinese recognition of Silla, as well as diplomatic relations and trade. In spite of frequent invasions, revolts, and changes of dynasty, Korea has remained a unified, independent country until modern times.

The United Silla Period lasted from 668 until 918. The capital remained at Kyongju, but there were now five secondary capitals scattered throughout the peninsula. The Sinification of Silla that had begun before unification increased rapidly following the takeover of Paekche and Koguryo, each of which already had a well-organized Chinese-style bureaucracy long before their conquest by Silla. Silla now needed that kind of centralized bureaucracy in order to administer the much larger area and population that had come under its control. The Silla king wisely rewarded the surviving aristocracy of Paekche and Koguryo who had assisted in the expulsion of the T'ang armies with court ranks or government posts.

The annual tribute missions to the T'ang court ensured closer contact with China than had been possible in the past. The T'ang Dynasty (618–907) was a glorious Golden Age in the history of China, a time of outstanding achievement in every area of cultural endeavor. Both Korea and Japan greatly admired T'ang culture, and both emulated it as closely as they could.

Chinese Buddhism was at its height during the T'ang Dynasty. Emperors and aristocrats lavished their support on Buddhist temples and monasteries, many of which became rich and powerful. United Silla Korea and Nara Period Japan (710–794) followed the T'ang example in their opulent patronage of Buddhism (see Cat. 8, 9). The overwhelming size of Tōdaiji Monastery in Nara attests to its generous support by Emperor Shōmu (724–748). The splendidly restored 8th-century Pulguksa Monastery and magnificent Sokkuram Grotto Temple near Kyongju attest to the lavish patronage of United Silla kings.

The Nara emperors and United Silla kings did not ignore secular splendor either. They built elegant T'ang-style palaces and surrounded themselves with T'ang-style luxury goods, some of which were imported from China, and many of which were made locally

based on T'ang prototypes. This pervasive imitation of T'ang culture was facilitated by the large number of Japanese and Korean Buddhist monks and lay students who went to China for study. Most of this Chinese-style elegance was, of course, limited to the capital cities; little of the imported luxury penetrated the Japanese or Korean countryside.

While the benefits of T'ang-style material culture in Korea were visible mainly around the capital district at Kyongju, T'ang-style bureaucratic administration reached throughout the United Silla Kingdom. Korea was divided into nine provinces, based on a Chinese model. The provinces were subdivided into prefectures, as was the practice in China. The provinces and prefectures were all given Chinese-style names in 757. A complex hierarchy of Chinese-style government bureaus administered the country on behalf of the king. Government officials received regular salaries computed in grain or in the yield of a given acreage, based on the importance of their posts. There were two basic and equal categories of government officials; civil and military. Army installations were systematically set up in each province.

However, United Silla ignored one significant aspect of Chinese bureaucracy, the civil-service examinations. During the T'ang Dynasty, the examination system became an important means of selecting educated and talented men for the huge bureaucracy that was necessary to run a country the size of China. The examinations were open to everyone, although they naturally tended to favor the upper classes, who had a better opportunity to acquire the elaborate formal education in the Confucian classics necessary to pass the examinations. In Korea, by contrast, government appointments were made almost solely on the basis of aristocratic birth. At the other end of the social scale, the Korean peasants who worked the land to support the government were condemned by birth to the status of serfs.

Toward the end of the 8th century, serious difficulties overtook the United Silla Kingdom, and the 9th century, the final century of Silla rule, was a time of utter chaos. In the wake of several uprisings, the last legitimate Silla king was murdered in 780. A series of twenty kings followed in quick succession, none of whom came from the direct royal line. Each was a puppet placed on the throne by one or another of the squabbling factions at court. Assassinations and coups became routine. The capital district at Kyongju was laid waste.

Meanwhile, Korea's peasants had been taxed beyond endurance to support the greedy aristocracy. The serfs who worked the estates of the nobility and the slaves who labored in the government factories were also badly treated. The result was a series of peasant rebellions and the flight of thousands of serfs from the estates to which they were bound; in desperation many of them became brigands.

Even Buddhism, once considered the guardian of the state, now began to cause trouble. Lavish donations of goods and land by the aristocracy had made some of the Buddhist sects very rich. Many commoners became monks to avoid military service and farm labor. Noblemen often took the tonsure to escape court intrigues. The number of monks swelled dramatically. Many of the monasteries became huge, powerful establishments. Seeking additional power, some of them began to meddle in government affairs. During the 9th century, the king found it necessary to curtail the power of the monasteries and confiscate much of their land. At about the same time, Buddhism in China was dealt a blow from which it never recovered: Between 841 and 845, a mad T'ang emperor seeking Taoist immortality destroyed 44,600 Buddhist monasteries and defrocked 260,000 monks and nuns. Only the Ch'an (Zen) sect escaped persecution; its personal, contemplative approach kept it from becoming a nuisance to the government.

By the end of the 9th century, the peasant rebellions had spread throughout Korea, and the situation was out of control. In 901, a Buddhist monk named Kungye founded a kingdom of his own in north Korea and called it Later Koguryo. Kungye's father was a Silla king, but his mother was a lowly concubine. Considered outside the royal line, Kungye entered the Buddhist priesthood, a common practice at the time. After establishing the Later Koguryo Kingdom, Kungye set up a T'ang-style administration, but unfortunately he became a terrible tyrant. He was deposed by one of his own military officials, who took the throne for himself in 918, thus marking the end of the United Silla Period and the beginning of the Koryo Dynasty.

THE KORYO DYNASTY

The name of the Koryo Dynasty was formed with the first and last of the three Chinese characters with which "Koguryo" is written. The Western name "Korea" derives from "Koryo." The Koryo Dynasty lasted from 918 to 1392. It began when one of Kungye's generals, Wang Kon, seized the throne of Later Koguryo for himself in 918. In 935 the last king of United Silla capitulated. He was granted one of Wang Kon's daughters in marriage and given a high post in the new government. With this shrewd move, Wang Kon absorbed the United Silla bureaucracy smoothly into his own regime.

Wang Kon built his capital at Kaesong (also called Songdo), near the west coast of Korea, slightly north of the Han River estuary, not far from Seoul, the present capital of South Korea. Seoul itself was designated a secondary Koryo capital (Southern Capital), as were P'yongyang (Western Capital), which had been the capital of Lo-lang and Koguryo, and Kyongju (Eastern Capital), the former capital of Silla.

Kaesong was laid out in the grand manner with a rectangular grid of broad streets and avenues dominated by a huge royal palace in imitation of Ch'ang-an, the great capital city of T'ang China. Kaesong became one of the most splendid cities of the world in its day. The roofs of the palace were covered with expensive celadon porcelain tiles that glistened in the sunlight like blue-green jade.

Just as the Koryo kings copied Ch'ang-an when laying out their capital city, so they also imitated T'ang administrative structure when setting up their government bureaucracy. In 958 a Chinese-style civil service examination system was put into operation, but since class consciousness is much stronger in Korea than in China, the examinations were open to commoners in theory only.

Koryo emulation of T'ang forms lasted long after the fall of the T'ang Dynasty itself. Following the collapse of T'ang in 907, China was plunged into a half century of chaos, called the Five Dynasties Period (907–960) after five regimes in North China that followed each other in rapid succession. South China broke up into ten different kingdoms during this period. China was unified again under the Sung

Dynasty in 960. Korean contact with China was not as close in Sung times as it had been during the T'ang. Two powerful Tartar kingdoms stood between Korea and Sung China, the Khitan (Liao Dynasty) and the Jurched (Chin Dynasty).

Orthodox Buddhism in China was effectively and permanently destroyed by the imperial persecution of 841–845. However, the situation in Korea was quite different. Buddhism flourished more than ever under the ardent official patronage of Koryo Dynasty kings (see Cat. 11). Wang Kon, the founder of the dynasty, was a devout Buddhist. He is usually called King T'aejo; Koryo kings, as well as those of the succeeding Yi Dynasty, are traditionally referred to by their posthumous titles, as was the practice in China. In the *Ten Injunctions,* promulgated for the benefit of his successors, T'aejo emphasized the fact that the prosperity of the dynasty depended on the divine protection of the Buddha. Under the lavish patronage of the Koryo kings and aristocracy, leading monasteries once again became rich and powerful. Many acquired vast estates of farmland, the true measure of wealth at the time.

The great monasteries rivaled the royal court as centers of learning and art. One of the notable cultural achievements of the Koryo Dynasty was the production of a set of wood blocks for printing the *Tripitaka,* the complete collection of Buddhist sacred texts. Each block was carved with the Chinese characters for one page of text. The blocks have survived—all 81,137 of them—in the repository of the Haeinsa monastery on Mt. Kaya in South Korea.

Shamanism was maintained alongside Buddhism in Korea, just as Shintō was in Japan. King T'aejo's *Ten Injunctions* admonished subsequent Koryo kings to continue the observance of Shamanist rituals as well as Buddhist ones. Inevitably, Shamanist and Buddhist beliefs commingled. By the time of the Yi Dynasty (1392–1910), most Korean Buddhist monasteries had subsidiary buildings for the worship of important Shamanist deities, particularly Sanshin, the Mountain Spirit (see Cat. 30).

When the various Buddhist sects arrived in Korea from China, they were already somewhat adulterated by Chinese beliefs, especially Taoist ones. According to Taoist geomancy, for example, buildings must be positioned so as to be in harmony with the forces of nature. Many Buddhist monasteries were built on high mountains to the northeast of cities or palaces to protect them from the evil influences that emanate from that direction.

Buddhism in Korea declined considerably during the Yi Dynasty since Confucianism was the religion favored by the court. Sharply curtailed by the Yi kings, Korean Buddhism survived as a kind of folk religion in which Buddhist, Taoist, and Shamanist elements were intermingled.

Sung Dynasty Chinese emissaries to the Korean court remarked in their journals about the sharp disparity between the elegant luxury of the Koryo aristocracy and the wretched poverty of everyone else in Korea. The peasants' grain taxes and periodic mandatory labor supported the aristocracy in high style but left little for the peasants themselves. Below the peasants in the social hierarchy was a large class of laborers and slaves who worked as servants for the aristocracy or toiled in government mines and factories. As early as the 12th century, oppression of peasants and slave laborers by the aristocracy resulted in rebellions. Feuding factions at court created further disorder. In 1170, the military officials responsible for guarding the palace killed the civil officials at court and installed a different king on the throne. The remainder of the 12th century was marred by continuous civil war.

Racked by internal difficulties, the Koryo Dynasty also faced serious threats from outside. In 1011, the Khitan Tartars (Liao Dynasty) invaded Korea and overran the capital. The Jurched Tartars (Chin Dynasty) conquered North China in 1126 and forced Korea to pay heavy tribute.

In the 13th century, an even more awesome force appeared at Korea's northern border: the Mongols. They invaded the peninsula in 1231 and attacked the capital. The king capitulated and agreed to recognize Mongol suzerainty. However, after the withdrawal of the Mongol troops, he moved his capital to Kanghwa Island, just off the west coast near the estuary of the Han River, a location that could be more easily defended against Mongol attack. The move infuriated the Mongols; they retaliated by ravaging the entire Korean peninsula for the next quarter century. In 1258, Korea was annexed to the Mongol Empire. In 1279, the Mongols completed their conquest of China, where they established the Yuan Dynasty (1279–1368), with its capital at Peking. Koryo kings were henceforth forced to live in Peking part of the time.

Devastated by the brutal Mongol occupation, Korea was further strained by two attempted Mongol invasions of Japan. In 1274, and again in 1281, the Mongols sent huge fleets of warships to conquer Japan. The attacks were launched from Korea, which was forced to furnish the ships, the provisions, and some of the troops. Fortunately for Japan, the two Mongol armadas were both wrecked by fierce storms near the coast of Japan just after the fighting started. The Japanese credited their native Shintō deities for saving Japan from the Mongols and named the storms *kamikaze* (Divine Winds).

But Korea's external problems did not end there. In retaliation for the invasions, Japanese pirates (*wakō*) took advantage of the weakened condition of Korean coastal towns and raided them continuously throughout the late 13th and 14th centuries, ravaging the coastal districts and driving the inhabitants inland, while completely disrupting Korean shipping. In desperation, some Koreans became pirates themselves.

In 1368, the overextended Mongol Empire collapsed and was replaced in China by a native dynasty, the Ming (1368–1644). The Koryo Dynasty, having suffered such heavy Mongol domination, was unable to survive for long after the fall of the Yuan. The more progressive factions at the Koryo court were anxious to form an alliance with the new Ming Dynasty. The more conservative factions, unfortunately, insisted on remaining loyal to the Mongols. Korean troops were therefore sent to attack Ming forces in Manchuria. The commanding general, Yi Song-gye, realizing the absurdity of this undertaking, ordered his troops to return to the capital instead. He took over the government in 1388 and proclaimed himself king in 1392, marking the end of the Koryo and the beginning of the Yi Dynasty.

THE YI DYNASTY

The Yi Dynasty lasted over five hundred years, from 1392 to 1910, perhaps the longest continuous regime in the history of the world. Recent Korean publications and the gallery labels in the Korean National Museum refer to the Yi Dynasty as the Choson Period, based on the fact that the first Yi king received permission from Ming Dyansty China to name his regime after the earliest Korean state, Choson (3rd century B.C.–108 B.C.).

The Yi capital was built at Seoul and remained there throughout the dynasty. Today, Seoul is the capital of South Korea. Its two Yi royal palaces, the Kyongbok Palace (begun in 1395, rebuilt in 1867) and the Ch'angdok Palace (begun in 1396, rebuilt during the 19th century) survive as impressive examples of Ming-style palace and garden architecture. Yi Dynasty philosophical, literary, artistic, and administrative forms imitated as closely as possible those of Ming Dynasty China. Just as Silla and Koryo had copied T'ang, Yi ardently copied Ming, often becoming more orthodox and conservative than the Ming Chinese themselves.

Yi Song-gye, like other Koryo and Yi kings, is usually referred to by his posthumous title, T'aejo ('Grand Progenitor'). Immediately after founding the Yi Dynasty, he established formal tributary relations with Ming China. Korea agreed to send annual embassies to the Ming court bearing monetary tribute in return for recognition, protection, and trade. Throughout history, China has considered this its normal type of relationship with neighboring countries.

The two distinguishing characteristics of Yi Dynasty Korea were close imitation of Ming Dynasty China and the ascendancy of Confucianism, which became the official religion of the Yi Dynasty, as well as the philosophical basis for Yi administration. Buddhism was severely proscribed. Shamanism, with an admixture of Buddhism, Taoism, and Confucianism, survived as the religion of the common people.

Confucius was a great Chinese philosopher and teacher whose traditional dates are 551–479 B.C. ("Confucius" is the Latin version of his Chinese name and title, K'ung-fu-tzu, "Master K'ung.") What has survived of his ideas and teachings is contained in the *Analects (Lun yu)* written down by his disciples and their followers. The *Analects* consists primarily of answers to questions, each preceded by "The Master said—" Confucius conveyed moral precepts rather than abstract philosophy. His teachings emphasized loyalty and responsibility to one's family—especially to one's parents—as well as to one's ruler. Confucius defined the proper behavior for each type of human relationship: between a son and his father, a husband and his wife, a man and his brother, a subject and his king, one state and another, and so forth (see Cat. 52).

The Confucian social hierarchy consisted of heaven, earth, king, parents, teacher, and the individual. The king and his officials were supposed to behave righteously toward their subjects and venerate their ancestors, the earth, and heaven. According to Confucian ideals, a nation would be peaceful and prosperous if appropriate relationships were maintained between its various levels of society.

As the centuries passed, Confucianism became a powerful force in Chinese life, but many disparate ideas were added to the original ethical precepts of Confucius and his disciples. By the Sung Dynasty (960–1279), Confucianism had evolved an elaborate cosmology, a mystical side unrelated to the teachings of Confucius himself and borrowed largely from Taoism. Taoist cosmology recognized a basic unity behind the diverse functions of the universe, yet viewed everything in terms of duality: positive/negative, male/female, light/dark, and so forth. The myriad activities of the universe derive from the interaction of *yin* and *yang,* the negative and positive principles. The pair of intertwining commas on the Korean flag (and a constant design motif on utilitarian objects in Korea) is the ancient Chinese graphic representation of interacting *yin* and *yang* (see Cat. 88).

The complex, developed form of Confucianism is called "Neo-Confucianism" to distinguish it from the teachings of the Master himself. Neo-Confucianism acquired all the trappings of a religion, complete with Confucian temples and elaborate rituals, in which ancestor worship played an especially important part. Neo-Confucianism was synthesized and codified by Chu Hsi (1130–1200). Chu Hsi School Neo-Confucianism hardened into an intimidating orthodoxy in the late Sung Period that was handed on to the succeeding Yuan (Mongol) Dynasty. It took root in Korea at the time of the Mongol domination during the late Koryo Dynasty, and it went on to become virtually the state religion of the Yi Dynasty.

Yi rulers attached even more significance to Neo-Confucian ideals than the Chinese did. Yi insularity and conservatism helped to preserve many Confu-

cian rituals and other practices in Korea long after they fell into disuse in China. Among Neo-Confucian ideals, none was more important than that of the superior man, the Confucian sage, who brought his wisdom to perfection through learning and the cultivation of righteousness, selflessness, and filial piety. According to this ideal, human nature has the potential for such development if guided and inspired by correct Confucian behavior and principles. The sage advises the king, and the king rules his subjects justly.

Elaborate Confucian rituals involving music and processions were performed on specific days of the year at the royal palace or at Confucian temples in Yi Dynasty Korea. In addition, each individual, from king to commoner, was responsible throughout the year for maintaining the practice of ancestor worship, the most important Confucian ritual in every Yi Dynasty Korean household. On the anniversaries of the deaths of ancestors for several generations back, a spirit tablet—a rectangular plaque with the name of the deceased written or carved on it—was placed on an altar in the household shrine and the ancestor was venerated (see Cat. 35). Only the men in the family participated in this ritual. The status of women in the Yi Dynasty was low, their main responsibilities being to bear sons and care for their husbands and parents.

Confucianism's hold on Yi Dynasty Korea was ensured and perpetuated by the fact that the Confucian classics were the main subject matter of the government examinations, just as they were in China. Appointment to high government posts, as well as the land and prestige that went with the position, depended on success in the examinations. The situation in Korea was exacerbated by the fact that the government examinations, plus all the long study and preparation necessary to pass them, were in Chinese. This tended to stifle creativity on the part of the Korean intelligentsia and promote strict adherence to orthodox Chinese teachings.

The ascendancy of Confucianism in Yi Dynasty Korea was accompanied by a corresponding decline in Buddhism. T'aejo, the first Yi king, was himself a Buddhist. Nevertheless, he reacted against the political and spiritual corruption into which late Koryo Dynasty Buddhism had fallen. Swayed by his Confucian-trained advisors, he withdrew official government support from the Buddhist church and canceled the tax exemptions of the monasteries. He also prohibited the construction of new monastery buildings and curtailed the repair of existing Buddhist structures. T'aejo's son, T'aejong, the third Yi king, went further: he dismantled all but 250 of the Buddhist monasteries in Korea and appropriated their land for the crown. Persecution continued under T'aejong's son, Sejong, the fourth Yi king: he banished Buddhist monks from the capital; decreed that the seven Korean Buddhist sects must merge into two; and reduced the number of monasteries to only 36, whose population of monks he limited to 3,700. Following these persecutions, Buddhism in Korea survived as a sort of folk religion with a large admixture of Taoist and Shamanist elements.

Yi Dynasty Korea really had four religions—Confucianism, Buddhism, Shamanism, and Taoism—although no one was actually aware of the fourth. Taoism, unlike the other three, had no temples or shrines of its own in Korea. Nevertheless, Taoist ideas and Taoist symbolism permeated Korean life at every level. Neo-Confucianism took much of its cosmology from Taoism. Korean Buddhism and Korean Shamanism borrowed heavily from Taoism. Even more significant were the ubiquitous symbols, auspicious or protective, that served as the principal motifs on all the household objects in every Korean home; this symbolism was all Taoist in origin.

Buddhism, Confucianism, and Shamanism met the need for institutional religion at the various levels of Korean society. Similarities in beliefs and practices between Shamanism and Taoism made Koreans receptive to Taoist themes, while at the same time eliminating their need for institutional Taoism.

The philosophical Taoism taught by the founder of Taoism, Lao-tzu (b. 604 B.C.), had little impact on Korea. However, religious Taoism, founded by Chang Tao-ling (b. A.D. 126), thoroughly permeated Korean culture. Chang Tao-ling promoted Lao-tzu's classic, the *Tao Te Ching*, as the paramount Taoist scripture. He also advocated solitary meditation in the mountains in order to attain spiritual enlightenment, as recommended by Lao-tzu. However, Chang Tao-ling went well beyond Lao-tzu in teaching that longevity, and even immortality, could be achieved by the use of magic potions. Religious Taoism acquired a pan-

theon of deities and ecstatic rituals as well as the magic elixirs. All this is quite similar to Korean Shamanism and was thus easily absorbed into Korean culture. In China, religious Taoism provided a necessary antidote to the pious decorum of Confucianism. In Korea, this role was filled by Shamanism, which took over much of the lore of religious Taoism. Korea's four religions were considerably intermingled. Most Koreans were nominally Buddhists, yet they routinely invoked Taoist spirits to repel evil or attract good fortune, and they regularly engaged the services of *mudang* (shamans), while at the same time practicing ancestor worship and other Confucian rituals.

The rigid Confucian social structure of Yi Dynasty Korea divided society into four classes: royalty, the aristocracy, commoners, and the "low born." The king and the court nobility constituted a relatively small group. Beneath them was a large class of scholar officials, called *yangban*, who ran the extensive government bureaucracy. *Yangban* were the landed aristocracy, the elite of Yi society, both intellectually and economically. Only *yangban* normally received the elaborate classical Chinese education necessary to pass the government examinations and obtain high official positions. *Yangban* usually held these posts and lived in the capital or other large cities, but they owned much of the land on which the farmers toiled, since only *yangban* were permitted to own land. The *yangban* class had two equal categories: civil officials and military officials—indeed, the literal meaning of *yangban* is "two groups." Membership in the *yangban* class became hereditary.

Social mobility was virtually nonexistent during the Yi Dynasty, as class consciousness had always been strong in Korea. The Yi government set up and effectively maintained a rigid social hierarchy. Each person was locked into the class to which he was born, and he was expected to follow his forebears' occupation. There was a wide gap between the wealth, education, and refinement of the *yangban* class and the relative poverty of everyone beneath it.

Between the *yangban* and the commoners was a very small "middle class" (*chungin*), consisting of low-ranking government officials, doctors, engineers, and court artists. Commoners (*yangmin*) formed the largest class. Yi society was agricultural; farmers made up the majority of the population. Most of them worked on farms owned by absentee-landlord *yangban* or by the government. They were allotted a small share of the crop from the land on which they worked; the rest went to the landowner and to the government as taxes. Artisans were below farmers in the official hierarchy. Merchants, who were few in number, ranked below artisans, since contempt for money and profit making was a standard Confucian pose.

Below the commoners was a large "low-born class" *(ch'onmin)*, considered outside the social order because it contributed little or nothing toward maintaining society. The "low-born class" consisted of servants, slaves, workers in government mines and factories, butchers, tanners, Buddhist monks and nuns, shamans, *kisaeng* (female entertainers similar to Japanese *geisha*), prostitutes, actors, and fortune-tellers. Butchers and tanners were excluded from society because they violated the Buddhist prohibition against taking life, yet Buddhist monks and nuns were relegated to the same outcast group!

The 15th century, the first full century of Yi rule, was a time of vigorous intellectual activity in Korea. The *yangban* class strove diligently and enthusiastically to master classical Chinese literature, history, philosophy, calligraphy, and painting. One of the great cultural achievements of the Yi Dynasty was the use of movable type for printing. Each letter (in this case, each Chinese character) was carved on the end of a small block of wood only slightly wider than the letter itself. The pieces of type were set one above another to print a line of text. The type was then reused indefinitely in other combinations. This method was much faster and less laborious than the earlier method of carving all the characters for an entire page of text on the surface of a single large woodblock. Movable type was probably invented in China, but its first extensive use anywhere in the world was in early 15th-century Korea.

The extraordinarily long five-hundred-year tenure of the Yi Dynasty would seem to suggest a high degree of stability and tranquillity. Alas, such was not the case. After its first glorious hundred years of unity, strength, energy, and achievement in the 15th century, the Yi regime was racked by the same internal dissent and external pressure that had destroyed the Koryo Dynasty. The 16th century was bad; the

17th, 18th, and 19th centuries were worse. It is all the more remarkable, therefore, that the Yi regime survived for such a long time. The Confucian-oriented bureaucracy was extremely conservative, and perhaps Korea was too weakened by continuous internal squabbling and intermittent invasion to undertake a change of government.

The principal internal problem was factionalism: Groups within the government struggled with one another for supremacy. Officials alligned with losing factions were purged and sometimes executed. Endless factional disputes drained the government of its energy, efficiency, and responsiveness. The principal external problem was invasions by the Japanese and the Manchus (Ch'ing Dynasty China, 1644–1912).

The warlord Toyotomi Hideyoshi consolidated Japan under his rule in the late 16th century after two-hundred-fifty years of continuous civil war. With no more worlds to conquer at home, he decided to invade China, which seems absurd, given its size and population. However, Hideyoshi was an extremely shrewd ruler. He probably wanted to keep his generals and their armies busy lest they be tempted to rebel against his regime.

Hideyoshi tried to form a military alliance with Korea against China. Korea understandably remained loyal to its great mentor, Ming China. Hideyoshi reacted by invading Korea in 1592 with 160,000 troops. Crippled by factional disputes, the Yi government was totally unprepared for the invasion. The Japanese quickly captured Pusan, Seoul, and P'yongyang, then went on to ravage the whole peninsula. The Ming Dynasty dispatched an army across the Yalu River to attack the Japanese invaders from the north.

Admiral Yi Sun-sin (1545–1598), Korea's greatest military hero, attacked the Japanese by sea in the south, destroying the fleet that was supplying and reinforcing their troops. Admiral Yi invented the "turtle ship" *(kobukson)*, the world's first iron-clad warship. The armored roof above its upper deck resembled the shell of a turtle and protected the sailors and fighting men on board from the enemy's cannons, muskets, and arrows. Admiral Yi's fleet consisted of 149 ships, of which 43 were turtle ships.

The Japanese retreated to the southern tip of the peninsula late in 1593 and tried to negotiate a truce with the Chinese. The talks dragged on for three years, since each side behaved as if it were the victor. Hideyoshi became impatient and attacked Korea with a new army of 140,000 troops in 1597. The Korean government had stupidly stripped Admiral Yi of his rank through jealousy and factional intrigue, but it quickly reinstated him to defend Korea against the new Japanese invasion. Hideyoshi died in Japan of natural causes in 1598. Upon learning of his death, his commanders in Korea, realizing the folly of their undertaking, sailed for home.

Admiral Yi once again attacked the Japanese fleet, causing great damage, although he himself was killed in the engagement. His memorial at Asan near the hot-spring resort of Onyang is among the most impressive shrines in Korea. His war diaries have survived at Hyonch'ungsa, a Buddhist temple, and have been translated into English. His turtle-ship fleet became a frequent subject of Yi Dynasty screen paintings. Such screens functioned as talismans to repel evil spirits from a household in the same way that Admiral Yi's fleet repelled the Japanese from Korea.

Tokugawa Ieyasu, formerly one of Hideyoshi's leading generals, defeated the forces loyal to Hideyoshi's son at the battle of Sekigahara in 1600. In 1603 Ieyasu had the emperor name him *shōgun* (military dictator) of Japan. Ieyasu reestablished diplomatic relations with Korea in 1606. However, Korea's troubles were far from over. The Ming Chinese soldiers who had come to Korea's aid ravaged the peninsula almost as badly as their Japanese enemies had. The expense of sending a large army to Korea weakened the Ming government, itself racked by serious factional disputes. Troops who would normally have been stationed in North China and Manchuria to protect China from the Manchus had been diverted to Korea to fight the Japanese.

In 1627, the Manchus invaded northwest Korea and forced the Yi government to renounce the Ming Dynasty. In 1636, one hundred thousand Manchu troops overran the entire Korean peninsula. In 1637, they forced Korea to become a tributary state to the Ch'ing (Manchu) Dynasty. In 1644, the Manchus completed their conquest of China, and the Ming Dynasty collapsed. The Ch'ing Dynasty lasted from 1644 to 1912.

Instead of recovering from the Japanese and Manchu invasions, Korea remained crippled by factional strife and rampant corruption in the government. Corrupt officials absorbed more and more of the taxable farmland into their own tax-free estates, increasing the tax burden on the already over-taxed peasants and decreasing government revenue. The government became too impoverished to store grain against droughts and floods, resulting in severe famines followed by devastating epidemics. Many peasants were forced to become bandits. There were major peasant rebellions in 1811 and 1862.

A visitor to Korea today is impressed by its abundance of Christian churches. Even small towns often have them. Many Koreans turned to Christianity for solace during the troubled times of the late Yi Dynasty. Korean Christianity remains viable today, having survived the Japanese annexation. Roman Catholicism was brought to Korea from Peking in the second half of the 18th century. The Ch'ing emperors permitted a Catholic presence in China and even employed an Italian Jesuit priest, Guiseppe Castiglione (1688–1768), as court painter. Chinese, and later French, missionaries spread Catholicism in Korea, where it was called *sohak* (Western learning). The Confucian-trained officials of the Yi bureaucracy regarded it as subversive. It challenged their authority by teaching love of God rather than loyalty to king, family, and ancestors. A few Korean scholars were attracted to Christianity by the Western scientific knowledge that came along with it. But severe government persecutions of Christianity in 1801, 1839, and 1866 forced Korean converts to practice their new religion in secrecy.

Throughout the 18th century, Korea was at peace with its neighbors. China enjoyed a century of prosperity under the K'ang-hsi (r. 1662–1722) and Ch'ien-lung (r. 1736–1796) emperors. Korea continued to maintain its tributary relationship with the Ch'ing Dynasty. Korea carried on a limited trade with Japan through the Japanese feudal lord of Tsushima, the island in the straits between Korea and Japan. Korea also sent several large diplomatic and cultural missions to Japan. The Korean envoys' processions, especially the details of their clothing, so different from that of Japanese, were carefully recorded by Japanese artists at the time. Otherwise, Korea pursued a policy of national isolation. So did Japan under the Tokugawa shoguns (the Edo Period, 1603–1868).

The external calm of 18th-century Korea was not matched by the internal situation. Destructive factionalism within the government bureaucracy continued unabated. Shifts in power from one of the major factions to the other and back again during the 18th century cost the lives of some four thousand officials. To make matters worse, toward the end of the 18th century, a new external threat appeared from the West. French and English ships began visiting the Korean peninsula demanding trade relations. Korea resisted as best it could, fighting skirmishes on Kanghwa Island with the French in 1866, the Americans in 1871, and the Japanese in 1875.

During the 19th century, Korea was in a state of near collapse. Each king was intentionally placed on the throne while still a boy, enabling regents and their backers to wield control. Through this device, the Kim clan and the Min clan took power. The feuding factions of the previous century were reduced to a minor role in the government. The Ch'ing Dynasty sent a resident official to Seoul; through him China interfered directly in Korean politics.

Korea's economic woes were worse than ever. The continuing transfer of taxable farmland to the tax-exempt estates of corrupt officials reached the point where the meager portion of the crop allotted to the peasants who grew it was insufficient to feed them adequately, and the remainder was insufficient to support the government. Natural calamities added to the people's misery: floods destroyed crops and caused famines, which were followed by epidemics.

Foreign pressure on Korea to open its doors to trade and diplomatic relations now became intense. Korea was no longer in any condition to resist. The Yi government signed a commercial treaty with Japan in 1876 and another with the United States in 1882. The 1876 treaty marked the beginning of a gradual Japanese takeover of Korea that culminated in the 1910 annexation.

The isolationist policy of the Tokugawa shoguns was also broken by foreign pressure. Commodore Matthew Perry sailed from the United States to Japan in 1853 with a fleet of sail-and-steam warships bearing a letter from President Millard Fillmore demanding the opening of Japanese ports to foreign ships for water and supplies. Perry returned for an answer in 1854 with seven warships. Japan had no coastal defenses or modern weapons of any kind, leaving her no choice but to sign the treaty. England, Russia, and Holland soon negotiated similar treaties with Japan.

The humiliation of being at the mercy of foreigners led to the overthrow of the Tokugawa regime. Administrative control was restored to Emperor Meiji and a European-style parliamentary government. Japan turned itself overnight from an isolated, backward, feudal country into a powerful modern industrial nation. During the Meiji Period (1868–1912), Japan fought two wars involving Korea. The Sino-Japanese War (1894–1895) began when Korea, unable to cope with desperate gangs of bandits, asked China to send troops and restore order. Japan insisted on sending troops also, in accordance with a treaty it had signed with Korea in 1885. The Chinese and Japanese troops clashed; war was declared between China and Japan. China had very few modern weapons; Japan had plenty, including a fleet of battleships. Japan easily won the war. The Chinese fleet surrendered to the Japanese. Russia, Germany, and France supervised the signing of the peace treaty.

The Russo-Japanese War (1904–1905) began when the Japanese fleet blockaded the Russians at Port Arthur, on the tip of the Liaotung peninsula in the Yellow Sea between Korea and China. The Russians sent troops into Korea from the north, and the Japanese from the south; several battles were fought. The Japanese drove the Russians back across the Yalu River into Manchuria, then out of Port Arthur, then out of Mukden, Manchuria. The Japanese fleet annihilated the Russian fleet and won the war. The United States supervised the signing of the peace treaty. Five years later, Japan incorporated Korea into the Japanese Empire. The Japanese annexation of Korea lasted from 1910 until the end of World War II in 1945.

PROLOGUE

THE UNIQUENESS OF KOREAN ART

Korean art is rich and diverse, as a glance through this catalog will suggest. It is an art with which few Westerners are familiar. Even those of us who have had some exposure to Far Eastern culture have tended to regard China as a vast and overwhelming civilization of which the arts of Japan and Korea were provincial imitations. This view is not only unfair, it is inaccurate. Japanese art and Korean art are as different from Chinese art, and from each other, as are the languages and personalities of the three peoples.

Chinese art has, of course, been a major influence on Japanese and Korean art, and a great deal of direct imitation has taken place. In Japan, artistic developments have usually followed a cyclical pattern, with periods of enthusiastic borrowing from China followed by periods of assimilation and restatement in Japanese terms. In Korea, Chinese influence has been much more pervasive and continuous, partly because of Korea's geographic proximity to China. Japan was able to separate itself from the outside world during periods of self-imposed isolation simply because it is an island nation.

Official art in Korea, that is, the art of the royal court, the powerful Buddhist monasteries, and the scholar bureaucrats, strove to be as correct, and therefore as Chinese, as possible. In Korean folk art, on the other hand, one finds a truly indigenous artistic expression, one that is quite distinct from the art of China. This indigenous Korean artistic expression is characterized by directness, ruggedness, and unpretentiousness. Once one learns to recognize them, one can also find it in the more official forms of Korean art, in spite of the heavy overlay of Chinese style they bear.

Thirty years ago, one often heard Japanese art called a mere imitation of Chinese art. Since that time, Japanese art has been so extensively published in the Western World that almost no one would make such a statement today. Although Korean art has been avidly admired and collected in Japan since the 16th century, it remains relatively unknown in the West.

Even today, one hears Korean art dismissed as a mere imitation of Chinese art. Ironically, the one type of Korean art that *has* been admired in the West *was* based closely on Chinese models: Koryo Dynasty celadon porcelain (see Cat. 13–21). Koryo celadon was an official art form; the best pieces were made for use in the royal palace, and only the aristocracy could afford it.

Koryo celadon has been collected by European, British, and American museums and private collectors for about a hundred years. The Western world responded readily to this ware because it was similar to the Sung products from which it derived. Chinese celadon has been part of the Western tradition since the 16th century, when shiploads of Ming Dynasty export ware began to reach Europe, finding its way into nearly every princely house. Koryo celadon seems attractive to us because it fits comfortably into this tradition.

The other reason why Koryo celadon has been virtually the only form of Korean art to be collected in the West is that its beauty is very apparent, rich and real, sometimes even profound. Nevertheless, it is an obvious kind of beauty, elegant and easily admired. The beauty of other forms of Korean art is much more challenging to Westerners. It is a rugged kind of beauty, never obvious, never merely pretty, and it represents the true artistic expression of the Korean people. Fortunately, The Brooklyn Museum's collection of Korean art is quite comprehensive; it contains a full range of divergent types, from official to folk art.

The rich diversity of Korean art makes it difficult to generalize about its characteristics. Nearly all the rules one attempts to formulate turn out to have many exceptions. Still, it does have certain unique characteristics that distinguish it from the art of its giant neighbor and mentor, China, and it accurately reflects the personality of the people who produced it.

Koreans are tough, and they are justifiably proud of being so. They have survived and often prospered in a harsh environment of bone-chilling winters and sweaty, hot summers, in a country where much of the land is solid rock, a country whose history is filled with hardship.

During the Korean War (June 25, 1950–July 27, 1953), Communist North Korean troops with Russian T-34 tanks swept through South Korea. They were finally stopped at the Naktong River near Taegu, just above the southern tip of the peninsula. Seoul was reduced to rubble. Yet today, only thirty years later, Seoul is a splendid, large, modern city of skyscrapers and high-rise apartments, broad avenues and parks, a fine international airport, excellent hotels, and sprawling shopping malls overflowing with the latest electronic gadgets. Koreans used to eat poorly, dress poorly and work long and hard just to survive. Now, the countryside is laced with six-lane expressways filled with new cars, trucks, and busses. The "Miracle of South Korea" is entirely due to the talent, hard work, determination, wit, and spirit of the Korean people.

Koreans are direct. Their straightforward speech and independent manner are quite unusual in the Orient. Together with their adventurous spirit, this has earned them the nickname, the "Irish of Asia." The assertiveness of the Korean personality is matched by the assertiveness of Korean cooking, notable for its bold flavors, usually spiced with more fiery hot chili peppers than Western palates can tolerate—and lots of garlic, whose taste and aroma are everywhere in Korea.

Koreans are rugged, and so is their country. Koreans need to be rugged to survive Korean winters, with their icy Siberian winds. The land in the Korean peninsula is also rugged: low mountains, sparsely wooded, punctuated by huge chunks of solid granite, with rice paddies in the flat river valleys, surrounded by a magnificent, rocky, convoluted coastline.

Korean art displays these same characteristics. It eloquently expresses the qualities of the land and people who produced it. When free from the need to imitate Chinese models, Korean art abounds in vitality, directness, strength, joy, and a beguiling naiveté. One sees these qualities in the lively shapes and often outrageously bright colors of Korean folk paintings, for example. While Korean scholar paintings tend to employ the muted washes of Chinese literati paintings, other types of Korean painting often feature acrid harmonies of bold red, bright green, and deep blue that are completely different from the color schemes of Chinese and Japanese paintings.

The rugged charm, vigor, striking lines, perfect proportions, and handsome woods of Korean furniture are extremely impressive. One finds these qualities also in the bright, unpretentious richness of Korean lacquer, or in the informal strength and energy of Yi Dynasty ceramics. Unpretentiousness, directness, ruggedness, spontaneity, and joy are the qualities that give Korean art its compelling appeal as well as its uniqueness.

CATALOG

THE CHINESE COLONY
AT LO-LANG
108 B.C.–A.D. 313

1. Belt Hook

Bronze
H. 2⅜", W. 3⅝"
Chinese, Han Dynasty, 2nd century A.D., from
Lo-lang, Korea
Gift of Mr. & Mrs. Paul Manheim   69.125.11

The belt hook was a standard Chinese garment fastener during the Eastern Chou Period (770–221 B.C.), the Ch'in Dynasty (221–206 B.C.), the Han Dynasty (206 B.C.–A.D. 220), and on into the Six Dynasties Period (A.D. 220–581). A stud on the back of the body of the belt hook engaged a hole in one end of the belt; the hook engaged a ring, sometimes of bronze, sometimes of jade, attached to the other end of the belt. Since it was a separate part, the ring is almost invariably missing today. Chou Dynasty belt hooks tended to have a spoon-shaped body tapering into a hook terminating in a mythical animal head. Han Dynasty belt hooks often represented an entire animal, with the hook protruding from its chest, as we see here.

The crisp simplification and stylization of this horse, with his arching, close-cropped mane, are extremely sophisticated and appealing. They remind one of ancient Greek depictions of horses. In fact, there may be a distant connection. Greek art influenced the art of Scythia and, through it, had some impact on the Scytho-Siberian art of Central Asia. Certain elements of Scytho-Siberian style, and especially the horse motif, were adopted by the Chinese at the beginning of the Han Dynasty, when they abandoned their clumsy war chariots in favor of the cavalry techniques of their Central Asian nomad enemies.

The full, rounded forms and alert posture of this horse convey a feeling of power and energy. The surface of the bronze has a handsome apple-green burial patina; some tomb earth adheres to the surface. Bronze belt hooks were prominent among the luxury goods placed in the tombs of deceased aristocrats, who were expected to continue using them in the spirit world. The present example comes from the Han Dynasty Chinese colony at Lo-lang in northwest Korea (108 B.C.–A.D. 313). This belt hook was probably imported from China; numerous nearly identical examples have been excavated in China itself. But this belt hook may have been cast by an immigrant Chinese craftsman living in the Lo-lang colony.

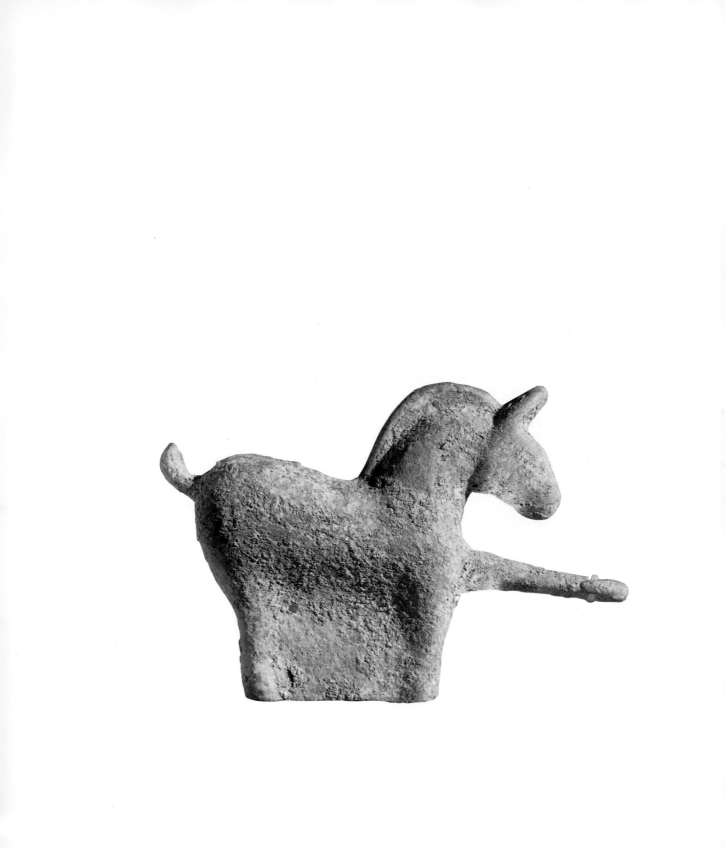

THE KAYA CONFEDERACY
A.D. 42–562

2. Jar (Kimhae Type)

Gray stoneware
H. 10¼", W. 10½"
Kaya, 3rd–4th century
Gift of Robert Anderson   82.171.8

Kaya was a confederation of tribes occupying the central portion of the southern coast of Korea, with Silla to its east and Paekche on the west. Karak was the largest principality within the Kaya confederacy. The capital of Karak was at Kimhae, across the delta of the Naktong River from the modern city of Pusan at the southeastern tip of the Korean peninsula. Tombs of the Karak aristocracy in the vicinity of Kimhae have yielded a rich variety of luxury goods, objects that were interred with the dead warrior chieftains to serve them in the spirit world: iron armor and helmets, bronze horse trappings, a gilt-bronze crown, gold earrings, and quantities of gray pottery.

Kaya pottery is of two basic types. The earlier type, made in the 3rd and 4th centuries, consists primarily of large, spherical storage jars like this one. They are so characteristic that scholars, dealers, and collectors refer to them simply as Kimhae jars. The later type of Kaya pottery, made in the 5th and 6th centuries, consists primarily of bowls, cups, or jars having tall, hollow, perforated bases, (see Cat. 3)

The present jar is typical of the Kimhae type in having a textured surface. In this case, the texture was beaten onto the soft clay with a paddle wrapped in matting made of twisted cords. Jars like this were coil built, in much the same way as American Indian pottery. The nearly completed jar was placed on a potter's wheel; the neck and lip were thrown from the upper coils of clay. This forming process is called coil-and-throw. It was the standard forming technique for globular jars during the Kaya and Silla periods. It is entirely feasible to throw a jar this size from a lump of clay centered on the potter's wheel, but the old coiling technique, in existence long before the potter's wheel was invented, continued to be used for round jars; it had become a tradition. Modern Korean *kimch'i* jars are made by coiling, but for a different reason—they are simply too large to throw on a potter's wheel.

The texture on the surface of the present jar, and on Kimhae jars in general, had become an intentional decorative effect but was originally a by-product of the forming process. After the potter finished joining the coils to form the jar, he beat the surface with a wooden paddle to make the walls thinner and more uniform, while his other hand held a wooden block inside the jar at the point where the paddle struck the outside, so as to maintain the shape of the jar and prevent it from collapsing from the beating. The paddle was originally carved with a pattern or wrapped with cord to prevent it from sticking to the wet clay. In time, the texture impressed on the clay surface by the textured paddle came to be admired for its visual propertes.

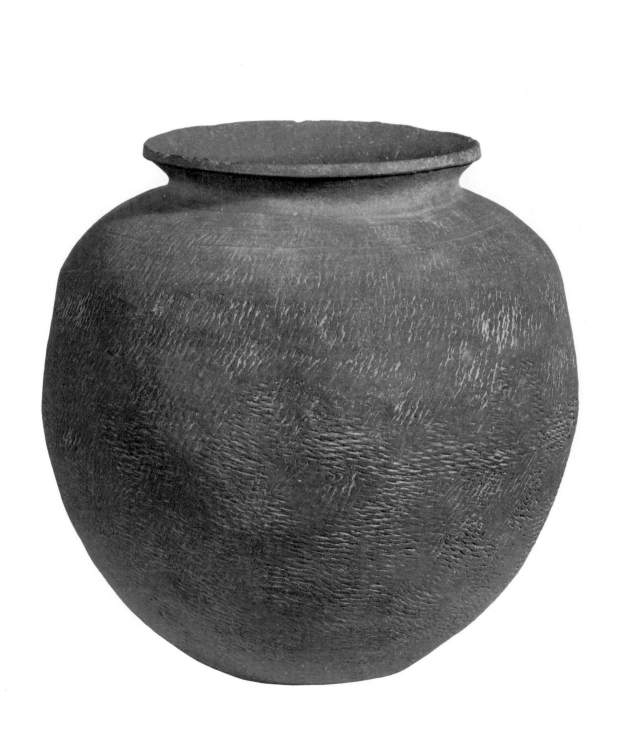

3. Pedestal Jar

Gray stoneware with deposits of natural ash glaze
H. 7½", W. 6½"
Kaya, 5th–6th century
Gift of Nathan Hammer   74.61.8

The characteristic Silla Period ceramic type was a gray-black stoneware pedestal bowl, a vessel supported on a tall, hollow, flaring, and perforated base (see Cat. 5). However, archaeological evidence seems to indicate that this ceramic type developed in the Kaya area first and was subsequently adopted by Silla. Sue Ware, the dark-gray pottery of the Tumulus Period in Japan (300–552) is nearly identical to 5th–6th-century Kaya and Silla pottery, from which it clearly derives. The dominant Yamato clans of Tumulus Period Japan were close relatives of the Kaya people, having migrated to Japan from the Kaya area. Kaya was called Mimana by the Japanese, who maintained a colony there from the middle of the 4th century until 562, when Kaya was conquered by Silla.

The present jar originally had a domical lid with a central knob; the jar's lip was obviously intended to fit within the rim of a lid. A very similar Kaya pedestal jar with strap handle in the Korean National Museum still retains its lid. The combed decoration on the Brooklyn jar is typical of 5th–6th-century Kaya and Silla pottery but, like the ware itself, as well as the pedestal-vessel type, probably originated in Kaya and was adopted by Silla.

Because of two major innovations, the potter's wheel and the kiln, 5th–6th-century Kaya and Silla pottery was technically advanced compared to the earthenware of the Neolithic and Bronze-Iron Age that preceded it. Whereas the earlier ware was somewhat uneven and restricted in form due to being coil built, the Kaya-Sila ware was thrown on a fast wheel, giving it thin, even walls and permitting complex, sophisticated vessel shapes. Neolithic and Bronze-Iron Age earthenware was baked in an open fire in a shallow pit, leaving it brittle and porous. Kaya-Silla pottery was tough and completely nonporous; it was fired at high stoneware temperatures in efficient, large, single-chambered kilns built on the slopes of hills to provide a good draft for the fire.

The dark, olive-colored, lustrous surface on the shoulder of the present jar is natural ash glaze. Wood ash from the fire was carried through the kiln chamber by the draft and deposited on the horizontal surfaces of the pots, and on the vertical surfaces facing the draft. The silica in the ash formed a rudimentary glaze on those surfaces. The intentional glazing of ceramic wares must have developed from this; potters learned to mix wood ash with water and sand and apply this preparation to pots before firing.

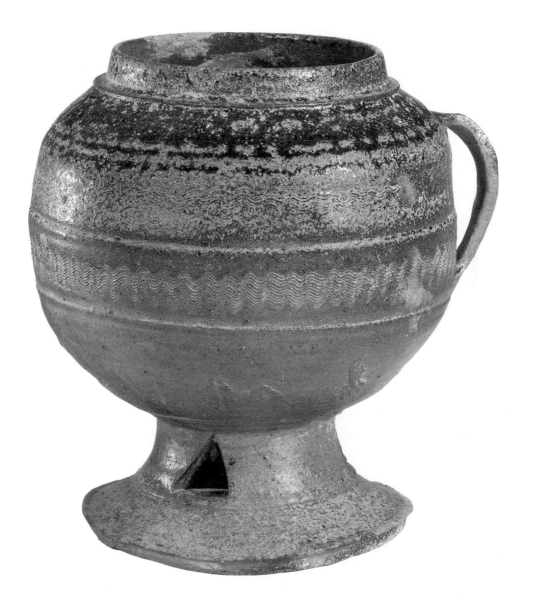

THE SILLA PERIOD
313–668

4. Kuan Um (Avalokitesvara)

Gilt bronze
H. 4¼", W. 1¾"
Silla Period, first half of the 7th century
Lent by Dr. Ralph Marcove   TL1984.194

The three and a half centuries between the fall of Lo-lang in 313 and the unification of Korea by Silla in 668 is called The Three Kingdoms Period because the northern half of the peninsula was ruled by the Koguryo Kingdom, the southwest quarter by the Paekche Kingdom, and the southeast quarter by the Silla Kingdom. Buddhism was introduced into each kingdom by Chinese monks and received enthusiastic state support, although the old native Shamanist beliefs were not abandoned. As in early Japan, the rulers of the three kingdoms were eager to acquire the advanced material culture of China. Embracing Buddhism was seen as a way of facilitating this. The traditional dates for the introduction of Buddhism are 372 for Koguryo, 384 for Paekche, and 528 for Silla.

Buddhism was first brought to China by missionaries from India in the 1st–2nd century. Buddhism was subsequently adopted as a state religion by the T'o-pa Tarters, who conquered northwestern China in the late 4th century and held it until the middle of the 6th century. Buddhism spread from there to other parts of China and on to Korea. Emissaries from the Paekche Kingdom introduced Buddhism to Japan in 552.

Indian missionary monks and Chinese Buddhist pilgrims returning from India introduced several different sects of Buddhism into China. Chinese missionary monks, or returning student monks who had gone to China for study, brought these various sects to Korea and Japan. The Pure Land Sect became by far the most popular because it made salvation very easy for the ordinary believer. Instead of earning one's own enlightenment (Buddhahood) by selfless acts and rigorous spiritual discipline throughout countless incarnations, the believer had only to utter the formula "Praise be to Amitabha Buddha" in good faith at least once during his lifetime, and he would be reborn in the Western Paradise (The Pure Land) after he died.

Avalokitesvara (Chinese: Kuan-yin; Korean: Kuan Um; Japanese: Kannon) is the most compassionate, and therefore the most popular, of the Bodhisattvas. Bodhisattvas are the savior figures of Buddhism, beings who have postponed their own salvation (Buddhahood) until all sentient beings in the universe have attained theirs. Bodhisattvas work diligently and constantly to bring about the salvation of believers. Avalokitesvara is the main Bodhisattva associated with Amitabha, the Buddha of the Western Paradise, and may usually be identified by a diminutive seated figure of Amitabha in the front of his diadem. That small figure is absent or obliterated in the present image of Kuan Um. However, the Bodhisattva is positively identified by another attribute, the *kalasa* (flask) held in his right hand; it contains the nectar of compassion. The *Lotus Sutra* describes the Western Paradise of Amitabha Buddha; chapter twenty-five deals with Avalokitesvara in particular. The first great flowering of Pure Land Sect Buddhism in Korea took place during the first half of the 7th century. Many sculptures of Amitabha, and especially of Avalokitesvara, were made at that time.

The style of the present image reflects 5th–6th-century Chinese prototypes of the Six Dynasties (Northern Wei) Period in its dematerialized body, prominent head and hands, and the swallow-tail drapery falling on either side of the legs. However, the columnar stance and the fuller forms of the legs reflect Chinese Buddhist sculpture of the Northern Ch'i (550–577) and Sui (581–618) Dynasties.

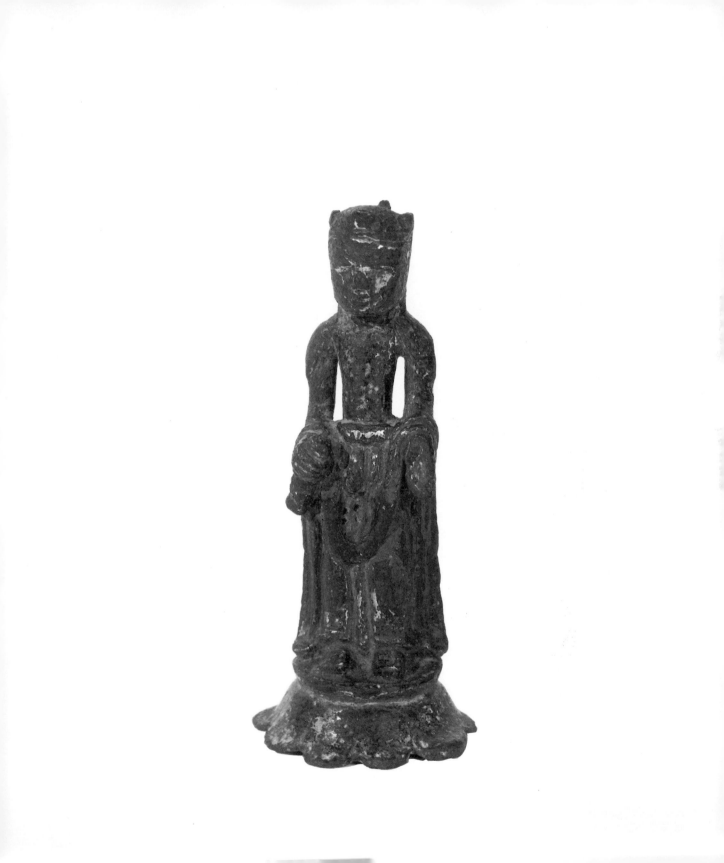

5. Pedestal Bowl with Cover

Gray Stoneware
H. 7½", W. 5½"
Silla Period, 5th–6th century
Gift of Sir George Sansom   40.519 a&b

Large, hemispherical earthen burial mounds were erected for deceased Silla kings. Somewhat smaller ones were built for other important members of the Silla aristocracy. At ground level beneath the center of the mound was a stone-lined burial chamber. The body was placed in a coffin near the center of the burial chamber, wearing finery that included jewelry made of gold and jade. The burial chamber was filled with all sorts of luxury goods meant to serve the dead warrior chieftain in the spirit world. We know a great deal about the material culture of the Silla Kingdom simply from the objects excavated from the tombs of its leaders: gold crowns, gold earrings, gold belts, jade jewels, steel swords, armor, bronze horse trappings, bronze mirrors, and pottery. Even the more modest Silla tombs were furnished with quantities of gray-black pottery.

The most prevalent and characteristic vessel type among Silla burial pottery is the pedestal bowl with cover, seen here. Vessels of this type were presumably used to warm and serve hot food at banquets. The lid lifts off and turns upside down to become another bowl, its central knob serving as the bowl's foot. Surrounded by such vessels, the tomb's occupant could continue to enjoy elegant banquets in the spirit world. Pedestal bowls are also prevalent in Sue Ware, the gray-black pottery of Japan's Tumulus Period (300–552). The mound tombs that gave this period its name are similar to those of Kaya and Silla, and their contents of luxury goods are nearly identical to Kaya and Silla prototypes, since the Yamato clans were related to the Kaya people.

The present vessel is somewhat unusual in retaining its original lid. Silla pedestal bowls coming on the art market in recent years have usually had no lid at all, or else a mismatched lid from another bowl. Brooklyn's example is also unusual in having bold incised designs on its surface. One is tempted to see a rudimentary landscape in these designs, with the sawtooth bands becoming mountain ranges and the "arrowheads" becoming trees. It is more likely, however, that this triangular zigzag pattern filled with close-set, parallel, diagonal lines is abstract and was originally symbolic, and that it derives from similar ornaments on cast-bronze artifacts from Korea's Bronze-Iron Age. The decoration on the loop of a horse-shaped *Belt Hook* in the Kyongju National Museum is almost identical to that on the Brooklyn *Pedestal Bowl*.

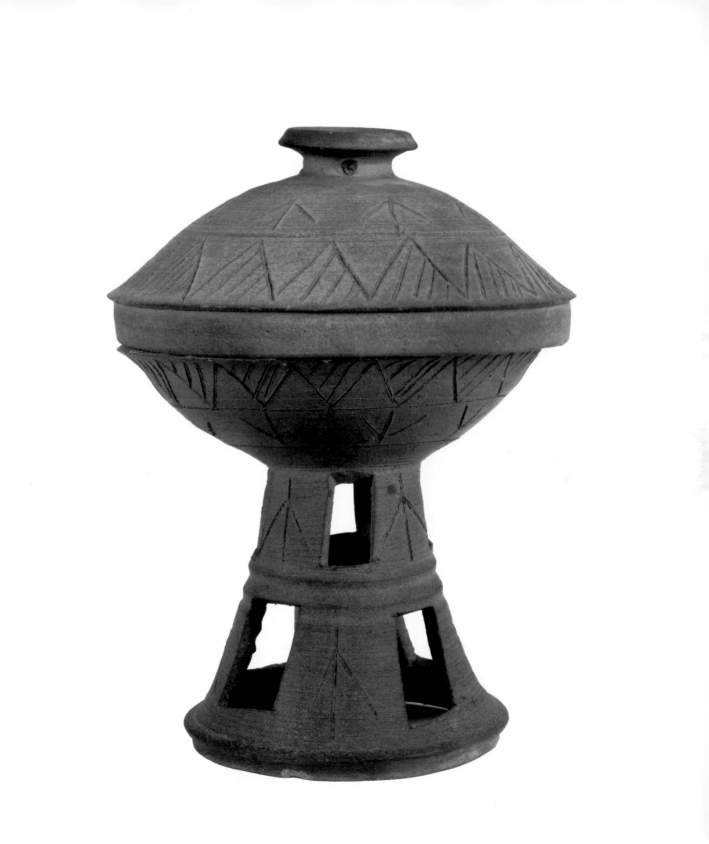

6. "Jingle-Bell" Libation Cup

Gray stoneware with deposits of natural ash glaze
H. 6½", W. 3½"
Silla Period, 5th–6th century
Gift of Mr. & Mrs. Roger Elliot and Mr. & Mrs. Jack
Ford, In Memory of Jean Alexander   85.114.2

The characteristic Kaya/Silla pottery pedestal bowl
with cover (see Cat. 5) derived from a Chou Dynasty
(1027–221 B.C.) Chinese vessel, the *tou*. The *Libation
Cup* we see here has a tall, perforated stem like that
of a pedestal bowl. However, in this case the stem
expands into a perforated globular bell having two
hard clay pellets rolling around inside to produce a
sound. Fired in an efficient, sloping kiln, Silla gray-
black stoneware vitrified sufficiently to resonate
when struck, although it cannot ring like a bell; only
porcelain can do that.

Attached spherical jingle bells appear frequently
on horse fittings and other cast-bronze artifacts of
Korea's Bronze-Iron Age. Such jingle-bell ornament
is typical of the animal-style bronze art of nomadic
warrior tribes who roamed the steppes and forests
of Central Asia, Mongolia, and Manchuria. Various
groups of these nomads were among the ancestors
of the Korean people, as we have seen. The early
culture of Korea was a blend of nomad elements and
Chinese-derived elements; this *Libation Cup* illustrates
the fact perfectly.

Pottery vessels with fanciful shapes like this attest
to the skill and confidence of Silla potters. Complex
and thin-walled forms such as this were borrowed
from metalwork and were difficult to render in clay.
Silla pottery vessels with unusual shapes, including
a famous ewer in the form of a horse and rider,
can be seen in various museums in Korea but are
extremely rare in America and Europe. The turned
ridges, simple combed decoration, and deposits of
natural ash glaze on this *Libation Cup* are typical of
Silla pottery in general, and of the Kaya pottery that
slightly preceded it (see Cat. 3).

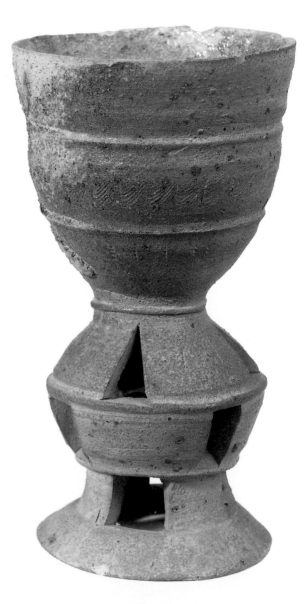

7. Pair of Earrings

Gold
H. 3⅛″, W. ¾″ each
Silla Period, 5th–6th century
Anonymous gift   83.195 a&b

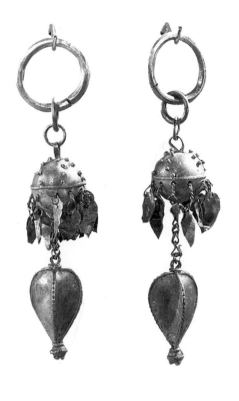

Of all the splendid luxury goods deposited in Silla tombs, the most spectacular are the personal adornments made of gold. Gold crowns, gold belts, gold necklaces, gold earrings, gold bracelets, and gold rings have been found, as well as fragments of clothing made of cloth woven with gold threads.

The most abundant objects in this precious hoard are pairs of gold earrings. Men and women both wore them. Several pairs have been excavated from the tomb of a single individual, so it appears that Silla aristocrats owned many pairs, more than one of which were buried with them. Nobles of the Koguryo Kingdom and the Paekche Kingdom also wore earrings, but the largest quantity and generally the best quality have been recovered from Silla Kingdom tombs.

Earrings were worn by some women in Han Dynasty China, but the Chinese regarded their use as a barbarian custom. Chinese records mention that the Koguryo aristocracy wore earrings.

The uppermost ring on every Silla earring has a narrow slit through it, as we see here. This slit may have engaged the lobe of the wearer's ear, which may have been specially pierced for that purpose, but the slit is always quite narrow, so perhaps an additional element, such as a tied piece of string, was originally used to attach the earring to a pierced ear.

The leaf-shaped spangles and heart-shaped finials of the present earrings are typical of Silla earrings in general. The studded, hollow globes also appear in other examples, sometimes as the sole element of the pendant portion.

The technique of granulation was used sparingly here to produce the studs on the upper halves of the globes. Granulation means decorating a gold surface by the application of multiple, tiny, spherical beads of gold. This fascinating goldsmith's technique seems to have been invented in Mesopotamia around the 18th century B.C. It spread to Persia, then to Greece and Etruria, then across the silk-trade routes through Central Asia to China. Han Dynasty Chinese brought the technique to their colony at Lo-lang in Korea. It was used to good advantage on a famous gold buckle unearthed from one of the tombs there. Many Silla earrings were lavishly decorated with granulation.

THE UNITED SILLA PERIOD
668–918

8. Bul (Buddha)

Gilt bronze
H. 2⅞", W. 1⅜"
United Silla Period, 8th century
Gift of Dr. & Mrs. George Liberman   77.261

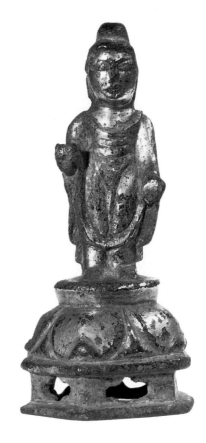

A tiny, gilt-bronze image like this was intended for the personal household shrine of a devout believer rather than for worship in a temple; it could even be carried with its owner on a journey. The ample proportions of the figure (the full, swelling forms of the face, torso, legs, and arms) closely reflect those of T'ang Dynasty (618–907) Chinese Buddhist images. The T'ang Dynasty was a Golden Age of cultural achievement in China. Nara Period (710–794) emperors in Japan and United Silla kings in Korea emulated T'ang styles as closely as possible. The annual tribute missions from United Silla to the T'ang court ensured close contact with China. As it did in early T'ang China, Buddhism received lavish state patronage in United Silla Korea.

The hands of Buddhist images usually assume specific symbolic gestures called *mudrā*. The identity of the deity is often indicated by the gestures of his hands. The particular combination of hand positions seen here is the most prevalent one on standing images of the Buddha in the Far East. It does not identify the specific Buddha represented by the image, however, since four different Buddhas are often shown with this combination of *mudrā*: Sakyamuni (the historic Buddha, Gautama, founder of Buddhism and an actual religious teacher and philosopher of India who died about 483 B.C.), Vairocana (the Cosmic Buddha), Bhaisajyaguru (the Buddha of Healing), and Amitabha (the Buddha of the Western Paradise).

In this *mudrā* combination, the right hand makes the gesture meaning "have no fear" (*abhayamudrā*): palm outward toward the worshiper, fingers and thumb together, extended upward. The left hand makes the gesture meaning "the Vows are fulfilled" (*varadamudrā*): palm outward toward the worshiper, fingers and thumb together, extended downward; it refers to the vows made by the Buddha to offer assistance, dispense favors, and grant desires to all sentient beings.

The upper half of the pedestal on which the present *Buddha* stands is in the form of an upside-down lotus having five petals. The lotus is an important Buddhist symbol; it refers to the purity of his teachings, which are like a lotus rising pure white above the muck in the bottom of a pond. The five petals here refer to the four directions of the compass and its center, suggesting the Buddha's dominion over the entire universe.

9. Yaksa (Bhaisajyaguru)

Bronze
H. 7⅛″, W. 2″
United Silla Period, 8th century
Frank L. Babbott Fund   74.165

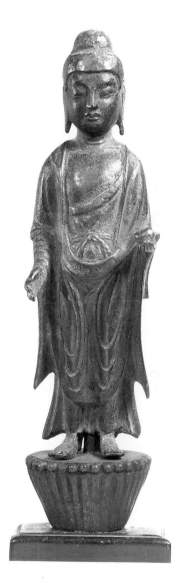

The identity of the specific Buddha represented by this image is indicated by the attribute (*laksana*) held in his left hand. It is a bowl (*pātra*), not the alms bowl often held by other Buddhist deities, but a medicine bowl or jar; it is sometimes depicted with its cover on, but here is shown with the lid removed. Bhaisajyaguru is the Buddha of Healing. His medicine bowl holds ointment to cure all the ills of mankind, and it is his identifying attribute. Sickness and injury being so common, Bhaisajyaguru was among the most widely worshiped of all the Buddhas.

The Sanskrit word *laksana* has another meaning besides that of a symbolic implement held by a deity. In the case of a Buddha, it also refers to the thirty-two signs that distinguish his anatomy from that of a mere human. Two of these thirty-two *laksana* are apparent on the present image. The hemispherical protuberance on top of the head (*ushnisha*) contains the Buddha's boundless consciousness and knowledge. The extended earlobes refer to the fact that Prince Siddhartha, the Buddha Sakyamuni before his enlightenment, wore the heavy earrings of an Indian prince.

The full, if not to say plump, face of this image is a stylistic element derived from T'ang Dynasty Chinese Buddhist sculpture (see Cat. 8). Here the style is based on that of the early T'ang Period: the body has not yet developed the ponderous massiveness characteristic of late T'ang Buddhist sculpture. This *Yaksa* could pass for a late 7th-century Korean sculpture, except that the figure is hollow and was cast with two large, oval-shaped openings on the back of the body and another on the back of the head. This feature is typical of 8th-century Korean bronze images but not of 7th-century ones.

Iconography, style, and technique aside, this little bronze figure of Bhaisajyaguru is an extraordinarily powerful work of religious art. The alert and compassionate expression of the face plus the welcoming gesture of the right hand express perfectly the caring and healing capacities of the Buddha of Medicine. The face of this image conveys a profound spirituality.

10. Bowl and Cover

Stoneware with deposits of natural ash glaze
H. 4⅜", W. 5¼"
United Silla Period, 8th–9th century
Gift of Sir George Sansom   40.721 a&b

The form of this *Bowl* is more sophisticated than the somewhat angular forms of 5th–6th century Silla pottery. The tall, perforated pedestal (see Cat. 5) has disappeared, replaced with a flaring footring. The dynamic, swelling, and harmonious shape of this *Bowl*, like so much in the high culture of the United Silla Period, reflects the pervasive influence of T'ang Dynasty Chinese forms.

The technique, however, is a direct continuation of earlier Silla methods: gray-black stoneware pottery with incised and impressed decoration and deposits of natural ash glaze. T'ang pottery was much more advanced technically: buff pottery covered with intentional, applied glazes either clear or in various colors, including amber, green, and blue. Often three different colored glazes were used on the same piece, creating an extremely striking decorative effect. T'ang potters also made a hard, high-fired, porcelaneous white ware. United Silla pottery was technically primitive by comparison.

Aside from the T'ang-inspired shape, the decoration of this covered *Bowl* distinguishes it from a 5th–6th-

century Silla piece. Instead of horizontal bands of combing or sparse, simple incised designs, the entire exterior surface of the vessel is covered with a textured pattern of impressed dots within partial circles, the design perhaps meant to suggest the scales of a dragon. The dragon is a frequent and auspicious motif in the Far East (see Cat. 69). As with the combed or incised designs on 5th–6th-century Silla pottery, these circle-and-dot designs were stamped into the leather-hard surface of the clay before drying and firing.

The impressed decoration on United Silla pottery is thought to have contributed to the development of slip-inlaid decoration on Koryo and Yi Dynasty ceramics (see Cat. 17, 61). The technique of slip inlay, which became a Korean specialty from the 12th century onwards, consists of painting a thick application of white slip (liquid clay) over impressed or incised designs, letting it set leather hard, then scraping all the white clay off the gray clay surface, leaving the white remaining as inlay in the recessed designs.

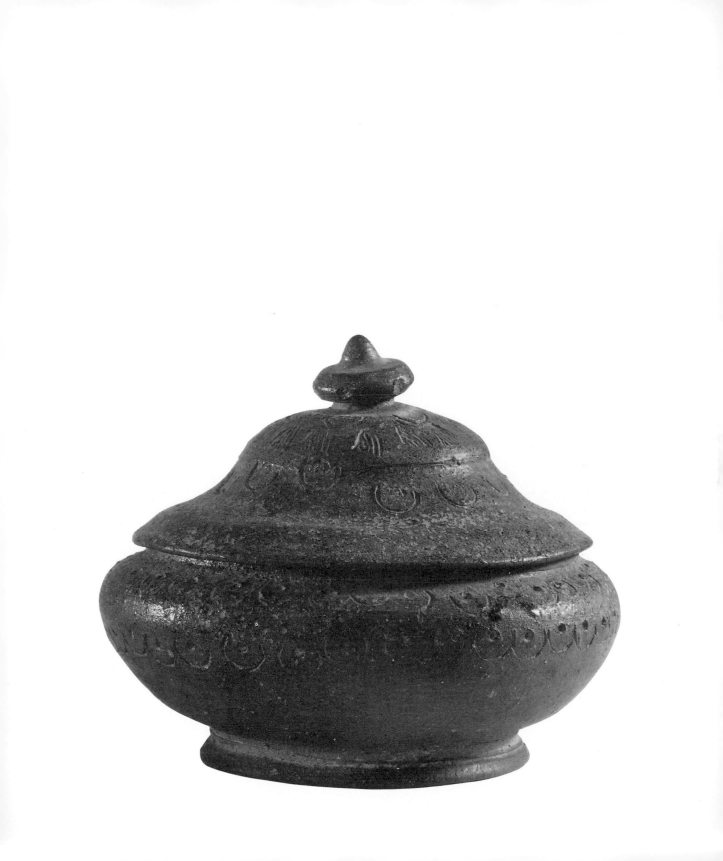

THE KORYO DYNASTY
918–1392

11. Amit'a (Amitabha) Triad

Hanging-scroll painting; ink, color, and gold on silk
H. 51¼", W. 32¼" exclusive of mounting
Koryo Dynasty, 14th century
Gift of Prof. Harold Henderson   61.204.30

A large, elegant Buddhist painting like this would have been a major icon in a prosperous Buddhist temple. The most characteristic type of icon painting used by the Pure Land Sect is seen here. Amitabha and his two Bodhisattva assistants are shown gliding through the sky, coming to Earth to carry the soul of a newly deceased believer back to the Western Paradise. The lotuses supporting the feet of the three deities are borne along on little clouds. This theme is understandably a very comforting one to a devout Buddhist. Paintings of this subject were sometimes mounted on small, three-panel screens to be placed at the bedside of a dying believer so he could feel himself being transported to the Pure Land.

The Bodhisattva at the right, holding the *kalasa* (flask) in his right hand, is Avalokitesvara (see Cat. 4). The Bodhisattva at the left is Mahasthamaprapta; he is a manifestation of Amitabha's spirtual wisdom, just as Avalokitesvara is a manifestation of Amitabha's mercy.

The present painting was acquired in Japan during the 1950s. Its Japanese lacquered-wood storage box has an inscription on the lid attributing the painting to Chang Ssu-kung, a Chinese artist of the Sung Dynasty (960–1279). Very few Koryo Dynasty Buddhist paintings have survived. There are only about five in public collections in the United States and one in Europe. None are known to have survived in Korea. Lee Byung-chull, founder of the Ho-am Art Museum, recently purchased a Koryo Buddhist painting in Japan and brought it back to Korea for his museum.

Most, perhaps all, of the extant Koryo Dynasty Buddhist paintings were at one time preserved in Buddhist temples in Japan. These paintings reached Japan from Korea during the 13th through the 16th centuries, by trade or as booty from Japanese pirate raids on Korean coastal towns or from Hideyoshi's invasions of Korea in 1592 and 1597.

Koryo Buddhist paintings preserved in the storehouses of Japanese Buddhist temples were nearly all ascribed to the Sung Dynasty of China, as in the case of the present painting. Such misattribution is not as ridiculous as it might sound, however. Korean Buddhist paintings of the Koryo Dynasty were based closely on Sung Dynasty Chinese prototypes. Only in recent years have Korean and Japanese scholars begun to attribute the extant Koryo Buddhist paintings correctly to Korea.

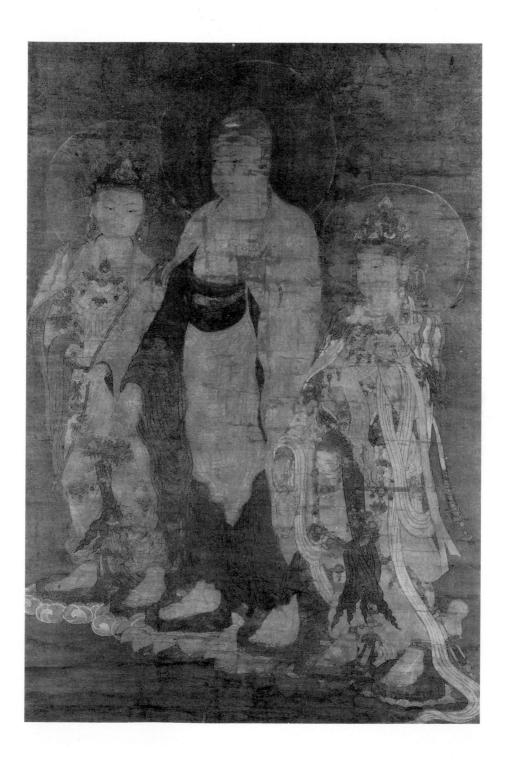

12. Ewer

Stoneware
H. 9⅞", W. 8¼"
Koryo Dynasty, 11th–12th century
Gift of Sir George Sansom   40.722

The Koryo Dynasty is famous for its celadon porcelain (see Cat. 13), but celadon was expensive and only the aristocracy could afford it. The everyday, workhorse ceramic ware of the Koryo Dynasty was unglazed gray-black stoneware, a direct continuation of Silla and United Silla pottery. The techniques remained the same as before, but the shapes changed drastically. As with so much of Koryo Dynasty culture, the models were Chinese wares of the Sung (960–1279) rather than the T'ang Dynasty.

The present *Ewer* was formerly attributed to the Silla period simply because it is made of gray-black stoneware instead of celadon porcelain. But the shape, with its delicate, recurving spout and stately, balanced proportions, is a Sung-derived shape that simply did not exist in Silla or United Silla times. Antique dealers in the United States still usually call this kind of ware "Silla."

The incised design of lotus petals forming a band around the lower body of this *Ewer* is another indication of its Koryo date. Whether incised, carved, or slip inlaid, this border design is common on Koryo celadon (see Cat. 14) but virtually nonexistent on United Silla ware.

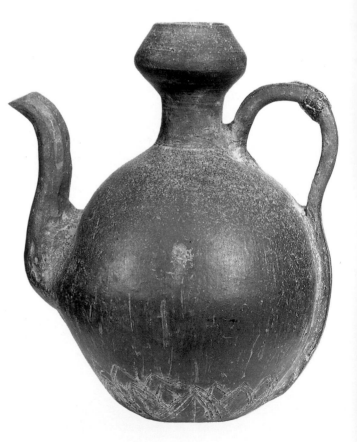

13. Ewer

Celadon porcelain
H. 9¼", W. 7⅞"
Koryo Dynasty, 11th–12th century
1916 Museum Collection Fund   17.24

Throughout the world, the most famous art form, indeed the most famous product, of old Korea is celadon porcelain. Celadon is a high-fired, porcelaneous ware having a gray clay body covered with a translucent, greenish feldspathic glaze. The green color of the glaze results from the presence of iron oxide fired in a reduction kiln (one in which only a limited amount of oxygen is available during firing). The semitransparent, greenish glaze on the light-gray clay body yields the typical gray-green color of celadon, which ranges from olive through gray-green to an almost turquoise blue green. The latter color is considered the most desirable and occurs only on the best pieces. Chinese and Korean connoisseurs named it "kingfisher blue" after the brilliant, iridescent plumage of this small bird.

"Celadon" is the Western term for a ceramic ware that was developed in China at the beginning of the Sung Dynasty (960–1279) and introduced to Korea by Chinese potters in the 10th–11th century. The East Asian term for "celadon" is composed of two Chinese ideograms meaning "blue green" and "porcelain," respectively. The origin of the European term "celadon" is uncertain but the following explanation seems the most plausible: by the 16th century, Chinese celadon porcelain was being imported into Europe, where it became a fashionable luxury item. During the 16th century, the celadon reached Europe in Portuguese ships; in the 17th century, Dutch and English ships joined the trade. Astree's lover Celadon in Honore d'Urfe's romance *L'Astree*, wore a green cape. The play was extremely popular, and its hero's name may have been borrowed for the newly fashionable green porcelain imported from Ming Dynasty China.

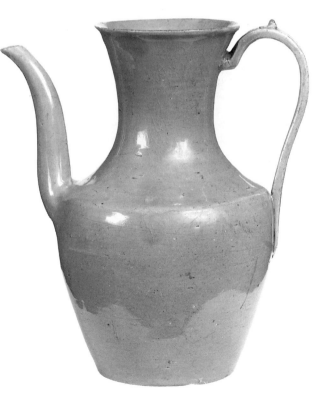

14. Ewer

Celadon porcelain
H. 15", W. 8⅞"
Koryo Dynasty, 12th century
Museum Collection Fund   57.141

This *Ewer* is one of the great treasures of The Brooklyn Museum. It dates from the 12th century, when Korean celadon porcelain was at its peak of excellence. The glaze on the *Ewer* is the most desirable color, the legendary "kingfisher blue." It is a rich, elegant bluish-green, not heavy and opaque, but delicate, subtle, and translucent. The shape of the *Ewer,* based on that of a calabash gourd, is sensuous, flowing, and perfectly proportioned. The gourd theme has been picked up by the gracefully arched handle, whose shape suggests three gourd vines twisted into a braid and tied with a string. The loop of "string" was meant to receive a silk cord whose other end was fastened to a similar loop on a tiny celadon stopper, which is now missing. The delicate, recurved spout echoes the curve of the handle. The surface of the spout is cut into subtle lengthwise facets.

The decoration fits and enhances the form perfectly. It depicts a lotus blossom, with a lotus-petal border below and drifting clouds above. The clouds have been rendered so as to suggest the heads and stalks of *pulloch'o* (Chinese: *ling chih*), the mythical Sacred Fungus of Taoism, a kind of magic mushroom that grows in the Land of the Immortals and bestows eternal life on those who eat it. The *pulloch'o* motif was an auspicious symbol of longevity in Korea; it appeared frequently in the decoration of household objects as well as in paintings.

The technique employed in decorating the present *Ewer* consists mainly of incised designs, that is, lines engraved in the surface of the leather-hard clay prior to glazing and firing. However, a little of the clay surface above or below some of the outlines has been carved away to make the leaves or petals stand in low relief against the surrounding background. Thus the technique should properly be called "incised-and-carved decoration." The blue-green glaze takes on a darker color where it runs thick in the recesses of the engraved lines and carved depressions, heightening the design, which reads as darker blue green against the lighter blue-green background.

The lotus was an important Buddhist symbol signifying the purity of the Buddha's teachings (the flower rises pure white or pure pink above the muck at the bottom of a pond). The lotus motif was not confined to Buddhist ritual objects; it became a frequent decorative motif on secular objects as well.

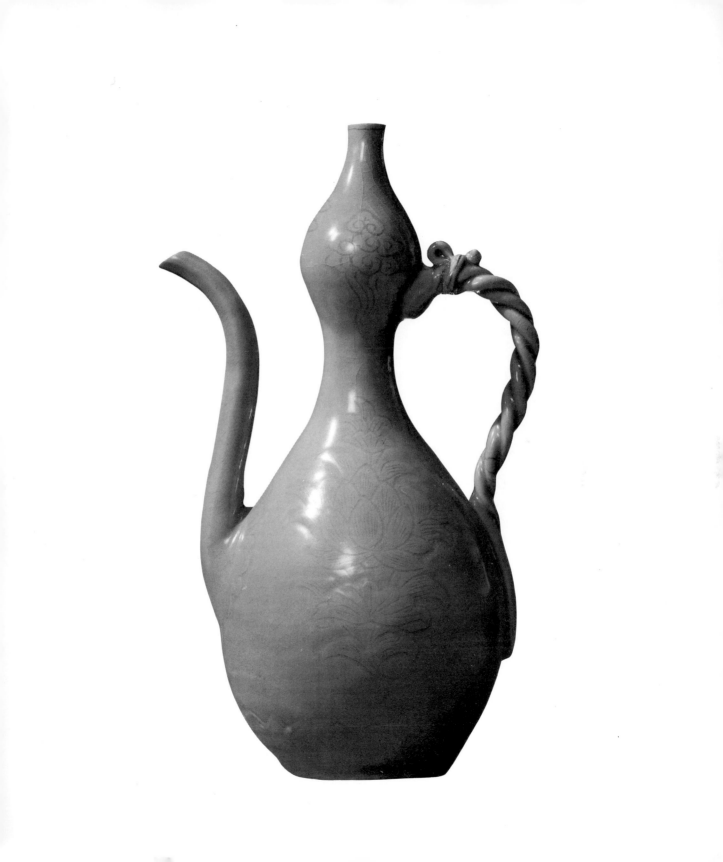

15. Ewer with Lid

Celadon porcelain with white and black slip decoration
H. 9⅞", W. 9½"
Koryo Dynasty, first half of the 12th century
Gift of Mrs. Darwin R. James III   56.138.1 a&b

This magnificent wine vessel is the most famous Korean work of art in The Brooklyn Museum. It has been illustrated in books and articles published in England, Japan, and Korea, as well as in the United States. Its lustrous glaze is the "kingfisher blue" color found on only the best 12th-century celadons. Its powerful, swelling body is boldly incised and carved with a design of overlapping lotus petals framing leaf sprays. The handle is in the form of a lotus stalk bound at the top with reeds. The lid is in the shape of an upside-down lotus flower. The lid knob is in the form of a lotus blossom just unfurling from the bud. A butterfly is modeled in relief on the back of the lid. A vine leaf appears on top of the handle. The butterfly and the leaf each originally supported a small loop to hold each end of the silk cord attaching the lid to the handle.

In addition to the strong, elegant shape, the striking incised designs, and the exquisite glaze color, this rare vessel is notable for another decorative element: touches of white slip accenting its ornamental motifs. Prior to applying the glaze, the potter used the point of a brush to touch on dots of white slip (liquid clay) in rows along the edges of the leaf sprays as well as on the lotus petals of the lid knob. A coating of white slip was painted on the butterfly and the vine leaf; the butterfly's eyes were touched with dots of black slip.

This kind of restrained and restricted use of painted white slip to augment incised decoration seems to have been an important step in the development of slip-inlay techniques by Korean potters during the first half of the 12th century (see Cat. 17). Simple linear decoration painted in white slip under the glaze appears on a few celadons from Sung Dynasty China: a Lung-ch'uan celadon bowl excavated in Korea has delicate, widely spaced radiating lines of painted white slip combined with a lobed rim to suggest the petals of a flower. The discovery of this Sung bowl in Korea, incidentally, verifies the fact that actual pieces of Chinese celadon, as well as celadon production techniques, were brought from China to Korea. For some reason, the Chinese soon abandoned slip-decorated celadon, while the Koreans developed slip inlay into a national speciality.

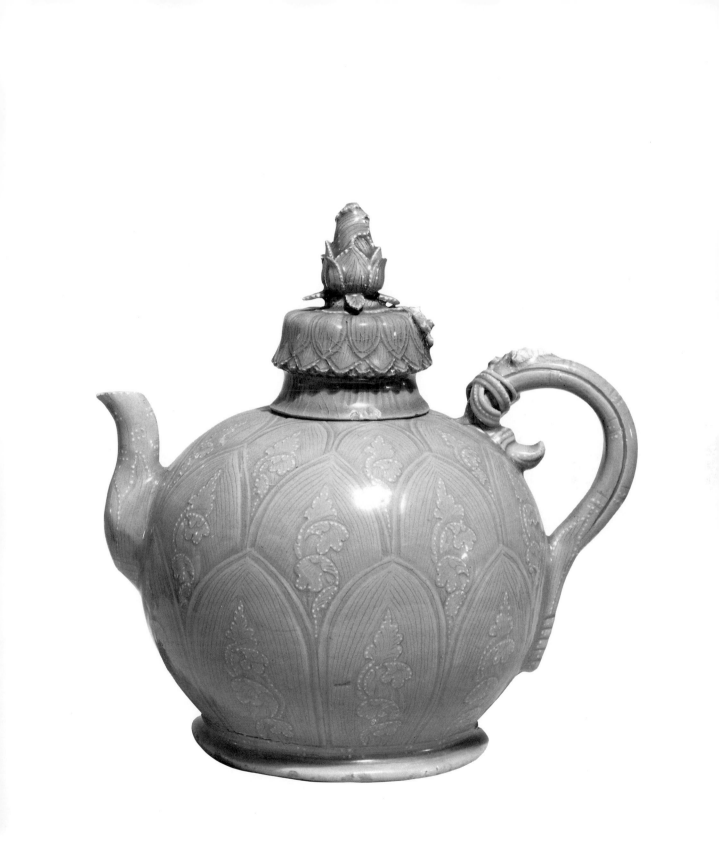

16. Prunus Vase

Celadon porcelain with white slip decoration
H. 13¼", W. 7¼"
Koryo Dynasty, first half of the 12th century
Gift of Miss Antoinette Kraushaar   76.43

This handsome *Vase,* with its lyrical design of
small, scudding clouds, is a great rarity: its decoration
consists of painted white slip. Like the dots of white
slip accenting the incised decoration on the preceding *Ewer* (see Cat. 15), painted white slip designs
such as we see here seem to have been a necessary
step in the development of slip-inlaid decoration
during the first half of the 12th century in Korea.

With slip inlay, the design was either impressed
(stamped) or incised into the surface of the leather-
hard clay, then painted over with white slip (liquid
clay); after the slip set leather hard, it was scraped
away to the surface of the pot, leaving white clay
inlaid in the surrounding gray clay. Slip inlay was a
more complex and expensive process than painting
the design in white slip. However, slip inlay
produced more satisfactory results: the white clay
was thicker and therefore appeared more uniform,
whiter, and more opaque through the glaze. In the
case of painted slip, if it was thinly applied, the
background gray showed through it in places; if it
was thickly applied, it looked lumpy under the
glaze. Koryo potters soon abandoned painted white
slip decoration in favor of slip-inlaid decoration. Slip
painting was revived later in the Koryo Dynasty for
a different style of decoration: underglaze iron-oxide
brown-black painted designs of floral sprays
inspired by Chinese Tz'u-chou Ware (see Cat. 21)

The shape of the present *Vase* is a splendid example
of one of the classic Koryo celadon vessel shapes,
the *maebyong* (Chinese: *mei p'ing*), literally "Plum
vase," considered ideal for displaying a single
branch of blossoming prunus (plum, apricot, peach,
cherry, or almond). This form of vase originated in
Sung Dynasty China. The Chinese version is generally more cylindrical, however. By constricting the
lower half of the vase, Korean potters emphasized
the swelling, globular form of the upper half, making
the proportions of the vase seem less stable but more
dynamic and powerful than the Chinese prototype.

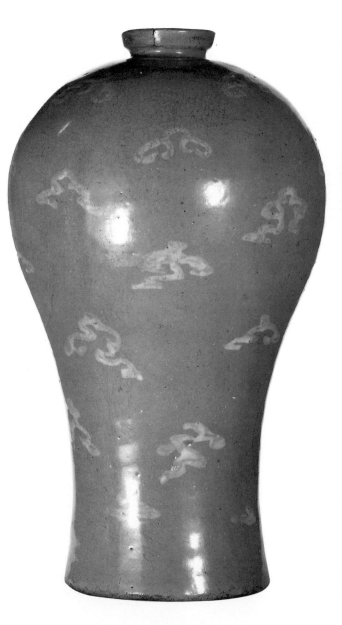

17. Wine Cup and Cup Stand

Celadon porcelain with slip-inlaid decoration
H. 2³/₁₆", W. 3⅛" cup; H. 1⅛", W. 4⅞" stand
Koryo Dynasty, 12th century
1916 Museum Collection Fund   17.26 a&b

The decoration on this elegant little *Cup and Stand* is a classic example of fully developed slip-inlay technique. The horizontal line below the rim was incised, as were the black leaves and stalk of each chrysanthemum plant. The key-fret border was impressed, one segment at a time, using a carved ceramic stamp; each chrysanthemum was also impressed with a carved stamp. White slip (liquid clay) was applied generously with a large brush over the border pattern and the flower; black slip was similarly painted over the leaves and stem. After it set leather hard, the slip was scraped away, leaving the white-and-black design inlaid in the gray clay surface. Then the glaze was applied, by dipping the vessel quickly into a large vat of liquid glaze, rotating it to ensure an even coating, and allowing the excess to run off. The glaze on this particular *Cup and Stand* fired a handsome blue-gray color. Slip-inlaid decoration on Koryo celadon was quite sparing at first, as here; later, the designs gradually occupied more and more of the vessel surface.

Painted-slip decoration preceded and probably influenced the development of slip-inlaid decoration (see Cat. 15, 16). The inlay technique produced a more uniform and brilliant white, causing the painted-slip technique to be abandoned. Slip-inlay was used in China, but only very rarely. Its stylistic derivation in China may have been from the inlaid metalwork of the T'ang Dynasty (618–907). Korean potters seem to have developed slip-inlay independently around the middle of the 12th century. The technique quickly became a national specialty. Slip-inlay decoration is the Korean potters' unique contribution to ceramic art. Koryo slip-inlaid celadon declined somewhat in quality during the 13th, and especially the 14th century, but slip-inlay technique was revived in the succeeding Yi Dynasty (1392–1910) in the form of overall patterns (Punch'ong Ware, 15th–16th century, see Cat. 61).

The stamped and incised decoration on typical

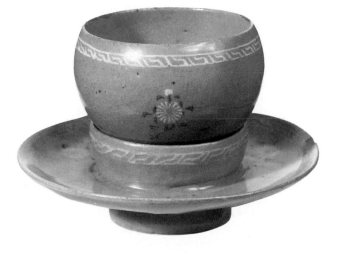

gray-black pottery of the United Silla Period (see Cat. 10) may have been instrumental in the development of Koryo slip-inlaid decoration. United Silla pottery recovered from tombs sometimes has light-colored earth imbedded in the designs as a result of burial. This effect may have inspired Koryo potters to brush liquid clay into the incised and stamped designs on their celadons.

The Korean term for slip inlay is *sanggam*, but the word also means "inlay" in general. Bronze inlaid with silver, and black lacquer inlaid with mother-of-pearl were other Koryo Dynasty specialties; the design motifs were much the same as those on inlaid celadon. Mother-of-pearl inlaid lacquer has continued to be a famous Korean product until the present day (see Cat. 86). Inlaid decoration in any medium appealed strongly to Korean taste.

18. Wine Bottle

Celadon porcelain with slip-inlaid decoration
H. 11¾", W. 7¹/₁₆"
Koryo Dynasty, 12th–13th century
Gift of Paul Manheim   67.199.3

This wine-bottle shape, with an ovoid body tapering gracefully into a tall, flaring neck, is one of the classic vessel shapes of the Koryo Dynasty. It occurs frequently in bronze (see Cat. 23) as well as celadon, and also in ordinary gray-black pottery.

The decoration on the present *Bottle* is typical of fully developed slip-inlaid celadon. The same designs appear over and over on other 12th–13th century examples. We have already encountered a white chrysanthemum with black leaves and stem (see Cat. 17). On the shoulder of this *Bottle*, where the body becomes the neck, we see a row of small stamped-and-slip-inlaid circles suggesting a string of beads with three hanging tassels, as if a necklace had been hung around the neck of the bottle. The three single chrysanthemums on the belly of the *Bottle* are each enclosed in two incised circles within a border of stamped *ju-i* scepter heads, the latter a common border design on Koryo celadons.

The *ju-i* scepter was an ancient Chinese ritual implement. It had a long, lightly S-curved handle and an inverted, ornamental, trefoil head. The *ju-i* scepter was originally a symbol of the Buddha and his doctrines, often held by the images of certain Buddhist deities. Later, *ju-i* scepters of jade or cloisonné were presented to honored Chinese laymen as tokens of esteem and good wishes (the two ideograms with which *ju-i* is written mean "as you wish"). The three-lobed head of the *ju-i* scepter was also equated with the mythical Taoist Sacred Fungus.

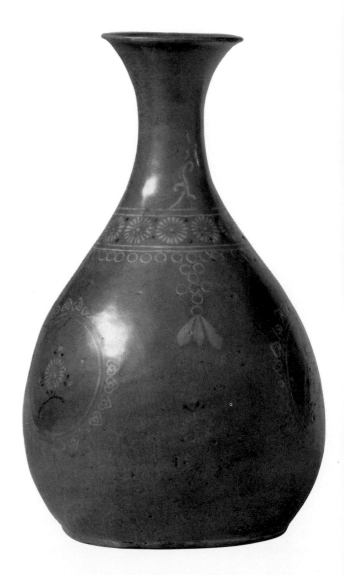

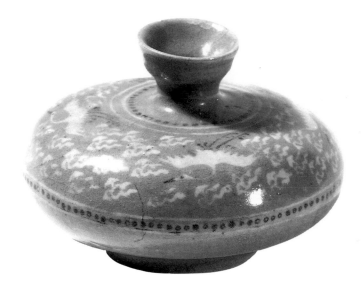

19. Oil Bottle

Celadon porcelain with slip-inlaid decoration
H. 2¼", W. 3⅜"
Koryo Dynasty, 12th–13th century
Gift of David James in memory of his brother,
William James   54.10.10

Slip-inlaid decoration on Koryo celadons was quite sparing when the technique first developed but became more exuberant as time went on, occupying more and more of the available surface, especially on small pieces, as we see here. This kind of tiny, squat bottle with a short neck and galleried mouth was used for cosmetic oil; it was a standard item in celadon toilet sets made for the ladies of the Koryo aristocracy. The complex pattern of small-scale, slip-inlaid designs filling much of the visible surface on a small piece like this creates a rich, jewellike effect.

The subject of the decoration here is cranes flying among clouds. Like the Sacred Fungus, the crane was an old Chinese Taoist symbol of immortality and became a popular motif in Korea (see Cat. 70). Manuchurian cranes, whose adults are about five feet tall when standing fully erect, could formerly be seen in large numbers all over Korea, Japan, and northeastern China. Today, only a few small flocks have survived in certain remote areas.

Since early times, the Chinese considered cranes the companions and messengers of the Taoist Immortals, who were said to fly back and forth between China and the Isles of the Blest (in the Eastern Sea) on the backs of cranes. Here, the auspicious symbolism of longevity and immortality is carried even further: the trefoil heads of the little scudding clouds on this *Oil Bottle* refer to the three-lobed heads of the Sacred Fungus.

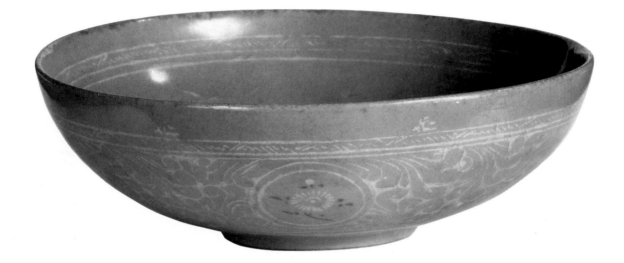

20. Bowl

Celadon porcelain with slip-inlaid decoration
H. 2¾", W. 7⅞"
Koryo Dynasty, 12th–13th century
Gift of the executors of the estate of Colonel Michael
Friedsam   32.886

The exterior of this *Bowl* displays a variation on the slip-inlay technique known as reverse inlay, in which the background portion of the design is carved out and filled with white slip. The elements of the design thus consist of gray clay surface surrounded and defined by a white-slip background. The gray clay appears greenish or bluish through the celadon glaze.

Reverse inlay was used for the floral arabesque pattern covering most of the exterior of this *Bowl*. Set within that pattern are four rondels enclosing chrysanthemum sprays done in regular white and black slip inlay. All the designs on the interior of the *Bowl* are rendered in regular slip inlay rather than reverse inlay. The decoration on the interior consists of five clusters of three pomegranates surrounding a central circle enclosing a sixth pomegranate cluster. The central circle has a border of *ju-i* scepter heads (see Cat. 18).

Both the exterior and interior have upper borders composed of paired horizontal lines with an undulating vine-scroll design between them. The exterior shows the late 12th–13th-century tendency to fill up more and more of the surface with inlaid designs.

The pomegranates decorating the interior of the *Bowl* were an especially auspicious motif. The pomegranate was an old Chinese Taoist fertility symbol: its many seeds suggested numerous progeny. The Chinese believed that a man achieved a certain immortality by siring many sons and grandsons. A wife's principal duty was to bear male children. The pomegranate was also a symbol of wealth: it was shaped like a moneybag and the seeds inside looked like jewels. In spite of all the symbolic meaning that accrued to it, this fruit was not native to China; it was introduced from South Asia in 126 B.C. Pomegranates, with their dual symbolism, became popular design motifs in Korea, appearing frequently on paintings and household utensils.

21. Prunus Vase

Celadon porcelain with black-slip decoration
H. 8¾", W. 6"
Koryo Dynasty, 13th–14th century
Gift of Mr. & Mrs. Robert Fomon   78.199

The reader will recall that the use of painted white-slip decoration on Koryo celadon seems to have preceded and influenced the development of slip inlay (see Cat. 16). Once the inlay technique was fully developed, painted white-slip decoration was abandoned. Painted black-slip decoration, on the other hand, became quite fashionable in the 13th and 14th centuries, although the technique seems to have been used as early as the end of the 11th century. The designs were painted with brownish-black slip (liquid clay containing iron oxide) before applying the celadon glaze.

Iron-painted celadon has a completely different look than the white-painted variety (see Cat. 16). The designs are larger, bolder, more spontaneous, and more energetic. Black-painted Koryo celadon decoration was obviously inspired by Tz'u-chou ware, a widespread northern Chinese ceramic ware with a buff-colored clay body and vigorous dark-brown iron-painted decoration. Tz'u-chou ware was produced throughout the Sung (960–1279) and Yuan (1279–1368) dynasties and well into the Ming (1368–1644). The exuberant floral sprays and chrysanthemum-petal border on this *Prunus Vase* clearly reflect its Tz'u-chou prototypes.

Iron-painted Koryo celadons from the 13th–14th century usually have a coarse, olive-gray, or olive-brown glaze, as we see here. The kilns that produced this ware were not capable of achieving the more refined blue-green, gray-green, or gray-blue celadon glaze colors. Also, the clay was less carefully sieved and the throwing and trimming were less skillful. The Mongol devastation of 13th-century Korea had taken its toll. Compare the clumsy potting, coarse clay, and dull olive glaze of this *Prunus Vase* to the elegance and refinement of a 12th-century example (see Cat. 16).

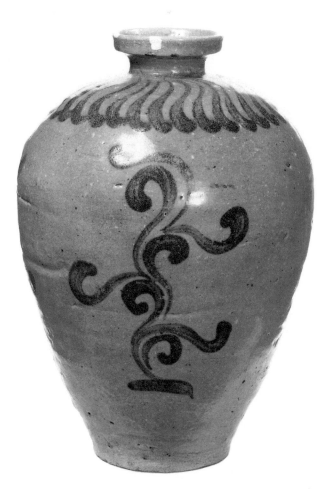

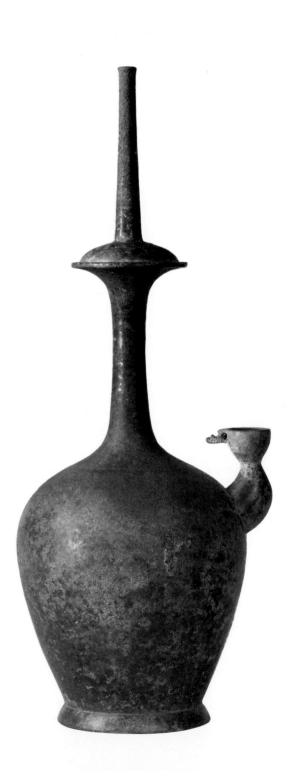

22. Kundika (Buddhist Ritual Water Sprinkler)

Bronze
H. 14½", W. 4⅞"
Koryo Dynasty, 12th century
Gift of Paul Manheim   74.27

The *kundika* (Korean: *chong-byong*) was a form of
kalasa (flask), the characteristic attribute held by
Avalokitesvara containing the nectar of compassion
(see Cat. 4, 11, 27, 28). Originally an Indian ritual
vessel, the *kundika* became a standard Koryo Dynasty
vessel type. It occurred frequently in celadon
porcelain as well as in bronze. Since extant examples
owe their survival to having been deposited in
tombs, Korean *kundika* either had a symbolic function
in connection with the spirit world, or they had
become secular luxury items as well as ritual vessels.

In its Buddhist context, a *kundika* contained the
water (or nectar) of life. The water was poured
through the vessel's tubular finial and refilled
through the covered spout on the shoulder. The
faithful worshiper was enjoined to become a
receptacle for the Buddha's Doctrine in the same
way that the *kundika* was a receptacle for the water
of life. In the Far East, paintings of Avalokitesvara
sometimes depict a *kundika* holding a willow branch.
Avalokitesvara used this willow branch to sprinkle
the nectar of compassion on his worshipers.

The filling spout on a Koryo *kundika* normally has
a hinged caplike lid. The lid is missing from the
present example, but the remains of its hinge may
be seen at the back of the filling spout. The graceful,
elegant lines of this *Kundika* seem entirely appropriate
to its use in stately Buddhist rituals. The surface of
the bronze was originally polished bright but has
developed a handsome gray-green patina from
burial in a tomb.

23. Wine Bottle

Bronze
H. 12½", W. 7"
Koryo Dynasty, 13th century
Gift of Dr. & Mrs. Robert Dickes   74.159.2

Here is a typical bronze example of the classic Koryo wine-bottle shape; we have already seen it in celadon (see Cat. 18). Bronzes like this were deposited in the tombs of the Koryo aristocracy, along with celadon porcelain, so that the deceased could continue to enjoy their use in the spirit world. Like the *Kundika* (see Cat. 22), this *Wine Bottle* was polished bright when it was new but has now developed a light-green patina from burial.

The technique employed in the manufacture of this *Wine Bottle* was entirely different from that of the *Kundika*. The *Kundika* was cast; the *Wine Bottle* was spun. Spun bronze involved mounting a small bronze cylinder on a lathelike device and drawing the malleable metal out to its final shape while it spun at high speed. This technique permitted thinner walls, making the vessel considerably lighter than its cast counterpart, thus requiring less bronze. The present *Bottle* was made in four sections, which were then brazed together. The lowest section is like a bowl with a high foot ring; the next section is cylindrical; the two upper sections are conical. The three joints between the sections have been accented with incised lines to articulate visually the surface of the *Bottle*. The uppermost section, the mouth of the *Bottle*, was cast rather than spun; it has slightly thicker walls than the other sections. The bottom of the *Bottle* consists of a round, flat bronze disc brazed inside the top of the foot ring.

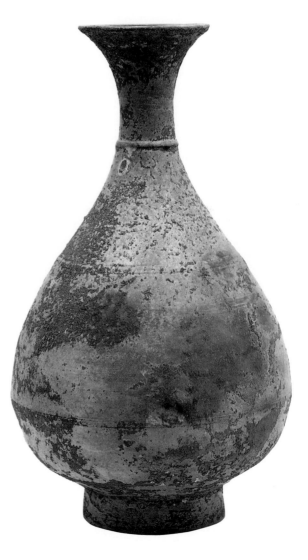

24. Ewer

Bronze
H. 10¼″, W. 8⅞″
Koryo Dynasty, 13th century
Purchase   74.163.3

Once again we find a vessel shape in bronze that we have seen before in celadon porcelain (see Cat. 13). With minor variations, Koryo vessel shapes became standardized; they were part of the distinctive Koryo Dynasty sense of form.

A ewer like this one, whether bronze or celadon, originally came with a matching bowl that corresponded to the shape of the lower half of the ewer. When not in use, the ewer nestled snugly in the bowl; when it was used, water from the ewer was poured into the bowl, for mundane purposes such as washing the hands and face.

Like the bronze *Wine Bottle* (see Cat. 23), the body of this *Ewer* was made of spun bronze. The spout was cast and brazed to the shoulder of the vessel. The straplike handle was hammered from a strip of bronze and riveted to the body and neck of the ewer. The lid and its knob, which is in the shape of a lotus bud, were cast. The lid is hinged to the top of the handle.

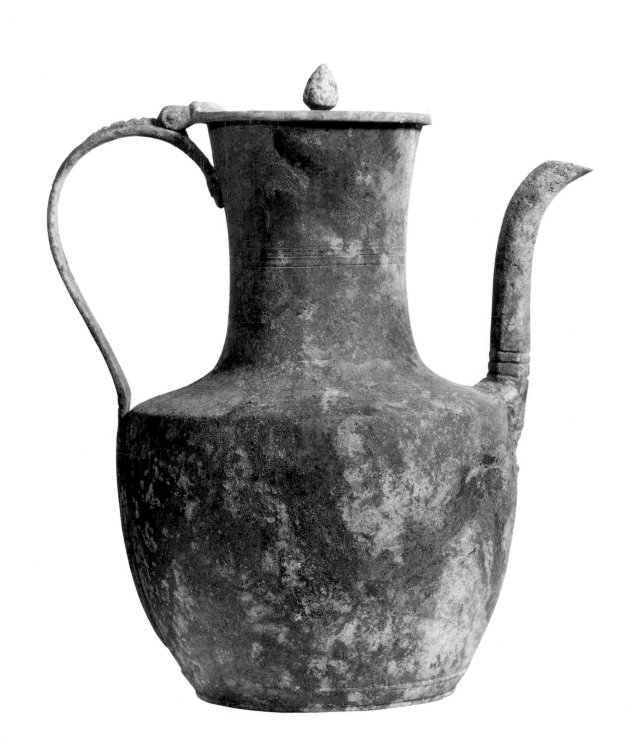

25. Mirror

Bronze
Diameter 5⅛″
Koryo Dynasty, 11th–12th century
Purchase   75.65.1

This *Mirror* was deposited in a Koryo Dynasty tomb, and was not excavated until recent times. Thus, like most ancient Chinese, Korean, and Japanese bronze mirrors, it has a dark-green burial patina. When new, its silvery yellow-white surface was polished bright; the reverse side, which is perfectly flat and smooth, formed an excellent reflecting surface. The hemispherical boss in the center of the obverse side has a transverse opening for the loop of a braided silk tassel that served as the mirror's handle. Bronze mirrors were essential items in the toilet sets of aristocratic ladies. The mirror was supported by a lacquered wood stand while the lady applied her makeup.

Quantities of ancient bronze mirrors have survived in China and Korea because of the custom of placing them in tombs. As with other luxury goods so deposited, the mirrors were meant to be used by the dead in the spirit world. In the case of the mirrors, however, there was also a special, magical reason for burying them with the dead: Because mirrors reflect images and light, from early times Taoists believed that they had the power to radiate light for eternity, thus magically illuminating the interior of the tomb.

The design cast in relief on the obverse of this particular *Mirror* also involves magic. The scene suggests longevity, and even immortality, for the mirror's owner. The female figure seated at the left is Hsi Wang-mu (Korean: So Wang-mo), Queen Mother of the West and the Queen of the Fairies (female Taoist Immortals); she is also the ancient Chinese Taoist Goddess of Immortality. She lives forever, ageless and beautiful, in her palace somewhere deep in the Kunlun Mountains of Central Asia. Phoenixes act as messengers and steeds for her and her fairies (see Cat. 72).

The peach trees in Hsi Wang-mu's orchard bear fruit every three thousand years; it takes another three thousand years for the magic peaches to ripen. Every six thousand years, Hsi Wang-mu holds a banquet for the Taoist Fairies and Immortals at which they partake of the magic fruit. Eating a Peach of Immortality bestows three thousand years of life (see Cat. 73) The clusters of leaves above Hsi Wang-mu on this *Mirror* represent the magic peach trees in her orchard.

The male figure standing at the right is Tung Fang-so, a legendary advisor to the third Han emperor, Wu Ti (r. 141–87 B.C.). Tung Fang-so is said to have found his way to Hsi Wang-mu's palace and stolen one of the Peaches of Immortality, which he ate, causing him to live three thousand years. The rockery below the two figures on the *Mirror* suggests the lofty peaks of the Kunlun Mountains; the scudding clouds in the border suggest the Abode of the Immortals.

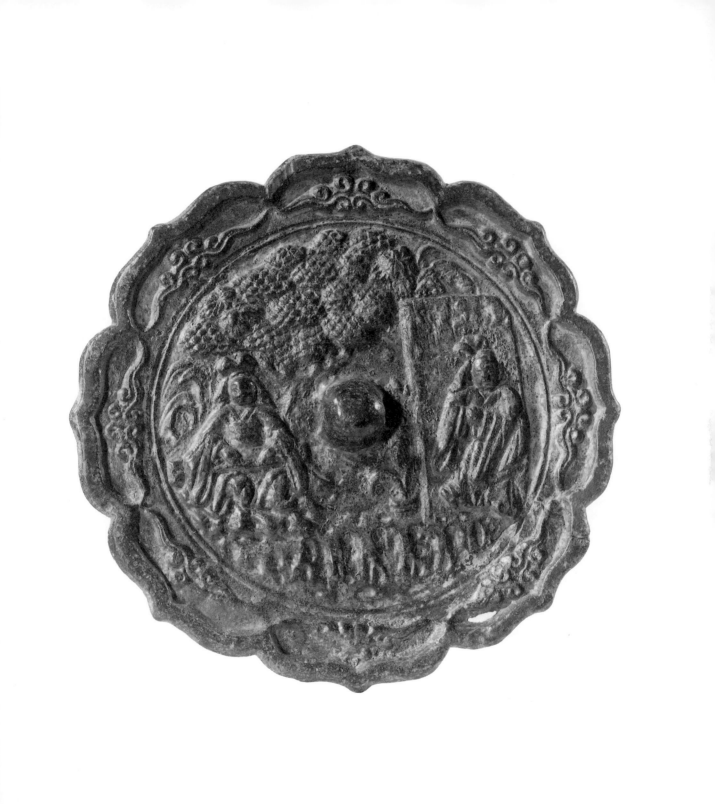

26. Mirror

Bronze
Diameter 5¾"
Koryo Dynasty, 12th–13th century
Purchase   75.65.2

The design cast in relief on the obverse of this *Mirror* depicts a ship sailing on a stormy sea. Three male figures, one of whom holds a sword aloft, stand in the bow of the ship. Five slightly smaller figures stand in the stern near the steering oar. A large dragon arises from the sea to confront the ship. Mythical fish swim at the upper left and the right. Clouds of spray cap the surging waves. At the top, above the ship's banner, is a four-character inscription in archaic seal-style script: *huang pi ch'ang ch'on* (clear, vast, luminous heaven).

While an exact interpretation of the nautical myth depicted on this *Mirror* is not possible today, certain observations may be made about the scene. The figure with the sword looks as if he were about to smite the dragon. This is unlikely, however, since in the Far East the dragon is benevolent, unlike his Western counterpart, who is the embodiment of evil slain by St. George. The Far Eastern dragon dwells in a palace at the bottom of the sea and in the storm clouds of the sky. He brings the rain that is essential for the crops (see Cat. 33). The dragon on this *Mirror* is probably assisting rather than threatening the figures in the ship.

A magic boat ferries the souls of the dead across to the spirit world; that may well be the theme depicted here. The dragon may be guiding and protecting the boat of souls on its way to the spirit world.

Since there seem to be eight figures on the ship, the motif may also refer to the Eight Immortals. The Chinese, with their predilection for numerical categories, codified the Taoist Immortals theme as "The Eight Immortals" (*pa hsien*). There were, of course, countless other Taoist Immortals. They were said to dwell on P'eng Lai, the mythical Islands of the Immortals in the Eastern Sea. The Eight Immortals were singled out from the others because of their special magic powers.

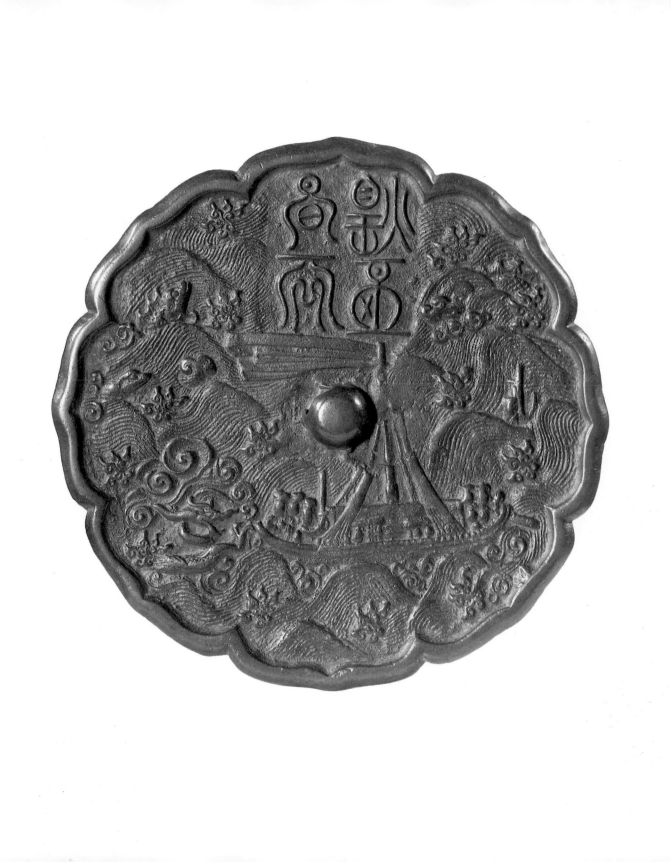

THE YI DYNASTY
1392–1910

27. Amit'a (Amitabha) Triad

Hanging-scroll painting; ink, color, and gold on silk
H. 36 5/16", W. 20⅞" exclusive of mounting
Yi Dynasty, 16th century
Source unknown   X715

This triad consists of a seated Buddha and two standing Bodhisattvas. The main deity is Amitabha, the Buddha of the Western Paradise of the Pure Land Sect (see Cat. 11). The Bodhisattva at the lower right is Avalokitesvara (Korean: Kuan Um), identified by the small figure of Amitabha on his diadem, and by the *kalasa* (flask) in his right hand (see Cat. 4). Avalokitesvara is the most compassionate, and therefore the most widely worshiped, of the Bodhisattvas. In the standard Amitabha triad of the Koryo Dynasty and later, the two Bodhisattvas were Avalokitesvara and Mahasthamaprapta, the manifestations of Amitabha's mercy and wisdom, respectively (see Cat. 11).

The present painting varies the standard formula by replacing Mahasthamaprapta with another Bodhisattva, Ksitigarbha (Korean: Chi'jang). Ksitigarbha is the patron of travelers, the Buddhist St. Christopher. Granite images of him stood along old country roads. More importantly, however, Ksitigarbha is the Bodhisattva who rescues the damned from Hell, the savior of dead children in particular. He uses the iron monk's staff in his right hand to batter down the gates of Hell. The flaming jewel in his left hand lights the way out of the underworld. Ksitigarbha came to be widely worshiped. By the beginning of the Yi Dynasty, he often took the place of Mahasthamaprapta in Amitabha triads.

Ksitigarbha is the only Bodhisattva depicted as a Buddhist monk. Other Bodhisattvas wear the elaborate drapery and ornate jewelry of an Indian prince, the imaginary garb of Prince Siddhartha (Sakyamuni Buddha before his enlightenment). Ksitigarbha wears the shaved head or close-cropped hair of a monk rather than the crownlike diadem of other Bodhisattvas. In the present painting, Ksitigarbha wears the complex drapery and necklace of a Bodhisattva, but he is often depicted in the simple robe of a monk.

The monk's staff held by Ksitigarbha is like the actual staffs Buddhist monks used to carry while walking out-of-doors. Such a staff has loose jingle rings on its finial; the sound they made was supposed to chase away insects in the monk's path lest he step on one and break his vows against taking life.

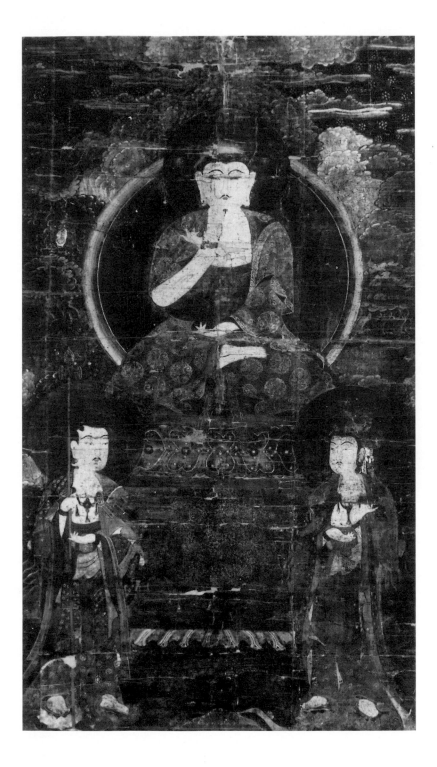

28. Amit'a (Amitabha) and The Eight Bodhisattvas

Hanging scroll painting; ink and gold on purple silk
H. 39", W. 32"
Yi Dynasty, dated in accordance with 1666
Gift of Mr. & Mrs. Herbert Greenberg   86.260.1

The central deity in this complex assemblage is once again Amitabha, the Buddha of the Western Paradise (see Cat. 11, 27). Here, Amitabha is surrounded by a group of eight Bodhisattvas in accordance with *The Eight Bodhisattva Mandala Sutra*. A *sutra* is a Buddhist sacred text. A *mandala* is a mystic diagram. A Buddhist *mandala* is usually a magic arrangement of Esoteric Buddhist deities who have specific spiritual and cosmic functions. A *mandala* symbolizes certain processes of the universe or assembles certain mystical forces to fulfill a worshiper's needs. *Mandalas* were thought to possess potent spiritual and magical power. Korean paintings of Amitabha and The Eight Bodhisattvas first appeared in the late Koryo Dynasty.

Avalokitesvara and Mahasthamaprapta, the two Bodhisattvas who normally accompany Amitabha (see Cat. 11), stand at either side of his dais, Avalokitesvara to the right, holding a *kalasa* (flask), Mahasthamaprapta to the left, holding a book. To the right of Avalokitesvara is Samantabhadra, a Bodhisattva of Wisdom, holding a five-colored cloud scepter. To the left of Mahasthamaprapta is Manjusri, another Bodhisattva of Wisdom, holding a lotus stalk supporting a book. In the second row, to the right of Amitabha's halo, is the Bodhisattva Maitreya (the Buddha of the Future). To the left of Amitabha's halo

is the Bodhisattva Ksitigarbha, wearing the close-cropped hair of a monk and carrying a monk's staff (see Cat. 27). At the far right and far left in the second row are Vajragarbha and Vijnesvara, two little-known Tantric Bodhisattvas, each holding a sword.

Supported by clouds in the upper right and upper left corners, on either side of Amitabha's lotus canopy, are two groups of eight figures with shaved heads and monk's robes. They are The Sixteen Arhats, the principal disciples of the Buddha. Leading the right-hand group of eight Arhats is a Buddha triad consisting of Sakyamuni, the historic Buddha, accompanied by two Bodhisattvas.

There is a dedicatory inscription in the rectangular panel below Amitabha's pedestal. About two-thirds of the inscription is effaced, but enough remains to provide some significant information: The painting was commissioned and dedicated in the cyclical year Pyong-o of the Son-chong era (equivalent to 1666). It was dedicated to Hyon-chong, the eighteenth king of the Yi Dynasty (r. 1660–1674). The donor, whose nom de plume was Sang-un, expressed his desire to "become a main pillar." The dedication to King Hyon-chong explains why gold was used for most of the lines in the painting; gold paintings were normally a prerogative of the Korean royal family.

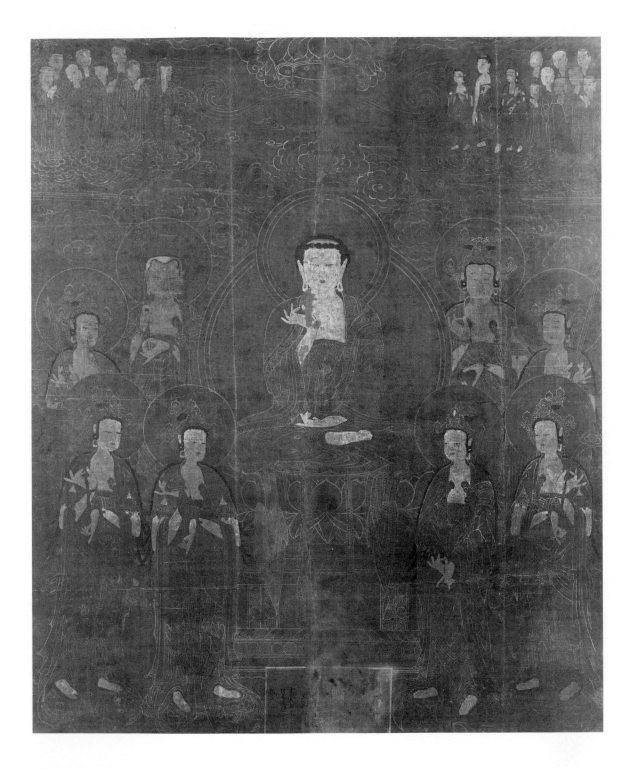

29. Amit'a (Amitabha) with Six Bodhisattvas and Two Arhats

Hanging-scroll painting; ink and color on silk
H. 31¾", W. 35¼"
Yi Dynasty, 18th century
Gift of Mr. & Mrs. Herbert Greenberg   86.260.2

Here Amitabha, the Buddha of the Western Paradise, is surrounded by four of The Eight Bodhisattvas who accompanied him in the preceding painting (see Cat. 28). Avalokitesvara, holding a *kundika* (ritual sprinkler), stands to the right of Amitabha's throne; Mahasthamaprapta occupies the corresponding position to the left. The Bodhisattva at the lower right bears no identifying attributes but is probably Maitreya, the Buddha of the Future, who is often paired with Ksitigarbha (see Cat. 28). Ksitigarbha stands at the lower left, identified by his shaved head and monk's staff. Flanking Amitabha in the second row are two monks, Ananda and Kasyapa, the Buddha's favorite disciples. On either side of Ananda and Kasyapa are two Bodhisattvas having no identifying attributes.

The Buddha and Six Bodhisattvas in this painting also represent Ch'il Song, The Seven Star Spirits. Confucianism was the official state religion of the Yi Dynasty. Although the government persecuted Buddhists severely, Buddhism survived in Korea as a kind of folk religion with a large admixture of Shamanist and Taoist elements. Although Korea had been a Buddhist country since the 4th–6th centuries, the Korean people had never abandoned their indigenous religion, Shamanism, which, in turn, had absorbed much from Chinese Taoism. Although Taoism, unlike Confucianism, had no temples or shrines of its own in Korea, it maintained a powerful influence on Korean religious beliefs and superstitions. Many of its deities were adopted by Shamanism and by Korean Buddhism. Taoist symbols in the form of animals, plants, mythical creatures, and abstract motifs, appeared constantly in Yi Dynasty household paintings and as ornaments on utilitarian objects (see Cat. 70).

The precincts of large Yi Dynasty Buddhist temples often included three subsidiary shrines, in addition to the main image hall and various other buildings. Each of these three side shrines (*sam song kak*) was dedicated to a Shamanist deity who had been adopted by Korean Buddhism: San Shin (The Mountain Spirit) (see Cat. 30), Tok Song (The Lonely Saint), and Ch'il Song (The Seven Star Spirits). Tok Song, whose name literally means "self-cultivation," was a Chinese Taoist saint adopted by Korean Shamanism and later embraced by Korean Buddhism. He epitomizes the Taoist ideal of attaining spiritual perfection, advanced age, and, perhaps, immortality, through the practice of solitary self-cultivation in remote mountain forests.

Like Tok Song, The Seven Star Spirits were Taoist deities assimilated by Korean Shamanism and subsequently by Korean Buddhism. A painting such as the present one would have been the main image in the Ch'il Song Kak (Seven Star Shrine) of a large Buddhist temple. In this context, The Buddha and Six Bodhisattvas also represents The Seven Star Spirits. The Seven Stars are those of Ursa Major, the Big Dipper, which is visible throughout the year from the northern hemisphere. Several other stars and constellations were deified by Chinese Taoists, but the Big Dipper was the most important because it was thought to bestow good and bad luck.

Buddhist paintings of The Seven Star Spirits usually represent them as a Buddha flanked by Six Bodhisattvas, as we see here. According to the teachings of Mahayana Buddhism, Sakyamuni, the historic Buddha, was preceded by seven earlier Buddhas, one in each of seven earlier cycles of time. In Korea, The Seven Buddhas of the Past were equated with The Seven Star Spirits.

Korean shamans (*mudang*) also employed Seven Star Spirit paintings, which were among the magical paraphernalia kept in *mudang* houses and used in shaman rituals (*kut*), usually performed outdoors. Shamanist paintings of Ch'il Song normally depict The Seven Star Spirits as gentlemen in imaginary Chinese Taoist costumes rather than as Buddhas and Bodhisattvas. Some Shamanist paintings depict the Seven Stars as women dressed in the distinctive costumes of *mudang*; most Korean shamans were women. The most basic Shamanist representations of The Seven Star Spirits are arrangements of seven small discs, or else five-pointed stars, in the positions occupied by the Big Dipper's stars, with a line connecting each disc to the next.

Seven was considered a lucky number in the Far

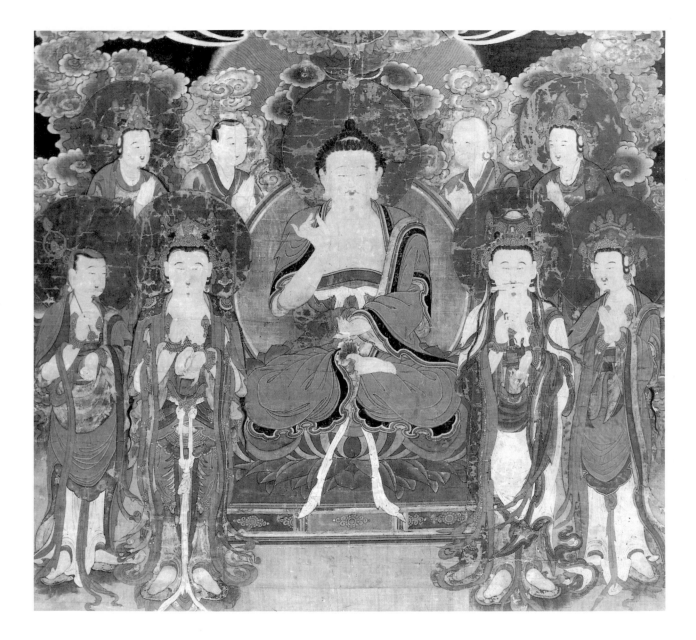

East. The Big Dipper's seven stars were paralleled by the seven "stars" of the face: two eyes, two ears, two nostrils, and a mouth. A person's destiny was thought to be controlled by The Seven Star Spirits. It was therefore important that a Korean Buddhist pay his respects and make a monetary offering in the Seven Star Shrine inside the compound of a Buddhist temple. It was equally imperative that a Shamanist believer stay on good terms with The Seven Star Spirits through the intercession of a *mudang*.

30. San Shin (The Mountain Spirit)

Hanging-scroll painting; ink and color on silk
H. 34″, W. 24½″ exclusive of mounting
Yi Dynasty, 19th century
Purchase　84.145

The Mountain Spirit was the most popular deity in the pantheon of Korean Shamanism. During the Yi Dynasty, his popularity forced Korean Buddhism to adopt him into the Buddhist pantheon. Buddhism had always tended to accommodate certain local, non-Buddhist deities; this flexibility is one of the reasons why Buddhism has spread over such a wide area and endured for so long.

As we have seen, The Seven Star Spirits and The Lonely Saint were Chinese Taoist deities absorbed into Korean Shamanism and then borrowed by Korean Buddhism (see Cat. 29). Two of the three side shrines in the precincts of large Yi Dynasty Buddhist temples were dedicated to The Seven Star Spirits and The Lonely Saint, respectively. The third and most important side shrine was dedicated to The Mountain Spirit. In addition to the ones within Buddhist temple compounds, thousands of independent Mountain Spirit Shrines were located throughout Korea, especially at sacred sites like the Diamond Mountains, where they often perched on top of cliffs. Since The Mountain Spirit was the most popular Shamanist deity, *mudang* (shaman) houses also maintained paintings of him.

Whereas The Seven Star Spirits and The Lonely Saint were of Taoist origin, and certain other Shamanist deities were of Taoist, Confucian, or Buddhist origin, The Mountain Spirit was a pure Korean Shamanist deity. However, his great popularity did not result from his being native; it resulted instead from his capacity to bestow children. A Yi Dynasty wife's first duty was to bear male children. A barren wife was disrespected or even rejected by her husband and his family. The fault was always assumed to be hers. If she had trouble conceiving, she went to a Mountain Spirit Shrine and prayed earnestly to The Mountain Spirit to grant her a baby. If the problem continued, she would hold a vigil at the shrine night and day, a one-hundred-night vigil being the most severe, recommended only for extreme cases. The Mountain Spirit had a second popular function: granting long life. Worshipers placed coins in his offering box to assure his help in achieving a long and happy life.

The Mountain Spirit is usually depicted as an old man with a white beard, as we see here. He is usually shown seated beside a pine tree accompanied by his messenger, the Tiger. He often holds a walking staff and fan, in this case a banana-leaf fan. The Mountain Spirit is often accompanied by two perpetually youthful attendants called *Dong-ja* (see Cat. 58). Here one holds a peony, a symbol of feminine beauty and sexuality; the other holds a pomegranate, a symbol of abundant progeny.

When The Mountain Spirit was shown wearing a crown, he represented Tangun. According to Korean mythology, the ancestor of the Korean people was a great hero named Tangun, the grandson of Hananim, the Creator and Supreme Ruler of the Universe. Tangun traditionally founded Korea in 2333 B.C. When Tangun died, he turned into The Mountain Spirit.

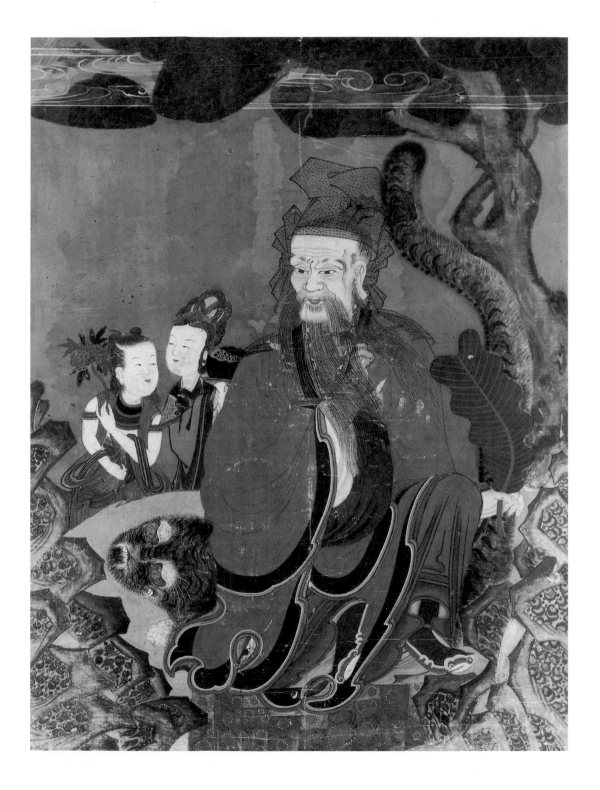

31. O Bang Jang Kun (The Five Guardian Generals)

Hanging-scroll painting; ink, color, and gold on silk
H. 57", W. 40"
Yi Dynasty, 19th century
Purchase   80.76

We have noted that The Seven Star Spirits were Chinese Taoist deities appropriated by Korean Shamanism and later borrowed by Korean Buddhism (see Cat. 29). The Mountain Spirit was a pure Korean Shamanist deity adopted by Korean Buddhism (see Cat. 30). The Five Guardian Generals were the reverse: Shamanist deities derived from Buddhist ones. The Five Guardian Generals were the most powerful of the many guardian spirits in Korean Shamanism. They protected believers from evil influences emanating from the five directions, that is, the four cardinal directions plus the center.

The Five Guardian Generals are The Blue King (Chong Je) of the East, The White King (Paik Je) of the West, The Red King (Chu Je) of the South, The Black King (Hyon Je) of the North, and The Yellow King (Hwang Je) of the Center. The Five Generals were usually depicted as a group rather than singly, and they were often accompanied by other deities, as they are here. They usually wore imaginary Chinese armor, as in the present painting, but they were sometimes shown in Chinese Confucian attire, or Chinese Taoist costume, or even the Indian skirts and scarves of Buddhist deities.

The Five Guardian Generals derive from The Four Heavenly Kings, whom they closely resemble. The Four Heavenly Kings were directional Guardian Generals prominent in the iconography of Chinese, Korean, and Japanese Buddhism almost from its inception. The Four Heavenly Kings were frequently represented in sculpture as well as in paintings. They wore imaginary Chinese armor. Their function was to protect the Buddha, Bodhisattvas, and worshipers from the forces of evil emanating from the four directions.

The Five Guardian Generals simply added a fifth guardian to protect the center. The names of The Five Guardian Generals were different from those of The Four Heavenly Kings. The names and colors of The Five Guardian Generals were based on an ancient series of Chinese Taoist guardian spirits called The Animals of the Four Directions. This series of mythical guardian animals was mentioned in the I Ching. Many Taoist beliefs and practices found their way to Korea due to increasing Sinification during the Three Kingdoms Period. The finest extant representations of The Animals of the Four Directions are in Korea rather than China: magnificent wall paintings in 6th–7th-century Koguryo Kingdom tombs in North Korea.

The Animals of the Four Directions are The Blue Dragon of the East, The White Tiger of the West, The Red Phoenix of the South, and The Black Tortoise of the North (entwined by a snake). Each is derived from a constellation in its respective direction of the sky. These four cardinal spirits were considered crucial in the geomancy of a building site and are still invoked for this purpose today in China and Korea. The four main gates of a Korean palace bore depictions of their respective spirit animals to protect the palace from evil influences. The four spirit animals were also critical in the selection of a proper tomb site, which must have a Blue Dragon Ridge (or at least hill) on the east, a White Tiger Ridge on the west, and access from the south (north is the direction of honor).

In the present painting, The Five Generals are accompanied by a figure in imaginary Taoist costume to the right of the central General and another in imaginary Confucian costume to the left of the central General. The two figures probably represent Lao-tzu and Confucius, the founders of Taoism and Confucianism. Confucius holds his book, the Analects. Above the center General are two unidentified Bodhisattvas, one holding a lotus, the other a stylized peony. On either side of the Bodhisattvas are youthful attendants, two females to the right, three males and a female to the left.

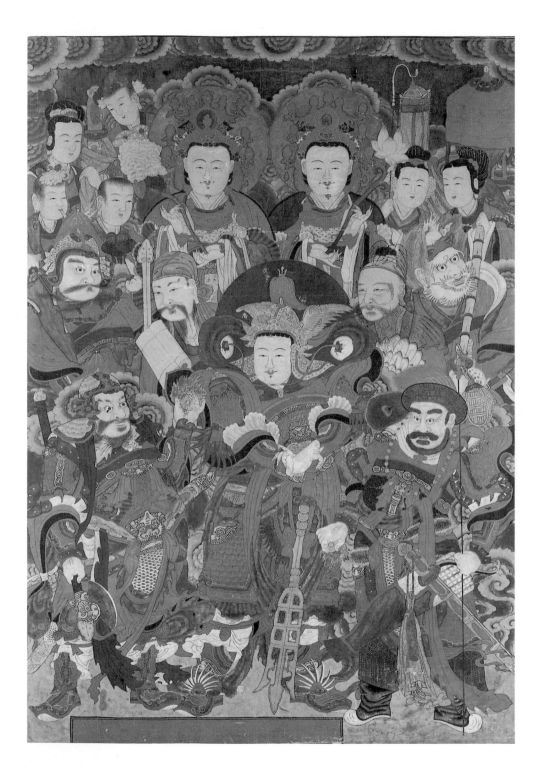

32. Three *Mudang* (Shamans) and a Tiger Performing a *Kut* (Shaman Ritual)

Hanging scroll painting; ink and light color on paper
H. 24⅞", W. 30¾" exclusive of mounting
Yi Dynasty, 19th century
Gift of Mr. & Mrs. Allen & Susan Dickes Hubbard
86.264.2

A few of the extant Shamanist paintings in Korean collections depict the shamaness herself, deified as The *Mudang* Spirit. A small number of other surviving paintings depict *kut* (shaman rituals), but the present painting is the only example I know of in which a tiger participates in the *mudang* dance. The tiger actually seems to be levitating, and he is not an ordinary tiger. This Tiger is The Messenger of the Mountain Spirit, and a potent guardian spirit in his own right (see Cat. 54).

Most Korean shamans were women, although the profession was not limited to them. The hat worn by each *mudang* in this painting is a characteristic type of shaman headgear. It has a close-fitting, hemispherical crown; a broad, flat brim; a chin strap of large beads; and a long peacock tail feather swinging from the metal finial on the center of the crown. One *mudang* holds an oversize folding fan (in the closed position). The other two hold paddlelike ritual implements. Tridents and folding fans were the standard implements used in shaman rituals. During a *kut*, which may last anywhere from an hour or so to as long as several days, the *mudang* dance themselves into an ecstatic trance in which they mystically become one with the spirit being invoked.

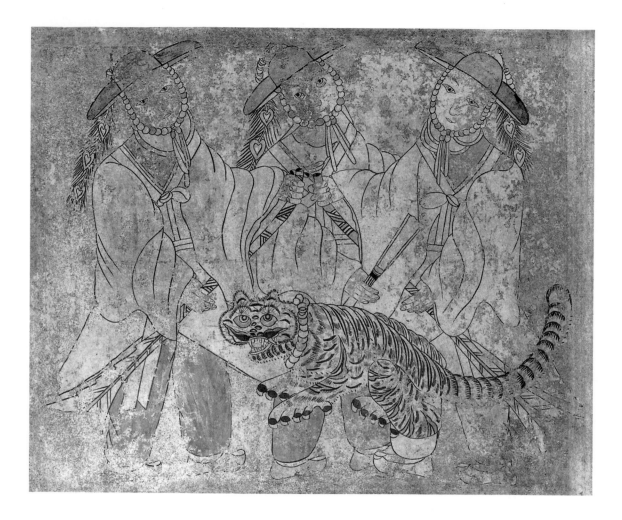

33. Rain Dragon

Hanging-scroll painting; ink and color on paper
H. 35⅜", W. 27¼", exclusive of mounting
Yi Dynasty, 18th century
Gift of Mr. & Mrs. Burton Krouner   82.133

During a drought, Korean shamans invoke dragons to bring rain. The rain-supplication ritual is one of the most ancient and important *kut* (shaman rituals). *Mudang* dance in front of a Rain Dragon painting and make animal-blood offerings to the Rain Spirit personified by the dragon. *Mudang* rain holes, cuplike depressions carved in boulders, were meant to receive these offerings and are found throughout Korea.

The dragon is the best-known and perhaps the most ancient mythical creature in the Far East. Like most of the other imaginary animals in Chinese mythology, the dragon is of Taoist origin. Dragons decorate the surfaces of bronze ritual vessels from the Shang (1523–1028 B.C.) and Chou (1027–256 B.C.) dynasties, often in conjunction with the Thunder Pattern, a squared-spiral design derived from ancient pictographs for clouds, lightning, and thunder. Chinese depictions of dragons reached their full, familiar form during the Han Dynasty (206 B.C.–A.D. 221); they were transmitted to Korea through the Han trading colony at Lo-lang (108 B.C.–A.D. 313). Although Taoist in origin, the dragon became associated with all four Korean religions: Buddhism, Confucianism, Taoism, and Shamanism.

The Far Eastern dragon is awesome but benevolent, unlike the Western dragon, who is the embodiment of evil, the serpent in the Garden of Eden, the symbol of Satan slain by St. George. In China and Korea, a dream about a dragon is the most auspicious of dreams: If a man dreams of a dragon, he will achieve success: if a woman dreams of a dragon, she will bear a son who will be a virtuous man.

The dragon is a water spirit who controls oceans, rivers, lakes, rain, and floods. He lives in the Dragon Palace at the bottom of the sea or among the clouds in the sky. When a rainstorm occurs, it is because a dragon is ascending to the sky. He sometimes takes human form as The Dragon King, who is also called The Water Spirit or the Dragon Spirit, depicted as an old man with a white beard, who is often shown riding a dragon. The Dragon King and The Mountain Spirit are sometimes paired in Shamanist paintings that symbolize their dominion over mountains and seas. As we have seen, the tiger is the messenger of The Mountain Spirit (see Cat. 30). Similarly, the tortoise is the messenger of the dragon and communicates between the Dragon Palace at the bottom of the sea and mortals on land. The tiger and the dragon, the two most powerful spirit animals, are often paired in *pujok,* paper talismans pasted on the doors or walls of Korean houses to ward off evil spirits.

The dragon is frequently shown pursuing, or clutching in one of his front claws, the Flaming Pearl (a magic jewel from the sea symbolizing wisdom and immortality). Immortality was primarily a Taoist consideration; wisdom was more of a Confucian theme. In a Confucian context, the dragon came to symbolize Heaven, as well as the virtue and authority of a king (see Cat. 69). As a royal symbol, the dragon was often painted yellow; as a rain symbol, he was usually painted blue. They were a predominant theme in the architectural decoration and ritual paraphernalia of Korean royal palaces and Confucian temples. A five-clawed dragon in China or Korea was usually, but not always, restricted to royal use. Other depictions of dragons showed only four claws, or even three, on each foot. A scroll painting of a dragon was often hung in a man's study to suggest his role as a virtuous head of the household.

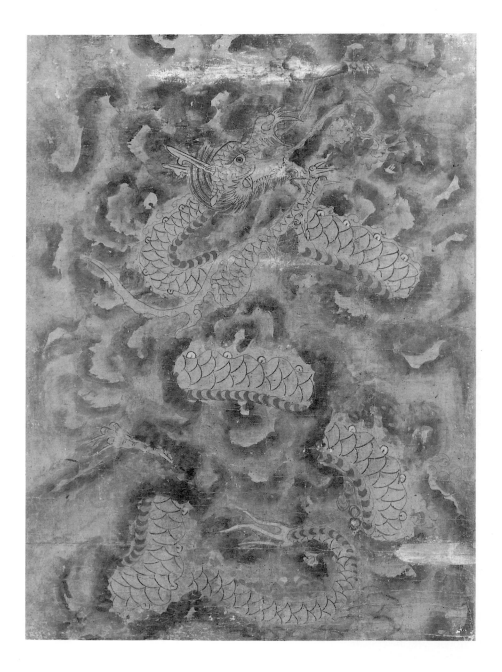

34. Kam Mo Yo Je Do (Spirit Shrine)

Hanging-scroll painting; ink and color on paper
H. 67 5/16", W. 56 ⅝"
Yi Dynasty, dated in accordance with June, 1811
Purchase   86.25

The paintings we have considered thus far have been religious, either Buddhist or Shamanist. They were icons, objects of veneration and spiritual contemplation in Buddhist temples of Shamanist *mudang* houses. They were aids to worship and meditation, as well as the focus of religious rituals. Such paintings were never displayed in ordinary homes; to do so would have been unthinkable.

Spirit Shrine paintings, on the other hand, were specifically intended for use in Yi Dynasty homes. An ancestral shrine was an integral part of every Korean house. Confucianism, the state religion of the Yi Dynasty, held that ancestor worship was the primary duty of every Korean family, who were morally obliged to worship their ancestors for at least three generations back. A wealthy household maintained a separate room, or even a separate building, as an ancestral shrine. The room was equipped with special furniture and utensils for the rituals of ancestor worship: altar tables and offering stands, as well as a small but very high chair that served as a throne for the ancestor's spirit, whose presence was indicated by a wooden tablet inscribed with the ancestor's posthumous name. During the ceremony, the spirit tablet was placed on the tall chair or on an altar table

in front of an ancestor portrait of the deceased (see Cat. 35). Lacking such elaborate paraphernalia, or the room to house it, a family of modest means used a Spirit Shrine painting instead.

Kam Mo Yo Je Do means "Shrine Where the Ancestors Come When Worshiped." The space between the open doors of the tile-roofed shrine in the painting was left blank. On the anniversary of an ancestor's death, a slip of paper inscribed with his posthumous name was pasted temporarily on the blank space.

The present *Spirit Shrine* painting is larger than the usual household variety, and the ancestors' names are permanently inscribed in gold on the large, red spirit tablet in the doorway where the blank space would have been. This painting commemorates royal ancestors. The tablet is inscribed with the spirit names of a former king and queen. The ink inscription in the lower right corner of the painting includes a date: the sixth month of the sixteenth year of the Chia-ch'ing era. Chia-ch'ing was the fourth emperor of the Ch'ing Dynasty; he reigned from 1796 to 1820. This yields a date of 1811 for the painting. It was standard practice to inscribe Chinese reign dates on 18th- and 19th-century Korean paintings, since Korea maintained close tributary ties to China at the time.

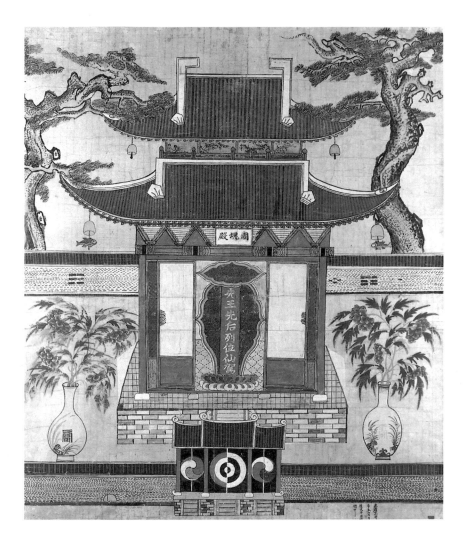

35. Portrait of Chief Minister Mun Suk-kong

Hanging-scroll painting; ink and color on silk
H. 28½", W. 20¼" exclusive of mounting
Yi Dynasty, 19th century
Gift of Dr. & Mrs. John Lyden   86.271.7

At the royal court and in government buildings, portraits of kings and important officials served a significant purpose. According to Confucian theory, the portrait of a virtuous man has an important didactic function: it inspires correct moral behavior in those who view it. State portraits thus constituted an official art serving the interests of the government in maintaining the status quo.

The three-line inscription at the upper right of the present painting reads: "Portrait of Chief Minister Mun Suk-kong, name Ik-mo, pseudonym Chong-kyon-yo." The one-line inscription below reads: "Respectfully inscribed by his seventh-generation descendant, Sang-hak, in the last ten days of the month, during Autumn, in the fifty-seventh cyclical year." The year cycle recurs every sixty years. "Mun Suk-kong" is the posthumous name of Han Ik-mo, who was born in 1703 and became Chief Minister in 1772.

Chief Minister Mun wears a court robe and an official belt indicating his court rank. He wears a black-lacquered horsehair-gauze court cap, whose shape is another indication of his court rank. The chief minister's face is drawn with unusual skill and sensitivity. One feels that the portrait is a good physical likeness and reveals something of Mun's personality as well. In fact, the portrait was probably painted well after the chief minister's death. The

artist probably never saw him or knew him. Such was usually the case with Chinese and Korean ancestor portraits, which tended to be perfunctory. They were virtually mass-produced to meet the demand, ancestor worship being a moral duty of every citizen.

Still, the extraordinary sensitivity of the present portrait would seem to suggest that it is based on sketches made from life. Perhaps this painting was done as a court portrait while Mun was still alive rather than the usual ancestor portrait painted after his death. The drawing and brushwork are of the highest quality, unusually so for an ancestor portrait. The artist was obviously talented and well trained. He must have been a court artist, a professional painter employed by the Bureau of Painting (To-hwa-so). Korean court painters, unlike Korean scholar painters and Chinese court painters, were not permitted to sign their work. They were called upon primarily to paint ancestor or court portraits, commemorative pictures of important ceremonies and major historical events, and decorative, symbolic screens for the royal palace, government buildings, or Confucian temples. Yi Dynasty court painters came mainly from the *chungin* class, a small class below the scholar officials and above the commoners, made up of minor government officials, doctors, scientists, engineers, and translators.

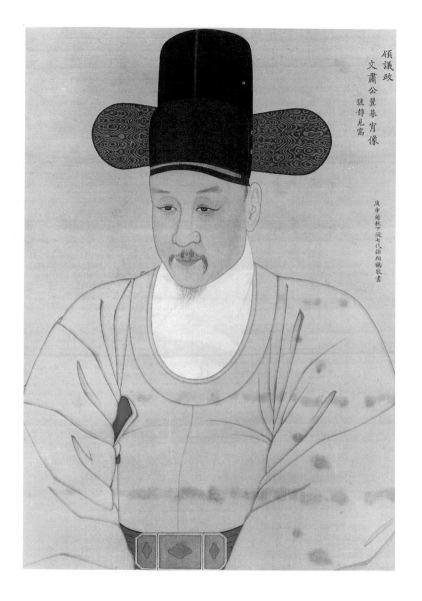

領議政
文肅公翼恭肖像
號靜見寓

庚申菊秋下澣七代孫相鶴敬書

36. Kuo Tzu-i's Banquet

Six-panel screen painting; ink and color on silk
H. 79½", W. 142½"
Yi Dynasty, 19th century
Gift of John Gruber   84.251

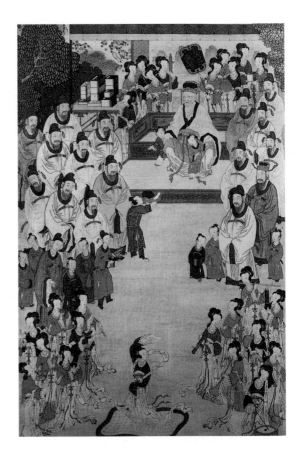

This magnificent screen is one of the finest examples of large-scale Korean court painting in any American or European collection. Within the limitations of the court style (thin, even lines filled in with bright, flat color), the high quality and decorative splendor of this screen are unsurpassed. The theme is a perfect expression of the Confucian ideals prevailing at the Yi court: a loyal, hard-working official, justly rewarded by his monarch, enjoying a bountiful old age.

Kuo Tzu-i (697–781) was a T'ang Dynasty Chinese general, a paragon of Confucian virtue whose loyal service was amply rewarded by the four successive emperors he served. For thirty turbulent years, General Kuo was "The Pillar of the Empire," suppressing revolts within China while keeping the barbarian hordes outside at bay. T'ang military strength was insufficient to defend China's northern and western borders against fierce Central Asian nomads, so Kuo manipulated them by playing one tribe off against another. An endless series of revolts within China kept Kuo busy fighting the insurgents as well. Against overwhelming odds, General Kuo brought China safely through a series of major crises.

Emperor Ming Huang expressed his gratitude by bestowing the title of Prince on General Kuo. The general had eight sons and seven sons-in-law who rose to prominence in the government. Kuo Tzu-i lived to be eighty-four. He was eventually blessed

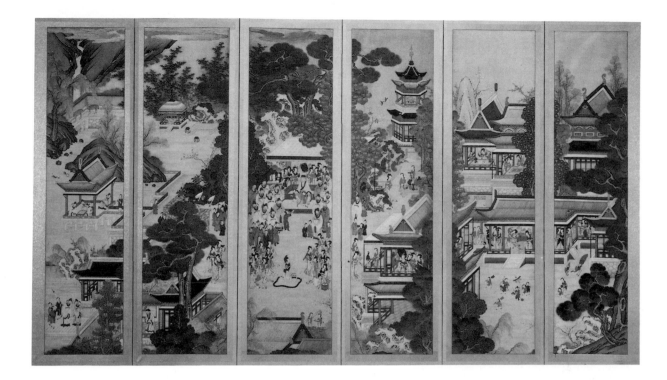

with so many grandchildren and great-grandchildren that he could no longer distinguish them, so he merely nodded when each child stepped forward to pay his respects. Instead of depicting General Kuo in the heat of battle or leading his victorious troops, this screen shows him enjoying the privileges of a well-earned retirement.

We see the happy old gentleman attended by his sons and daughters, surrounded by their many children, enjoying the performance of a dancing girl amid the pavilions and gardens of a fanciful Chinese palace. The elegant figures wear imaginary T'ang Dynasty costumes. The garden is filled with lakes, trees, bamboo, exotic rocks, deer, peacocks, cranes, and mandarin ducks. Attendants perform music or prepare food and drink while gentlemen play chess, ladies dance, and children parade their hobby horses.

Court paintings such as this employed the finest available materials. The painting surface is silk; Korean screens were normally painted on paper or linen. Brilliant mineral color was used lavishly. Called *tang-chae* (Chinese colors), the mineral pigments were quite costly; many of them had to be imported from China. Expensive mineral colors were used much more sparingly, if at all, on more ordinary Korean screens.

The lighter, more transparent colors one sees here and there on this screen are vegetable dyes rather than mineral pigments. Both types of color used animal-glue or fish-glue binders and were mixed with water prior to being brushed onto the surface of the cloth or paper. Once the paint set, it was no longer water soluble.

37. Scholar Contemplating a Cascade

Traditionally attributed to Yi Chong (1578–1607)
Album-leaf painting mounted as a hanging scroll;
ink on silk
H. 11¼", W. 10⅞" exclusive of mounting
Yi Dynasty, 16th century
Purchase 75.130

Most Korean court painters worked in two basic modes. The first employed thin, even outlines filled in with relatively bright colors. This mode was used for portraits (see Cat. 35) and compositions involving groups of figures (see Cat. 36). The other mode was ink-monochrome painting, using a variety of short, strongly modulated brushstrokes and graded areas of ink wash. Color was sometimes added, but it was light color, consisting of dilute washes of vegetable dyes. The ink-wash mode was used primarily for landscape paintings, like the present one, or for paintings of bamboo, plum blossoms, or grass orchids (epidendrum).

Scholar Contemplating a Cascade is traditionally attributed to Yi Chong (1578–1607). Several generations of Yi Chong's family were professional artists in the Bureau of Painting, starting with his grandfather, Yi Sang-jwa (act. mid-16th century). Yi Sang-jwa was originally a slave in the household of a scholar official, but he developed such phenomenal artistic skill that the king appointed him to the Bureau of Painting. After the king's death, Yi Sang-jwa was selected to paint the king's ancestor portrait, the highest honor that could be accorded to a court painter.

Yi Sang-jwa's grandson, Yi Chong, was brought up to be a painter; he was trained from early childhood in the use of a brush. By the age of ten he had become a competent landscape painter and was also skilled at figure subjects. When he was eleven, Yi Chong decided to become a Buddhist monk. He joined a monastery in the Diamond Mountains, an area famous for its spectacular granite pinnacles (see Cat. 43). He continued to paint throughout his short life. He was noted for his independent ways and difficult personality, painting only when and what he wanted to, turning down commissions from powerful persons if they did not suit him. Most of his surviving pictures are small landscapes like this one. He died at the age of twenty-nine.

Korean ink-wash paintings of the 16th century are extremely rare outside major museums in Korea. Only a handful have reached the West, usually by way of Japanese collections. Most of these have been misidentified as Chinese, since they follow Chinese models quite closely. Shimada Shujirō has been active in reattributing many of them to Korea.

The present painting skillfully perpetuates the style and subject matter of the Southern Sung Academy. The Sung court was forced to flee south to the city of Hang-chou in 1126, when the Jurched Tartars conquered North China. The Southern Sung period lasted from 1127 to 1279. A new style of landscape painting was developed by Ma Yuan and Hsia Kuei, two great artists at the Southern Sung Imperial Painting Academy.

During the Yuan Dynasty (1279–1368), the Ma-Hsia style was kept alive by painters in the port city of Ning-po and elsewhere. In the Ming Dynasty (1368–1644), the Ma-Hsia style provided the basis for a new painting style developed by artists of the Che School. Ming Dynasty China exerted tremendous influence on Yi Dynasty Korea, and the Che School was the major source for 15th- and 16th-century Korean landscape painters. *Scholar Contemplating a Cascade* follows the Ma-Hsia/Che style quite closely. However, the relative flatness and spatial ambiguity, as well as a slight awkwardness in the brushwork, mark this painting as Korean rather than Chinese.

The seal in the upper left corner reads: "To Chung-kyon In" (The Seal of To Chung-kyon). This is not a known art name of Yi Chong. The placement of the seal suggests that it was added later. When a Chinese, Korean, or Japanese artist impressed his seal on a painting, he usually integrated it with the composition instead of stamping it in a far corner.

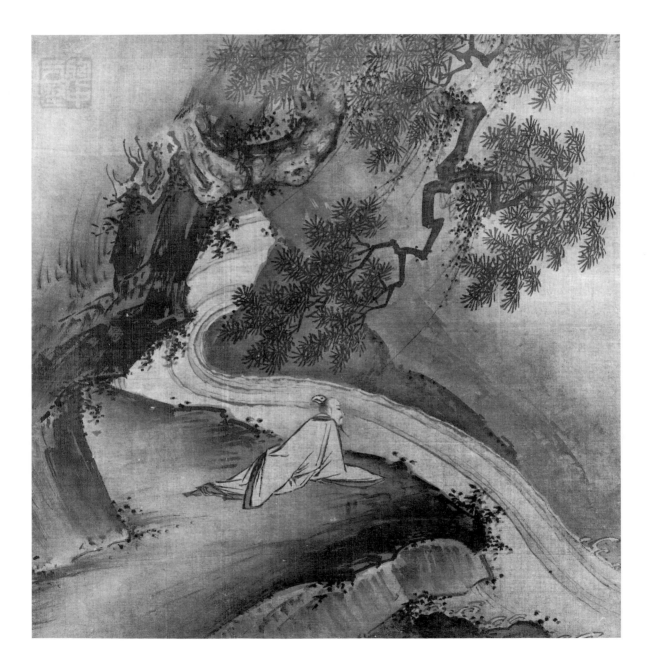

38. Landscape and Poem

By Kim Myong-kuk (act. first half of the
17th century)
Fan Painting; ink on gold leaf on paper
H. 8½", W. 11" exclusive of mounting
Yi Dynasty, 17th century
Gift of Dr. & Mrs. Robert Dickes   74.81.2

The Che School was one of the two major sources for early Yi Dynasty landscape painting (see Cat. 37). The other major source was the Northern Sung landscape tradition. This seems anomalous, since the Northern Sung style had become passé in China with the development of the Southern Sung style, which was the basis for the Che School style. However, the old Northern Sung style did not die out in North China when the Sung court fled to the South in 1126. The Northern Sung landscape tradition continued to flourish in North China throughout the Chin (1126–1234) and well into the Yuan Dynasty (1279–1368).

Because of physical proximity and trade between North China and Korea, the Northern Sung landscape tradition perpetuated in the Chin Dynasty exerted strong influence on Korean landscape painting until as late as the 17th century. Korea was cut off from direct land contact with Southern Sung China by the Jurched Tartars, so the Southern Sung style did not penetrate Korea until after China was reunified by the Mongols. Because of Korean emulation of the Ming Dynasty, it was primarily through the Che School that the Southern Sung style finally became a major source for Korean landscape painters, side by side with the old Northern Sung style.

Many early Yi Dynasty landscape paintings actually combined these two seemingly antithetical styles. The hybrid style that resulted is not as awkward as one might expect. In fact, this hybrid style proved instrumental in the development of 15th-century ink-wash landscape painting in Japan. It is reflected in the work of Shūbun, a Zen painter-monk who was one of the most influential Japanese artists of his day. Shūbun visited Korea in 1423–1424 to obtain a complete set of printed Buddhist scriptures for his monastery's library. During his stay in Korea, Shūbun was profoundly impressed by Korean ink-wash landscape painting. The Korean hybrid style influenced Shūbun's own style, and he in turn passed it on to a whole generation of Japanese artists.

Landscape and Poem is a 17th-century Korean interpretation of the Southern Sung landscape style as transmitted by the Che School in the Ming Dynasty. The Northern Sung tradition emphasized verticality: nearby crags and peaks filled the picture from top to bottom, blocking a view into the far distance and leaving little of the format unfilled. The Southern Sung tradition did just the opposite, as we see here. It emphasized the horizontal by means of level, continuous mountain ridges in the distance. The view extended to infinity, suggesting the continuity of a vast universe. Much of the format was left empty. The blank paper (or silk, or, in this case, gold leaf) stood for water (supporting the two sailboats on the lake) and sky (the area above the mountains). It also suggested mist-filled atmosphere infusing the deep pictorial space.

When painting landscapes, Kim Myong-kuk employed the style of the Che School. The Che style continued to be the main current of Korean landscape painting in the 17th century, but it became increasingly abbreviated and mannered. Many of Kim Myong-kuk's surviving works are small-scale pictures, album-leaf or fan paintings. This one is a fan (not the folding fan, which was invented in Japan during the 9th–10th century and subsequently became popular in China, but a traditional Chinese nonfolding fan, whose short bamboo handle splayed out as thin stationary ribs to support the oval paper surface). The handle and ribs were removed from the present fan painting when it was mounted flat and framed.

Kim Myung-kuk was one of the most famous Korean artists of the 17th century. He was a court painter (a member of the *To-hwa-so*, the Bureau of Painting), yet we know almost nothing about his life.

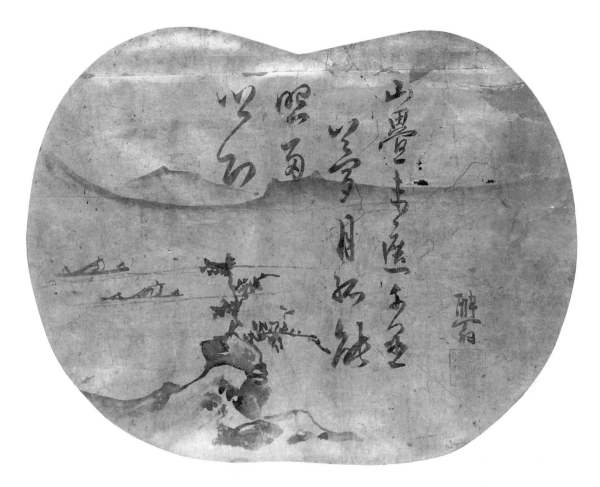

This suggests that he may have been a commoner rather than a member of the professional class to which most court painters belonged. In spite of his apparently humble origin, he gained the admiration and trust of the king. In 1636 and again in 1643, he was dispatched to Japan with Korean envoys on important diplomatic missions. Kim Myong-kuk's paintings were much admired by the Japanese military aristocracy at the court of the Tokugawa *shōgun*. The Japanese commissioned so many Kim Myong-kuk paintings that most of his surviving oeuvre is in Japan. In recent years, the Korean National Museum has been buying Kim Myong-kuk paintings back from the Japanese.

The artist's signature appears at the lower right of this fan painting: Ch'ui-ong (Drunken Old Man, one of his art names). Below the signature is one of the artist's seals; another follows the poem. The poem was inscribed by Kim Myong-kuk himself; he may have composed it, or he may have quoted it from some Chinese or Korean poet. The couplet reads:

Even overlapping mountains cannot prevent
    a dream from traveling a thousand miles.
The solitary moon can illuminate myriad views.

39. Po-dae (Pu-tai)

By Kim Myong-kuk (active first half of the 17th century)
Hanging-scroll painting; ink on paper
H. 20½″, W. 10⅝″ exclusive of mounting
Yi Dynasty, 17th century
Gift of Mrs. Robert van Roejen   59.26

Po-dae (Chinese: Pu-tai) was a household god, a God of Good Fortune. He was said to be an incarnation of Maitreya, the Buddha of the Future, and to have been a Buddhist monk who lived in China during the 6th century A.D. His name means "cotton-cloth bag." He was usually represented with a big cloth bag slung over his shoulder, as he is here. His treasure bag contained precious things that brought happiness and success to his devotees.

Kim Myong-kuk is best known for eccentric figure paintings rather than landscapes (see Cat. 38). His mythical Taoist and Buddhist figures were executed in a bold, rough, abbreviated style with a small number of exaggerated calligraphic brushstrokes suggesting the form of an entire figure.

The rough, free, fluid brushwork of Kim Myong-kuk's figure paintings no doubt contributed to the legend of his excessive fondness for wine. So did his choice of "Drunken Old Man" as an art name. The signature at the lower left of the present painting reads: Ch'ui-ong ("Drunken Old Man"). The seal below the signature reads: Kim Myong-kuk In (The

Seal of Kim Myong-kuk). It was said that Kim Myong-kuk loved to drink and frequently painted while drunk. Prospective patrons hoping to commission paintings were advised to bring gifts of wine when they came to visit him. Since early times in China it was traditional to say that certain poets, painters, and calligraphers—especially those who worked in a free style—did their most inspired work while drunk.

Kim Myong-kuk's figure paintings were enormously popular in Japan. They reminded the Japanese of the legendary Zen eccentrics painted by Japanese artist monks from the 14th century on. Kim Myong-kuk's figures sprang from the same source: Southern Sung Ch'an (Zen) figure paintings by artist monks like Liang K'ai and Mu-ch'i. This tradition was brought to Japan by Zen monks who went to China for study. The Southern Sung Ch'an figure painting tradition was transmitted to Korea by Ming Dynasty Che School artists, just as was the Southern Sung Academy landscape tradition.

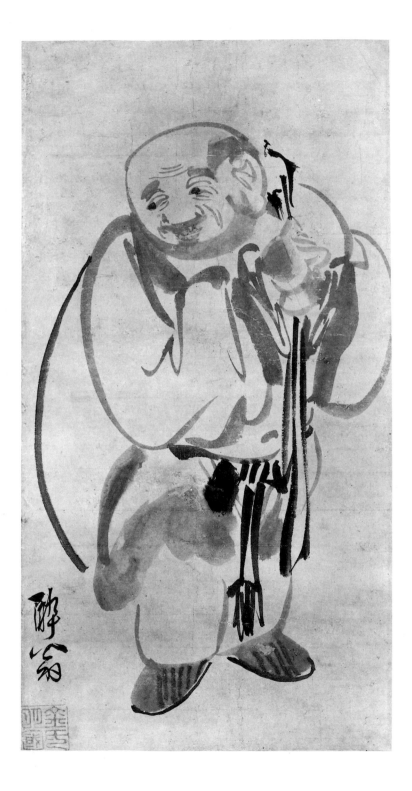

40. Grapevine
Hanging-scroll painting, ink on paper
H. 26″, W. 12¾″ exclusive of mounting
Yi Dynasty, 16th century
Lent by Dr. John Lyden   TL1986.442

While some Chinese painters were capable of treating all types of subject matter, others tended to specialize in one category, such as landscape, or figures, or birds and flowers. It was not unusual for an artist to specialize in an even more narrow subject, such as bamboo, or grass orchids (epidendrum). One famous artist, the monk Tzu-wen, specialized in grapevines. His work was so celebrated in later centuries that an entire tradition of grape paintings in ink evolved from it. The Tzu-wen grape-painting tradition was very influential in Korea and Japan as well as in China. Grapevines became a popular subject with many Korean artists, including folk painters, court artists, and scholar painters. Ink-wash paintings of gnarled vines, coiling tendrils, tattered leaves, and clusters of plump grapes have remained a frequent subject of Chinese, Korean, and Japanese paintings throughout the centuries since Tzu-wen developed this motif in the mid-13th century.

Tzu-wen is usually known by his art name, Jih-kuan. Little is recorded about his life. He came from Hua-t'ing in Kiangsu Province and lived in the Ma-nao monastery in Hangchou. The Ch'an (Zen) monasteries of Hangchou, the capital of the Southern Sung (1127–1279) Dynasty, were renowned centers of art and learning as well as spiritual training. Many of the monks were poets, calligraphers, or painters, and some combined all these skills. Tzu-wen was famous for his grass script (calligraphy in cursive, running style) as well as his paintings of grapevines. He usually inscribed each painting with a poem of this own composition. His calligraphy complemented the expressive gestures of the vines and leaves in the painting. As with so many Chinese artists who worked in a loose, free style, Tzu-wen was said to have been unusually fond of wine.

Grapes were not native to East Asia. The cultivation of grapes was introduced to China from South Asia in 126 B.C. Like bamboo, and grass orchids, grapes lent themselves well to expressive treatment in ink-wash paintings. The grapevines provided an opportunity for a virtuoso display of ink-monochrome technique. The ink wash was graded from light to dark on the plump grapes to suggest their three dimensional volume. The ink was also variegated on the complex, flat, tattered shapes of the leaves. The vines themselves, with their gnarled, angular stalks and curling tendrils, offered an opportunity for expressive linear gestures.

tional symbolism.

The present painting has a sturdy ruggedness, awkward angularity, and spatial flatness that readily distinguish it from a Chinese painting of grapes. Like so many Korean paintings, this picture possesses an absolutely charming naiveté, as well as great strength and dignity.

Grapevine is so close in style to the painting *Grapes* by Sin Sa-im-dang in the Chun Hyong-pil collection that the two could be by the same hand. Sin Sa-im-dang (1512–1559) was one of the few women among well-known Korean artists of the past. Her father was a poor but respected Confucian scholar. Unlike other Korean women of her day, she learned to read and write classical Chinese, studied the Chinese classics, and became a skilled calligrapher and painter. She also excelled at the more womanly arts of sewing and embroidery. She married a young government official and bore four sons, the third of whom, Yi Yul-gok (1536–1584), was one of the greatest Korean statesmen and scholars of the 16th century.

As a painter, Sin Sa-im-dang was said by critics of her day to be a rival of An Kyon (b. 1418), one of Korea's most famous landscape painters. Sin Sa-im-dang was proficient at landscape, but the artistic speciality for which she became famous was bird-and-flower painting. Her flower pictures often included butterflies. Grape paintings, for which she became especially well known, were a subspeciality within the bird-and-flower category.

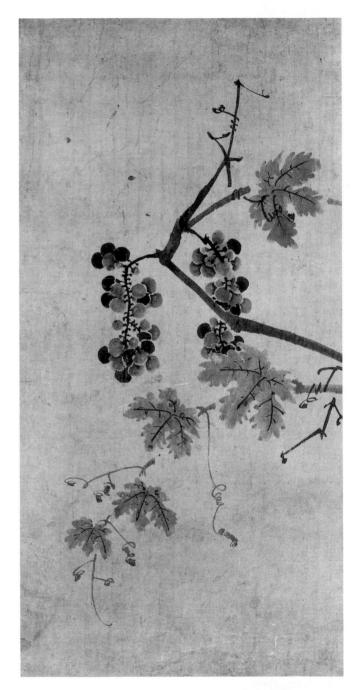

41. Landscape: Boating on the Lake

Fan-shaped album-leaf painting; ink and light color
on linen
H. 8¾", W. 15" exclusive of mounting
Yi Dynasty, 18th–19th century
Purchase   75.125.14

Toward the end of the 17th century, an altogether different Chinese painting tradition gradually became influential in Korea. It was literati painting (the paintings of scholar artists and literary men). By the 18th century, literati painting had become a major Korean tradition; it continues to be a viable and significant style of painting in Korea today (see Cat. 100).

According to the theories of Chinese literati painting, an artist must express his own lofty spirit and noble sentiments in his pictures and capture the essence of the subject but avoid realistic or obviously skillful drawing. Professional painting was not considered art because an artist who was forced to please a patron in order to sell his work was not free to express his own mind. Also, professional artists generally lacked the classical literary education that would permit them to combine painting, calligraphy, and poetry in their work. Many literati artists in China, did however, rely on their paintings for a livelihood; they simply accepted monetary "gifts" in exchange for their pictures.

In terms of style and technique, literati artists created paintings by the additive application of numerous small brushstrokes rather than lines, clear-cut strokes, or continuous areas of wash. Ink was the primary medium; when color was present, it was usually limited to dilute washes of indigo (bluish, cool) and red ocher (reddish-brown, warm). Landscape was the major theme: not the observed landscape of nature, but an idealized landscape of the scholar artist's mind, the sort of place where he would like to retire—a small, isolated cottage among mountains and streams, with trees and a bamboo grove nearby. In the bird-and-flower category, literati artists made a specialty of bamboo, grass orchids (epidendrum), plum blossoms, and chrysanthemums.

In Korea, the best literati paintings were produced by professional painters (court artists who were members of the Bureau of Painting) rather than as an avocation of the scholar-official class in keeping with the Chinese ideal. Many *yangban* must have tried their hands at literati painting, since painting, along

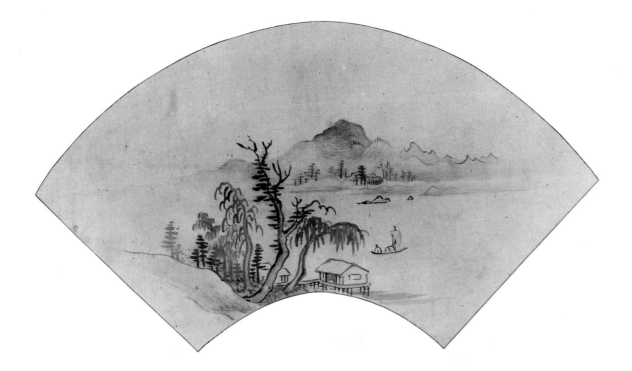

with calligraphy, literature, and history, were traditional accomplishments of the scholar-official class in China upon which the Korean one was based. Unfortunately, the technique of literati painting was easily imitated by real amateurs, often with disastrous results. However, the fine points of the style were difficult to master. Even the most talented Korean literati painters were unable to recreate the subtleties of brushwork, the treatment of pictorial space, or the philosophical depth of their Chinese models.

The introduction of the literati painting style to Korea in the late 17th century, and its great popularity there during the 18th and 19th centuries, were due to the influence of a late Ming Dynasty painter, art critic, and theorist named Tung Ch'i-ch'ang (1555–1636), and to the dissemination of woodblock-printed Chinese painting manuals, such as the *Mustard Seed Garden* (first edition 1679–1701) in Korea.

Tung Ch'i-ch'ang codified Chinese painting theory and criticism in an entirely arbitrary but extraordinarily influential way that relegated professional painters to an imaginary "Northern School," and to the status of mere artisans, while literati painters were elevated to an imaginary "Southern School." By Tung Ch'i-ch'ang's day, most of the more talented painters in China were working in the literati style anyhow. These scholar artists were also the art critics of their day. Led by Tung Ch'i-ch'ang, they praised their own style of painting and condemned other styles as nonart.

Among the painting styles consigned to the non-art "Northern School" were the Southern Sung Academy tradition and its Ming Che School successors, the prime sources for 15th–17th-century painting in Korea. Among the artists assigned to the superior "Southern School" were the 10th-century painter Tung Yuan, the scholar artists of the Northern Sung Dynasty, the Four Great Masters of the Yuan Dynasty, and the Wu School of the Ming Dynasty. *Landscape: Boating on the Lake* is a distant but charming and lyrical Korean reflection of landscapes by Shen Chou (1427–1509), the founder of the Wu School.

42. Bamboo

Hanging-scroll painting; ink on silk
H. 50¾", W. 13" exclusive of mounting
Yi Dynasty, 19th century
Gift of Robert Anderson   84.244.13

Bamboo had long been a favorite subject for Chinese painters of all schools, but literati artists were particularly fond of bamboo. The stalks and leaves provided an ideal vehicle for virtuoso ink brushwork. The brush, ink, water, and paper used for ink paintings were exactly the same as those used for calligraphy, so it was relatively easy for a Chinese scholar official, educated in the classics and expert at calligraphy, to become an ink bamboo painter. Literati symbolism was associated with the bamboo theme: bamboo bends before the wind, just as the Confucian scholar bends before adversity, but it never breaks.

The ink used in Far Eastern calligraphy and painting was in the form of an ink cake (also called an ink stick), a rectangular (or sometimes round) block of hard ink made of pine-soot carbon mixed with fish-glue or animal-glue binder. The ink stick was ground on the surface of a slate ink stone, which had a depression at one end to hold some water, until the desired water-and-ink mixture was achieved. The mixture was applied to the paper with a brush. Once the ink set, it was no longer water soluble.

In the literati painting tradition, even more than other schools of Far Eastern painting, the artist frequently wrote a poem on his painting. The poem's theme, of course, corresponded to the subject of the painting. Ideally, the poem would have been the painter's own composition, but a well-selected quotation from a poet of the past was acceptable.

The five-line poem on the present painting reads:

Silent bamboo is reflected on the northern window of the retired scholar's studio.
Jade-colored moss and blue indigo plants bask in the shade, enjoying the harmony of this secluded retreat.
The wind-bell in front of the bed-screen tolls the passing of two months in this pavilion beyond compare.
Spring branches and new grass stir the memories of an old man after a stroll in the mountains.
Leaving public affairs behind, I sit down to contemplate the graceful beauty.

The painting/poem is signed: I-tang Ko-sa (The Gentleman of Moral-Principles Pavilion). I-tang is the painter's art name. His surname, Cho, is given in the first seal.

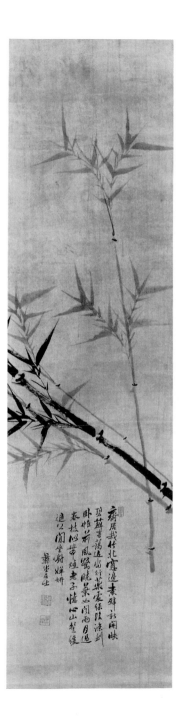

43. Myong-kyong Tae (Bright-mirror Pinnacle) in the Diamond Mountains

By Kim Ch'ang-up (1658–1721)
Hanging-scroll painting; ink and light color on paper
H. 21¾", W. 12⅝" exclusive of mounting
Yi Dynasty, early 18th century
Gift of Dr. & Mrs. Charles Perera   84.141.10

The Diamond Mountains (Kumgang San) cover an area of 160 square kilometers near the east coast of Korea, some 60 kilometers north of the thirty-eighth parallel. Since early times, the Diamond Mountains have been one of the most important pilgrimage sites in Korea, not only because of the breathtaking natural scenery but because the area is sacred to Buddhism, Shamanism, and Taoism.

The name Diamond Mountains is Buddhist in origin: *San* means "mountain," while *Kumgang* is the Korean pronunciation fo the two Chinese characters used to translate the Sanskrit word *vajra*, "diamond thunderbolt." A *vajra* is a Buddhist ritual implement and the attribute of certain Buddhist deities, whose adamantine qualities it suggests. The twelve thousand famous, needlelike rock spires in the Diamond Mountains suggest *vajras* and the magic powers with which this implement is associated. Koreans also equate the peaks in the Diamond Mountains with the mountains in the Buddha's Paradise. Many Buddhist temples were built in the Diamond Mountains.

In Taoist terms, Koreans equated the Diamond Mountains with the Islands of the Immortals. The wild ginseng that grows in the Diamond Mountains suggested *pulloch'o*, the Sacred Fungus eaten by Taoists to obtain immortality (see Cat. 70). Taoist adepts in ancient China practiced solitary asceticism and meditation in deep mountain forests in order to achieve spiritual well-being, long life, and magic power. Thus Taoist mountain mysticism and Taoist concepts of longevity and immortality came to be associated with the Diamond Mountains.

It is in terms of Shamanism, however, that the Diamond Mountains played their most important role in the spiritual life of the Korean people. Many of the twelve thousand granite pinnacles in the Diamond Mountains resemble human figures or animals such as tigers or dragons. It is easy to see why these rocks became a focus for animistic beliefs. Hananim, the Shamanist Creator, imbued mountains, rocks, trees, and animals with portions of his spirit, making them sentient. Thus it seems quite natural that a spirit-dwelling rock may assume the form of a warrior, a monk, a mother holding her child, a tiger, or a dragon. Mountain worship is a significant aspect of Shamanism and the Mountain Spirit is the most popular Shamanist deity (see Cat. 30). Korean animistic beliefs go back to Neolithic times. Along with Shamanism itself, they were brought to Korea by early peoples from the mountains, forests, and grasslands of Central Asia, Mongolia, Manchuria, and Siberia.

Paintings of the Diamond Mountains were especially appropriate during the Tan-O Festival. Tan-O, the fifth day of the fifth month in the old lunar calendar, is one of The Four Happy Occasions,' the four major annual festivals of Korea. During Tan-O, Koreans honor the spirits and ask their help in achieving good health, long life, harmony, and success. Throughout Korea, *mudang* (shamans) perform special *kut* (shaman rituals) to propitiate important local spirits such as the Dragon King of the Han River flowing past Seoul. Many powerful spirits dwell in the Diamond Mountains, so paintings of the Diamond Mountains came to be associated with the Tan-O Festival.

The three-character inscription at the upper right of the present painting names the great rock spire in the center of the picture: Myong-kyong Tae (Bright-mirror Pinnacle). It was usual for Korean paintings of famous views in the Diamond Mountains and elsewhere to include the name of the site. The seal here records the name of the artist.

Kim Ch'ang-up was born into the scholar-official class. His father, Kim Soo-hwan, became a prime minister. The young Kim excelled in poetry, calligraphy, and painting. He specialized in literati-style landscapes. His painting style, and his choice of actual Korean scenery (*chin-gyong,* "real views") rather than imaginary Chinese scenery, were based on the work of his friend Chong Son. Kim Ch'ang-up kept a record, the *Yeonheng Diary,* when he and his brother traveled to Peking as part of an official Korean mission in 1713. On this trip the Kims introduced Chong Son's paintings to the Chinese court.

Chong Son (1676–1759) was the first Korean artist to create a truly national style of landscape painting, as opposed to merely imitating Chinese models. Chong Son came from an impoverished scholar's family. He was appointed to the Bureau of Painting. In his younger years, Chong Son, like other late-17th-century Korean court painters, based his landscapes on Chinese examples from the two major Ming Dynasty painting traditions, the academic Che School and the literati Wu School. Chong Son and other Korean artists sometimes combined elements from these two traditions in a single painting.

In his maturity, Chong Son turned away from the imaginary views of idealized Chinese scenery that had been the subject of Korean landscape paintings. He began to paint recognizable views of actual Korean scenery instead. He traveled the length and breadth of Korea painting famous scenic views; the Diamond Mountains became his favorite theme. When Chong Son included human figures in his mature landscapes, the figures wore Korean dress for the first time, unlike the imaginary Chinese scholars who populated earlier Korean landscape paintings.

Two important new Korean painting traditions sprang from Chong Son's work. The first was the depiction of native Korean landscapes. The second was the genre painting tradition that became fashionable in the second half of the 18th century: scenes of Koreans engaged in everyday Korean activities.

Bright-mirror Pinnacle follows Chong Son's lead in its style as well as its subject matter. The long, bold strokes outlining the crags and clustered granite pinnacles are based on Chong Son's mature style. The two gentlemen sitting in conversation on the square boulder beside the rapids are wearing Korean dress.

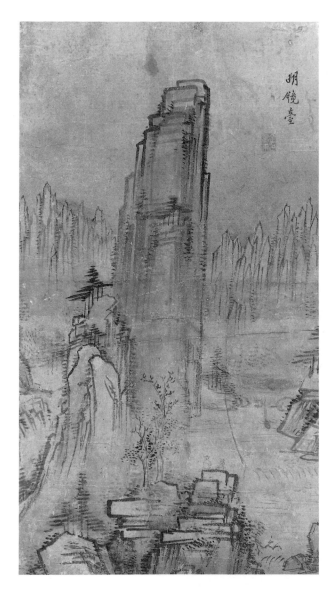

44. Young Scholar on His Way to His First Official Post

Hanging-scroll painting; ink and light color on silk
H. 10⅝", W. 15½" exclusive of mounting
Yi Dynasty, 18th century
Purchase   75.125.12

Chong Son often depicted Korean figures wearing Korean attire within his landscape paintings. This was a major departure from earlier landscape paintings in Korea, which were inhabited by idealized Chinese figures wearing Chinese costume. Once Chong Son had made this breakthrough, other Korean artists followed his lead. The present landscape is done in Chinese style, with a mixture of Che School and literati painting elements. The "axe-cut" texture strokes on the rocks derive from the Southern Sung landscape-painting tradition by way of Ming Che School interpretations. The horizontal, oval-shaped dabs of ink repeated rhythmically to suggest foliage are a standard feature of the literati style. But the real subject of this splendid little painting is the procession of figures making their way along the mountain road. They are all wearing typical Korean attire.

The subject of the painting represents the happiest moment in the life of a Korean scholar official. The young man has just passed the government civil service examinations and is on his way to another province to begin work at his first official post. He is accompanied by his five retainers. Two of them play flutes and joyfully dance along the road ahead of the young official on his horse. The retainer leading the procession carries a sword, an indication that the young man is a military rather than a civil official.

A young scholar on his way to assume his first appointment is the key event in the Peaceful Life *(Heng Nak To)* theme frequently represented on Yi Dynasty screens. Cheap, folk art versions were produced for the homes of commoners. Even though they had little chance of becoming scholar officials, commoners respected and admired learning and high office. The screen's function was edifying and didactic in the best Confucian tradition. The screen also lent an air of refined elegance to the room in which it stood. More expensive versions of *Heng Nak To* screens graced the houses of the scholar officials themselves.

A Peaceful Life screen celebrates the happiest events in the successful life of an idealized scholar official. Typically, the first panel depicts the child's first birthday party. The second panel shows the young man's wedding procession. The third panel depicts him celebrating one of the annual Korean festivals. The fourth panel shows him traveling to assume a high government post (the subject of the present painting). The fifth panel depicts him celebrating his sixtieth birthday surrounded by his children and grandchildren. The sixth panel shows him happily attended by a large retinue of lesser officials and servants.

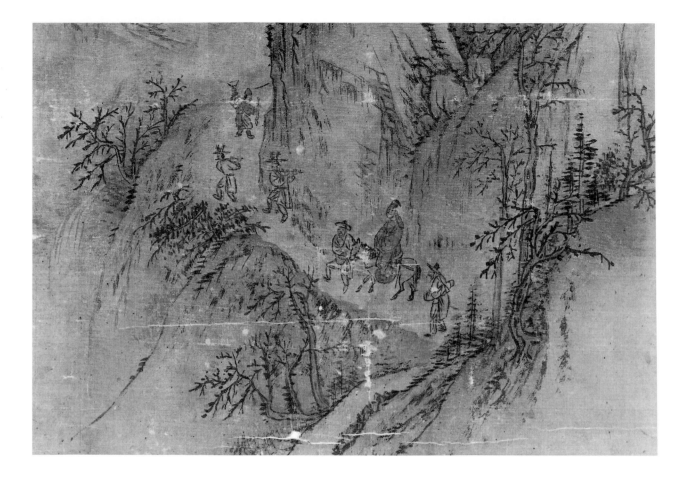

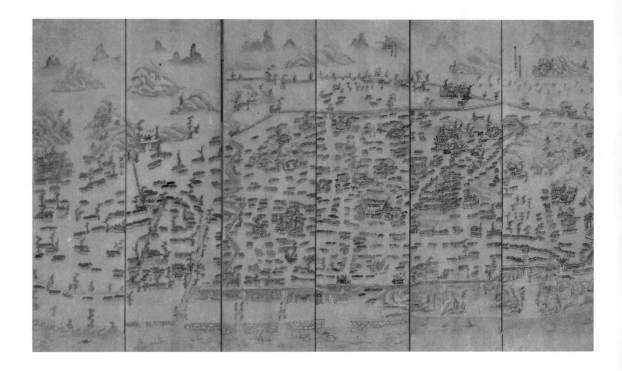

45. The City of P'yongyang

Twelve-panel screen painting; ink and color on linen
H. 48", W. 162" exclusive of mounting
Yi Dynasty, 19th century
Lent by Dr. Ralph Marcove   TLI983.230.1

Chong Son's innovative depictions of recognizable views of actual Korean scenery ultimately led to representations of vast panoramas such as we see here. The subject of this screen is the walled city of P'yongyang and its environs, with tiny inscriptions naming each important building, mountain peak, river, island, or scenic spot.

P'yongyang, now the capital of North Korea, has a long history. Wang-hsien, the capital of the Han Dynasty Chinese trading colony of Lo-lang (108 B.C.–A.D. 313) was located at P'yongyang. The capital of the Koguryo Kingdom was moved to P'yongyang from Kungnae in 427 and remained there until Silla conquered Koguryo in 668. During the Koryo Dynasty

(918–1392), P'yongyang was one of the three secondary capitals of Korea, the main capital being at Kaesong.

The following are some of the interesting features of the city identified by inscriptions on the screen: P'yongyang Song (P'yongyang Castle), reconstructed several times from the late Koguryo Period (7th century) to the late Yi Dynasty (18th century). Walls divided the castle into four sections. The Northern Keep, the highest, was last rebuilt in 1714. The Inner Keep, last rebuilt in 1624, is a reduced version of an earlier one. The remaining area of the earlier Inner Keep is now called the Middle Keep. The large area to the south of the Middle Keep is called the Outer Keep and is crisscrossed by a rectangular grid of roads.

Yongmyong-sa (Yongmyong Temple) was originally built by royal decree in 392 on the site of the second palace of the Koguryo Kingdom. It was one of nine Buddhist monasteries in P'yongyang. During the Yi Dynasty, Yongmyong-sa became one of the thirty-six

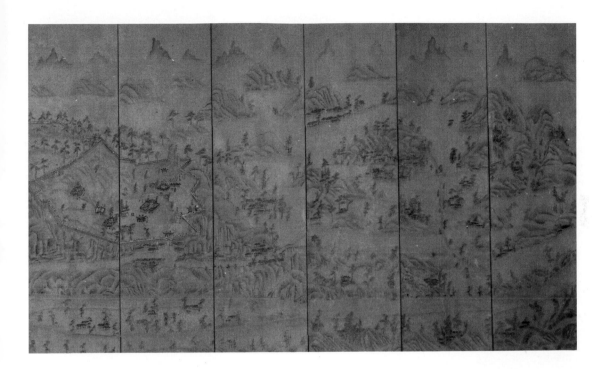

Korean monasteries of the Son Sect (Chinese: Ch'an; Japanese: Zen).

Tangun-chon (Tangun Shrine), was built during the reign of Sejong (1418–1450), the fourth king of the Yi Dynasty, for the worship of Tangun and Wang Kon (founder of the Koryo Dynasty) as national ancestors. Tangun is the mythical progenitor of the Korean people; according to tradition, he founded the Korean state in 2333 B.C.

Pu-pyok Lu (Floating Jade Pavilion), located on Ch'ong-lyu Pyok (Clear Stream Cliff) to the east of Mt. Kum-su near Mo-lan Peak, was one of the celebrated "Eight Views of P'yongyang." The Pavilion stood like floating jade beside the Tae-tong River. It was originally built about a thousand years ago as a subsidiary structure of the Yongmyong Monastery. In the 12th century, King Yejong instructed Yi An to rename the structure "Floating Jade Pavilion."

The Eight Views of P'yongyang concept derives from a long tradition that began in 11th-century China with paintings of The Eight Views of Hsiao and Hsiang. The Hsiao River, a tributary of the Hsiang, itself a tributary of the Yangtze, joins the Hsiang River just before the latter empties into Lake Tung-t'ing, in the Ling-ling District of Hunan Province. This area has been celebrated since early times for the scenic beauty of its streams, lakes, hills, trees, and mists. The Eight Views of Hsiao and Hsiang were a series of imaginary landscapes involving seasonal phenomena and times of day, all meant to evoke poetic moods. There was no fixed order in the series. The titles were: "Clearing after a Storm in the Mountain Village," "Evening Bell from the Distant Temple," "Returning Sails on the Distant Bay," "Night Rain at Hsiao-Hsiang," "Evening Glow over the Fishing Village," "Autumn Moon over Lake Tung-t'ing," "Wild Geese Coming down on a Sandbar," and "Evening Snow on the River."

The Eight Views of Hsiao and Hsiang enjoyed a

considerable vogue during the Sung Dynasty but fell into disuse in China when the academic Sung landscape painting tradition was replaced by the literati landscape painting tradition in the 13th–14th century. However, Korean and Japanese versions, substituting famous local scenic views for the imaginary Chinese ones, were quite popular in the 18th and 19th centuries. In Korea the series usually involved the scenery of a specific part of the peninsula, for example, "The Eight Views of the East Coast," "The Eight Views of the West Coast," "The Eight Views of the South Coast," "The Eight Views of Cheju Island," "The Eight Views of Seoul," or "The Eight Views of P'yongyang."

The present screen painting has twelve panels to accommodate its panoramic subject. Korean screens usually had eight panels, although ten-panel screens were not uncommon. Korean screens were nearly always single screens rather than pairs, whereas Japanese screens, which are more familiar to Westerners, usually consisted of a pair of six-panel screens.

The most typical type of Korean screen painting had a separate composition on each panel (see Cat. 49). In Japanese screens, the composition usually continued across all twelve panels of the pair. A few Korean screens had continuous compositions (see Cat. 36). In the present screen, the panoramic view necessitated a continuous composition.

46. Genre Scenes: Agriculture and Household Industries

Pair of hanging-scroll paintings; ink and light color on silk
H. 48½″, W. 13¼″ each, exclusive of mounting
Yi Dynasty, 19th century
Gift of Robert Anderson   84.244.8 & .9

Chong Son's innovative pictures of actual Korean scenery established a new tradition of landscape painting in Korea. Another important new painting tradition evolved indirectly from Chong Son's work. The figures wearing Korean attire that Chong Son inserted into many of his landscapes paved the way for the Korean genre painting of the second half of the 18th century and later–"genre" means the depiction of ordinary people engaged in everyday activities.

The present two scrolls were originally two of eight panels on a screen, the characteristic type of Korean screen with a separate but related painting on each panel. Six of the panels have been destroyed or lost; these two were remounted as a pair of hanging scrolls.

Agriculture and Household Industries was a popular Korean painting subject in the 18th and 19th centuries. The theme is Confucian: honorable peasants working diligently to support themselves and the state. In the agrarian society of the Yi Dynasty, agriculture was paramount. Farmers stood just below the court nobility and land-owning scholar bureaucrats in the social hierarchy, well above artisans and merchants. In the home of a commoner, an Agriculture and Household Industries painting provided a didactic exhortation as well as the celebration of a familiar way of life. In the home of a scholar official or nobleman, such a painting expressed respect for the occupation upon which the national economy was based. Agriculture and Household Industries paintings were filled with delightful, realistic depictions of local customs, costumes, building types, utensils, and scenery.

According to historical records, Sejong (1418–1450), the fourth king of the Yi Dynasty, commissioned the first Korean paintings of agricultural scenes, thereby establishing the precedent for a long tradition. Other 18th–19th century Korean Agriculture and Household Industries paintings typically depict the same activities we see in this pair of scrolls: tilling, planting, harvesting, silkworm cultivation, spinning, and weaving. The present paintings include an additional edifying subject: children attending class at the village school.

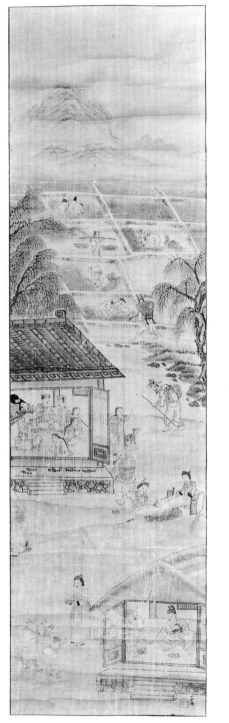
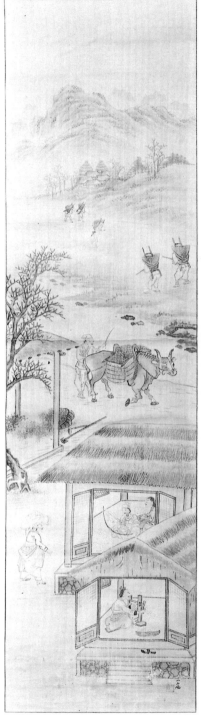

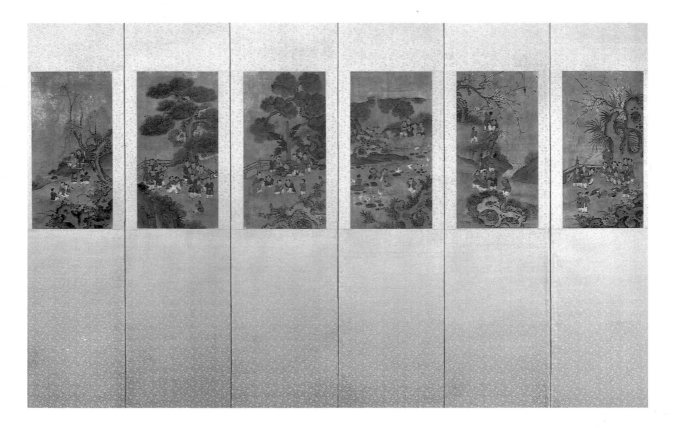

47. *Baekjado* (One Hundred Children)

Six-panel screen painting; ink and color on paper
H. 24⅜″, W. 13″ each panel, exclusive of mounting
Yi Dynasty, 18th–19th century
Gift of Mr. & Mrs. Allen & Susan Dickes Hubbard
86.264.1

While the Agriculture and Household Industries subject (see Cat. 46) was Confucian, One Hundred Children was a Taoist theme. Since early times, the Chinese liked to create numerical categories and associate them with magic power and symbolic meaning. Among these mystical categories, "one hundred" and "ten thousand" were auspicious numbers signifying abundance. Screen-paintings of One Hundred Children were popular in 18th–19th-century Korea. The screens usually had eight panels. Twelve or thirteen children were depicted on each

panel, for a total of one hundred. Two of the original eight panels of the present screen are missing.

A *Baekjado* screen was especially appropriate for display in the bedroom of a newly married couple. The screen's purpose was more than decorative. It was meant to inspire the bride to conceive: Seeing a hundred children on the screen in the bedroom every day, she could hardly fail to bear children of her own. Boys were preferable, so all one hundred children on the screen are boys. A Yi Dynasty wife's first duty to her husband and his family was to bear male children.

Baekjado screens were also displayed at first-birthday parties. In China, Korea, and Japan, a child is considered one year old at birth. The traditional Korean first-birthday party was held one hundred days after the baby's birth. The delay was necessitated by the high rate of infant mortality during the Yi Dynasty.

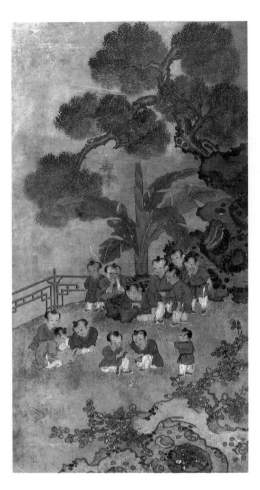 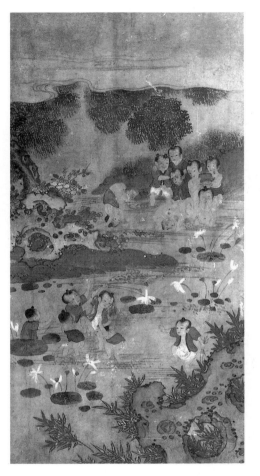

The first-birthday party was a joyous event. Friends and neighbors joined the family celebration and brought lavish gifts.

Unlike the hard-working peasants in Agriculture and Household Industries paintings, who wore ordinary Korean clothing (see Cat. 46), the little boys in One Hundred Children screens wore imaginary Chinese court costumes. The setting in which they pursued their elegant pastimes was not an ordinary Korean household; it was an imaginary Chinese palace garden, with pavilions, balustrades, trees, flowers, streams, ponds, and exotic garden rocks.

Depicting the children as members of the Chinese court nobility was meant to symbolically ensure achievement by the actual children of the household.

Chinese, Korean, and Japanese screens, hand-scrolls, and painting-albums "read" from right to left, the opposite of the Western method. This is based on the fact that the vertical lines of Far Eastern writing progress from right to left. The princely pleasures enjoyed by the little boys on the present screen consist of: a cock fight, gathering branches of blossoming plum, bathing in a lotus pond, watching a baby chick, wrestling, fishing.

48. Hunting Scenes

Two panels from an eight-panel screen painting; ink
and color on linen
H. 46½", W. 16" each, exclusive of mounting
Yi Dynasty, 19th century
Lent by Dr. John Lyden   TL1986.40.4&.5

Screen paintings of hunting scenes were considered
especially appropriate for the quarters of military
officials. Most Yi Dynasty military officers were
members of the land-owning scholar-official class.

The finest Yi Dynasty hunting screens were painted
by court artists for the royal family or high-ranking
government officials. The present panels, while well
drawn, lack the sophistication of court artists' work.
As for technique, expensive mineral colors were
used very sparingly, and hemp cloth was used rather
than silk. These scenes were probably painted for a
middle-level official. Folk-painting versions of the
subject are marked by unskilled brushwork and
more naive treatment; they were painted by itinerant
artists for use in the homes of commoners. Like most
Korean screen-painting themes, hunting scenes were
available to all but the lowest classes of society.

Korean hunting screens traditionally depict gallop-
ing horsemen armed with spears, bows, swords,
matchlock guns, and falcons, chasing after tigers,
bears, wild boars, deer, rabbits, and game birds.
Surprisingly, the hunters on these screens wear
Mongol costume rather than Korean or Chinese
attire. The landscape setting is meant to suggest the
barren plains, sandy hills, and desolate mountains of
Mongolia. Given the animosity the Koreans had for
these people after their brutal occupation of Korea in
the 13th century, it seems odd that the horsemen in
Korean hunting screens are shown as Mongols.

However, Mongol Hunters had been a traditional
subject of Chinese paintings for several centuries. The
tradition began with Ch'en Chu-chung, a Southern
Sung court artist active during the Chia-t'ai era (1201–
1204). Ch'en Chu-chung was a court artist of the
Imperial Painting Academy in Hang-chou. The Sung
court had fled south in 1127 when North China was
conquered by the Jurched Tartars. Northern and

southern China were both conquered by the Mongols
in 1279.

Even though they were enemies, the Chinese
greatly admired the equestrian skills of the Tartars
and Mongols. The nomads were expert horsemen
since early times. Their derring-do in hunting and
fighting on horseback was legendary. By the 3rd century B.C., the Chinese were forced to abandon their
cumbersome war chariots and adopt the cavalry
techniques of their nomad enemies.

Ch'en Chu-chung became famous as a painter of
horses. He was compared to Han Kan, the most
famous horse painter of the T'ang Dynasty. Ch'en
Chu-chung usually depicted horses in the setting of
a Mongol hunt or encampment. The paintings proved
so popular that they became the basis for a tradition.
This became a standard treatment for the hunting
theme in Chinese painting.

Romantic fascination with the exotic played a considerable role in the popularity of such paintings.
Ch'en Chu-chung and other artists of his day liked to
illustrate "The Eighteen Songs of Wen Chi." These
poems were said to have been written by Lady Wen
Chi, a Chinese noblewoman captured by the
Hsiung-nu Tartars in A.D. 195. She was carried off to
Mongolia, where she lived for twelve years as the
wife of a Hsiung-nu chieftain, for whom she bore
two children. Her poems expressed her sorrow at
having to leave her Tartar husband and children when
she was finally ransomed and returned to China.
The chieftain had treated her with great kindness
and became despondent over losing her. Paintings
based on Wen Chi's poems were fashionable in China
from the early 13th century onward. The artists took
delight in depicting the costumes, tents, banners,
weapons, horse trappings, and other exotic paraphernalia of the Tartars and Mongols.

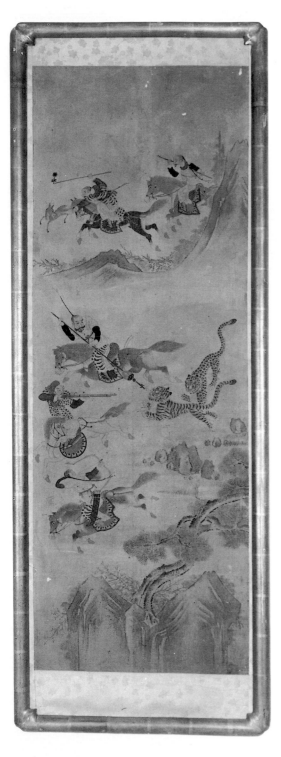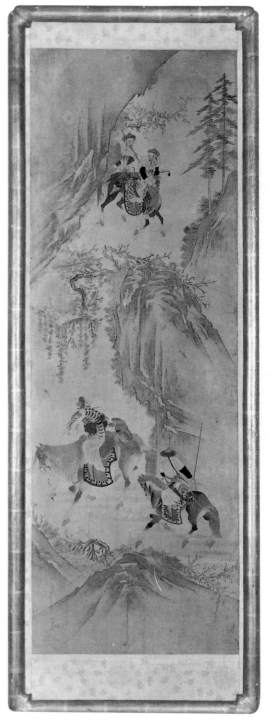

49. *Hwacho* (Birds and Flowers)

Ten-panel screen-painting; ink and color on linen
H. 47¾", W. 11¾" each panel, exclusive of mounting
Yi Dynasty, 19th century
Lent by Mrs. Peter Durgin   L76.2

Korean Buddhist paintings (see Cat. 11, 27, 28, 29) were painted by highly trained artist monks. Painter monks endured long, rigorous spiritual discipline as well as lengthy apprenticeships in Buddhist painting techniques. Those who failed to complete the training sometimes became itinerant artisans who painted and repainted the elaborate, brightly colored decoration on the columns, beams, brackets, and eaves of Buddhist temples. Exposed to the weather, this decoration required almost constant renovation.

Korean court paintings (see Cat. 35, 36, 37, 38, 39, 40, 47) and the finest Korean literati (scholar) paintings (see Cat. 41, 42) were executed by highly trained professional artists who belonged to the Bureau of Painting. Their patrons were the court nobility and the land-owning scholar bureaucrats.

Korean folk paintings, on the other hand, were produced for commoners (farmers, artisans, and merchants). The present screen, and the other Yi Dynasty paintings to follow, are folk paintings (see Cat. 50, 51, 52, 53, 54, 55, 56). The professional painters who produced them were completely different from the artists who belonged to the Bureau of Painting. Folk painters were itinerant artisans who traveled from village to village. They were called "passing guests" because they lodged at a villager's house while painting whatever pictures his family needed. When a folk painter finished his work for one family, he moved on to another house in the village. When he had painted all the pictures the village required, he moved on to another village. Folk painters used much cheaper materials than court artists, and had much less formal training. Toward the end of the Yi Dynasty, itinerant resident folk painters were gradually replaced by artist peddlers who displayed their pictures for sale in the village square and painted pictures to order on the spot.

Their wandering, independent existence gave Korean folk painters a kind of artistic freedom. The highly traditional, conservative nature of Yi Dynasty society resulted in a standardization of folk-painting functions and themes. However, the anonymous folk artists painted these stock themes in infinitely varied, personal, and unself-conscious ways. Their work has a compelling directness, energy, and naiveté.

Korean folk paintings enhanced everyday life in several ways: as bright, joyous decoration, as auspicious symbols, and as talismans. Until modern times, the latter functions were as important as the first. The symbolism had a practical, magical purpose: attracting good fortune and repelling evil. Most of the subjects of Korean folk paintings were intended to promote long life and good fortune or to offer protection against evil spirits.

Prior to the 20th century, the meanings of the various symbols were understood, indeed taken for granted, by Koreans of all classes. The symbols consisted of mythical creatures as well as certain animals, birds, fish, plants, objects, and ideograms. The symbolism was derived from animism, the belief that animals, birds, trees, mountains, rocks, and blades of grass are imbued with sentient spirits. Most of the symbolism in Korean folk art came from Taoism. Korean Shamanism evolved from the same early sources as Chinese Taoism. Shamanism provided a deeply felt belief in animism that gave Taoist symbols great immediacy in Korea.

During the latter part of the Yi Dynasty, screen paintings were used by all but the poorest class of Korean society, from the royal court and the scholar officials to the farmers, artisans, and merchants. Screen paintings were displayed in the main rooms of most Korean houses. Koreans were continually surrounded by screen paintings. Hanging-scroll paintings, door-panel paintings, transom-panel paintings, and horizontal-scroll paintings were also displayed in Korean homes, but screen paintings were more ubiquitous.

In a purely physical sense, Korean screens helped keep drafts away from the occupants of the house, who sat on small cushions on the floor. Avoiding drafts was an important consideration in Yi Dynasty houses. Korea is extremely cold in the winter. Snowfall is generally light, but an icy wind from Siberia howls through the land, chilling everything in its path. Thick, weighted felt hangings were placed over

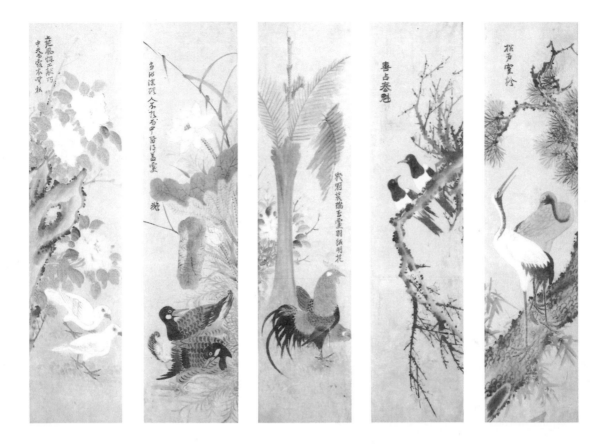

the interior side of windows specifically to stop drafts.

Because of the bitter cold, Korean houses had few windows. The large areas of unbroken wall space provided an ideal setting for screen paintings. During the winter, screens created a cozy sense of enclosure within a room. They also provided paintings of flowers during the season when flowers do not bloom. In the summer, screens standing in front of windows were folded up and put away. The windows were opened for a view of the blossoming trees and shrubs in the garden beyond the veranda.

Hwacho (Birds and Flowers) screens were the most prevalent type of Korean screen paintings. The Birds and Flowers category of painting subjects was established early in the history of painting in China. The category includes small animals, insects, and woody plants, as well as birds and flowers proper.

Korean *hwacho* screens nearly always depict the animals and birds as pairs. Each pair of animals or birds serves as a symbol of happy marriage and marital fidelity. A *hwacho* screen could be used in almost any room of a Korean house but was especially appropriate for the wife's bedroom or sitting room.

The subjects and inscriptions of the ten panels of the present screen are as follows (from right to left):

A pair of cranes on the trunk of a pine tree, inscribed, "A pine tree lifts the cranes on high." Cranes are the companions, messengers, and vehicles of the Taoist immortals and thus symbolize longevity and immortality. Pine trees also symbolize longevity because they live many years, resist harsh weather, and stay green through the winter (see Cat. 70).

A pair of magpies on the branch of a blossoming plum tree, inscribed, "Magpies announce the first sign

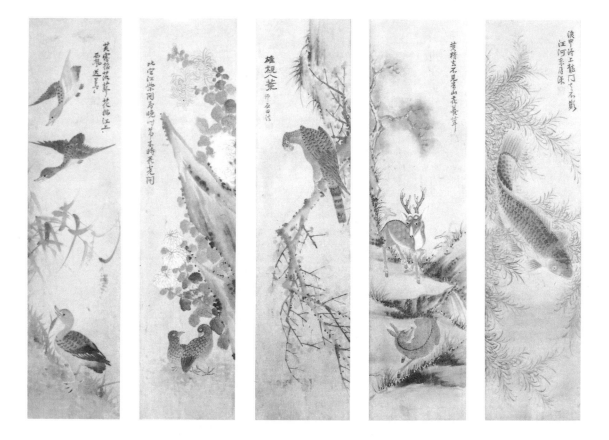

of spring." Magpies are the messengers of The Village Spirit and often bring good tidings (see Cat. 54).

A rooster and hen beside a banana plant, inscribed, "The tall crown (of the banana plant) is adorned with jade; the (rooster's) red plumage rivals the brightness of the flowers." A rooster is a symbolic household guardian. A painting of a rooster wards off evil spirits, just as a rooster's crowing at dawn drives away the spirits of the night.

A pair of ducks beside lotus plants, inscribed, "Unnoticed by all, the lotus becomes an umbrella for ducks in the rain." Ducks mate for life and so became symbols of fidelity and marital bliss (see Cat. 59).

A pair of white doves beside peonies and garden rocks, inscribed, "In the royal garden, the elegance is pleasing and the layout is skillful, but the rain and dew belong to everyone." Peonies are symbols of feminine beauty and female sexuality; upright

garden rocks suggest male potency (see Cat. 53).

A carp swimming among river grass, inscribed, "When a carp swims upstream past Dragon Gate, his pleasure turns the Sok-chong River to spray." Carp symbolize courage and perseverance because they leap over waterfalls and swim through rapids on their way upstream to spawn (see Cat. 56).

A pair of deer beside a pine tree, inscribed, "Where Sacred Fungus and mysterious rocks are found, flowers on the blue mountain make a deer's antlers grow." Deer are companions and messengers of the Taoist Immortals; they symbolize long life and immortality (see Cat. 70).

A hawk on a blossoming plum tree, inscribed, "The hawk sees all national boundaries." Hawk paintings are talismans against fire, flood, and wind (see Cat. 55).

A pair of quail beside chrysanthemums and garden rocks, inscribed, "When red and purple flowers blossom at the end of spring, 'tis the season when flying flowers (the quail) bloom."

A pair of wild geese flying above a third goose standing beside reeds, inscribed, "When the rose-mallows sway and the China-grass flowers are full, the west wind on the river brings the wild geese." Wild geese mate for life and so became symbols of happy marriage and marital fidelity (see Cat. 59).

The painter's seal appears after each inscription; it bears his art name, Yu-ryong (The Sound of Lapis Lazuli Jewels).

50. *Hwacho* (Birds and Flowers)

Four panels from an eight-panel screen; scorch on paper
H. 38¾", W. 11¾" each, exclusive of mounting
Yi Dynasty, 19th century
Purchase   75.65.3-.6

Birds and Flowers was the most prevalent subject of 18th–19th-century Korean screen paintings (see Cat. 49). Some screens were done in techniques other than painting. One alternate technique was embroidery. Embroidered screens are still used as household decoration in Korea today. Another technique was wood-block printing, either black and white, or with color added by hand over block-printed outlines. The latter type is almost indistinguishable from paintings. Yet another technique was pyrography ("scorched pictures"), which was quite popular in Korea during the latter part of the Yi Dynasty. The four panels we see here were originally part of an eight-panel pyrography screen.

Pyrography "paintings" seem to be unique to Korea. Called *indu kurim*, pyrography consists of pictures drawn on paper with a heated metal stylus whose dull point scorches lines on the surface. In China the technique was used to decorate small bamboo objects such as folding-fan frames. In Korea *indu kurim* was used to decorate bamboo items such as fan frames, brush holders, cups, arrow quivers, combs, and tobacco pipes, as well as to draw pictures on paper.

Like the pictures themselves, the poetic inscriptions on the present panels were scorched rather

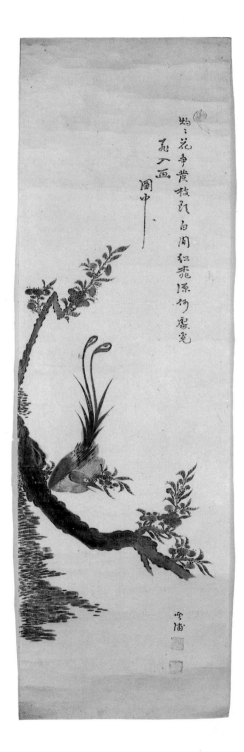

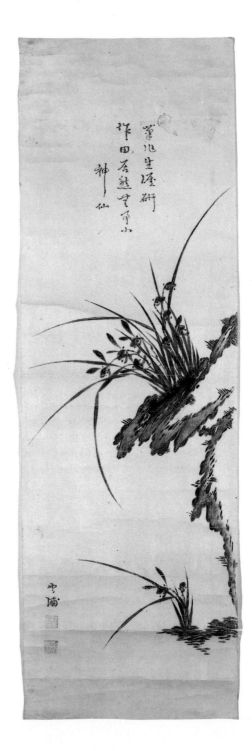

than written with a brush and ink. The subjects and the inscriptions are as follows:

A wagtail on the branch of a blossoming peach tree, inscribed, "Flaming blossoms compete with each other. Branches droop like combed hair. Where can I find the Peach Blossom Spring beside the white stream? Look, it has jumped into my painting!" *The Peach Blossom Spring* was a well-known story by a famous Chinese poet of the Six Dynasties Period, T'ao Yuan-ming (365–427). It concerned a fisherman who accidently discovered a hidden valley where everyone lived in blissful harmony. After the fisherman returned to his own village, he was never able to find the hidden valley again.

Grass orchids (epidendrum) growing on a cliff, inscribed, "Orchids spend their lives cultivating fields. Living without troubles, they are really little Immortals." Here the epidendrum serve as metaphors for retired scholars or Taoists, living in the bosom of Nature.

A kingfisher and lotus, inscribed, "When the color of the midnight moon fills the pond, red lotus buds quietly exude a subtle fragrance." The lotus is an old Buddhist symbol of purity (it rises pure white or pure pink from the black muck at the bottom of a pond). The kingfisher is admired for his brightly colored, iridescent plumage.

A bush-warbler, chrysanthemums, and a garden rock, inscribed, "Under the round window, two stalks of chrysanthemum have already bloomed. My house is the home of chrysanthemum-mindedness." Chrysanthemums have been admired by the Chinese, Koreans, and Japanese since early times.

Each panel is signed (in pyrography) with the artist's pen name, Un-p'o (Cloud-beach).

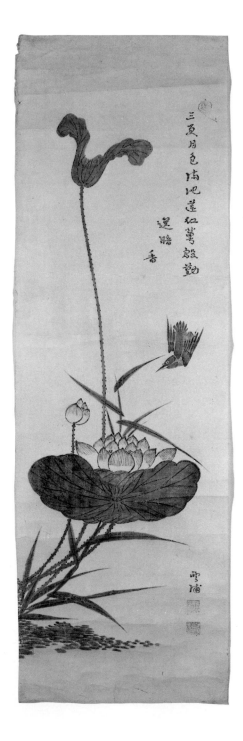

51. *Ch'aekkori* (Books and Scholar's Utensils)

Six-panel screen-painting; ink and color on paper
H. 39⅛", W. 10⅝" each panel, exclusive of mounting
Yi Dynasty, 19th century
Gift of H. O. Havemeyer   74.5

While the symbolism implicit in Birds and Flowers screens (see Cat. 49, 50) is Taoist in origin, Books and Scholar's Utensils is a Confucian subject. *Ch'aekkori* screens were still-life paintings of furnishings from an idealized scholar's study. The word *ch'aekkori* means "books and scholarly paraphernalia." Paintings of this subject were usually eight-panel screens with separate arrangements of Chinese-style books and scholars' accoutrements on each panel. Most of the books were depicted closed and stacked in slipcases, so *ch'aekkori* screens are often called "book-pile screens" in English.

Ch'aekkori screens were unique to Korea, although they were based on a Chinese decorative-arts motif called "precious things," which consisted of imaginary bronze vessels, porcelain vases, jade scepters, polished coral, and the like, sometimes including books. Similar luxury items normally accompany the books and scholars' utensils depicted in *ch'aekkori* screens. The scholars' utensils usually include writing brushes, ink stones, ink sticks, water containers, rolls of paper, and stone or ivory seals.

Since playing the *ch'in* (Chinese zither) was one of the polite accomplishments cultivated by an ideal Confucian gentleman, zithers were often depicted on *ch'aekkori* screens. Other luxury items frequently depicted include eyeglasses (for reading), fans, tobacco pipes, and the utensils for preparing steeped green tea: teapot, small cups, and charcoal brazier. Motifs from Birds and Flowers screens occasionally found their way into Books and Scholar's Utensils screens: peonies, chrysanthemums, epidendrum, or lotus, (shown potted or in vases), peaches or pomegranates (in a bowl), or pairs of goldfish (in a glass bowl).

A *ch'aekkori* screen was considered ideal for display behind the desk in a scholar's study, where it conveyed an air of dignity, luxury, and reverence for scholarship. Folk-painting screens of Books and Scholar's Utensils were popular in commoners' homes as well. An elaborate Confucian education and the luxury goods illustrated in *ch'aekkori* screens were not available to most commoners, but the sense of gentility and the Confucian ideal of self-improvement conveyed by these screens were appreciated by commoners as well as scholar officials. *Ch'aekkori* were also meant to instill scholastic diligence in the children of the household.

The present screen seems to have been all too successful in achieving this goal: The children of the household have written pencil and crayon graffiti consisting of Chinese ideograms all over the screen! One frequently encounters children's graffiti on Korean folk-painting screens. These screens were not treasured as great works of art; they were used as everyday household furnishings. When they wore out, they were thrown away, and new ones were commissioned from an itinerant painter the next time one came through the village.

Like most other types of Korean screen paintings, *ch'aekkori* also functioned as talismans. A Books and Scholar's Utensils screen displayed in the home was supposed to promote virtue and harmony in the household, just as the observance of proper Confucian moral responsibilities by persons of all classes was supposed to ensure harmony in the state.

Earlier and more usual versions of *ch'aekkori* screens depicted separate arrangements of books and utensils against plain backgrounds on each panel. A bold variation of this treatment appeared toward the end of the Yi Dynasty. The variant type had a continuous composition across the eight panels of the screen. The books and utensils were arranged on the shelves

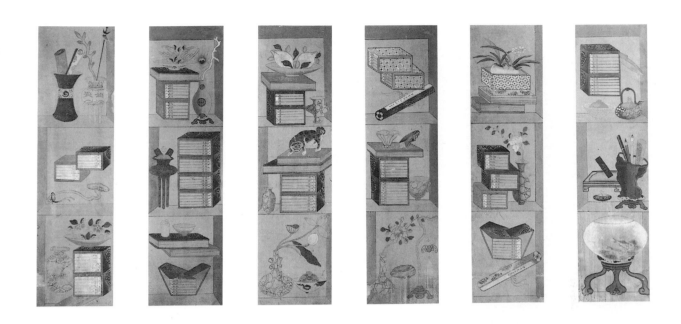

of a continuous bookcase. The shelves and compartments of the bookcase were rendered in exaggerated perspective. The perspective was not Western-style one-point perspective. It was reverse perspective, the type used in China since the T'ang Dynasty (618–907) or earlier.

The perspective and three-dimensional shading in "bookcase *ch'aekkori*" could have come from Western art indirectly, by way of China. Father Giuseppe Castiglione (1688–1768), an Italian Jesuit painter, went to China in 1715 and remained there until his death.

He served as court painter to the Ch'ien-lung emperor and took a Chinese nom de plume, Lang Shih-ning. His paintings were immensely popular in China. They combined Chinese technique and subject matter with Western perspective and modeling in light and shade. Castiglione and his Chinese pupils had hundreds of followers. His style even influenced the designs on late 18th-and 19th-century Chinese porcelain and other decorative arts. Reflections of his style were probably transmitted to Korea on Chinese decorative objects.

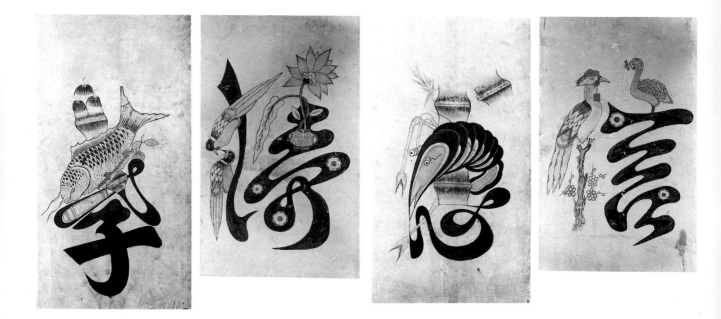

52. *Munjado* (Pictorial Ideographs: "The Eight Virtues")

Seven panels from two different eight-panel screens;
ink and color on paper
H. 30¼", W. 16½" each, exclusive of mounting
(77.97.1–.4)
H. 18", W. 11⅛" each, exclusive of mounting
(TL1986.183.1–.6)
Yi Dynasty, 19th century
Gift of Arthur Wiesenberger   77.97.1–.4
Lent by Dr. John Lyden   TL1986.183.1–.6

Korea has had its own phonetic alphabet, *hangul* (also called *onmun*), since 1443, when it was invented by the scholar official Chong In-ji at the command of King Sejong. Nevertheless the prestige of Chinese ideographs remained very strong in Korea. During the Yi Dynasty, men of learning wrote with Chinese characters; this was one of the attainments upon which the *yangban* class prided itself. *Hangul* was used by women and the lower classes. Modern written Korean is usually a mixture of Chinese characters and *hangul*. Throughout the Yi Dynasty, inscriptions on paintings were in Chinese. This was even true of folk paintings. Commoners who were illiterate in Chinese still had respect and admiration for Chinese learning.

Munjado screens superimposed depictions of symbolic animals, birds, fish, plants, and even narrative scenes onto Chinese ideographs. *Munjado* conveyed "The Eight Virtues," that is, the eight cardinal principles of Confucian morality. Each

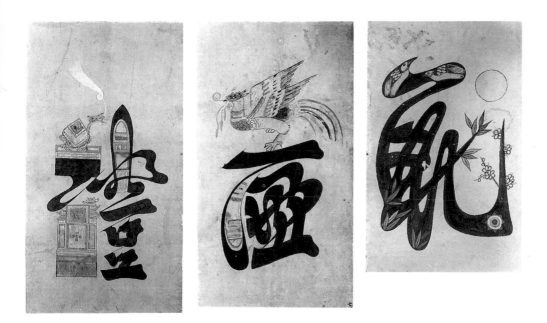

principle was represented by a single Chinese ideograph on each panel of a screen. It was a convenient coincidence that the number of cardinal principles was the same as the number of panels in the usual Korean screen.

The Eight Virtues (P'al Dok) represented the paramount principles of Confucian morality. In traditional order, they were: Filial Piety (honor one's parents), Brotherly Love (love one's siblings), Loyalty (be loyal to king and state), Sincerity (be trustworthy), Benevolence (do good), Duty (perform one's duty), Honor (uphold honor), and Humility (be humble and modest). Combining panels from two incomplete sets, the series shown here is complete except for "Duty."

There were two basic types of *munjado* screens. In the first and more common variety, depictions of symbolic animals, birds, fish, plants, or objects were substituted for certain strokes of the ideographs, for example, a fish in place of the four brushstrokes comprising the lower half of the character for "loyalty," or a bird in place of the upper stroke of the right half of the character for "trust." While the virtues for which the ideographs stand were Confucian, the symbolism of the pictorial embellishment was Taoist.

In the second type of *munjado* screen, narrative scenes involving groups of figures performing exemplary acts were superimposed upon the strokes of the ideographs, the strokes having been written extra wide to accommodate them.

53. Wedding Screen
Four panels of the original eight-panel screen-painting;
ink and color on paper
H. 69⅜", W. 76"
Yi Dynasty, 19th century
Gift of Robert Anderson   84.244.11

Korean Wedding Screens always depicted peony plants in full bloom, sometimes accompanied by garden rocks. They were magnificently decorative and luxurious. Their foremost function was to provide the setting, visual as well as symbolic, for a traditional Korean wedding ceremony. Wedding Screens were taller and wider than other Korean screens. On each of the eight panels was a nearly identical composition of gigantic peonies painted in outrageously bright colors and arrayed from top to bottom. The overall effect was one of ostentatious splendor; the feeling of richness and abundance was almost overwhelming.

Koreans call the peony "the queen of flowers." Peonies provide spectacular natural beauty in the courtyard of nearly every Korean home. The peony was traditionally regarded as a symbol of wealth, happiness, nobility, purity, spring, love, feminine beauty, and female sexuality. In full bloom, surrounded by an abundance of leaves, it was considered an auspicious harbinger of good fortune.

During the Yi Dynasty, weddings usually took place outdoors, in the main courtyard of the house. The ceremony was performed in front of a Wedding Screen; the screen was an essential accessory. A family too poor to own or buy one borrowed a screen from a more affluent family in the village. After the ceremony, the Wedding Screen was placed in the bride and groom's bedroom. The sexual symbolism of the screen's subjects was highly significant. The peonies suggested the bride's beauty and sexuality; the garden rocks suggested male potency.

The present *Wedding Screen* has lost four of its original eight panels. It includes a lotus (second panel from the right) among the traditional peonies. The lotus here symbolizes a bride's purity.

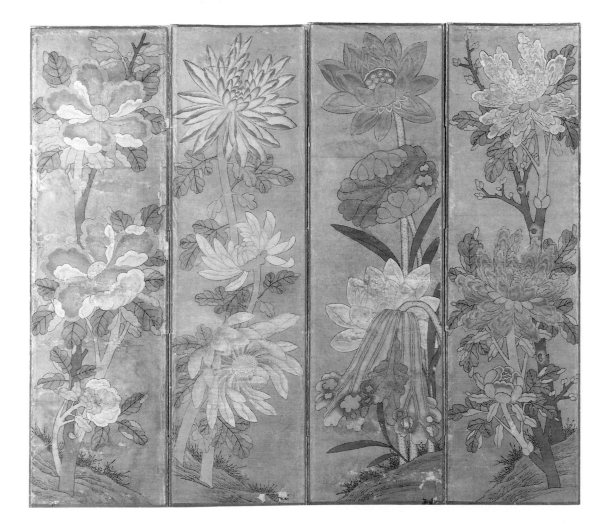

54. Tiger and Magpie

Hanging-scroll painting; ink and color on paper
H. 34¼", W. 16½" exclusive of mounting
Yi Dynasty, 19th century
Lent by Florence Selden   L81.18

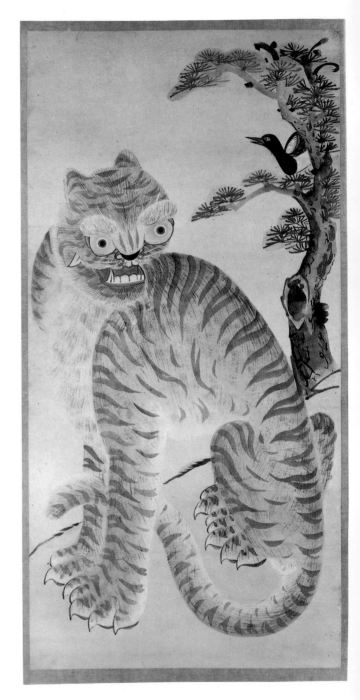

Siberian tigers (Panthera Tigris Altaica) used to roam the entire Korean peninsula, from the mountain forests in the northeast to the rugged seacoast of the southwest. The last recorded capture of a tiger in South Korea was in 1922; the species is probably extinct there today. There may still be a few tigers in the wilderness of the Mt. Paektu region in North Korea. The original habitat of the Siberian tiger included northeastern China and Siberia as well as Korea. Tiger claws, teeth, whiskers, and other parts were considered essential in certain Chinese and Korean folk medicines. In Korea, tiger bones were used to make a liquor called *hogolju*.

Tiger and Magpie paintings are among the most delightful of all Korean folk art. They were displayed in Yi Dynasty households at New Year's in order to protect the family against evil throughout the coming year. The tiger is the most powerful of the many evil-repelling animals in Korean mythology.

In a Tiger and Magpie painting, the tiger sits on his haunches looking angry and frustrated while the magpie chatters at him disapprovingly from the safety of a pine tree. Satirical humor is implicit in this juxtaposition: the magpie tormenting the tiger suggests commoners taunting corrupt and oppressive government officials.

On a less satirical level, the magpie is the messenger of the Village Spirit and is traditionally the bearer of good tidings. The tiger is the messenger of the Mountain Spirit. Paired with the tiger in a New Year's painting, the magpie portends good fortune for the coming year.

Visitors to Korea will understand why magpies are considered birds of good omen associated with villages. Korean magpies are huge black-and-white birds who seem almost tame in their wild state and prefer to live as close as possible to human habitation. If a row of tall trees stands beside a village, the magpies always choose the trees closest to the houses as the site for their gigantic nests.

55. Sam Jae Bu (Three-headed Hawk)

Amulet painting; ink on paper
H. 25″, W. 18″ exclusive of mounting
Yi Dynasty, 18th century
Purchase   85.170

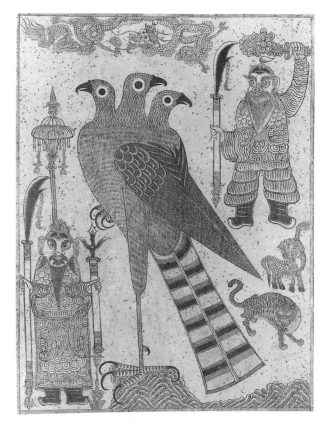

"*Pujok*" is the generic term for Korean amulet pictures, including those that invite good fortune as well as those that repel evil spirits. A subtype, *munbae* (door talismans), were hung on doors or gates to keep evil spirits out of buildings. *Pujok* were hung on walls, pillars, doors, ceilings, or storage chests. Smaller *pujok* were carried by individuals for protection away from home.

Pujok, like screen paintings, were used by Koreans of every class, from the royal family through the scholar officials to the farmers, artisans, and merchants. *Pujok* were subjected to rough use, displayed day in and day out, then discarded annually when new ones were hung up. Their magic power was only supposed to last for a year. Not many *pujok* have survived, but those that have are among the most delightful examples of Korean folk art.

Tan-O, The Festival of the Spirits, on the fifth day of the fifth month in the old lunar calendar, was one of the two traditional times to renew household *pujok*; the other was New Year's. For optimum magical efficacy, *pujok* were supposed to be printed or painted with red ink made from *chusa*, an expensive powdered stone imported from China for use in traditional medicine. *Pujok* were purchased from Buddhist monks, from *mudang* (shamans), or from fortune-tellers.

Even the king participated in the custom of renewing *pujok* during the Tan-O Festival. A large amulet painting of Chi U (Chinese: Chih Yu) was pasted on the entrance gate of the royal palace. Chi U is a mythical barbarian chieftain of ferocious mien who protects households against evil spirits and the nation against foreign invasions.

Most evil-repelling *pujok* depicted symbolic, or sometimes strictly mythical, animals, for example: tigers, roosters, dogs, or *haet'ae* (mythical lions). Good-fortune-inviting *pujok* depicted such things as the sun, the moon, stars, pomegranates, or one of The Four Animals of Good Luck: the dragon, phoenix, tortoise, and kylin.

The Three-headed Hawk (Sam Jae Bu) was a popular subject for *munbae* intended to be hung in the main doorway of a house to protect the occupants from misfortune. *Sam Jae Bu munbae* were traditionally renewed at New Year's so as to ensure protection throughout the coming year. The *Sam Jae Bu*'s three heads signify his special powers to guard against fire, flood, and wind, as well as his ability to bestow good forune for a period of three years. In the present painting, the Three-headed Hawk is accompanied by two Shamanist Guardian Generals, a dragon, a tiger, and a kylin.

56. Three Jumping Carp
Hanging-scroll painting; ink and light color on paper
H. 25¼", W. 15¾" exclusive of mounting
Yi Dynasty, 19th century
Gift of Mr. & Mrs. Burton Krouner   82.79

Carp were a very special and extremely popular subject in Yi Dynasty painting and decorative arts. Korean carp legends came for China, but the carp motif was more prevalent in Korea, perhaps because of the deep-seated Korean belief in Taoist/Shamanist animistic magic.

Carp have long been popular pets in China, Korea, and Japan. They grow quite large and become tame enough to eat out of one's hand. Brightly colored ones are especially prized and can be remarkably expensive today. Since carp were considered auspicious, fishermen who caught them were supposed to throw them back. Nevertheless, carp meat is a popular delicacy throughout the Far East, and carp soup is taken as a tonic to restore vigor.

Traditional carp symbolism was based on observed reality. Like salmon, carp swim upstream to spawn. They struggle against the current, fight their way through rapids, and leap over waterfalls along the way. In attempting to ascend waterfalls, they leap again and again until they either succeed or die. Because of this, carp came to signify courage, perseverance, endurance, vigor, and success. In Korea, a painting of a carp was hung in a boy's room to inspire these qualities in him.

According to an ancient Chinese legend, the carp in the Yellow River who managed to swim all the way upstream past the rapids at Lung Men (Dragon Gate) turned into dragons. Korean folk paintings of carp usually show them leaping out of the water, sometimes turning into dragons or becoming composite carp-dragons.

Beyond the edifying symbolism mentioned above, a Jumping Carp painting served a magical, Shamanist purpose in a Yi Dynasty household. When a Jumping Carp painting was hung on the wall above a bride's bed, it was supposed to cause her to dream of leaping carp, or of a dragon. Having dreamt this, she was supposed to give birth to a son who would be virtuous and successful. This magic function of Jumping Carp paintings cannot be overestimated, since bearing sons was a Yi Dynasty wife's highest duty.

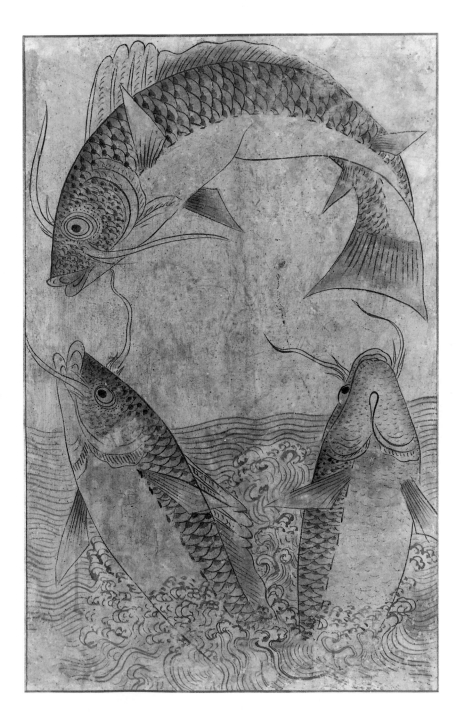

57. Tomb Guardian

Granite
H. 53", W. 14"
Yi Dynasty, 15th–16th century
Caroline A. L. Pratt Fund   85.18

Korea is a land of rocks. On nearly every mountainside, rugged masses of exposed granite swell up among the sparse covering of trees. The famous granite peaks partially surrounding the city of Seoul are typical of this phenomenon.

Koreans respect and enjoy rocks. Shamanist animism attributed sentient spirits to rocks, especially unusually shaped or unusually situated ones. Fantastic rocks became the subjects of local legends. The twelve thousand granite spires of the Diamond Mountains (see Cat. 43) are the best-known examples. Many such rocks were named according to their imagined shapes: tiger rock, dragon rock, demon rock, monk rock, old-woman rock, or even mother-holding-baby rock

Following long-standing practice in China, Koreans liked to place large rocks in strategic locations in their gardens (see Cat. 47). A garden rock was usually a craggy, upright, convoluted boulder, often perforated in several places, whose form suggested a mountain with grottoes, like the fairy peaks on the mythical Islands of the Immortals.

Since early times, Korean granite has proved an ideal architectural material. The buildings themselves were of wooden post-and-lintel construction with plaster walls and tile roofs, but large, rectangular blocks of granite were used for the foundation platforms. Monuments such as pagodas were often built entirely of granite. Tombs consisted of huge, hemispherical mounds of earth, but large granite blocks often formed a retaining wall around the base of the mound. The tomb chamber, at ground level beneath the center of the earth mound, was often lined with granite slabs.

Korean granite was also an excellent material for outdoor sculpture, tough enough to withstand the weather for centuries. Granite guardian figures and guardian animals stood near royal tombs. Granite pagodas and stone lanterns stood in Buddhist temple compounds. Commemorative tablets made of granite stood here and there in the countryside. Such a tablet usually consisted of a large, upright granite slab bearing an incised inscription and supported by a granite tortoise. Some of these tablets commemorated kings, but many of them commemorated virtuous villagers, humble, selfless men elected to this honor by members of their own villages after their deaths. Commemorative tablets were usually enclosed by small, tile-roofed, red-painted wood pavilions called "spirit houses."

This *Tomb Guardian* is typical of the standard type of Yi Dynasty granite guardian figure from the tomb precinct of a king or other important personage. Based on Ming Dynasty practice in China, a Yi Dynasty royal tomb had several pairs of large guardian figures and animals arrayed on either side of the Spirit Way, the avenue leading to the tomb. The figures or animals of each pair stood facing one another on opposite sides of the avenue. Silla Dynasty royal tombs employed similar granite figures, based on T'ang Dynasty Chinese precedent. Koryo royal tombs did likewise, following T'ang and Sung Dynasty Chinese examples.

The present *Tomb Guardian* represents a high-ranking court minister standing fully frontal in an attitude of reverence. He is a civil official rather than a military one. He wears Confucian court costume consisting of a full-length robe with pendant sleeves and a boxlike court hat. The toes of court shoes appear beneath the edge of his robe. A ceremonial apron indicating court rank hangs from his belt. His hands are clasped before his chest holding a wooden baton of office of the type carried at an audience with the king. A stone image such as this was meant to serve symbolically the deceased king as a loyal court minister in the spirit world.

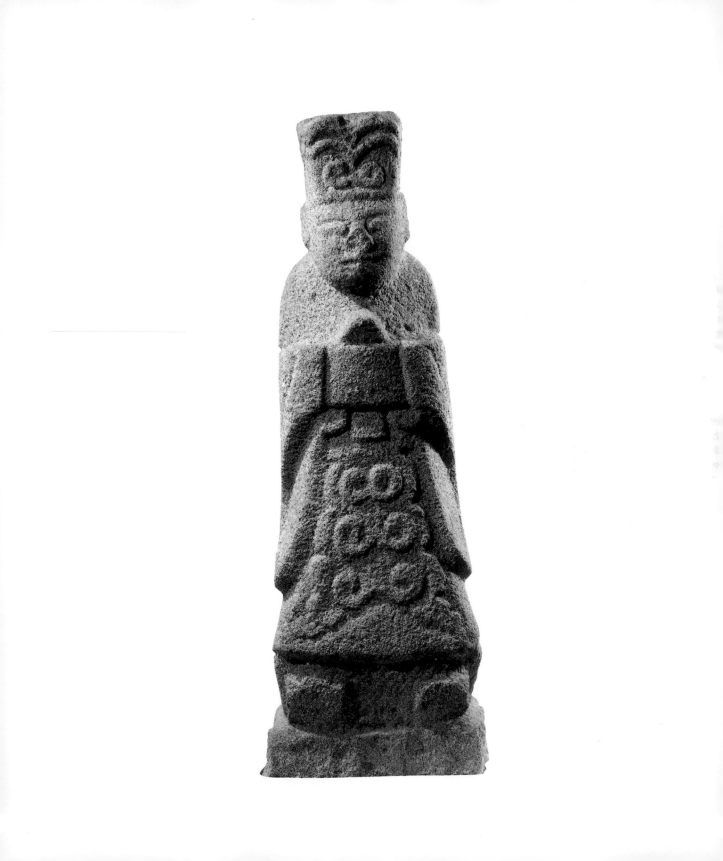

58. *Dong-ja* **(Altar Attendants)**
Pair of polychromed wood figures
H. 19″ (.1), 20″ (.2), W. 3½″ each
Yi Dynasty, 18th century
Gift of Dr. & Mrs. Stanley Wallace   83.174.1 & .2

These delightful painted wooden figures are splendid examples of Korean folk sculpture. A pair of *Dong-ja* like this usually stood on the altar table in front of a painting of The Mountain Spirit (see Cat. 30) or other deity in one of the subsidiary shrines of a Yi Dynasty Buddhist temple. Taoist in origin, *Dong-ja* were immortal youths who never aged. They usually wore imaginary Chinese court costume and plaited their hair in two balls on top of the head, in the fashion of noble children in T'ang Dynasty China.

The left *Dong-ja* in the present pair looks like a waiter with a white napkin over his arm carrying a tray of food with a domed cover. Actually the "tray" represents a porcelain bowl and the "cover" represents The Peach of Immortality (see Cat. 25), presented as an offering to whatever deity these attendants served.

The right *Dong-ja* in this pair holds a turtle with a head like a dragon. This is the mythical tortoise, the messenger of the Dragon King. Large sea turtles sometimes lived for several centuries, so the tortoise was an auspicious symbol of longevity offered by the *Dong-ja*. The tortoise was one of the *Shipjangsaeng* (The Ten Symbols of Long Life), which, singly or in groups, appeared frequently in Yi Dynasty paintings and decorative arts (see Cat. 70).

A tortoise entwined by a snake is one of The Animals of the Four Directions (Korean: *Sa Shin*), ancient Chinese Taoist guardian spirits mentioned in the *I Ching*: The Blue Dragon of the East, The White Tiger of the West, The Red Bird of the South, and The Black Tortoise of the North. The Tortoise is also one of the Four Animals of Good Luck (*Sa Ryong*): the dragon, phoenix, tortoise, and kylin.

Yi Dynasty geomancers continued to invoke The Animals of the Four Directions when selecting sites for buildings or tombs, but the *Sa Shin* were seldom represented in Yi art. The Four Animals of Good Luck, on the other hand, were frequent subjects of Yi Dynasty paintings and decorative arts. Hexagonal-diaper patterns, based on the natural markings of tortoise shells (for example, the pattern painted on the back of the tortoise held by this *Dong-ja*) also served as longevity symbols in China, Korea, and Japan.

The tortoise was among the most ancient of Taoist symbolic animals. Tortoise shells were used by Chinese diviners during the Shang Dynasty (c. 1500–1027 B.C.) to answer questions about future events by reading the cracks produced when a hot poker was applied to the back of the shell. The tortoise was sometimes shown carrying books, in reference to the legend about the tortoise who delivered the Eight Trigrams (magic writings) to Fu Hsi (Korean: Pok Hi), the primordial man. A huge stone figure of a tortoise was the standard support for a commemorative tablet in China and Korea.

Korean representations of the tortoise in any of his various mythical roles usually depicted him with the head and horns of a dragon to indicate that he was not a mere turtle. In either mythical or naturalistic form, the tortoise was an ubiquitous Yi Dynasty symbol of long life, good luck, and protection against evil. The tortoise's power to repel evil derives from his role as the guardian of the north among The Animals of the Four Directions. In this protective capacity the tortoise lent his form to Yi Dynasty wooden door latches.

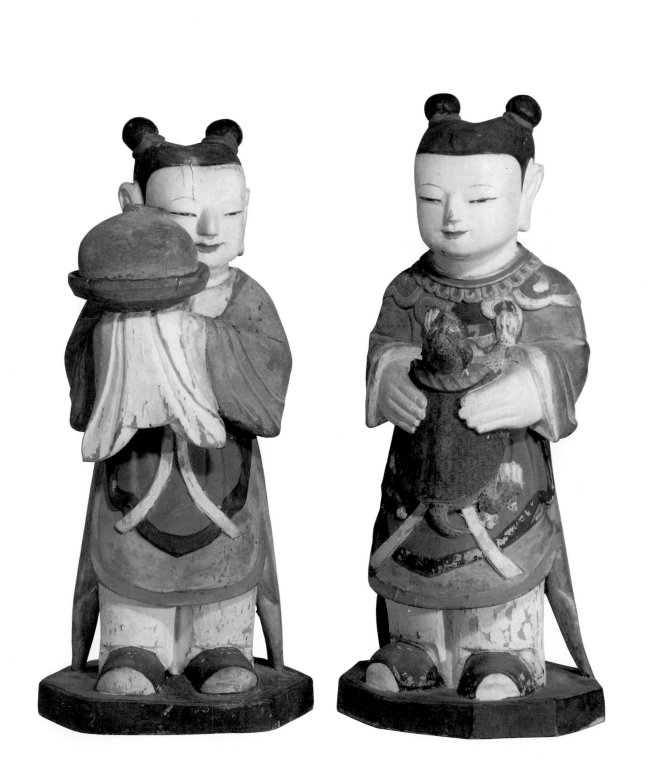

59. *Kirogi* **(Wedding Duck)**
Wood with traces of ink
H. 9½", L. 13½"
Yi Dynasty, 19th century
Gift of the Guennol Collection   86.140

Wild geese and mandarin ducks mate for life. The Chinese and the Koreans have used depictions of ducks or geese as symbols of fidelity and happy marriage since early times. Pairs of wild geese and ducks appeared frequently on Yi Dynasty *hwacho* (birds and flowers) screens (see Cat. 49).

A carved wooden duck or goose was an essential accessory at Korean weddings until Western-style weddings became fashionable in recent times. A Wedding Duck (*kirogi*) was a slightly less than life size, simplified wood figure of a duck (short neck) or a goose (long neck). Wedding Ducks were a nationwide Korean custom; the style of carving and painting varied from one district to another or even from one village to another. Some *kirogi* were rough and primitive, little more than a section of tree branch for a body and an upright stick for a head and neck. Other *kirogi* were more detailed. Some were simply stained dark brown; others were elaborately painted in bright colors. *Kirogi* made for the upper classes tended to be the more ornamental type, those for the lower classes the more primitive. Some *kirogi* were carved by professionals, others

were amateur work by local villagers or even by the groom himself.

The *kirogi* custom originally involved the use of a live wild goose. Wooden versions were later substituted due to the increasing difficulty of obtaining a live wild goose for the purpose.

Traditionally, the groom carried the *kirogi* to the house of the bride's family on the morning of the wedding. He placed it on a tray before the bride's mother and made a vow to be faithful to the bride for the rest of his life. The bride's mother symbolically offered some noodles to the *kirogi* to indicate her acceptance. The groom then returned to his own house carrying the *kirogi*. Sometimes the bride and groom held the *kirogi* during the wedding ceremony. The expression "feeding noodles to the goose" became a Korean euphemism for "marriage."

Many old *kirogi*, like the present one, are superb pieces of folk sculpture, warm and compelling in their directness and naiveté. The surface of the wood has taken on a rich, dark patina. The stylized form conveys the essence of the actual bird yet seems almost modern in its simplicity.

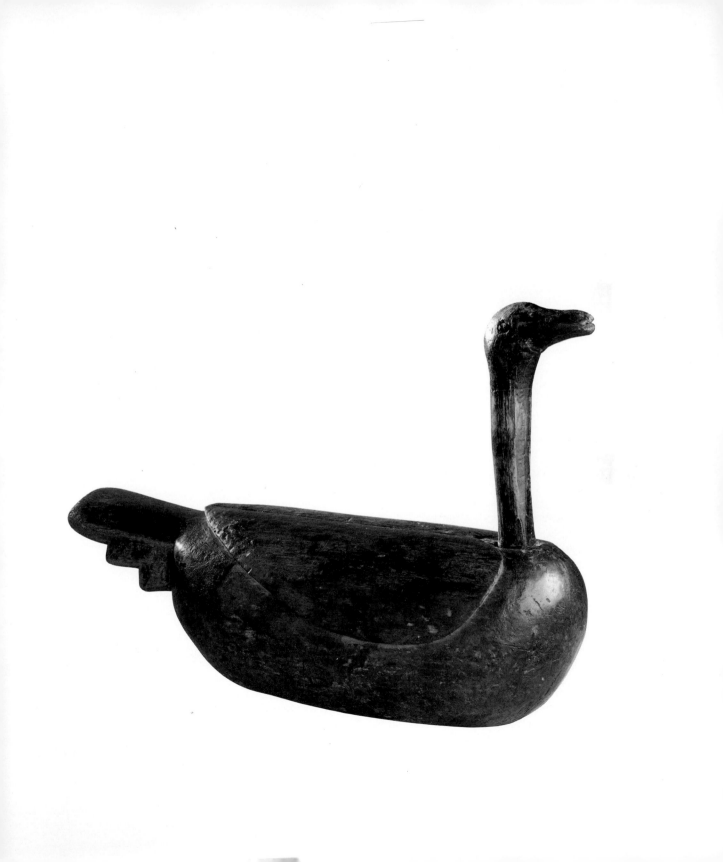

60. Prunus Vase
Transitional ware of inlaid celadon type
H. 10⅝″, W. 7″
Koryo-Yi Dynasty, late 14th–15th century
Lent by Dr. & Mrs. Robert Dickes   TL1984.355

Around the beginning of the Yi Dynasty, a rather abrupt change took place in Korean ceramics, an unusual phenomenon, since art styles, especially in the decorative arts, tend to change gradually, more or less independently of political developments. The change was from elegant, refined celadon porcelain, produced for the court and the aristocracy, to coarse, vigorous stoneware, produced for general use by commoners as well as for the court—the court pieces being only slightly less coarse.

This change took place at the end of the Koryo Dynasty and the beginning of the Yi Dynasty, between about 1350 and 1450. Some of the kiln sites in central and southern Korea have yielded shards and wasters of both late celadon and early *punch'ong* ware, indicating that the transition was accomplished smoothly, that is, without one tradition being destroyed and replaced by another.

A few rare pieces, greatly admired by connoisseurs in Japan, included elements of both the old tradition and the new; they are therefore called "transitional ware." The present *Vase* is a handsome and characteristic example of this type. The shape is an exaggeration of the classic Koryo *maebyong* (see Cat. 16); the upper portion has become slightly more bulbous. The glaze is a somewhat glassy late celadon glaze. The white-slip inlay technique is the same as that of inlaid Koryo celadons (see Cat. 18). However, the decoration has become more of an overall pattern. Koryo inlay designs such as lotus petals and *ju-i* scepter heads have been supplemented with space-filling patterns of parallel lines and stippled dots. The latter were primary elements of the new Yi Dynasty ceramic ware, *punch'ong* ware (see Cat. 61).

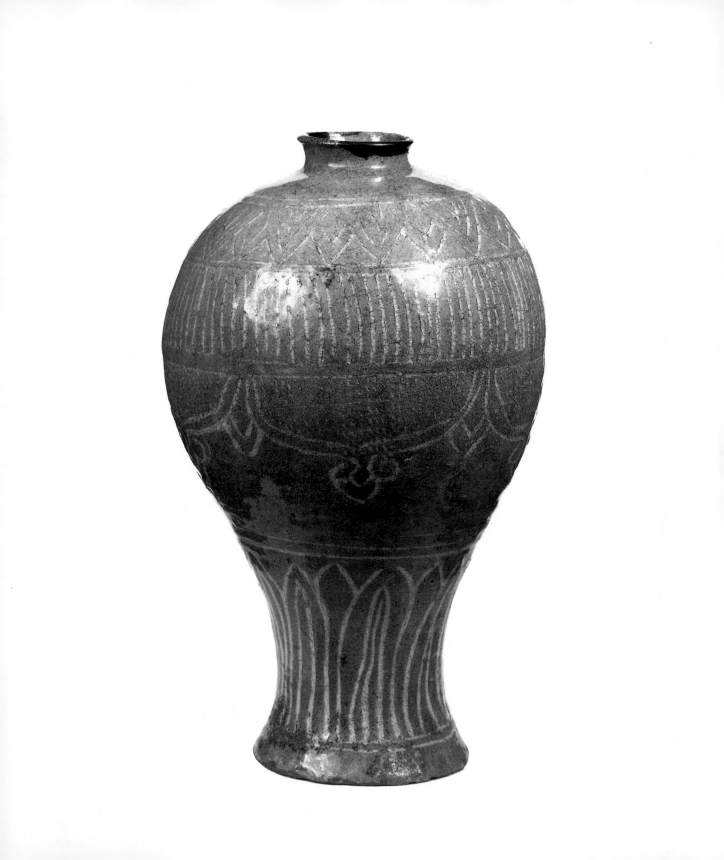

61. *Punch'ong* Ware Bowl

Glazed stoneware with inlaid-slip decoration
H. 3¼", W. 7½"
Yi Dynasty, 15th century
Gift of Paul Manheim   67.199.16

Punch'ong ware was the predominant Korean ceramic ware of the early Yi Dynasty, a period of two hundred years from the founding of the dynasty in 1392 until the Japanese invasions of 1592 and 1597. *Punch'ong* ware was produced in numerous kilns throughout central and southern Korea. Compared to Koryo Dynasty celadon porcelain, *punch'ong* ware is a coarse product. However, its strength and vigor often make up for its lack of refinement. It was produced in large quantities for everyday use by commoners, yet it cannot be called folk pottery, since it was also used at the royal court. The present *Bowl*, for example, has a two-character, inlaid inscription that reads *naesom*, the palace office in charge of food service. Yet the technical quality of this *Bowl* is hardly better than that of the average *punch'ong* ware used by commoners; the clay, the glaze, and the designs are the same. Koryo celadon was quite different, having been produced exclusively for the aristocracy.

A small amount of white porcelain, a very limited quantity of early blue-and-white porcelain, some rare black-glazed stoneware, and a few vessels with under-glaze iron-brown or copper-red painted decoration were produced during the early Yi period, but the overwhelming majority of ceramics from the first two centuries of the Yi Dynasty were *punch'ong* ware.

Punch'ong (Chinese: *fen ch'ing*) means "pale blue green." *Punch'ong* ware glaze is of celadon type. When thick enough and fired at the proper degree of reduction, it looks exactly like the Koryo celadon glaze from which it derives. However, the production of huge quantities of *punch'ong* ware for the masses precluded the precise firing control necessary to achieve blue-green celadon color. The gray clay used for *punch'ong* ware was very similar to the gray clay in Koryo celadon, but it was considerably coarser in texture.

The identifying characteristic of *punch'ong* ware was overall white-slip decoration. The decoration was produced in a variety of ways (see Cat. 62, 63, 64, 65, 66). The most typical kind was the stamped and inlaid type we see here. The designs were stamped (impressed) in the surface of the leather-hard clay after the *Bowl* was thrown and trimmed. Then white slip (liquid clay) was painted on liberally with a large brush. After the slip set, the surface was scraped free of slip, leaving the stamped designs filled with white clay in the surrounding gray clay surface. The technique was basically the same as that used for inlaid celadon but was done with much less care. The visual effect is quite different, however, because *punch'ong* ware has repeat patterns over most of the surface, while Koryo inlaid celadon has separate designs isolated in the blue-green ground. *Punch'ong* glaze sometimes developed a blue-green color where it ran thick, but normally was fairly transparent, so the gray clay usually looks gray through the glaze rather than blue green.

Punch'ong ware has been highly admired in Japan since the mid-16th century, when Japanese tea masters first selected *punch'ong* ware rice bowls for use as tea bowls in the Japanese tea ceremony. The Japanese term for *punch'ong* ware is *mishima* (also used for inlaid slip in general). The term *mishima* is often used by potters and collectors in the West as well.

The origin of the term *mishima* is obscure. It is thought to be derived from woodblock-printed almanacs sold at Mishima Shrine in Izu Province (modern Shizuoka Prefecture) during the 16th and 17th centuries. Mishima was the principal town of Izu Province; it was one of the fifty-three stations on the Tōkaidō highway between Edo (modern Tokyo) and Kyoto. Hiroshige's famous 1833 series of Tōkaidō prints included a depiction of the Shrine gateway in the view of Mishima. The Shrine almanacs were a *meibutsu* (famous local product) of Mishima. Travelers bought them as souvenirs and circulated them throughout Japan. The overall pattern of slip-

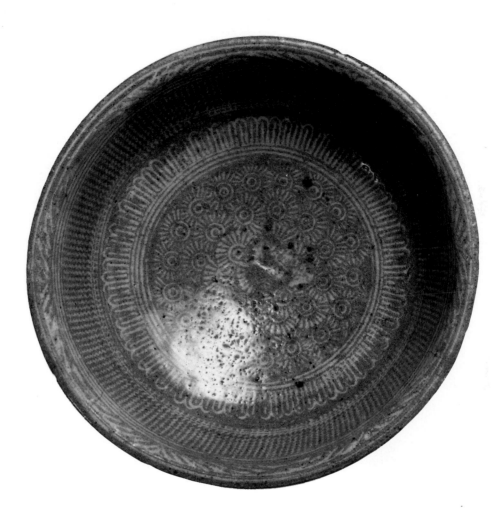

inlaid decoration on *punch'ong* ware was thought to resemble the vertical rows of minute ideographs on the woodblock-printed almanacs.

The designs on the present *Bowl* are typical *punch'ong* ware designs. One finds them repeated in various combinations on thousands of other bowls. The interior of this *Bowl* has a round central field filled with stylized, daisylike flowers suggesting the small, wild chrysanthemums that grow on Korean hillsides. Beyond the central field is a border of radiating petals. The sides of the *Bowl*, interior and exterior, have a continuous band of close-set vertical wavy lines known by the Japanese-derived term "rope-curtain pattern." The rim design, inside and out, consists of stylized grasses.

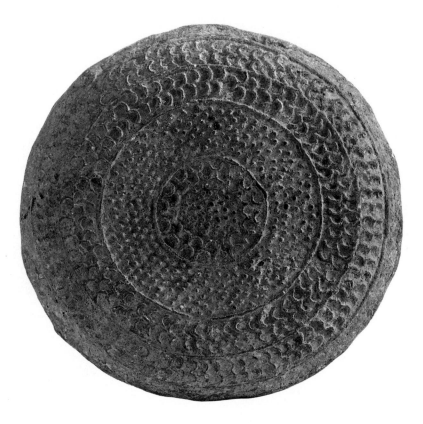

62. Mold for Inlaid-slip Decoration

Gray stoneware
Thickness at center ⅞", Diameter 3¼"
Yi Dynasty, 15th century
Gift of Robert Sistrunk   74.105

The chrysanthemums on the preceding *Bowl* (see Cat. 61) were stamped into the leather-hard clay individually, one flower at a time. The rows of large petals and wavy-line "ropes" were stamped with molds having four or five petals or "ropes" per mold. For small dishes and bowls, a single mold was used to stamp the entire interior design in one pressing. Then, white slip was brushed on, allowed to set, and wiped away, leaving the white clay inlaid in the gray ground. The present *Mold* is of this type; it is a rare example of an early Yi Dynasty potter's tool, perhaps the only one of its kind in the United States.

The raised designs on the *Mold* are typical *punch'ong* ware designs: patterns of dots and repeated U forms suggesting flower petals in the central rondel and dragon scales in the border. The same motifs appear on the opposite side of the *Mold* in a slightly different arrangement. The *Mold* is hollow and made of the same coarse gray clay as *punch'ong* ware itself, but without glaze or slip.

Similar but larger pottery molds were used to press the molded designs of peony petals and other motifs on the interiors of Koryo Dynasty molded celadon bowls. The bowl was thrown and trimmed in the usual way and then pressed onto the mold to produce the low-relief designs.

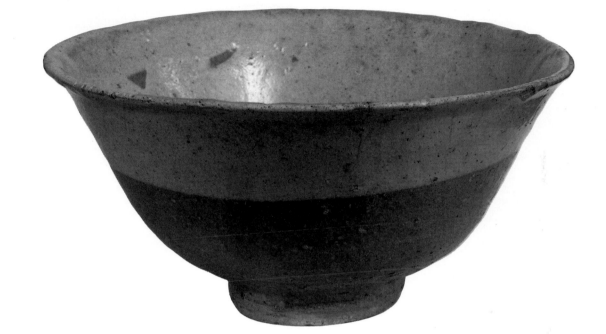

63. *Punch'ong* Ware Bowl (*Muji-hakeme* Type)
Glazed stoneware partially covered with white slip
H. 3⅜", W. 7⅛"
Yi Dynasty, 15th–16th century
Gift of John Lyden 82.184.1

It may seem odd that a Korean peasant rice bowl, devoid of decoration, is presented here as a work of art. Modern American potters undertand why: the Korean potter's direct and unself-conscious response to the clay was in complete harmony with his medium. In a bowl like this, clay was used as clay, with no extraneous decorative elements to get in the way, with no attempt to refine away the natural coarseness of the clay, allowing the clay instead to speak for itself.

There is also an historical reason why certain *punch'ong* ware bowls were celebrated as works of art. Japanese interest in folk art goes back to about 1920; Korean interest in folk art (as *art* rather than ethno-graphy) only goes back to about 1960. However, the artistic merits of Korean peasant rice bowls were recognized in Japan as early as the first half of the 16th century. The great tea master Takeno Jō-ō (1502–1555) selected certain Korean peasant rice bowls for use as tea bowls in the Japanese tea cermony. Prior to Jō-ō, Japanese tea-ceremony utensils had consisted of elegant, expensive Chinese luxury items such as Sung Dynasty celadon and Ming Dynasty carved lacquer. Jō-ō changed all that by selecting utensils that reflected the Zen Buddhist ideals on which the tea-ceremony aesthetic was based: profound spiritual beauty embodied in humility, frugality, and unpretentiousness. He selected rough, utilitarian ceramics from *punch'ong* ware kilns in Korea and rural kilns in Japan.

Because 16th–17th-century Japanese tea masters were the first to appreciate the aesthetic qualities of common *punch'ong* ware bowls, the designations they used for the different types of *punch'ong* ware have continued to carry considerable weight. Westerners and even Koreans use the Japanese terms for lack of a consistent Korean terminology.

The present *Bowl,* for example, is *punch'ong* ware of *muji-hakeme* type. *Muji* (literally, "no ground") is the Japanese term for "no design." *Hakeme* (literally, "the marks of a flat-edged brush") means "painted white slip with the brush marks showing" (see Cat. 64). The white slip on the present *Bowl* was applied by dipping the upper half of the bowl in a vat of liquid white clay, allowing it to fill the interior, then pouring off the excess. Because brushed white slip was preferred by the Japanese, this type was called "no-design brush mark," even though the slip was dipped on rather than brushed on.

Korean slipware, like most other slipware, stains easily from use. Numerous minute crackle fissures and pinholes in the glaze permit tea or soy sauce or other dark, thin liquids to penetrate the glaze and stain the white slip underneath. Due to the influence of the tea ceremony on the Japanese sense of beauty, the Japanese traditionally admire the effects of wear and age on objects. The stains acquired by slipware during years of use were a source of aesthetic pleasure to the Japanese.

64. *Punch'ong* Ware Bowl (*Hakeme* Type)

Glazed stoneware partially painted with white slip
H. 3", W. 7³/₁₆"
Yi Dynasty, 15th–16th century
Gift of Dr. & Mrs. Robert Dickes   82.173

Japanese tea masters' nomenclature for the various types of *punch'ong* ware is used in the West and in Korea as well as in Japan (see Cat. 63). This *Bowl* is a characteristic example of *hakeme,* a technique much admired and imitated in Japan. A *hake* is a flat-edged brush, as opposed to a *fude,* the usual writing brush, which comes to a point. The brush marks showing in the painted white slip on this type of *punch'ong* ware reminded the Japanese of paint applied with a *hake.* The brush used to apply this type of slip was not a *hake,* however, but a large, coarse, round brush made from the upper ends of rice straw.

The usual explanation for the use of painted slip is that slip does not adhere well when dipped on, but adheres better when brushed on. This theory seems faulty, since the slip on *muji-hakeme* bowls was dipped on and has usually adhered quite well (see Cat. 63). *Hakeme* has the advantage aesthetically, however. The linear tracks of the coarse brush give direction, gesture, energy, and vibrancy (gray showing through the white) to the brushed slip.

Hakeme has been extensively imitated by Japanese potters from the late 16th century until today. However, Japanese potters have never been able to achieve the sense of freedom, speed, and control in their brushed slip that even the most routine Korean examples display. The difference is that Korean potters were not striving for a visual effect but simply working quickly, spontaneously, and unself-consciously. Japanese potters imitated the technique, but their determination to achieve the visual effect prevented the spontaneous quality that makes Korean *hakeme* so appealing.

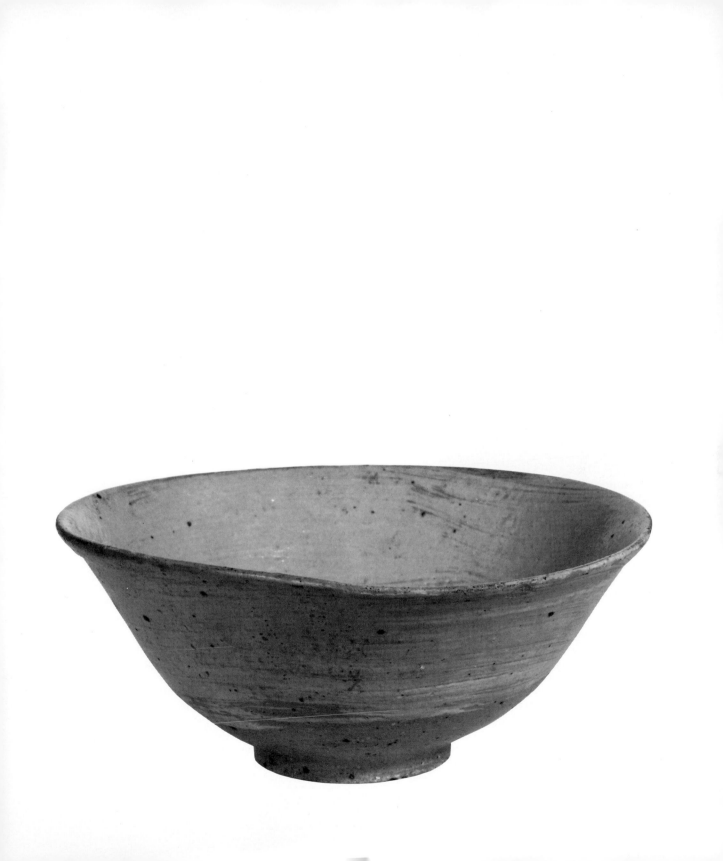

65. *Punch'ong* **Ware Wine Bottle (***Hori-hakeme* **Type)**
Glazed stoneware with white-slip decoration
H. 8⅝", W. 7"
Yi Dynasty, 15th–16th century
Ella C. Woodward Memorial Fund   75.61

This *Bottle* looks so modern that one is surprised to learn it was made five hundred years ago. As a work of ceramic art, it is unsurpassed. Form, decoration, color, and texture work together in perfect harmony. More bold and energetic than Koryo celadon, good *punch'ong* ware like this is the crowning achievement of the Korean potter's art. This fact is well recognized by modern potters in the West, and particularly in Japan, where this type of *punch'ong* ware has been very influential. Hamada Shōji (1894–1977), the great 20th-century Japanese potter, was an avid admirer and collector of early Yi Dynasty ceramics. Hamada often imitated the bottle shape we see here, thrown spherical, then gently pressed flat on two sides (called *henko* in Japanese). Through Hamad's work the *henko* shape entered the form vocabulary of contemporary ceramics in Japan and the West. Early in his career, Hamada also imitated this type of slip decoration.

Called *hori-hakeme* (carved *hakeme*), it involved painting the surface of the vessel with white slip, then carving away the slip to produce the design, here consisting of a bold peony blossom surrounded by a profusion of leaves, with a radiating chrysanthemum-petal border around the neck. The technique of carving decoration through slip to a contrasting clay beneath is known as "sgraffiato" in the West. It has been used independently in various parts of the world for many centuries. The inspiration for *hori-hakeme* decoration on *punch'ong* ware was certainly the sgraffiato decoration on certain types of Tz'u-chou ware in China.

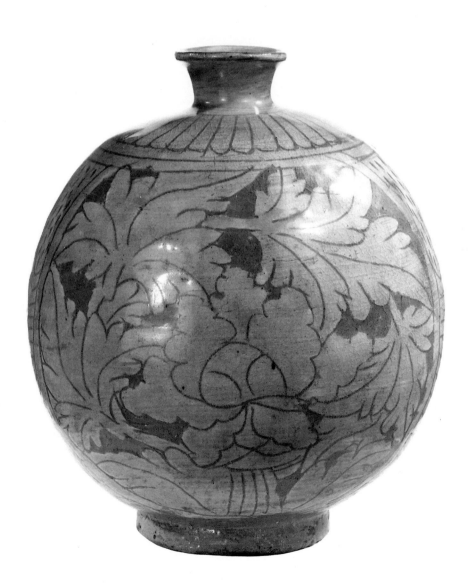

66. *Punch'ong* Ware Bowl (*E-hakeme* Type), Keryong-san Kiln

Glazed stoneware with painted slip decoration
H. 3⅛", W. 7"
Yi Dynasty, 15th century
Anonymous gift   83.32.5

In 1927 the Japanese ceramics scholar Nomori Ken excavated some of the kiln sites at Keryong-san. He uncovered the remains of more than twelve *punch'ong* ware kilns. They were situated near two villages in a valley among the eastern foothills of Keryong-san. This famous cluster of mountain peaks in south Korea has been celebrated since early times for its spectacular natural beauty. Keryong-san is about twelve miles west of the city of Taejon, which is roughly halfway between Seoul, on the middle of the west coast, and Pusan, at the southeastern tip of the peninsula.

Because of Keryong-san's magnificent scenery, King T'aejo, the founder of the Yi Dynasty, had originally intended to build his capital there. A census of Korean pottery kilns conducted for King Sejong in 1424–1425 recorded the Keryong-san kilns. It is believed that the kilns were founded by Buddhist monks who were forced to seek a livelihood when the new Yi government suppressed Buddhism in favor of Confucianism. Flourishing Buddhist monasteries at the foot of Keryong-san were forced to close at the beginning of the Yi Dynasty.

The Keryong-san kilns were active until the Japanese invasions of 1592 and 1597. At that time production ceased abruptly and was never revived. Some of the Keryong-san potters may have been among many villages of Korean potters abducted by the Japanese and forced to relocate in Kyūshū. The ceramics industry of Japan was permanently altered by the massive influx of Korean potters at the end of the 16th century.

Keryong-san kilns produced all of the different varieties of *punch'ong* ware; some of them also made white porcelain and black-glazed stoneware. However, the style for which Keryong'san is famous today consists of iron-black painted decoration over brushed white slip. The present *Bowl*, with its design of scrolling grasses, is a characteristic example. The spontaneous energy of the painted decoration reflects the vitality of the Korean people.

This style of Keryong-san ware is much admired in Japan, where it is designated *e-hakeme* ("*e*" meaning painted design, "*hakeme*" meaning "brushed white slip"). The painted designs are black rather than the brown of most other underglaze iron decoration. The color apparently results from manganese inclusions in the iron-bearing rock from which the black slip was prepared.

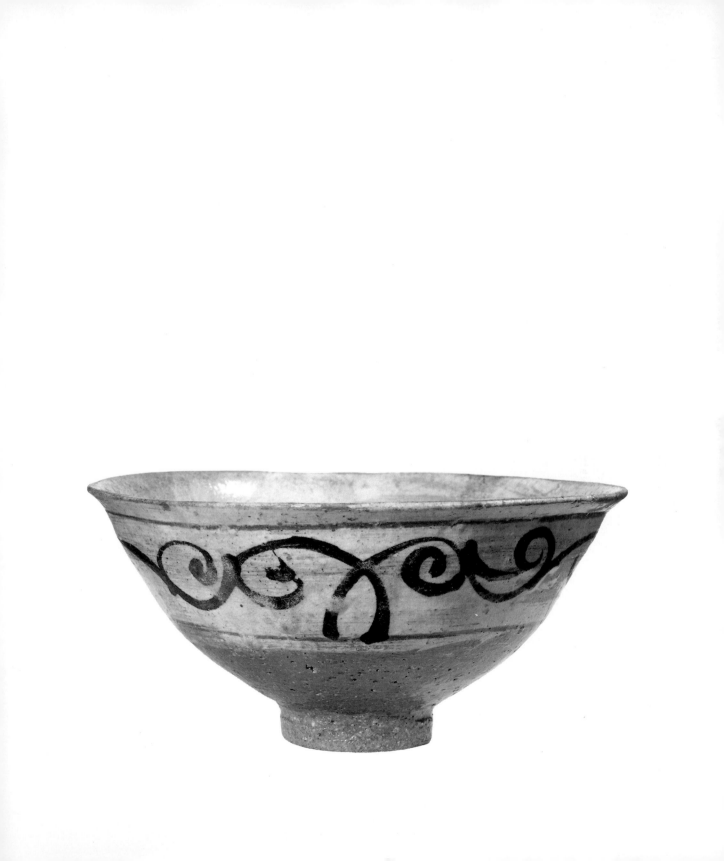

67. Storage Jar
White porcelain with a clear glaze
H. 11¾", W. 11"
Yi Dynasty, 17th century
Gift of John Lyden   84.262.8

The Korean ceramics industry was irrevocably changed by the Japanese invasions of 1592 and 1597. *Punch'ong* ware, the standard early Yi Dynasty ceramic type, went out of production altogether. When the ceramic industry was revived after the invasions, new styles came into vogue. The principal Korean ceramic ware of the 17th, 18th, and 19th centuries was blue-and-white porcelain. Highly refined blue-and-white was produced at government kilns for use in the royal palace. At the other end of the economic scale, large quantities of coarse, grayish blue-and-white were produced for use by commoners. Between these two extremes there was a range of technical and artistic quality. The painted designs on the less technically accomplished blue-and-white are often more lively and appealing than the relatively tight decoration on pieces made for palace use.

Along with blue-and-white porcelain, 17th–19th-century Korean kilns also produced plain white porcelain, brown-glazed ware, underglaze iron-painted ware, underglaze copper-painted ware, and vast quantities of plain, gray-glazed kitchenware.

The large white porcelain storage jars of the middle Yi Dynasty have long been admired by Japanese and Korean collectors. These big jars are like pieces of abstract sculpture. Their powerful, swelling forms have great presence; their slightly irregular lines make subtle sculptural gestures. Lacking ornament and having only their off-white color and semi-mat surface, these jars must succeed or fail on the basis of form alone.

These large white porcelain storage jars were made in two parts, an upper half and a lower half, thrown separately like two huge bowls, then joined rim-to-rim at the belly of the jar. The process is usually apparent in the jar's profile, as it is here. The glaze on these jars is slightly bluish where it runs thick. It has an orange-pink blush where it pulls thin or where oxygen has reached the clay through minute openings in the glaze. These subtle nuances of color add to the aesthetic appeal of these jars, even though they were unintentional on the part of the potter. Modern Japanese and Korean connoisseurs have raised a utilitarian 17th century vessel to the status of a work of art, and the judgment seems eminently deserved.

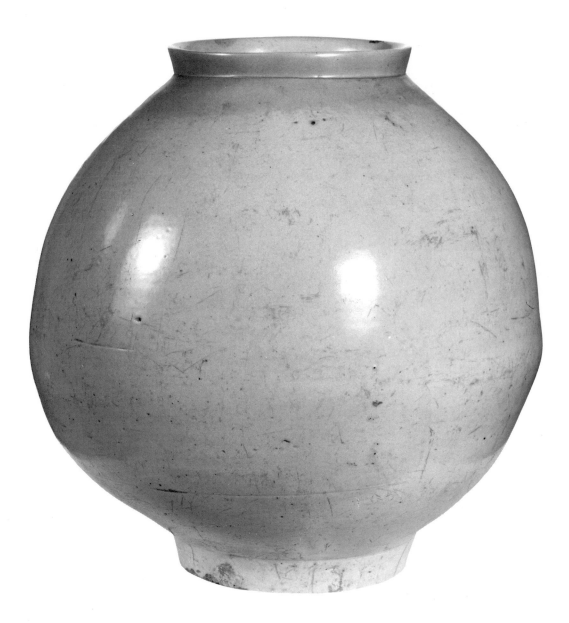

68. Storage Jar
White porcelain with iron-brown painted decoration
under a clear glaze
H. 12⅜", Diam 14⅝"
Yi Dynasty, 17th century
Gift of the Oriental Art Council   86.139

Iron-painted Dragon Jars are among the rarest and most spectacular Korean ceramics. Their powerful, swelling, dynamic shapes provide a perfect format for their eccentric, amusing, mysterious dragons. The ivory-white porcelain, blushing light bluish where the glaze runs thick, makes a perfect complement for the warm, brown-black, iron-oxide pigment, which burns reddish through the glaze in the places where it was painted most thickly.

These big storage jars were thrown in two halves, like two huge bowls, then luted together, rim-to-rim, at the belly of the jar. The technique tended to result in a diamond-shaped profile that is much more interesting than a mere globular shape. Japanese connoisseurs admire this profile and call it a *soroban-dama* (abacus bead) shape.

"Official" dragons on blue-and-white porcelain jars used for court ceremonies and Confucian rituals (see Cat. 69) were based closely on Ming Dynasty Chinese prototypes. These "official" dragons are more detailed, more fully realized, and more tangible than the "folk" dragon we see here. The "official" dragon is certainly awesome and majestic, but his very palpability makes him less mysterious, less the spirit creature he is supposed to be. The "folk" dragon on the present *Jar* is more imaginative,

more spiritlike. After all, no one has ever seen a dragon. I am tempted to think that a dragon would look more like the "folk" than the "official" version.

The present *Jar* was for utilitarian rather than ritual use. The dragon's function was to protect food inside the jar from evil spirits. The potters who made this *Jar* belonged to one of the lowest classes in Yi Dynasty society. They were extremely poor and were required to manufacture good, serviceable pots as quickly as possible just to eke out a living. Their pots were completely natural, direct, and spontaneous, free from any pretense or self-consciousness. The dragon is naive and whimsical, yet strangely moving, awesome, and spiritual. The clouds in which the dragon dwells, suggested by a few loose, wavy lines, are more compelling than the decorative ones on the "official" *Blue-and-White Jar*.

The irresistible freedom and naiveté of the iron-brown dragons has led some scholars to suggest that they were painted by children. The theory seems plausible. Because the potters were impoverished, every member of the family toiled in the workshop. Children were unable to perform the more physically demanding tasks of wedging clay, coiling, throwing, trimming, loading, or firing, but they were quite capable of painting the designs.

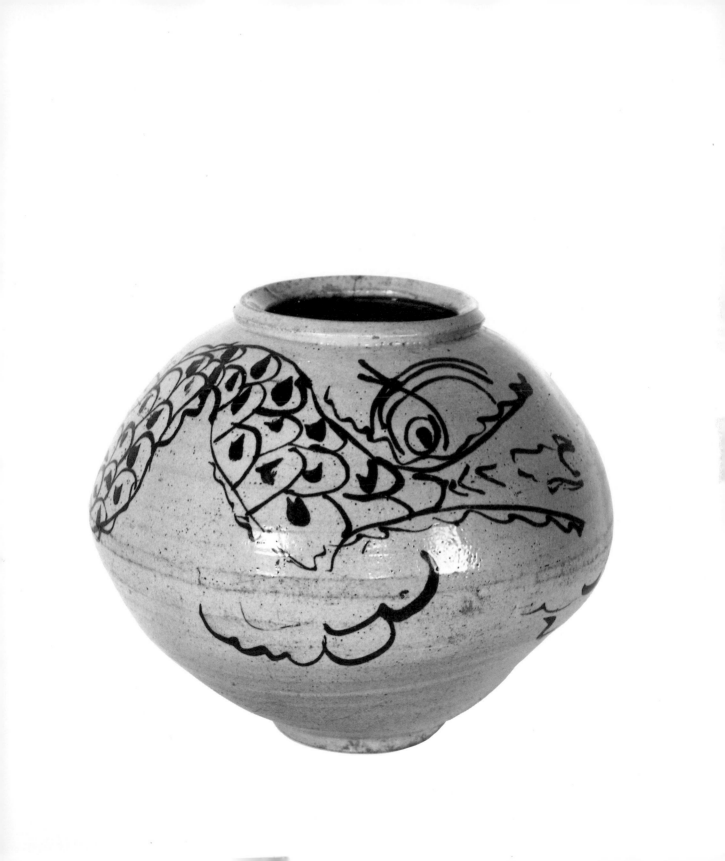

69. Blue-and-White Porcelain Dragon Jar

White porcelain with cobalt painted decoration
under a clear glaze
H. 20″, W. 13″
Yi Dynasty, 18th–early 19th century
Gift of Dr. & Mrs. Stanley Wallace   80.120.1

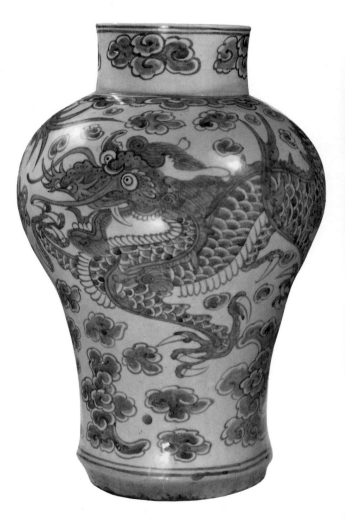

We have previously encountered the dragon in
his role as the Rain Dragon in a Shamanist rain-
supplication painting (see Cat. 33) and as an evil-
repelling Taoist spirit (see Cat. 68). Here we see the
dragon in a Confucian context, where he is a symbol
of Heaven, and of a virtuous king. The dragon was
an ubiquitous motif in the architectural decoration
and ritual paraphernalia of Korean royal palaces and
Confucian temples. Dragon jars like the present one
were made in pairs to stand before the altar of a
Confucian temple or in the throne room of a royal
palace. The dragon on this particular *Jar* has four
claws on each foot. In both China and Korea, the
image of a five-clawed dragon was usually reserved
for royal use, thus the present *Jar* was probably
intended for Confucian rituals.

The dragon is one of the *Sa Shin*, The Animals of
the Four Directions, ancient Chinese Taoist guardian
spirits mentioned in the *I Ching*: The Blue Dragon of
the East, The White Tiger of the West, The Red Bird
of the South (The Phoenix, see Cat. 72), and The
Black Warrior of the North (a Tortoise entwined by a
Snake). Each of these four spirit animals was based
on a constellation in its respective direction of the sky.

The dragon and the tiger (see Cat. 54) were paired
in Shamanist *munbae* (door talisman) paintings for Yi
Dynasty houses. A blue dragon and a white tiger
were pasted on the front door, the tiger to repel evil
spirits, the dragon to attract good fortune. In the
Taoist/Confucian cosmology of China, a dragon and
a tiger constituted a duality corresponding to *yang*
and *yin*. The dragon represented *yang*, the masculine,
positive principle in nature, characterized by activity,
light, heat, dryness, and height. The tiger represented
yin, the feminine, negative principle in nature,
characterized by passivity, darkness, cold, wetness,
and depth. *Yang* and *yin* combined and interacted in
all the myriad activities of the universe.

A dragon paired with a phoenix (see Cat. 72)
formed a similar *yang/yin* duality, with the phoenix
representing the feminine principle. The dragon and
the phoenix were symbols of the king and queen
respectively, or of the groom and bride at the
wedding ceremony.

70. Blue-and-White Porcelain Wine Bottle

White porcelain with cobalt painted decoration
under a clear glaze
H. 11¾", W. 6¼"
Yi Dynasty, 18th century
Gift of Stanley Herzman and Mr. & Mrs. Milton
Rosenthal   84.10

Korean screen paintings of *shipjangsaeng*, The Ten
Symbols of Long Life, were fairly common. It was
unusual, however, to depict all ten symbols on a
piece of porcelain. Due to the size and shape of the
vessel, only two or three of the symbols normally
appeared on a ceramic. The Ten Symbols were: sun,
clouds, water, rocks, deer, cranes, tortoises, pines,
bamboo, and Sacred Fungus. *Shipjangsaeng* is a Taoist
theme and came to Korea from China. Deer, cranes,
tortoises, pines, and Sacred Fungus, individually or
in various combinations, appeared frequently on
traditional Korean household objects, including
paintings, ceramics, lacquer, metalwork, wooden
utensils, bamboo ware, and embroidery.

Sun, clouds, water, and rocks appear to last
indefinitely, so they seemed appropriate as symbols
of long life. Deer were the companions and
messengers of the Taoist Immortals, auspicious,
sacred animals who always repaid favors. After a
mythical deer had lived a thousand years, its coat
turned gray; after fifteen hundred years, it turned
white; after two thousand years, its antlers turned
black and it became an Immortal, a Fairy Deer. When
depicted in pairs deer were symbols of conjugal bliss.

Cranes were also the companions and messengers
of the Taoist Immortals, as well as the mounts on
which Immortals flew to and from the Islands of the
Immortals (Chinese: P'eng Lai; Korean: Pong Nae) in
the Eastern Sea. Cranes were said to have magic
powers. By the age of six hundred years, cranes

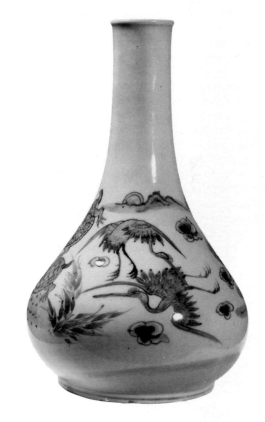

could subsist on water alone. At the age of two thousand, a crane turned black and became an Immortal. Cranes, like deer, were emblematic of a happy marriage. The female crane was very protective of her young and set a good example for human mothers.

The tortoise lived ten thousand years. The tortoise was the messenger of the Dragon King, who dwelt in the Dragon Palace at the bottom of the sea. Pine trees remain green throughout the year, resisting wind, rain, and snow. Bamboo stays green through the winter; it is hard and durable, bending before the wind but never breaking.

The Sacred Fungus (Chinese: *ling chih*; Korean: *pulloch'o*) was one of the most popular decorative motifs in the arts and crafts of Korea. The Sacred Fungus, or Fungus of Immortality, was a magic mushroom that grew in the Land of the Immortals. It bestowed eternal life on those who ate it. In ancient times, Chinese Taoist adepts searched the forests for Sacred Fungus. Many Taoists must have become intoxicated on hallucinogenic fungi; others perhaps died from eating poisonous mushrooms.

The Chinese emperor Ch'in Shih Huang Ti (246–210 B.C.) sent an expedition of three thousand men across the Yellow Sea to find the Islands of the Immortals and bring back some Sacred Fungus. The expedition never returned. Many Koreans believe it reached Korea and remained there, escaping Ch'in Shih Huang Ti's oppressive rule. The notion of Sacred Fungus was reinforced by an abundance of wild ginseng (*insam*) in the mountains of Korea. Korean ginseng was traditionally equated with Sacred Fungus. Ginseng root is still valued in China and Korea as a tonic thought to restore vigor and potency. Ginseng is a famous Korean product, but today much of the ginseng sold in Korea is grown in the north-central United States.

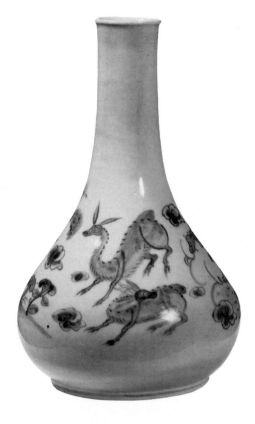

71. Porcelain Wine Bottle

White porcelain brushed with cobalt under
a clear glaze
H. 6″, W. 4¼″
Yi Dynasty, 18th century
Lent by Dr. John Lyden   TL1986.56.1

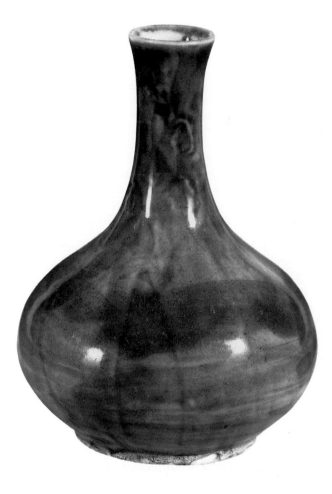

Blue-and-white ceramic ware, with cobalt-oxide painted designs covered with clear glaze, seems to have been invented in Iraq during the 9th century. The technique was imitated in Iran at the time on a very limited scale, since the cobalt mined in Iran seems to have been controlled by the regime in Iraq. For some reason, blue-and-white died out soon after its initial development. It was revived in the 11th–12th-century and spread throughout the Islamic world, where it has been widely used ever since.

The blue-and-white technique was brought to China from Iran in the 13th century as a result of the Mongol conquests. Iraq and Iran fell to the Mongols in 1219–1220. North China fell in 1222. The Mongols conquered the rest of China in 1279, putting them in control of the territory from Eastern Europe through Central Asia and China to Korea. Goods and ideas flowed across that vast area more freely than ever before.

There was a flourishing ceramic industry in north-central Iran during the 13th century. Blue-and-white was one of the standard decorating techniques used. The technique was brought from there to China in the 13th century. At first, the cobalt oxide was imported from Iran and referred to by the Chinese as "Mohammedan blue." But soon cobalt was being mined in China to meet the demand. Blue-and-white porcelain became the standard Chinese ceramic ware of the Ming Dynasty (1368–1644) and has remained popular in China ever since. The production of blue-and-white porcelain spread from China to Korea in the 15th century and from Korea to Japan in the early 17th century.

The present *Wine Bottle* is a rare type of Korean blue-and-white in which cobalt was brushed over the entire surface rather than on the design only. This type is called *ruri-yū* (lapis lazuli glaze) by Japanese connoisseurs. It was a Korean attempt to imitate Chinese blue monochrome porcelain of the K'ang-hsi reign (1662–1722), whose cobalt was either mixed into the glaze or blown onto the clay surface prior to glazing. The Korean blue monochrome looks smeared compared to the even blue of the Chinese pieces. Nevertheless, the uneven color and random patterns of the casual Korean brushwork give *ruri-yū* a sense of spontaneous vitality that the Chinese pieces lack.

72. Storage Jar
White porcelain with underglaze blue and red
painted decoration
H. 8⅞″, W. 6¾″
Yi Dynasty, 18th–early 19th century
1916 Museum Collection Fund   17.25

The phoenix was almost as ubiquitous in China
and Korea as were the dragon and the tiger. The Far
Eastern phoenix was not related to the Western one
except by name. In the West, it was a symbol of
resurrection (it rises anew from its own ashes).

The Far Eastern phoenix was a large, graceful, elegant bird said to appear in times of peace and prosperity and to dwell in lands with virtuous rulers. The
phoenix thus became a highly auspicious symbol. It
was said to nest in paulownia trees, so the paulownia
tree was also considered a good omen. The phoenix
was mythical, but the trees actually exist; paulownia
trees grow in the United States as well as Asia.

The Far Eastern phoenix had a rooster's head,
human eyes, a serpent's neck, a tortoise's back, bright
rainbow plumage, and a very long tail. The five colors
of its feathers represented the five virtues: upright-
ness, honesty, fidelity, justice, and benevolence.
Phoenixes were the messengers and mounts of Hsi
Wang-mu (Korean: So Wang-mo) and her retinue of
Taoist fairies (see Cat. 25).

In Korea, use of the phoenix motif was originally
restricted to royalty and high officials. During the
second half of the Yi Dynasty, the restriction was no
longer enforced. The present *Storage Jar* depicts a
phoenix flying among small clouds. Underglaze
copper red was used to supplement the cobalt blue.
Copper oxide was mixed with water and painted on
the vessel prior to glazing, just like cobalt blue or
iron brown. The copper-red color turned to muddy
gray if the firing was not controlled carefully; sometimes it simply blurred away under the glaze. When
all went well, however, the copper yielded a handsome color ranging from peach blossom pink
through deep red to blackish green. On the present
Jar, copper red was used effectively for the bird's
comb and for the dark accents on the clouds.

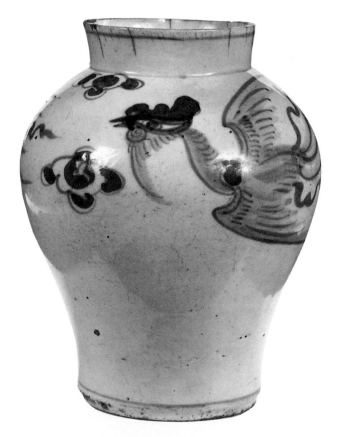

73. Porcelain Water Dropper in the Shape of a Peach

White porcelain with underglaze iron, cobalt, and
copper decoration
H. 4¼", W. 3½"
Yi Dynasty, 18th–early 19th century
Lent by Robert Anderson   TL1984.106.1

This jewellike porcelain utensil for a scholar's desk
is shaped like a peach, life-size, with a twig coiled
below as a footring. The twig extends up the front as
a small spout; a leaf from the twig is attached to each
side. Water droppers were made of either bronze or
porcelain, often in fanciful forms such as animals,
birds, or fish. A water dropper was essential in
preparing the ink used for writing and painting. An
ink cake made of pine soot carbon and animal-glue
binder was ground on the surface of a slate ink stone
having a shallow depression at one end to hold some
water, until the desired ink/water mixture was
obtained. A water dropper was used to replenish
water in the ink stone as it was used up.

The peach represented here is, of course, not an
ordinary peach. It is The Peach of Immortality, also
called The Fairy Peach, an ancient Taoist symbol of
longevity used frequently as an auspicious motif in
Korean arts and crafts (see Cat. 25).

As depicted in Chinese and Korean art, The Peach
of Immortality conveyed certain Taoist sexual symbolism related to the concept of immortality. According
to Taoist notions, a man achieved a kind of immortality by fathering many sons, who in turn sired many
grandsons. Potency was therefore seen as a means of
immortality. So it was that representations of The
Peach of Immortality tended to exaggerate its form so
that the cleft suggested a vulva and the pink tip suggested a nipple. Some artists and craftsmen intentionally turned this exaggeration into humorous parody.

The present *Porcelain Water Dropper* is something of
a technical tour de force in having all three underglaze
colors: cobalt blue (on the leaves), iron brown (on
the stem) and copper red (on the tip of the peach.)

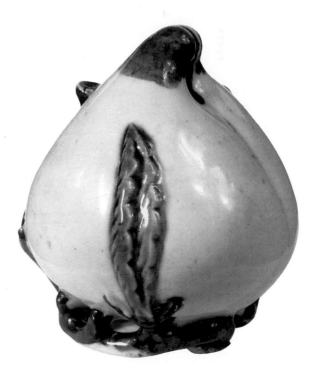

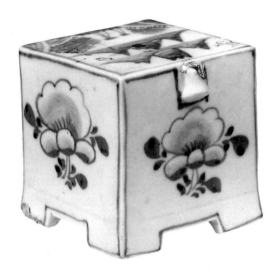

74. Blue-and-White Porcelain Water Dropper

White porcelain with cobalt painted decoration
under a clear glaze
H. 2¾″, W. 2½″
Yi Dynasty, early 19th century
Gift of Dr. John Lyden   79.273.2

Among the many fanciful shapes in which Korean water droppers were made (see Cat. 73), a square shape was fairly common. The standard square water dropper was low, however, usually about one-third the height of the present example. The foot at each corner, and the outline around each panel, give this little vessel great dignity. Its sides, top, and bottom were formed from flat slabs of clay. There is a tiny hole in the middle of the top to admit air, and a small spout high up on one side. The spout is shaped like a single joint of bamboo.

Each of the four sides has a bold, abbreviated rendition of a peony in full bloom. Peonies have been a favorite Korean motif since early times. On a *Wedding Screen* (see Cat. 53), peonies symbolized the beauty and sexuality of the bride. On this *Water Dropper*, the peonies symbolize abundance, wealth, happiness, and nobility of spirit.

The abbreviated landscape on top of the *Water Dropper* was one of the standard designs used by the official government kilns at Punwon-ni. It depicts the scenery of the area near the kilns: boats sailing on the Han River, with granite hills in the background.

75. Garden Seat

White porcelain with cobalt and iron decoration
under a clear glaze
H. 18½", W. 9¾"
Yi Dynasty, early 19th century
Gift of Mr. & Mrs. Herbert Greenberg   86.260.3

From a tiny porcelain *Water Dropper* for a gentleman
scholar's desk (see Cat. 74), we move to a large
porcelain *Seat* for a gentleman scholar's garden. Its
carved, openwork decoration depicts grapevines,
grape leaves, and clusters of grapes. The surface of
the grapes was painted with underglaze iron-brown
wash. Stylized "precious things" (coins, jewels,
treasure bags, and the like), a traditional Chinese
motif, were drawn in underglaze cobalt blue on the
border below the grapes.

Grapes were a popular subject in the paintings
(see Cat. 40) and decorative arts of Yi Dynasty Korea.
Ink-monochrome paintings of grapes first became
fashionable in China during the Southern Sung
(1127–1279) Dynasty. The 13th-century Chinese grape-
painting tradition was very influential in Korea and
Japan, as well as on subsequent generations of
Chinese artists. In Korea, court painters, scholar
painters, and folk painters all tried their hands at
grape painting.

The grape was not native to China, Korea, or
Japan. Its cultivation was introduced into China from
South Asia in 126 B.C.. Unlike most of the other
animal and plant motifs in Korean art, grapes had no
auspicious or protective symbolism.

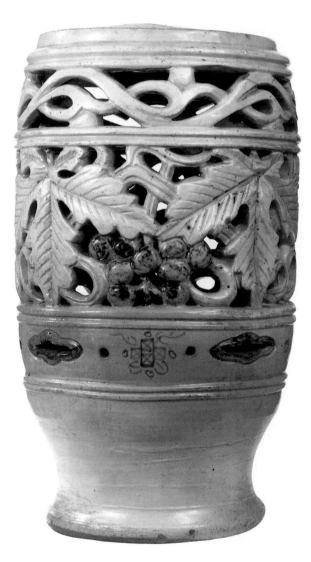

76. Blue-and-White Porcelain Jar

White porcelain with cobalt painted decoration
under a clear glaze
H. 5¾", W. 7¼"
Yi Dynasty, mid-19th century
Purchase   76.119

Blue-and-white porcelain was first produced in Korea during the reign of King Sejo (1455–1468). The cobalt was imported from China. A cobalt deposit discovered near the south coast of Korea in 1464 failed to yield sufficient mineral of usable quality, so cobalt continued to be imported from China for the duration of the Yi Dynasty. This made it an expensive commodity, especially during the 15th through the 17th century. A royal decree in 1461 restricted blue-and-white porcelain to use by the court and aristocracy.

The Japanese invasions of 1592 and 1597 disrupted ceramic production throughout Korea; many of the kilns were destroyed or abandoned. As late as 1618, official records indicate there were insufficient funds to import cobalt from China. In 1636 the Manchus invaded Korea in retaliation for Korea's stubborn loyalty to the Ming Dynasty (1368–1644). Korea was forced to become a vassal state of the Ch'ing Dynasty (1644–1912) established by the Manchus in China. Korean relations with China did not normalize again until about 1700. Korean porcelain production expanded rapidly during the 18th century.

The official Punwon porcelain kilns were a subsidiary of the Sa'ong-won, the government department responsible for preparing and serving food at the royal court. The Punwon kilns were established at Kumsa-ri in 1718 and moved to Punwon-ni in 1752. Punwon-ni is located near the confluence of the Han and the Pukhan rivers, some twelve miles east of Seoul. Boats sailing down the Han River with firewood for Seoul were required to pay a tax at Punwon-ni; this revenue helped support the government kilns.

The majority of the blue-and-white porcelain produced in Korea during the second half of the 18th and the 19th century came from the Punwon kilns. Their capacity was such that large quantities of ordinary blue-and-white porcelain for use by commoners were manufactured there each year after the government quotas of porcelain for royal and official use had been met. About two-thirds of the production at the Punwon kilns consisted of blue-and-white porcelain.

The present *Jar* is typical of official pieces made at the Punwon kilns in the 19th century. The color of the blue is quite good because by that time well-refined cobalt was being imported from China in quantity. The glaze is clear and glossy; the porcelain clay is pure white. However, by the middle of the 19th century, a certain slickness, stiffness, and artistic sterility had set in. The decline is especially evident in official pieces such as this one. Vessel shapes became somewhat mechanical, and the painted designs became rather stereotyped. The end came in 1883 when the Yi government concluded that the Punwon kilns were too expensive to maintain and cut off their state support. The kilns survived as a private enterprise, but porcelain technicians brought from Arita and Kutani in Japan introduced the ugly blend of Japanese and Victorian styles prevalent in Japanese ceramics at the time.

On the base of the present *Jar* is a two-character underglaze blue inscription: Un-hyon (Cloud Hill). The Un-hyon Palace in Seoul was the private residence of Prince Yi Ha-ung, better known by his title, Taewongun (Prince Regent). His son, King Kojong, the twenty-sixth monarch of the Yi Dynasty, was born in the Un-hyon Palace.

The prince regent directed sweeping reforms of government administration and national finances in 1863 that were designed to strengthen royal authority. Yi Ha-ung was adamantly opposed to foreign commercial interests that were infiltrating Korea at the time. In 1866 he ordered a severe persecution of Korean Catholics. France reacted by sending a fleet up the Han River to attack Seoul.

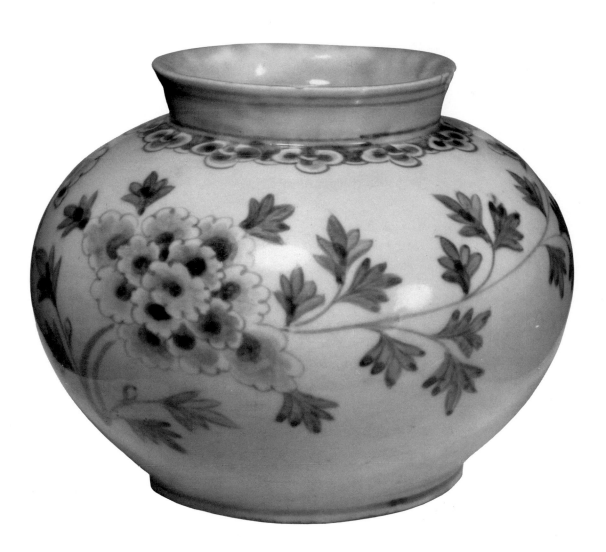

77. Honey Jar
Gray stoneware with a caramel-brown glaze
H. 8¼", W. 7¾"
Yi Dynasty, 19th century
Gift of Robert Anderson   84.244.5 a&b

This plebian brown-glazed *Jar* stands at the opposite pole in the 19th-century Korean ceramic hierarchy from the official *Blue-and-White Porcelain Jar* (see Cat. 76). Still, the brown *Jar* is a more aesthetically satisfying pot than the blue-and-white one. It is honest and unself-conscious. Its form is powerful and well proportioned. Its twelve facets, which were cut with a bamboo potter's knife, add a sculptural quality to its otherwise globular shape. The famous 20th-century Japanese potter Hamada Shōji (1894–1977) admired the cut facets on Korean ceramics and imitated them in his own work. Through Hamada, Korean-style faceting entered the work of several contemporary potters in the West.

In addition to their decorative effect, Korean facets had a utilitarian function. They made it easier to bind the jar with straw rope to hold the lid on tight and preserve the honey or other foodstuffs inside. Extra-tight packing is still called "honey packing" in Korea today. Faceting was also used on Korean wine bottles, but purely for visual effect. The walls of the vessel were thrown extra thick to allow the facets to be cut.

Black-glazed ceramic wares were first made in Korea in the early 12th century. Examples of Koryo Dynasty and early Yi Dynasty black-glazed ware are extremely scarce today. It has a rather thick glaze with very little luster. By the 18th century, Korean black glazes had become glossier and varied in color from reddish brown through olive brown to dark brown and black. The color derives from iron oxide and/or manganese oxide in the glaze, fired in an oxidizing kiln atmosphere (one in which an abundance of oxygen is available inside the kiln during firing).

During the 18th and 19th centuries, most of the black-glazed pottery made in Korea was utilitarian. It was produced by families of potters in small, remote pottery villages. When the local supply of clay or wood was exhausted, the village moved to another location. The principal product of these kilns was *onggi* (food-storage jars). *Onggi* came in various sizes, including extremely large ones; they were formerly used by every Korean family to preserve *kimchi* (pickled cabbage laced with hot chili pepper) and other foods during the winter months when fresh produce was not available. Today, refrigerators and industrial products like plastic and aluminum are rapidly replacing the once ubiquitous brown-glazed *onggi* jars.

Many of the *onggi* potters were Roman Catholics. Their low social status permitted them to move about more freely than other Yi Dynasty Koreans. Their isolation and anonymity made it possible for most of them to survive the severe government persecutions of Korean Catholics, which began in 1795 and continued until 1866. The last one was directed by Prince Regent Yi Ha-ung (see Cat. 76). Some of the *onggi* potters died as martyrs during the persecutions.

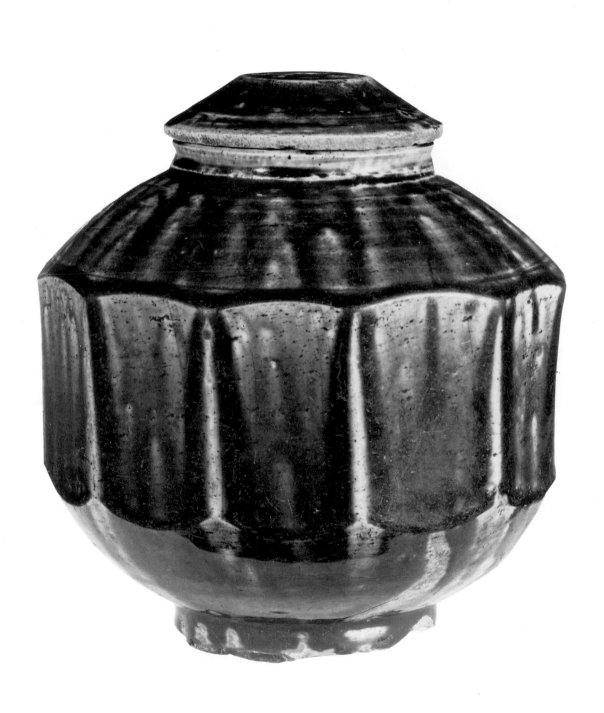

78. Three-level Chest *(Samch'ung Chang)*

Red and black lacquer on wood; zelkova burl panels;
brass fittings
H. 63⅛", W. 44¾"
Yi Dynasty, early to middle 19th century
George C. Brackett Fund　34.530

This magnificent *Chest* was made for the women's
quarters in the home of a member of the royal family.
The elaborate style, with a multiplicity of panels and
moldings, and the almost excessive exuberance of the
ornamental hardware, indicate that it was intended
for the women's quarters *(anch'ae)*. The strict tenets
of Confucianism required upper-class Yi Dynasty men
and women to maintain separate living quarters
within the same house. They ate separately and slept
separately, although husbands could visit their wives
during the night.

Chests decorated with red and black lacquer were
normally restricted to royal use. The edge of the
overhanging top of the present *Chest* is in red
lacquer. The main frame and most of the moldings
are in black lacquer, as are the five low panels across
the bottom. The frames of the upper and middle
pairs of doors are in red lacquer; so are the moldings
framing the openings for the lower two pairs of
doors, as well as the legs and stretcher.

The door panels, the fronts of the four small drawers
across the top, and the other main front panels are
zelkova burl wood with an oil finish. The complex,
swirling grain of zelkova burl suggested coiled
dragons to Koreans, so they called it "dragon wood"
(yong-mok). The side panels and back panels of this
Chest are made of pine and are undecorated. Korean
chests were always placed against a wall of the room,
so little attention was paid to the sides and back.

Unlike Japanese chests *(tansu)*, which were kept in
a separate fire-resistant storehouse *(kura)* behind the
garden, Korean chests were displayed prominently
in the main rooms of the house. Chests in the
women's quarters had elaborate designs, showy
woods, and ornamental fittings. Chests in the men's
quarters were more subdued in both style and
materials. A *chang,* the type of chest we see here, had
one or more levels within a single frame. Tall, two- or
three-level *chang* for clothing storage were the most
prevalent; this example is a three-level *(samch'ung)*

chang. As with nearly all Korean chests, each level
here consists of a single, boxlike compartment without any shelves, divisions, or drawers inside. The
interiors of most Korean chests were originally
papered. Certain *chang,* lower in height and quite
subdued in style, were used for storing books rather
than clothing. In either case, the folded clothing or
soft-cover, Chinese-style books were simply stacked
inside the empty compartment on each level of the
chest. *Chang* were used to store frequently needed
items, whereas *nong* (see Cat. 79) were meant
primarily for long-term storage of seasonal clothing.

Nearly all Korean chests had legs or removable
stands that supported them well above the floor.
The floors in the main rooms of Korean houses were
heated during the winter. The heating system, *ondol,*
was unique to Korea and completely different from
types of heating used in China and Japan. *Ondol*
worked on the same principal as modern radiant
(panel) heating, yet it was invented about a thousand
years ago. Korea is very cold in winter, especially the
mountainous northern part of the peninsula, where
Kaesong (Songdo), the capital of the Koryo Dynasty
(918–1392) was located. The *ondol* heating system was
developed in the capital and quickly spread throughout Korea. It had become standard in upper-class
Korean houses by the year 1200.

A stone and clay firebox was built into one outside
wall of the house at ground level, often adjacent to
the kitchen; the same firebox sometimes served as a
stove to heat the big iron cooking kettles. The space
between the stone-and-clay floors of the sitting and
sleeping rooms and the surface of the ground below
served as the flue for the firebox, conducting smoke
and heat under the rooms and heating their floors.
The earth surface beneath the house was sloped
upward slightly from the firebox to the chimney on
the other side of the house to provide a better draft
for the fire. Polished, oiled paper was glued to the
clay flooring, creating a smooth, shiny, tough floor

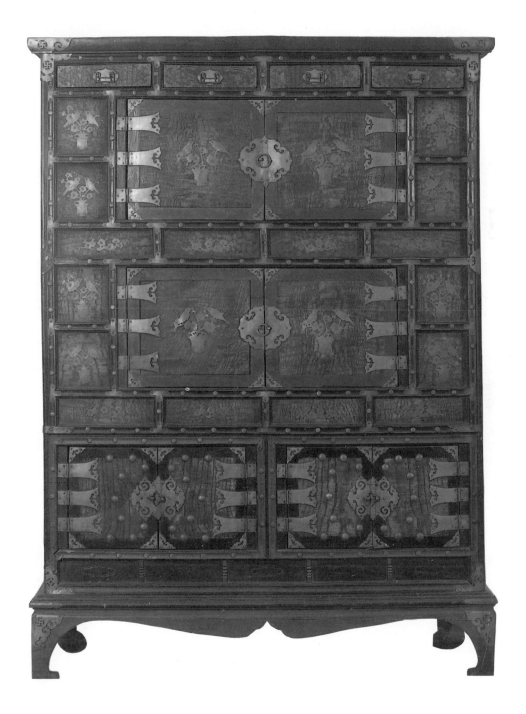

surface. *Ondol* floors remained warm and dry throughout the winter, unlike the cold, damp floors of traditional Chinese houses.

The brass fittings on the present *Chest* are unusually elaborate. The hinges, latch plates, drawer pulls, and corner fittings all have complex, ornamental open-

work. In addition, purely decorative brass plaques depicting potted plants and songbirds were applied to each main panel on the front. This extraordinarily uncommon feature, along with the red and black lacquer on the frame and moldings, indicates the *Chest* was made for royal use.

79. Two-unit Stacked Chest *(Ich'ung Nong)*

Lacquer inlaid with tortoise shell, on wood; brass fittings
H. 49⅜", W. 29½"
Yi Dynasty, 19th century
Gift of Dr. & Mrs. John Lyden   83.168.1 a&b

A *nong* is a Korean clothing chest consisting of two or more separate units (usually two) stacked on top of one another, an entirely different arrangement from a *chang*, which has one or more levels of compartments within a single frame (see Cat. 78). A *chang* was intended for frequently needed clothing, or sometimes books; a *nong* was meant for long-term storage of such items as seasonal clothing. The two units of a *nong* were nearly always identical and sometimes interchangeable. In the present example, the stand (legs and stretcher) is permanently affixed to the lower unit. Other examples have removable stands (see Cat. 80). A *nong* never had an overhanging top; it was composed of two simple, rectangular boxes. Each unit had a central pair of double doors. As with nearly all Korean chests, there were no shelves or drawers inside.

The present *Chest* must have been made for a member of the *yangban* class (the land-owning aristocracy). Colored lacquer, especially with inlay, was expensive; it was seldom used on anything larger than small boxes. If this *Chest* had been made for the royal palace, the dragons on its doors would have had five claws on each foot rather than four. The dragons are composed of tortoise-shell and brass-wire inlay on reddish-brown lacquer. Iron oxide was added to natural lacquer to produce this color.

The dragons on this *Chest* were meant to be viewed in a Confucian (see Cat. 69) rather than a Shamanist context (see Cat. 33). In Confucianism, the dragon was a symbol of Heaven and of a righteous king. The

eight Chinese characters inlaid along the stretcher of this *Chest* represent The Eight Virtues *(P'al Dok)* of Confucianism (see Cat. 52). From right to left: Filial Piety, Brotherly Love, Loyalty, Sincerity, Benevolence, Duty, Honor, and Humility.

The inlaid design on the upper center of each unit represents The Eight Trigrams, an ancient set of Taoist symbols suggesting patterns of change. The Eight Trigrams formed the basis for the *I Ching (Book of Changes)*, the most venerated and inscrutable of the Chinese classics. Taoism taught that only change itself was unchanging. The Eight Trigrams were employed in divination and geomancy. They were said to embody the metaphysical principles of the universe.

The Eight Trigrams consist of eight different combinations of three horizontal lines. Each line is either continuous or broken in the middle. The continuous lines are male *(yang)*; the broken ones are female *(yin)*. Each of the eight combinations is associated with certain specific phenomena, as follows: Three solid lines suggest Heaven, sky, father, strength, horse, south. One broken line above two solid lines suggests lake, marsh, mist, pleasure, satisfaction, goat, southeast. One broken line between two solid lines suggests fire, light, sun, brightness, elegance, pheasant, east. Two broken lines above a single solid line suggests thunder, moving, exciting, dragon, northeast. Two solid lines above one broken line suggests wind, wood, flexible, penetration, rooster, southwest. One solid line between two broken lines suggests water, moon, peril, difficulty, pig, west.

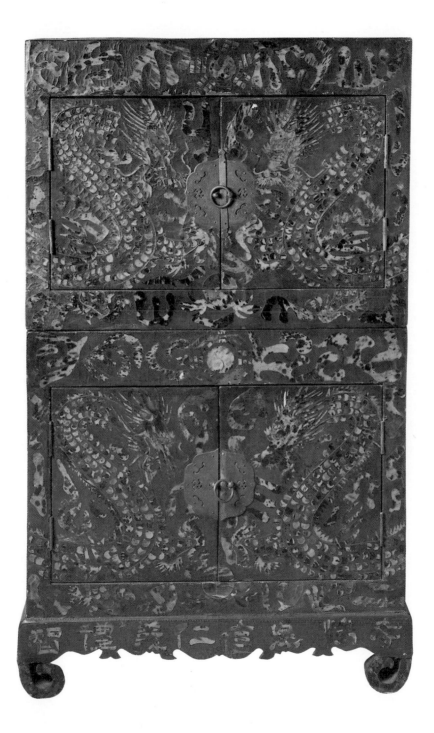

One solid line above two broken lines suggests mountain, resting, dog, northwest. Three broken lines suggests earth, mother, submission, ox, north.

The Eight Trigrams were said to have been invented by the legendary Chinese Emperor Fu Hsi in 2852 B.C. He based them on the markings on tortoise shells that were used for divination. Wen Wang (1231–1135 B.C.), the founder of the Chou Dynasty, wrote an explanation of The Eight Trigrams while he was in prison. Further interpretations written by his son Chou Kung were combined with Wen Wang's explanation to form the *I Ching*.

80. Two-unit Stacked Chest *(Ich'ung Nong)*

Split-bamboo basketry on wood; brass fittings
H. 48″, W. 33½″
Yi Dynasty, 19th century
Gift of Robert Anderson   84.244.3 a-c

The sides, top, and front panels of this *Chest* are covered with woven split-bamboo basketry. This is a highly unusual feature. Bamboo slats glued to the front surface of a chest in parallel rows were more common, but few examples have survived, since the bamboo tended to crack, warp, and detach due to changes in temperature and humidity.

Unlike the preceding *Nong* (see Cat. 79), this one has a detachable stand. However, the two units are still not interchangeable, as they are on some *nong;* the upper unit here has a row of four small drawers across the top.

The latch plates and hinges on this *Chest* are in the form of butterflies. They are made of yellow brass, the most common material for fittings on Korean furniture. Iron fittings were also used frequently (see Cat. 82). White brass fittings (brass having a high tin and nickel content) were sometimes used, especially on late pieces (those from the end of the Yi Dynasty and the beginning of the Japanese annexation).

Butterflies were often depicted on Korean *hwacho* (Birds and Flowers) screens, either painted or embroidered (see Cat. 49). Like the deer, geese, ducks, cranes, fish, and other creatures on *hwacho* screens, the butterflies were shown in pairs. The pairs of animals and birds were auspicious symbols of a happy marriage.

Butterflies were often represented in simplifed silhouette as brass fittings on Yi Dynasty furniture, where they had another auspicious meaning: longevity. The Chinese word for "butterfly" (tieh) was pronounced the same as a word that meant "seventy to eighty years of age" (the ideographs for the two words were, of course, altogether different). Homophonic symbolism like this was not unusual in China. Ironically, in China the butterfly symbolized long life, exactly the opposite of its meaning in the West, where it referred to the brevity of life.

Bats seldom appeared in paintings, but they were frequent motifs in the decorative arts of China and Korea. The conventionalized silhouettes of bats appear frequently as brass fittings on Korean furniture, especially as drawer pulls or drawer-pull plates. One also encounters the bat motif on blue-and-white porcelain, and as mother-of-pearl inlay on black or red lacquer, or as embroidery. Like the butterfly, the bat owes its symbolic meaning to a homophone in Chinese: the ideograph for "bat" was pronounced *fu,* the same pronunciation as another ideograph meaning "good fortune."

In Korea, swallows were also considered auspicious. Like magpies, swallows preferred to live in the midst of human habitation. They built their mud nests under the eaves of houses and darted about looking for scraps of food. Swallows were abundant in Korea; they came to be regarded as omens of success and prosperity. Swallows were seldom depicted in Korean paintings, but long, V-shaped hinges on Korean furniture suggested their forked tails and conveyed the auspicious meaning (see Cat. 78 for this type of hinge.)

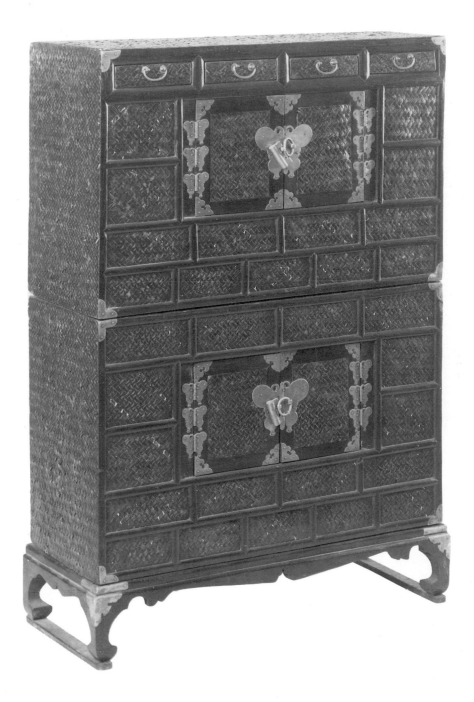

81. Chest *(Chang)*

Red lacquer inlaid with mother-of-pearl, on wood;
brass fittings
H. 32⅝″, W. 30⅜″
Yi Dynasty, late 18th–early 19th century
Lent by Mr. & Mrs. David Drabkin   TL1984.83 a&b

This type of low, single-level chest was called a
morijang (literally, "headside chest"). It was placed
close to the mat where a woman sat during the day
or slept during the night. A *morijang* was intended
for storing clothing needed frequently, such as
nightclothes. Most Korean furniture was built low, to
be accessible to a person seated on a cushion on the
floor. Notable exceptions were two- and three-level
clothing chests (see Cat. 78) and two-unit stacked
chests (see Cat. 79, 80).

No chairs were used in Korea until modern times.
(Royal thrones and high, narrow chairs for spirit
tablets used in ancestor worship were exceptions.)
Koreans sat on mats or cushions on the floor. In spite
of 20-century Western influence, they still prefer to
do so at least part of the time. This is somewhat
surprising, considering the pervasiveness of Chinese
influence on Korea, because chairs have been in
general use in China since the 8th century. Korea's
unique *ondol* heating system was no doubt part of
the reason. The *ondol* floor and the space just above
it were the warmest, coziest part of a Korean house
during the winter (see Cat. 78). The other reason was
simply preference. Though profoundly influenced by
Chinese culture, the Japanese also lived without
chairs until modern times.

The present *Chest* was probably built for the royal
family or a high-ranking member of the scholar-
official class. Colored lacquer and mother-of-pearl
inlay were very expensive. They were normally used
for small boxes. The red color of the lacquer on this
Chest resulted from cinnabar (mercuric sulfide)
mixed with the natural lacquer. Lacquer was made
from the juice of the Oriental sumac tree, which is a
different species from the American sumac, but the
sap of both is poisonous. Chinese, Korean, and
Japanese lacquer craftsmen gradually built up an
immunity to the toxin, which causes severe skin
irritation. Lacquer is messy stuff, difficult to work
with. It will not dry in a dry atmosphere, so a special

wet-room with ultra-high humidity was required.
Several coats of lacquer were normally applied, and
each coat had to be polished before the next one was
brushed on.

Mother-of-pearl inlay on lacquer has been a Korean
speciality for centuries and remains a popular luxury
item in Korea today. Several mother-of-pearl inlaid
lacquer boxes from the Koryo Dynasty have survived;
the earliest ones date from the 12th century. The
technique was brought to Korea from China. Shell-
inlaid lacquer flourished in China during the T'ang
Dynasty (618–907) and has been produced there ever
since. The technique appeared in China at almost
the beginning of lacquer working; examples from the
Shang Dynasty (ca. 1500–1027 B.C.) have recently
been excavated.

The mother-of-pearl inlay on the present *Chest* is
quite pictorial. Instead of the more usual formal
designs consisting of floral scrolls (see Cat. 86) or
geometric patterns, we find a series of fully realized
landscape vistas. These landscapes successfully
capture the soft, fluid, spacious feeling of ink-wash
paintings, yet they employ the hard, brittle medium
of pearl shell. Like the paintings on which they were
based, the landscapes on the *Chest* depict idealized
Chinese scholar sages enjoying imaginary lakeside
scenery of the sort to which a scholar official might
hope to retire some day. The upper front panel of the
Chest is inlaid with grapevines and squirrels, which
were also an ink-painting subject (see Cat. 40). The
inlay on top of the *Chest* depicts flowering plants and
a garden rock.

Much of the mother-of-pearl used for lacquer
inlay in China, Korea, and Japan actually came from
Okinawa. Pearl shell processed for such use was one
of the standard exports of the Ryūkyū Islands
(Chinese: Liu-ch'iu; Okinawa, the largest island of
the Ryūkyū chain, has given its name to the entire
archipelago). For five hundred years (1372–1879), the
Ryūkyūs were a nominally autonomous maritime

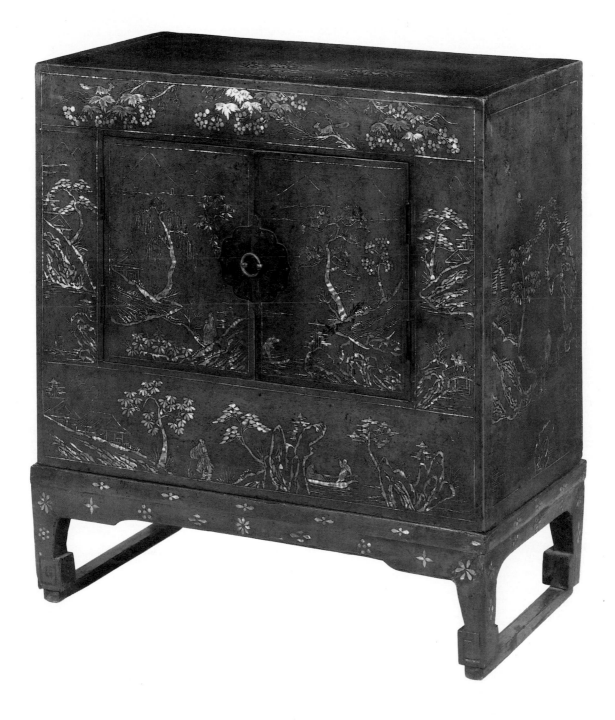

kingdom. Their location between the Pacific Ocean and the East China Sea was ideal for three-way trade with China, Korea, and Japan. They also provided a maritime link to the Philippines and Indonesia in the south. Okinawan merchant ships sailed as far as Southeast Asia and even to the Persian Gulf, where they made contact with Arab and Portuguese traders, among many others.

82. Chest *(Bandaji)*

Zelkova wood front, top, and sides; pine back; iron fittings
H. 25¾", W. 30"
Yi Dynasty, 19th century
Source unknown   X652.3

Chests with elaborate brass fittings and multipaneled fronts (see Cat. 78) and chests coated with red or black lacquer inlaid with mother-of-pearl (see Cat. 81) were meant for the women's quarters *(anch'ae)* of upper-class Yi Dynasty houses. Their decorative exuberance conveys a feeling of elegant gaiety. Furniture for the men's quarters *(sarang-ch'ae)* was much more sober in style, with simpler designs, more subdued woods, less lacquer, and relatively plain fittings, for which black-patinated iron often was used instead of brass. Chests for the men's quarters had quiet dignity, monumental strength, and surprisingly modern-looking lines. Here, the Korean furniture craftsman was at his best. His feeling for wood was unsurpassed. He let the material speak for itself in the most eloquent way. He selected, sawed, and planed the planks to take advantage of patterns in the grain, almost as if he were painting abstract pictures with wood. The iron fittings never concealed nor competed with the wood; they enhanced it with their contrasting color and texture.

Although he sometimes used natural (clear) lacquer, the Korean furniture craftsman usually gave his wood a rubbed oil finish. The oil brought out the richness of the color and grain and created a smooth, semimat surface. Perilla oil *(tul kirum)* was normally used. Perilla is a genus of Asiatic mint; the oil was derived from its nutlets. Several coats of oil were rubbed into the surface of the wood with a soft cloth.

The *bandaji* was the most common type of Korean chest. Almost every Yi Dynasty household owned one. Most *bandaji* were intended for storing clothing; a few were meant for books. The panel along the upper two-fifths of the front of a *bandaji* was hinged along the bottom and kept closed by a latch at top center. *Bandaji* means "half closing." Like other types of Korean chests, *bandaji* normally had no shelves, drawers, or dividers inside. Korean antique dealers and American collectors called *bandaji* "blanket chests," but in fact they were never used to contain blankets. The misnomer probably derives from the fact that sleeping mats were sometimes folded and stacked on top of a *bandaji* during the day when they were not in use.

Zelkova is the most beautiful of the many handsome woods used to make Korean chests. Zelkova is sometimes mistakenly called "elm"; it is similar in appearance and belongs to the same family, Ulmaceae. Zelkova, however, has more pronounced grain and more of an orange color than elm. Zelkova was prized for chests in Japan as well as Korea; Japanese call it *keyaki*, Koreans, *kwemok*.

Zelkova was expensive and was normally used only for the front panels of a chest; common woods such as pine were used for the top and especially for the sides and back. The present *Chest* was certainly a luxury item; thick planks of zelkova were used for the top and sides as well as the front. Only the back is made of pine. Korean chests were always placed against a wall, so the back was never seen. Korean furniture craftsmen often let the joinery show, as in the dovetail joints between the lower front panel and the sides here. This kind of unself-conscious directness is characteristic of Korean art in general.

Two of the motifs in the openwork decoration of

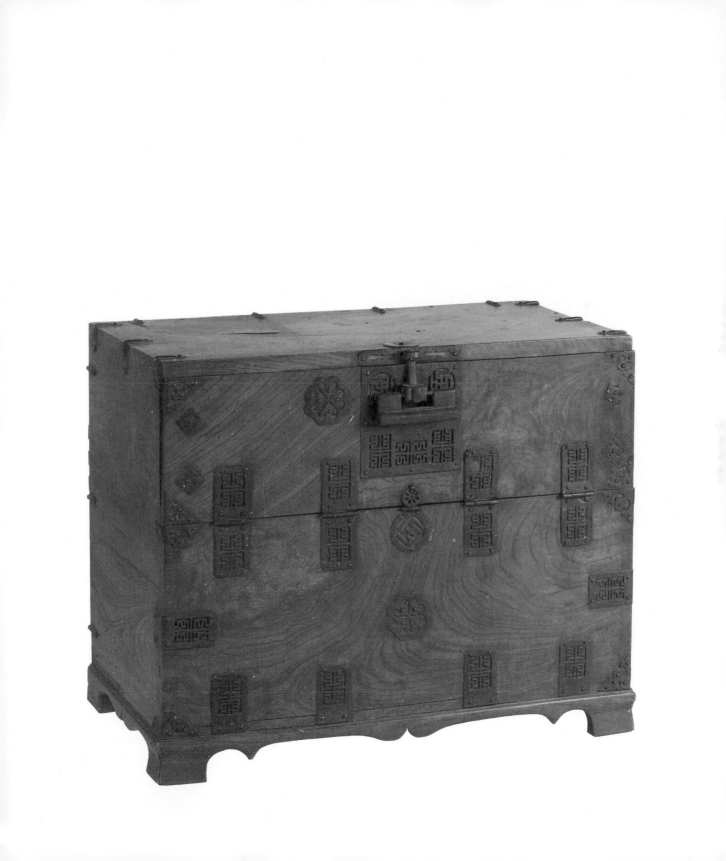

the hardware on this *Chest* appeared frequently on the fittings of Korean chests, in brass as well as in iron. The first was the key fret, or meander pattern. Key-fret designs were ubiquitous in the traditional decorative arts and architecture of China and Korea. The motif derived from an ancient Chinese design called the "thunder pattern," which was a repeat pattern of small, squared spirals. In the decoration on Bronze Age Chinese ritual vessels, the thunder pattern usually formed a background for depictions of spirit animals. The thunder pattern was based on archaic pictographs representing clouds and thunder. Its depiction on ancient ritual vessels expressed a desire to propitiate the spirits of nature, especially those involved with rain, which was so essential to early agriculture. The subsequent Taoist (and Korean Shamanist) Dragon-in-Clouds motif (see Cat. 33) evolved from ancient representations of spirit animals surrounded by thunder patterns, and they served the same purpose.

The second inanimate symbol that was especially popular for openwork decoration on the iron and brass fittings of Korean chests was the swastika. In Asia, the swastika was originally a Buddhist symbol. It represented the Cosmic Buddha at the center of the universe, with the universe revolving around him and constantly returning to the center, hence the four radiating spokes bent at right angles. In Korea, the swastika gradually became a secular symbol of harmony and happiness.

83. Rice Chest *(Ssal tuiju)*
Pine; iron fittings
H. 22″, W. 23⅝″
Yi Dynasty, 19th century
Lent by Dr. John Lyden   TL1986.40.3 a&b

The preceding chests (see Cat. 78–82) were intended to be used in the main rooms of upper-class Yi Dynasty homes. Such rooms had heated *ondol* floors. Rice chests, on the other hand, were meant to stand on the wood-floored veranda adjoining the kitchen. The veranda floor was on the same level as the *ondol* floors but was not heated. The kitchen floor was at ground level and made of packed earth.

Since they were kitchen furniture, rice chests were made of inexpensive wood, usually pine, and had a minimum of fittings, just an iron latch and latch plate. Some rice chests have subtle refinements, such as the bands of parallel grooves articulating the front panel and legs on the present example. The horizontal elements of rice chest frames extend outward at the upper corners, conveying an impression of architectural strength and solidity, like overhanging beams in a post-and-lintel building.

Access to the interior of a rice chest is through the front three-fifths of the top. The cover lifts forward and off when the latch is free. The latch is a hinged bar that drops through the front of the lid to engage a pair of loops on the upper front panel. A padlock was used to secure the loops and bar.

The underside of the removable lid of the present *Rice Chest* bears a three-character inscription written directly on the wood with a brush and ink: *cha-ri-pu* (literally, "self-illness-contracting amulet"). The inscription was a talisman meant to protect the family against illness and misfortune. Rice was the staple of the Korean diet. Rice chests were important symbolically as well as physically. The wife always kept the key to the rice chest, both for practical reasons and as a symbol of her authority within the household. A Yi Dynasty family's income was measured in rice.

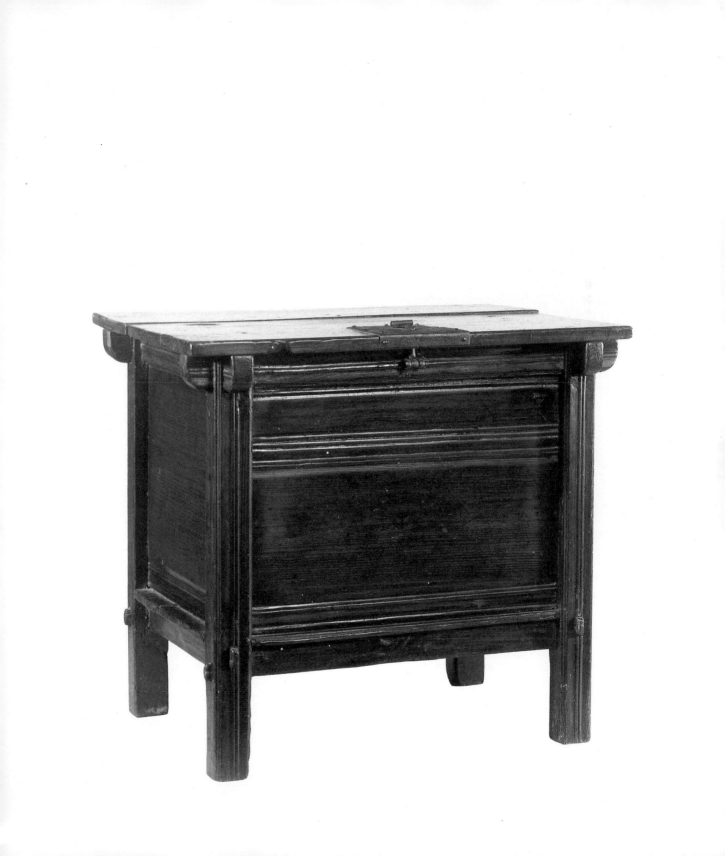

84. Scholar's Desk (*Ch'aeksang* or *Soan*)

Paulownia wood; brass fittings
H. 12″, W. 24½″
Yi Dynasty, late 18th–early 19th century
Gift of Dr. & Mrs. John Lyden   85.281.2

Chairs were not used in Korea until modern times. The master of the house sat on a large, thick, rectangular mat directly on the *ondol* (heated) floor. Guests sat on individual square cushions on the floor. The furniture was built low to accommodate persons seated on the floor (tall clothing-storage chests were an exception).

This little *Desk* is a splendid example of an essential piece of furniture for a Yi Dynasty gentleman. When the master sat on his mat, his back was toward a wall furnished with an array of stationery cabinets and display shelves. His small desk always stood in front of him, and an armrest was placed at his side. Book-storage chests were arranged along the side wall. An eight-panel screen painting stood directly behind the gentleman. The screen's subject had to be one that was considered appropriate for the men's quarters of the house, such as hunting scenes or a landscape. The colors in the painting were muted, or ink-wash alone was used. Screens for the women's quarters, on the other hand, used bright, joyous colors and usually had birds-and-flowers subjects.

This *Desk* has three small drawers in the upper register and one full-width drawer in the lower register. The small drawers are for reading and writing utensils such as eyeglasses, ink stones, and water droppers; the larger drawer is for writing brushes and rolls of paper.

Paulownia wood is quite soft, but it resists cracking due to changes in temperature and humidity, a problem that afflicts harder woods. Paulownia was ideal for small, essential pieces of furniture like this *Desk*. Paulownia wood is nearly white in its natural state; here, it has been stained dark brown with animal blood and given a natural (clear) lacquer finish.

The lines and proportions of this *Desk* are extremely handsome. It has a monumental presence belying its small size. The upturned ends of the top give the impression that the *Desk* is about to soar into flight. The same impression was conveyed by the upturned corners of the eaves on traditional Korean tile roofs. The upturned ends of desktops and book-chest tops had a practical purpose: to keep scrolls and brushes from rolling off.

The stepped-out stand of this *Desk* repeats the overhang of the top. The subtle curves of the legs echo the curves of the top; so do the scrolling contours of the stretchers between the legs. Unlike a Korean chest, which was always placed against a wall, a Korean desk stood in the middle of the room. The back and sides of a desk.were made of the same wood as the front, and they were given the same kind of finish.

The carved, fleur-de-lis ornaments on the lower drawer, sides, and back of this *Desk* are stylized representations of the Sacred Fungus (Chinese: *ling chih*, Korean: *pulloch'o*), one of The Ten Symbols of Long Life (see Cat. 70), and an ubiquitous motif on Korean paintings and household objects. Taoists believed that the Sacred Fungus bestows immortality on those who eat it. The trefoil tips of brass or iron fittings on Korean chests referred to the upper part of the Sacred Fungus. So does the carved, trefoil ornament we see here. It was fairly common, especially on book-storage chests. It was meant to be an auspicious symbol of long life and happiness for the gentleman who owned the *Desk*.

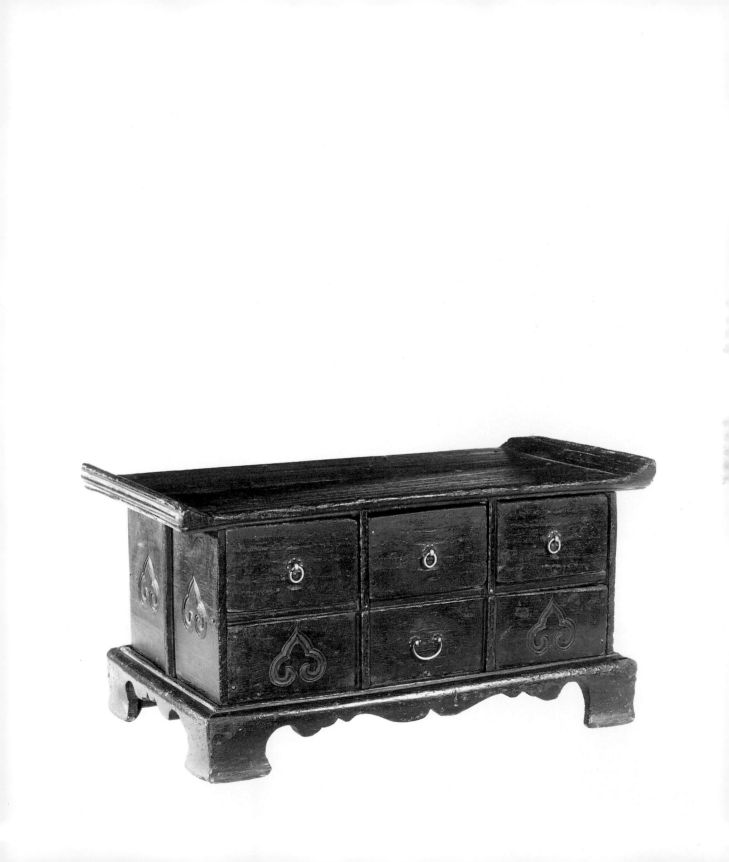

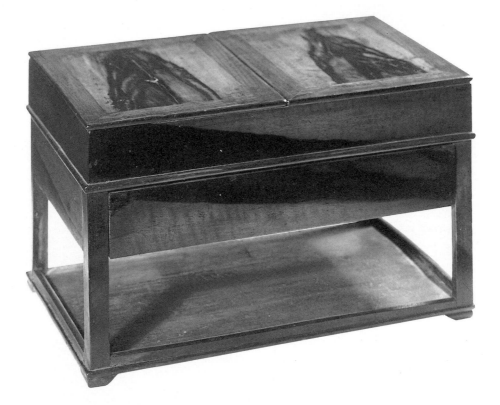

85. Ink-stone Box *(Yonsang)*
Persimmon wood and pine
H. 8⅝″, W. 14½″
Yi Dynasty, 19th century
Gift of Mr. & Mrs. John Menke   86.136

An ink-stone box usually stood beside a gentle-man's desk (see Cat. 84). Ink-stone boxes had two compartments in the upper section, each with a separate lid. One compartment was for the ink stone itself, the other for ink sticks and a water dropper. Below the pair of compartments was a full-width drawer for brushes. The open tray at the bottom was for rolls of paper. Every Yi Dynasty gentleman was supposed to be something of a scholar, calligrapher, and poet. Writing paraphernalia was therefore essential in his room.

Persimmon wood was prized for its dramatic two-tone grain. The furniture craftsman selected sections of two adjoining boards sawed from the same log to achieve the dark and light configurations on the nearly identical lid panels of this Desk; they were meant to suggest a landscape with steep mountains rising above the mist. For the front, side, and back panels, he reversed adjacent boards above and below to achieve a diagonal stripe of dark grain within light grain or light within dark. The effect is bold yet harmonious. Mirror-reversing neighboring or opposing panels—which allowed the grain patterns to repeat themselves in reverse—was a standard decorative technique for the multipaneled fronts of Korean chests. The technique was indicative of the Korean furniture craftsman's fondness for and inspired use of wood.

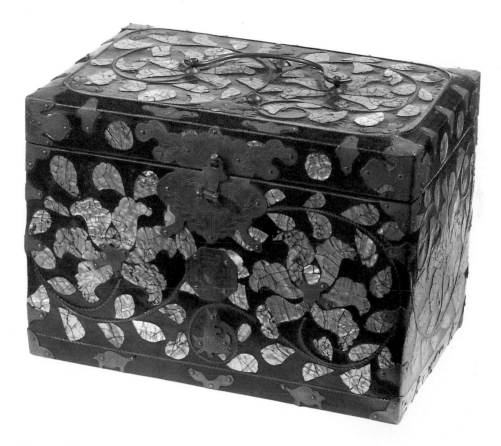

86. Jewelry Box *(P'ae-mul ham)*

Black lacquer and mother-of-pearl, over hemp cloth, on wood; brass fittings
H. 7½", W. 10¾"
Yi Dynasty, 19th century
Gift of Karel Wiest   81.59

This elegant box is a quintessential example of a characteristic Korean decorative technique: black lacquer inlaid with mother-of-pearl. Red and black lacquer were expensive; their use was normally limited to small items such as boxes and trays. Large chests finished in black or red lacquer inlaid with mother-of-pearl were the exception rather than the rule (see Cat. 79, 81). The Koreans often decorated red lacquer with inlaid mother-of-pearl (see Cat. 81), but black lacquer was more usual.

Modern trays, boxes, screens, and small tables done in red or black lacquer inlaid with mother-of-pearl are popular luxury items in Korea today. Black lacquer with mother-of-pearl inlay has been a well-known Korean speciality for centuries. Koryo Dynasty examples are extant, the earliest ones datable to the 12th century. The technique came to Korea from China, perhaps during the United Silla Period, which was profoundly influenced by the culture of T'ang Dynasty China. Lacquer inlaid with mother-of-pearl flourished in China during the T'ang Dynasty. Several T'ang examples have survived in the Shōsō-in storehouse at Tōdaiji, a Buddhist temple in Nara, Japan. They were deposited there by Emperor Shōmu's widow, Empress Kōmyō, in 756.

Shell-inlaid lacquer has had a long history in China. Examples dating from the Shang Dynasty (ca. 1500–

1027 B.C.) have been excavated. The earliest-known lacquer dates from Shang times, so shell inlay seems to go back to the very beginnings of the lacquerer's craft. Painted lacquer and lacquer inlaid with gold and silver were more prevalent than shell-inlaid lacquer during the Chou Dynasty (1027–221 B.C.) and the Han Dynasty (206 B.C.–A.D. 220). Lacquer inlaid with mother-of-pearl achieved prominence during the T'ang Dynasty (618–907) and remained in favor during the subsequent Sung, Yuan, Ming, and Ch'ing dynasties. Mother-of-pearl-inlaid Chinese lacquer of the Ming Dynasty (1368–1644) was a major source of inspiration for Yi Dynasty Korean lacquer.

The shell-inlaid designs on the front, back, top, and sides of this *Box* depict stylized peonies. Roped (twisted) brass wire forms the curvilinear stalks of the blossoms. Peonies have been a favorite Korean decorative motif since early times, incised or molded on the interior of 12th-century celadon bowls, painted on 18th–19th century blue-and-white jars, rendered in lacquer, stitched in embroidery, depicted in both ink-wash paintings and brightly colored folk paintings (see Cat. 53).

Koreans love peonies. They grow in the courtyard of nearly every house there. Peonies bloom in the spring, when nature renews itself with fresh leaves and grass, and they are among the largest and most luxuriant flowers. In Korea, peonies came to symbolize richness and abundance, wealth and happiness, nobility and purity, spring and sexual love. What could be more appropriate than peonies to decorate a lacquer box in which a wife kept her jewelry and incidentals?

87. Ox-horn *(Hwagak)* Document Box *(Soryu Ham)*

Back-painted ox horn, on wood; brass fittings
H. 5⅛", L. 16⅝"
Yi Dynasty, 19th century
Lent by Dr. John Lyden   TL1986.40.2

Bright, gay colors, dominated by an orange-red background, and lively bird-and-flower designs make painted-horn objects the most joyful of all Korean folk art. Painted-horn items were made for the women's quarters *(anch'ae)*, where loud colors and happy, auspicious motifs were the norm. Somehow the gaudy colors and multiplicity of designs on horn boxes never became vulgar or excessive, never overwhelmed the integrity of the harmonious, almost severe, rectangular forms of the boxes. This is true of Korean art and crafts in general; garish colors and crowded designs somehow remained subordinate to the forms of the objects on which they appeared.

Back-painted ox-horn *(hwagak)* was a characteristic Korean technique. The horn was soaked in warm water to soften it, then pressed into flat sheets, peeled in thin layers, cut into small rectangular panels, and polished to make it transparent. The designs were painted on what would become the reverse side of each panel, with the final lines and accents done first and the colors added on top of them, like Western or Chinese back-painted glass pictures. Each panel was glued to the box, painted side in. The horn formed a tough, lustrous surface and protected the painted designs from abrasion.

Typically, each panel on the present *Box* has its own separate composition, like an individual folk painting in miniature. With characteristic Korean

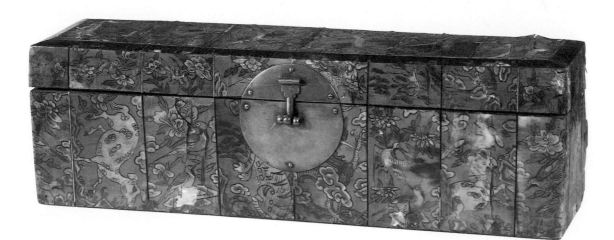

casualness, some of the paintings on the *Box* are horizontal and others are vertical. The brass latch-plate, which is original, was nailed right over the heads of the tiger and dragon!

The various designs on the *Box* constitute a virtual compendium of Korean folk-art motifs: peonies, lotuses, flowers, pairs of ducks and birds, a tiger, a dragon, cranes, deer, pine trees, rabbits, goats, and a male child. Most of these animals and plants are auspicious symbols. The tiger wards off evil. The dragon attracts good fortune. The cranes symbolize long life, as do the deer and the pine trees. The peonies suggest abundance and beauty. The lotuses stand for purity. The pairs of ducks and birds are emblematic of happy marriage. The male child is a joyous omen that the woman who owns the box will bear male children.

The shape and size of this *Box* indicate that it was a document box *(soryu ham).* The documents it contained would have been in the form of scrolls. The back-painted horn technique was more commonly used on boxes for women's incidentals, which were not as long and narrow as document boxes. Occasionally, larger pieces of furniture were covered with *hwagak.* The technique had one serious drawback: The horn panels tended to crack and curl due to changes in temperature and humidity, permitting moisture to damage the paintings underneath.

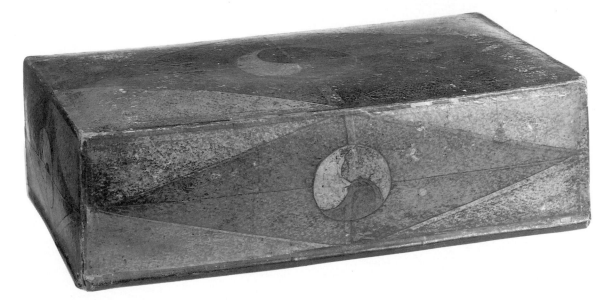

88. Stationery Box *(Mungap)*
Painted and cut paper, on papier-mâché
H. 4″, L. 13¼″
Yi Dynasty, 19th century
Gift of Dr. Kenneth Rosenbaum   84.203.10 a&b

Paper with painted and applied cut-paper designs was another characteristic Korean decorative technique. The paper was usually glued to papier-mâché to make small objects such as boxes; for larger items such as storage chests, it was glued onto wood. The paper surface was protected by an oil finish. The colors were predominantly bright red and yellow. The oil finish gradually darkened, making the colors look more muted.

These brightly colored, paper-covered items were made for the women's quarters of the house. The most typical pieces were sewing boxes, which were either high-sided square trays or deep, octagonal boxes with removable lids. The designs on the latter type were usually very similar to the designs on this *Stationery Box*. These designs were created with cut-paper appliqué, stenciled paint, and hand-applied paint.

The central motif on the top, sides, front, and back of this *Box* is a circle enclosing three curving, comma-shaped elements. This is a variant on the pair of circled commas representing *yang* and *yin*. The circled-comma symbol is called *t'aeguk* in Korean. It was originally an ancient Chinese Taoist device meant to suggest the operating principles of the universe. Two interlocking commas formed a circle. One comma represented *yang*, the male, positive principle; the other represented *yin*, the female, negative principle. The myriad activities of the cosmos derived from the interaction of *yang* and *yin*, which were opposite but mutual and inseparable. Turning together in a circle, the two commas symbolized endless cycles of movement and flux throughout the universe. Nothing was ever the same again; only change was unchanging.

The circled-comma motif was often combined with The Eight Trigrams (see Cat. 79). United in a single mystic diagram, these two sets of symbols formed a powerful talisman that was said to prevent misfortune, assure prosperity, and promote happiness. Understandably, this diagram appeared frequently in the folklore and decorative arts of China and Korea. The Eight Trigrams were usually arranged in a circle around the pair of commas. The South Korean flag uses a variant with the commas in the center of each side flanked by four of The Eight Trigrams, for a full complement of eight on the two sides of the flag.

89. Hatbox *(Kwansang)* and Hat *(Kat)*

Hatbox: black lacquer inlaid with mother-of-pearl, on papier-mâché; hat: black-lacquered horsehair mesh
Hatbox: H. 6¾″, Diam. 12¾″; Hat: H. 4¼″, Diam. 9¾″
Yi Dynasty, 19th century
Source unknown   Hatbox: X923.1 a&b; hat: X923.2

Until recent times, every well-dressed Korean man twenty years of age or older wore a hat *(kat)*. Modernization and Westernization have taken their toll on traditional Korean headgear, but an occasional elderly gentleman in the countryside still wears a *kat*. During the Yi Dynasty, the *kat* was worn indoors as well as out. If the wearer was a high official, he wore an official's cap *(t'ang-gon)* under his *kat*; the shape and material of the cap denoted his rank.

The form of the traditional Korean hat is very distinctive. There is nothing quite like it in China or Japan. It has a tall, cylindrical crown tapering slightly toward the top and a lightly arched brim of medium width. The brim did not encircle the forehead and temples like one on a Western hat. The crown has a short extension below the brim, so the hat sat well up on the head. Black silk ribbons tied under the chin kept it in place. Only a few traditional hatmakers have survived in Korea.

As an important article of daily attire, a gentleman's hat required an appropriately elegant box to store it in. The present *Hatbox* employs the characteristic Korean technique of black lacquer inlaid with mother-of-pearl (see Cat. 86). Here, the lacquer was applied on a papier-mâché core rather than on wood. The decoration includes several of The Ten Symbols of Long Life (see Cat. 70): deer, cranes, pine trees, bamboo, Sacred Fungus, sun, and clouds.

The circle in the center of the lid encloses a stylized form of the Chinese character meaning "long life." Around it are leafy branches bearing Peaches of Immortality (see Cat. 73), as well as flying cranes carrying peaches in their beaks. On the far side of the box are peonies (symbols of beauty and abundance), grass orchids (symbols of a gentleman scholar's nobility of spirit), and phoenixes (see Cat. 72).

90. Rectangular Tray Table *(Haeju-ban)*

Wood
H. 11″, L. 18¼″
Yi Dynasty, 19th century
Lent by Dr. John Lyden   TL1986.107.2

Because chairs were not used in Korea until modern times, daily activities such as eating, sleeping, reading, writing, and conversation took place at floor level. The master of the house sat on a large, rectangular mat in the sitting room of the men's quarters. His wife had a similar mat in her sitting room in the women's quarters. Guests and other members of the family sat on individual square cushions. The mats and cushions were placed directly on the heated *ondol* floor of each sitting room.

At night, sleeping mats, which had been folded and stacked on top of *bandaji* chests during the day, were spread on the *ondol* floors of the sleeping rooms located behind the sitting rooms in the men's and women's quarters. The husband did not normally see his wife during the day. He could visit her bedroom during the night.

The women of the household ate their meals in the women's quarters; the men ate in theirs. Small children remained in the women's area of the house. Each person was served his or her meal on an individual tray table while seated on a cushion or mat on the *ondol* floor of a sitting room. The standard size tray table we see here was used to serve a full meal. Smaller tray tables were used for drinks and snacks. Whereas Korean chests usually had an oil finish, Korean tray tables usually had a lacquer finish or a combination lacquer-and-oil finish to prevent spilled

food and beverages from staining the wood.

A swastika appears as a reticulated ornament on the supporting panel at each end of the present *Tray Table*. The swastika motif also appeared frequently in the openwork decoration of the brass or iron fittings on Korean chests (see Cat. 82), and in embroidered designs on Korean costumes and other textile items (see Cat. 98). Swastika designs developed independently in different parts of the ancient world. In China and Korea the swastika was originally a symbol of the Cosmic Buddha. Ming Dynasty (1368–1644) images of the Buddha, in both paintings and sculpture, were often emblazoned with a swastika on the Buddha's chest. Ming Dynasty China was the major source of influence for Yi Dynasty Korea. Yi Buddha images frequently had similar chest swastikas.

Confucianism was the state religion of the Yi Dynasty. Buddhism, its state support withdrawn, suffered occasional persecution by the government and declined rapidly. By the late Yi Period, the swastika motif had been largely secularized. Although most Koreans were probably still aware of its original Buddhist meaning, the swastika had become an ubiquitous ornament on household objects having no connection with Buddhism. The swastika simply became an auspicious symbol of harmony and happiness.

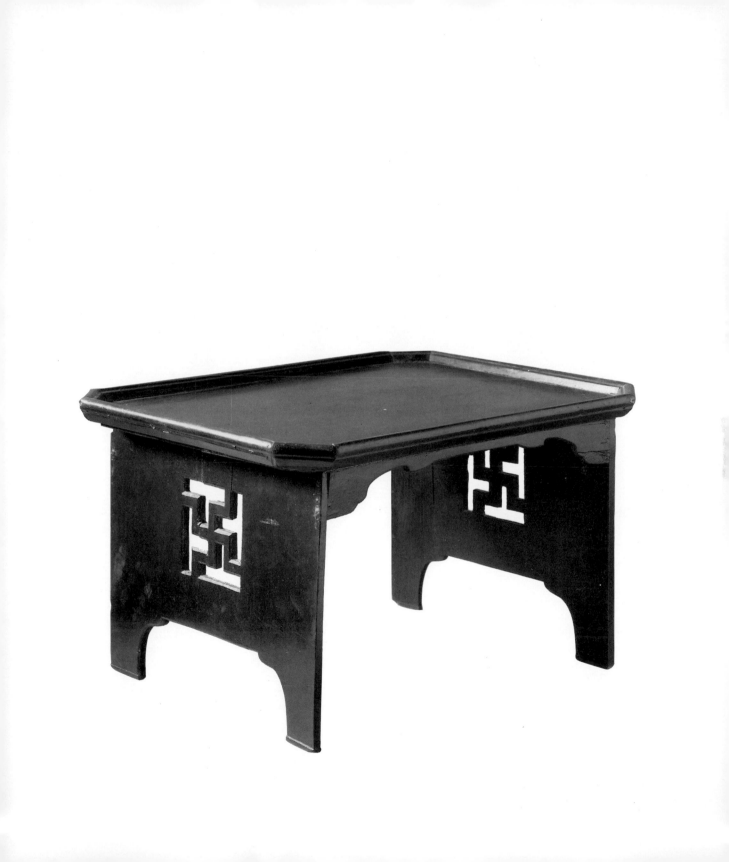

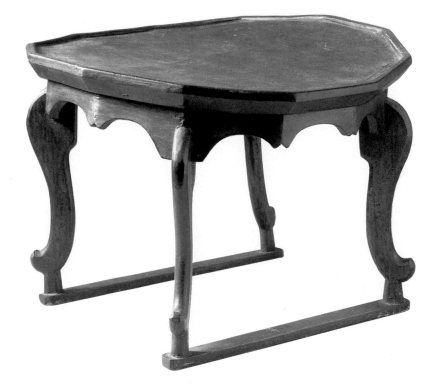

91. Tray Table *(Soban)*
Wood
H. 11″, Diam. 15½″
Yi Dynasty, 19th century
Lent by Dr. John Lyden   TL1986.107.3

Korea is hot and humid in summer but extremely cold in winter. The space immediately above the heated *ondol* floors in the sitting rooms or sleeping rooms of Korean houses was the warmest, most comfortable, most convivial place to be during the winter. Windows were few, and they were high on the walls to keep cold drafts away from people seated on the floor. During the summer, when the *ondol* floor was not heated, its smooth, shiny, oiled-paper surface was cool and pleasant to sit or sleep on. The lower part of the room remained cooler than the upper part.

Koreans ate their meals on individual tray tables while seated on cushions directly on the *ondol* floor (see Cat. 90, 92). Twelve-sided tray tables with cabriole legs were the most typical. The standard size we see here was used for full meals; smaller versions were used for drinks and snacks. The cabriole leg was called a "tiger leg" *(hochok)* in Korean.

The curve in the top of the present *Tray Table* was not the result of a subtle refinement in the design; the wood has simply warped quite badly. With characteristic nonchalance, Korean furniture craftsmen routinely used wood that was not adequately dried or seasoned. The dynamic lines, harmonious proportions, and solid workmanship of Korean furniture convey a satisfying sense of strength and reflect an admirably direct response to wood, so one scarcely notices the warping and cracks that often occurred. After all, the tendency to warp and split is an inherent characteristic of wood. Korean furniture is direct, natural, and rugged.

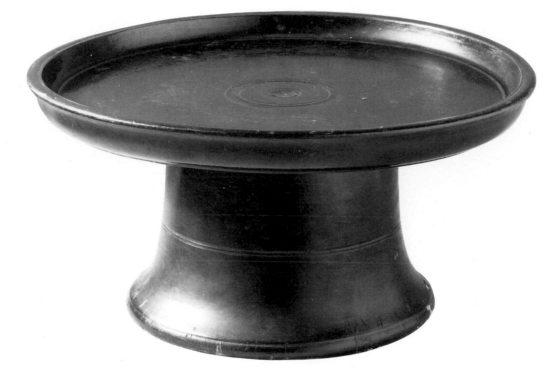

92. Round Tray Table *(Chaeban)*
Wood
H. 7½″, Diam. 15½″
Yi Dynasty, 19th century
Lent by Dr. John Lyden   TL1986.107.4

Korean craftsmen have been especially admired for their skills at wood turning. Cups, bowls, trays, tray tables, and other household items were made of turned wood. They were usually stained and finished with lacquer or lacquer and oil. Korean turned-wood objects develop a wonderfully mellow patina after years of use.

Wood turning is still a viable craft tradition in Korea today. One is startled to find that the craftsmen turn wood that has not been dried completely, wood that is almost green. One would expect objects turned from green wood to warp, split, and self-destruct. Yet somehow, Korean turned-wood items usually remain intact: there is some warping, but not

as much as one would expect, and some cracks inevitably appear but are usually not severe enough to interfere with function or visual appearance.

The present *Tray Table* has virtually no warping and only tiny radial cracks on the edge of the base. This is really quite remarkable; it attests to the skill and experience of the wood-turning craftsman who produced the *Table*. The tray portion and the tall, hollow pedestal are all turned from one large piece of wood. The lines and proportions are extraordinarily harmonious and pleasing, imbuing the piece with a sense of strength and grandeur, despite its simple, functional form. The pair of incised horizontal lines on the pedestal, three-fifths of the distance below the top, as well as the turned ring and small circle in the center of the top, serve to articulate those otherwise plain surfaces in a most appropriate way. This *Table* is a beautiful, simple, and functional object, like contemporary 20th-century design at its best.

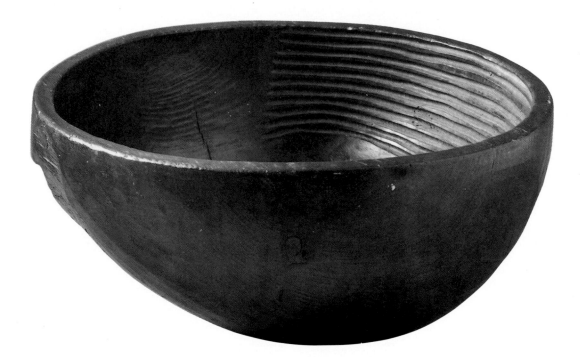

93. Rice-washing Bowl
Wood
H. 6¼", Diam. 16¼"
Yi Dynasty, 19th century
Lent by Dr. John Lyden   TL1986.107.1

Since it was a kitchen utensil, this large wooden *Bowl* is very informal, not as carefully shaped and finished as the preceding *Tray Table* (see Cat. 92), for example. Unlike the *Tray Table,* the *Bowl* was not turned on a lathe. It was chopped out and carved by hand from a large block of wood, using an adze, chisels, and draw knives. The tool marks were allowed to remain visible on the surface. Rice-washing bowls were rough, utilitarian vessels used in every Korean kitchen, yet they are aesthetically satisfying as well as perfectly suited to their mundane task. Even the most humble Korean wooden utensils have charm and dignity.

The Chinese, Koreans, and Japanese have always preferred white (polished) rice. In the past, beriberi sometimes resulted due to the thiamine in the brown hulls having been removed in the "polishing" process. Dietary customs are difficult to change. East Asians preferred the taste and consistency of white rice and associated brown rice with poverty and low social status.

After the rice had been harvested and hung on racks to dry, it was threshed with wooden flails and winnowed in shallow baskets to eliminate the chaff (the seed coverings of the rice grains and other debris). In Japan, the bran (the seed coatings on the rice grains) was removed by polishing machines operated by rice merchants. In Korea, housewives bought brown rice and polished it themselves with rice-washing bowls like the one we see here. The rice was mixed with enough water to form a heavy, thick, wet mass. The mix was kneaded up and down across the hard edges of the horizontal grooves on the inside of the bowl, like washing clothes on an old-fashioned washboard.

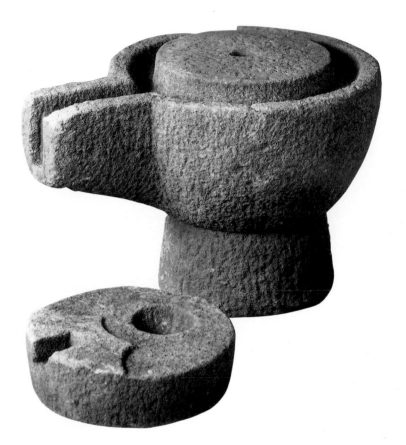

94. Hand Mill

Granite
H. 15¾", L. 19"
Yi Dynasty, 19th century
Lent by Dr. John Lyden   TL1986.40.1 a&b

The Korean peninsula is full of granite, and since early times, it has been used for the foundations of important buildings there. Korean granite also proved ideal for the construction of monuments such as pagodas, lanterns, and commemorative tablets. Tough and hard, Korean granite withstands the weather for centuries. Quantities of large-scale outdoor sculpture were also carved from it (see Cat. 57).

Here we see a household utensil made of granite, a *Hand Mill* for grinding rice or beans. The form is functional and the finish is rough, chisel marks

having been left on the surface. Still, there is such a sense of rightness about this *Mill*, such a feeling of inevitability, that one cannot help admiring it aesthetically. As in the case of Korean wooden objects, the granite has been worked in a remarkably direct and appropriate way.

The disclike grinding head fits onto the round grinding platform at the top of the mill. A short, stout wood dowel formed the axis. There is a slot on the upper edge of the grinding head for a wooden crank. Toward the opposite side of the top is a conical hole. Rice or dried beans were poured slowly through this hole as the grinding head was cranked round and round. The rice flour or bean meal fell into the groove around the grinding platform and moved along the spout until it dropped into a waiting container below.

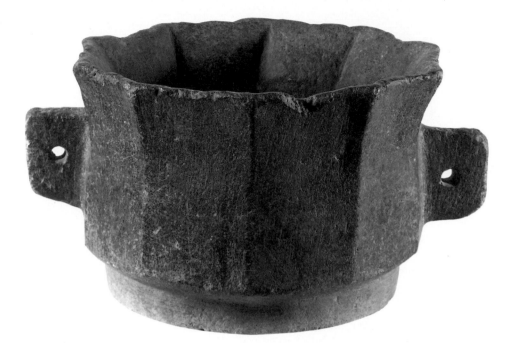

95. Small Brazier (Hand Warmer)
Slate
H. 6″, W. 11″
Yi Dynasty, 18th–19th century
Gift of Dr. John Lyden   82.50.11

Korean granite (see Cat. 57, 94), being extremely hard and tough, was ideal for architectural use, as well as for outdoor sculpture, and for utensils that had to endure rough service, like grinding mills. Granite working became a celebrated Korean craft tradition. There was also another well-known Korean stone-working tradition utilizing soft stone. Items for the scholar's desk, such as ink stones, water droppers, brush containers, paper holders, and incense burners, were made from soft stone. So were household objects such as braziers, hand warmers, pots, pans, casseroles, teapots, basins, flatirons, fulling blocks, and small boxes with lids, either round, octagonal, or rectangular.

Some of the more prestigious items (brush containers, water droppers, or covered boxes) were occasionally made from light-colored stone such as soapstone or alabaster. The more utilitarian items were made from dark-gray slate (pencil stone, black soapstone), which was almost black when its surface was polished smooth. The best ink stones were made from lavender-colored slate, the more ordinary ones from black slate.

The most characteristic product of this soft-stone craft tradition in the Yi Dynasty was the portable brazier (hand warmer) of dark-gray slate, such as we see here. Today these little fire pots are greatly admired by collectors in Japan as well as in Korea.

The shape, color, and texture of this *Small Brazier* have a compelling visual and tactile appeal. As with so many traditional Korean objects, the form and the material suited the object's function perfectly. Yet the aesthetic appeal goes well beyond mere functionalism. Subtle refinements of the *Brazier's* design, such as the exterior facets, the corresponding interior vertical grooves, and the slight upward curve of the handles, give it a simple elegance comparable to that of, say, contemporary Scandinavian furniture.

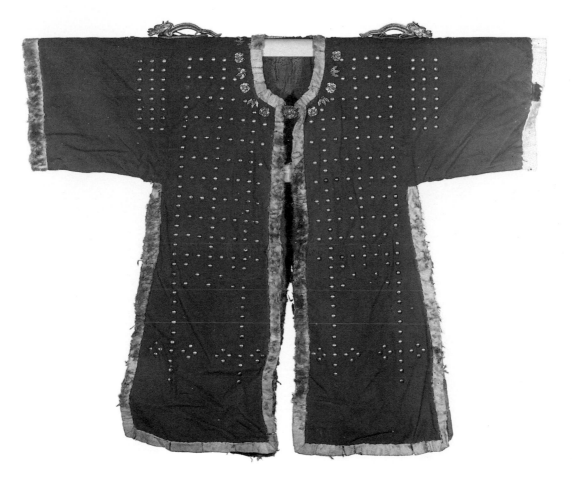

96. Suit of Armor for a Deputy Commander
(Tujong-gap)

Wool flannel lined with silk and edged with fur;
lacquered leather; gilt-copper fittings
Helmet: H. 32½″, W. 8″; Coat: H. 43″, W. 52″
Yi Dynasty, 18th–19th century
1913 Museum Expedition   X957.1 a&b

This elegant *Suit of Armor* was not meant to be
worn in battle. It was intended for the colorful
processions and other ceremonies held throughout
the year by the royal court. Although it incorporates
the finest materials and workmanship, this *Armor*
was strictly for show. The gilt-copper rivets arranged
in neat vertical and horizontal rows on the coat
and on the neck guards of the helmet are merely
ornamental. Their function on a suit of battle armor
would have been to secure small, overlapping steel
plates between the outer and inner layers of cloth.
The steel scales afforded protection against swords
and arrows. Likewise the helmet bowl, which would
have been made of steel on fighting armor, is made
of black-lacquered leather.

The various motifs depicted in the elaborate openwork gilt-copper fittings on the helmet are part of
the standard Yi Dynasty repertoire of auspicious
symbols. The dragon was a symbol of the king,
and of Heaven (see Cat. 69). When paired with the

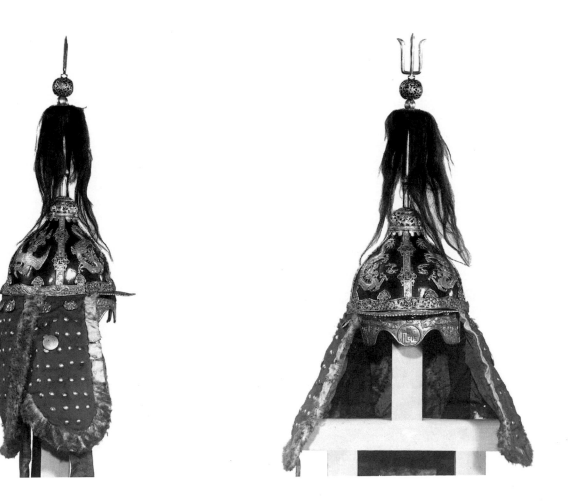

dragon, the phoenix was a symbol of the queen (see Cat. 72). The dragon protected the nation from calamity by repelling evil spirits, while at the same time inviting good fortune. The phoenix dwelt only in lands where there was peace and prosperity. The swastika, originally a Buddhist motif, became a secular symbol of success.

The Chinese ideograph on the nose guard of the helmet means "virtue," Confucianism's *summum bonum.* Shamanism was not ignored, however. The trident (on the helmet finial) is an attribute of Shamanist Guardian Generals (see Cat. 31). The central Guardian General in the painting holds a trident.

Moreover, his helmet has a red-plumed trident finial just like the one on this *Armor.* An iron trident is one of the standard implements used by *mudang* (Korean shamans) performing *kut* (shaman rituals).

The articulated, gilt-copper dragons forming the epaulets on this *Armor* are among the liveliest depictions of this creature to be found anywhere. They are magnificent sculpture in miniature; their dignity and energy belie their small size. Oak leaves, here represented by small, gilt-copper plaques around the neck area of the coat, were Yi Dynasty symbols of valor, an appropriate emblem for the costume of a military officer.

97. Helmet

Steel; leather
H. 19″, W. 8½″
Yi Dynasty, 18th century
1913 Museum Expedition   X957.5

Because the *Suit of Armor* (see Cat. 96) was made
for ceremonial use rather than battle, its helmet bowl
is lacquered leather. The bowl of the present *Helmet*
is made of steel; it was meant to be worn in battle. A
sturdy, ribbed band of steel riveted to the front and
back of the bowl provides vertical reinforcement. The
small visor, the hemispherical finial, and the tubular
plume socket are also made of steel. The intentional,
gray-black chemical patina on the steel helped
prevent rust and provided a handsome, dark finish.

The domical finial, the reinforcing bands, and the
visor are decorated with lotus-scroll designs in silver
damascening. The silver has tarnished a blue-black
color not unlike that of the surrounding steel, so the
decoration is now somewhat difficult to see. When
the silver was polished bright, its whiteness contrasted
sharply with the blue-black steel around it.

Damascening is the technique of decorating steel
with overlaid designs of softer metal of contrasting
color, usually silver or gold. The surface of the steel
was scratched with crisscross file marks wherever
the design was to appear. A strip or small sheet of
thin silver was hammered onto the surface. The
underside of the soft silver was forced into the burrs
and edges of the file marks by the hammering and
held the silver in place.

Damascening was used widely in the Arab world;
the term derives from the city of Damascus. The craft
of damascening also became a Korean specialty.
Household items, such as small covered boxes, portable braziers (hand warmers), candle stands, and
padlocks, were decorated by this process.

The neck guards of the present *Helmet* are made
of tough, gray leather lined with light-brown leather
and edged with snakeskin. They are decorated on
the outside with embroidered floral-scroll arabesques
in brightly colored silk thread that has now faded
somewhat.

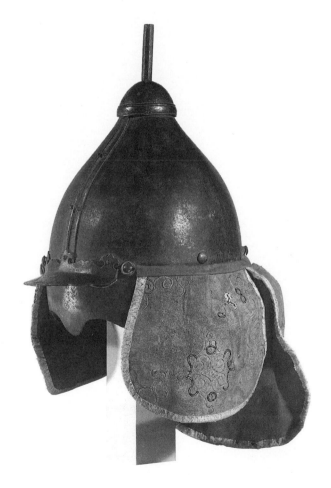

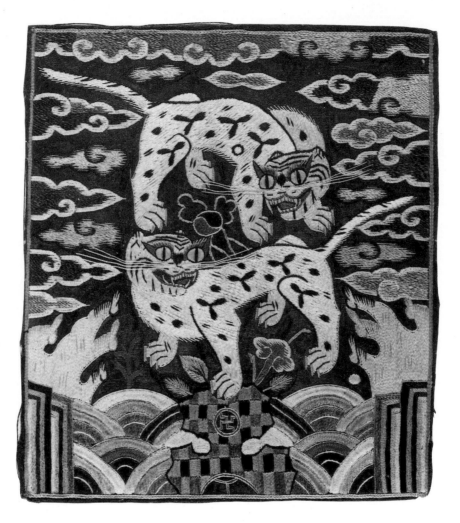

98. Two Pairs of Mandarin Squares *(Hyungbae)*
Silk embroidery
H. 9¼″, W. 8¾″ each (Cranes)
H. 7¾″, W. 7″ each (Tigers)
Yi Dynasty, 19th century
1913 Museum Expedition   X960.1&.2 (Cranes);
X903.1&2 (Tigers)

The art of embroidery is another famous Korean specialty. During the Yi Dynasty, robes, jackets, skirts, caps, purses, eyeglass cases, and pillow ends were often decorated with embroidery. But the most spectacular examples were embroidered screens. They were full-size, eight-panel screens, exactly like screen paintings except that they were embroidered

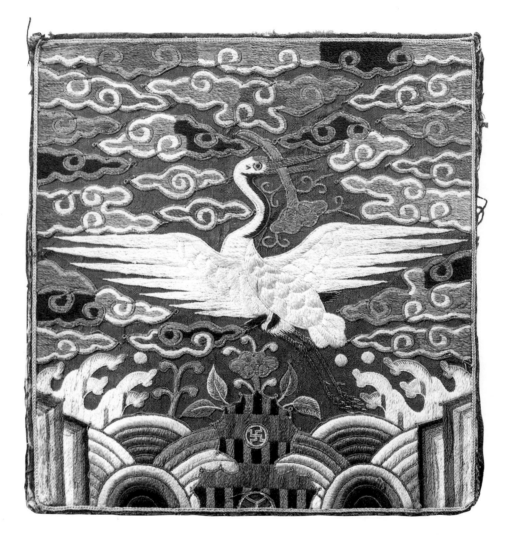

rather than painted, an extremely complex, time-consuming process. Birds and flowers were the most popular subject for embroidered screens, just as they were for painted ones (see Cat. 49). Elaborate compositions of figures in landscape settings were sometimes embroidered on screens.

Every high-ranking government official wore a pair of mandarin squares on his court robe, one on the chest and one on the back, following Ming Dynasty practice in China. Details of the designs indicated the court ranks and duties of the officials. Cranes indicated civil officials; tigers indicated military officials. Two cranes indicated a higher rank than one crane; two tigers did likewise.

MODERN KOREA
AFTER 1910

99. Mountain Landscape in Moonlight
By Kim Ki-chang (born 1914)
Ink and color on silk
H. 19¾", W. 21¾" exclusive of mounting
Dated in accordance with 1975
Gift of Dr. & Mrs. Peter Reimann   81.124

Kim Ki-chang is perhaps Korea's best-known living artist. He was born in Seoul in 1914. A childhood illness permanently impaired his hearing and speech; he communicates by exchanging written notes. At the age of sixteen, he became a pupil of the painter Kim Un-ho. During the 1930s, Kim Ki-chang's paintings won several important awards, including the coveted grand prize at the Choson Art Exhibition.

Soon after the end of World War II, Kim Ki-chang married Pak Nae-hyon, a leading artist in her own right. As is the custom in Korea, Pak retained her maiden name after their marriage. Kim and Pak held a number of joint exhibitions. After the Korean War, Kim Ki-chang began to show his paintings abroad as well as in Korea. His work has been exhibited in the United States, France, and Brazil.

Kim Ki-chang's painting style progressed from skillfully drawn, realistic figure paintings in the early 1930s through bold, free ink paintings of horses, figures, and landscapes in the 50s and 60s, to color abstractions in the late 60s, and on to calligraphic ink abstractions in the 1970s.

In the present painting, a pair of mandarin ducks, symbolic of happy marriage, fly among boulders, cliffs, and wind-blown pine trees, with blue mountain peaks in the distance and the moon rising at the upper left. The inscription at the lower right begins with a cyclical date equivalent to 1975, then the characters for "early spring," then Un Po (Mr. Cloud), one of Kim Ki-chang's art names. The upper seal reads, "Seal of Kim Ki-chang"; the lower one repeats his art name, Un Po.

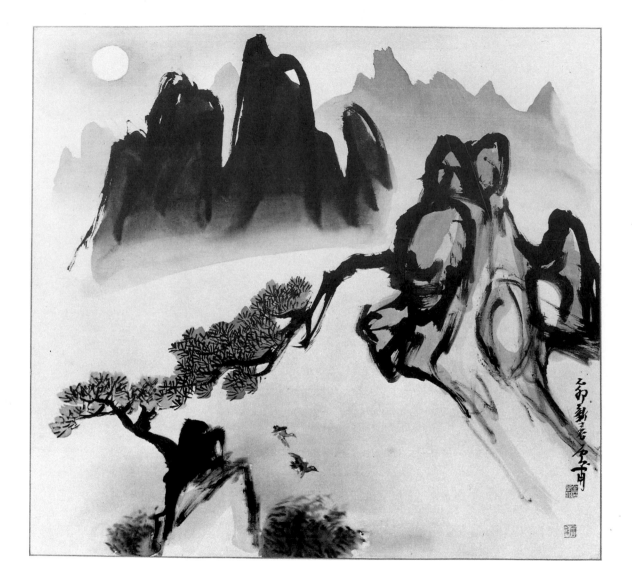

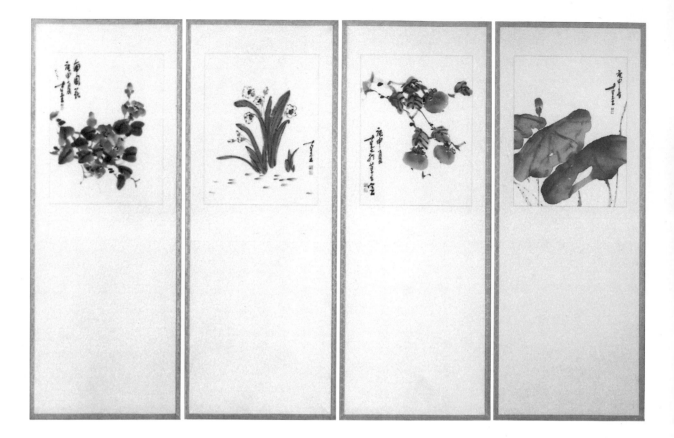

100. Flowers of the Four Seasons

By Park Sang-yol (b. 1923)
Eight-panel screen painting; ink and color on paper
H. 17⅞″, W. 13¾″ each painting, exclusive of mounting
Dated in accordance with 1980
Gift of Harold Glasser   82.176

Park Sang-yol was born in 1923 and currently lives in Seoul. He studied painting under Pae Lyom and Chang Wu-song. He works in the traditional literati style. In addition to numerous exhibitions in Korea, he participated in group shows in Tokyo and Osaka in 1976. He had a one-man show in the United States in 1977.

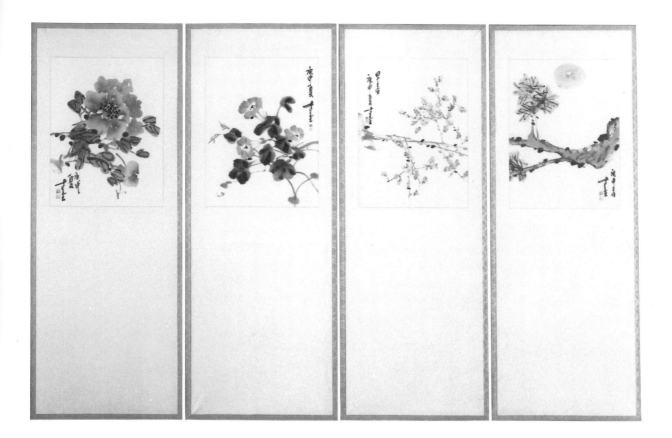

Reading from right to left in the customary manner, the subjects of the paintings on this screen are as follows: Pine Bough and Moon; Forsythia; Morning Glories; Peonies; Lotus; Persimmons; Daffodils; Camellias. Each painting is signed "Ko-tang," one of Park Sang-yol's art names. Each painting except the Daffodils bears a cyclical date equivalent to 1980. Two are inscribed "Spring"; five are inscribed "Summer." The Forsythia is inscribed with a title, "Early Spring." The Camellia likewise bears a title, "Flower of the Southern Provinces."

SELECTED BIBILIOGRAPHY

Choi Sunu
5000 Years of Korean Art
Seoul, Hyonam, 1979

Covell, Alan
Shamanist Folk Paintings: Korea's Eternal Spirits
Elizabeth, New Jersey, and Seoul, Hollym
International Corp., 1984

Covell, Jon
Korea's Cultural Roots
Salt Lake City and Seoul, Moth House and Hollym,
1981

Gompertz, G. St. G. M.
Korean Celadon and Other Wares of the Koryo Period
New York, Thomas Yoseloff, 1964

Gompertz, G. St. G. M.
Korean Pottery and Porcelain of the Yi Period
London, Faber and Faber, 1968

Kim Chewon and Lee Lena Kim
Arts of Korea
Tokyo, New York, and San Francisco, Kodansha
International, 1974

McCune, Evelyn
The Arts of Korea
Rutland and Tokyo, Tuttle, 1962

McCune, Evelyn
The Inner Art: Korean Screens
Berkeley and Seoul, Asia Humanities Press and
Po Chin Chai Co., 1983

The National Museum of Korea (ed.)
Folk Art of Korea
Seoul, The National Museum of Korea, 1975

The National Museum of Korea (ed.)
Masterpieces of 500 Years of Korean Painting
Seoul, The National Museum of Korea, 1972

Sayers, Robert
Potters and Christians: New Light on Korea's First
Catholics
Korean Culture 6 (2), 1985: 26–35

Wichman, Michael
Korean Chests: Treasures of the Yi Dynasty
Seoul, Seoul International Tourist Publishing Co.,
1978

Wright, Edward and Pai Man-sill
Korean Furniture: Elegance and Tradition
Tokyo, New York, and San Francisco, Kodansha
International, 1984

Zozayong (pseudonym of Cho Cha-yong)
*Guardians of Happiness: Shamanistic Tradition in Korean
Folk Painting*
Seoul, Emileh Museum, 1982

Zozayong
The Humor of Korean Tiger
Seoul, Emileh Museum, 1970

Zozayong
Introduction to Korean Folk Painting
Seoul, Emileh Museum, 1977

Zozayong
Spirit of the Korean Tiger
Seoul, Emileh Museum, 1972

COLOR PLATES

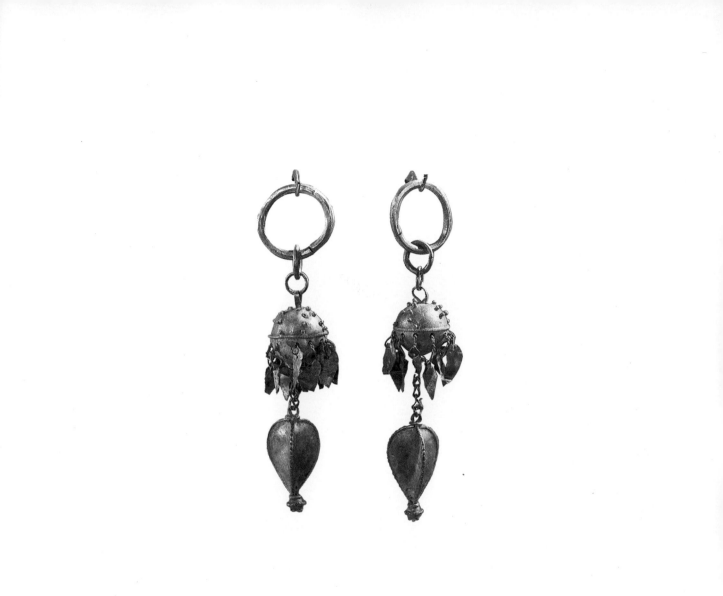

7. Pair of Earrrings

Gold
H. 3⅛″, W. ¾″ each
Silla Period, 5th–6th century
Anonymous gift   83.195 a&b

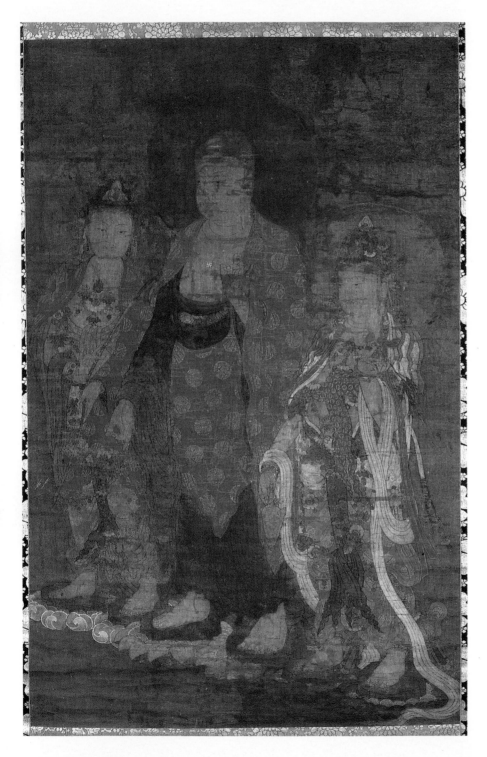

11. Amit'a (Amitabha) Triad
Hanging-scroll painting; ink,
color, and gold on silk
H. 51¼", W. 32¼" exclusive
of mounting
Koryo Dynasty, 14th century
Gift of Prof. Harold Henderson
61.204.30

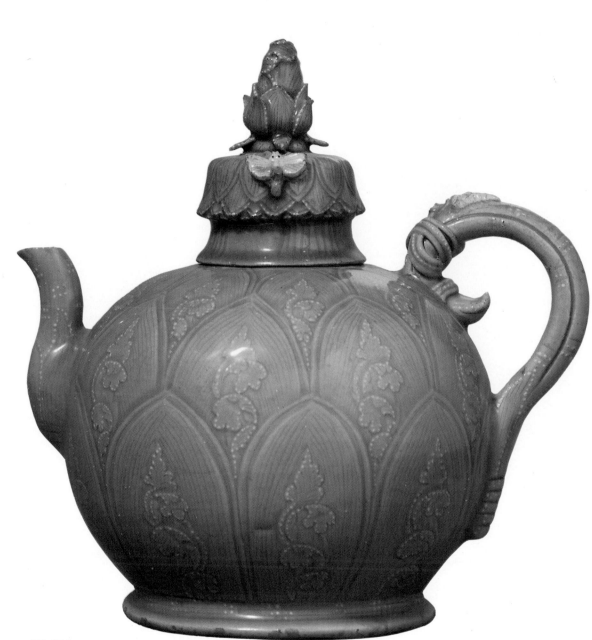

15. Ewer with Lid

Celadon porcelain with
white and black slip decoration
H. 9⅞", W. 9½"
Koryo Dynasty, first half of the 12th century
Gift of Mrs. Darwin R. James III   56.138.1 a&b

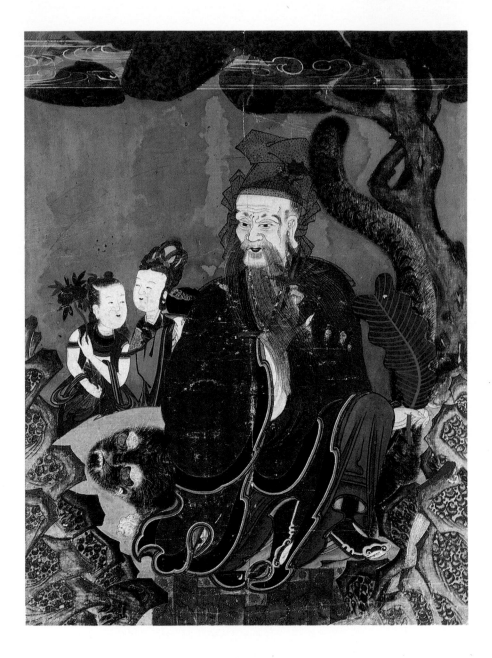

30. San Shin (The Mountain Spirit)

Hanging-scroll painting; ink and color on silk
H. 34″, W. 24½″ exclusive of mounting
Yi Dynasty, 19th century
Purchase   84.145

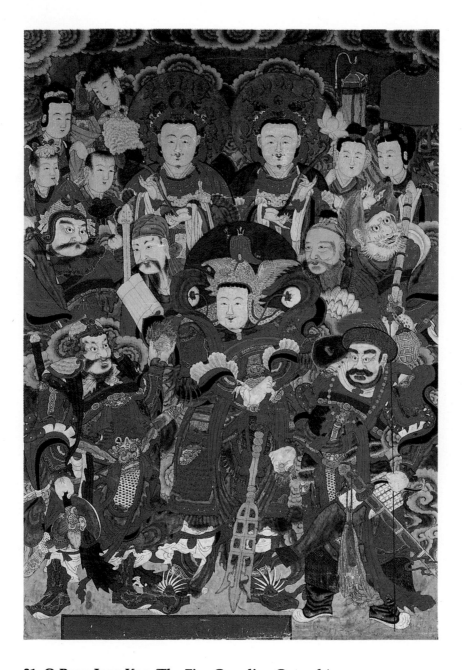

31. O Bang Jang Kun (The Five Guardian Generals)
Hanging-scroll painting; ink, color, and gold on silk
H. 57", W. 40"
Yi Dynasty, 19th century
Purchase   80.76

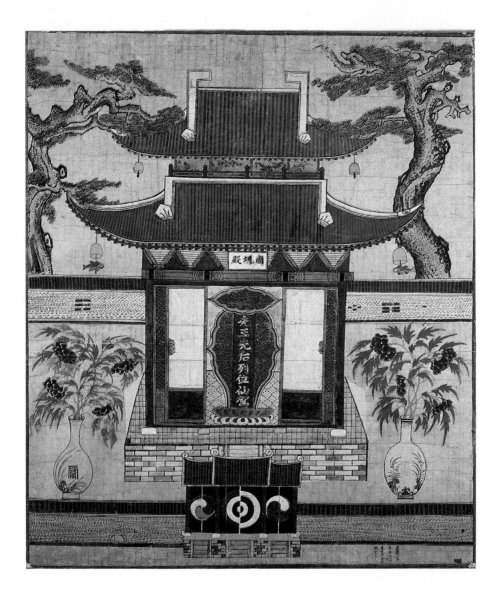

34. Kam Mo Yo Je Do (Spirit Shrine)

Hanging-scroll painting; ink and color on paper
H. 67 5/16″, W. 56 ⅝″
Yi Dynasty, dated in accordance with June, 1811
Purchase   86.25

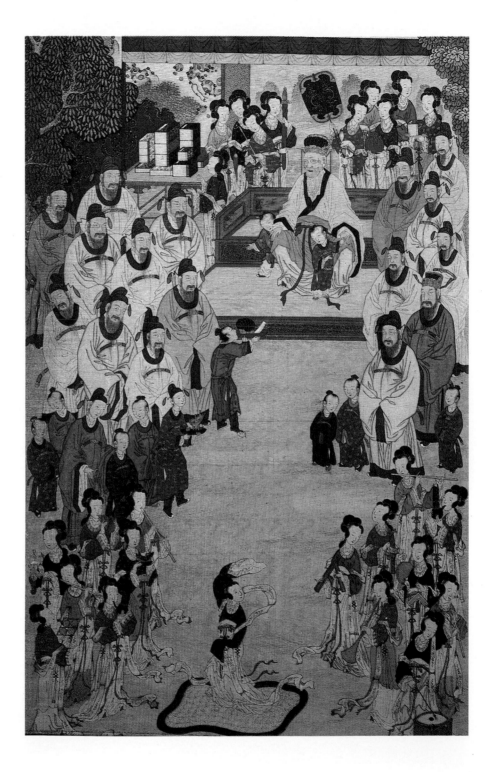

36. Kuo Tzu-i's Banquet

Six-panel screen painting;
ink and color on silk
H. 79½″, W. 142½″
Yi Dynasty, 19th century
Gift of John Gruber   84.251

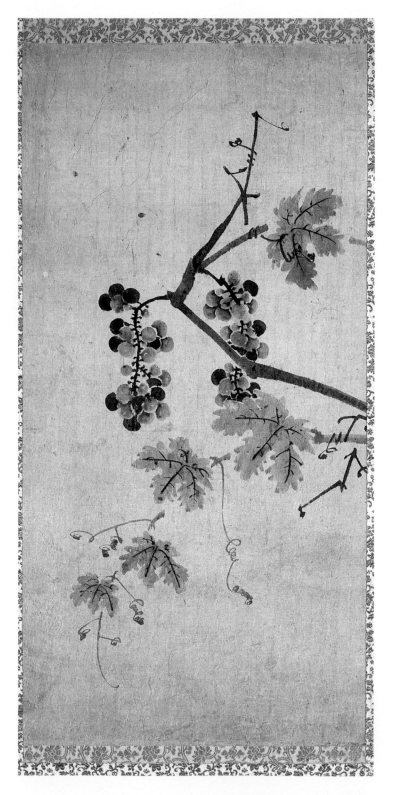

40. Grapevine

Hanging-scroll painting, ink on paper
H. 26″, W. 12¾″ exclusive of mounting
Yi Dynasty, 16th century
Lent by Dr. John Lyden   TL1986.442

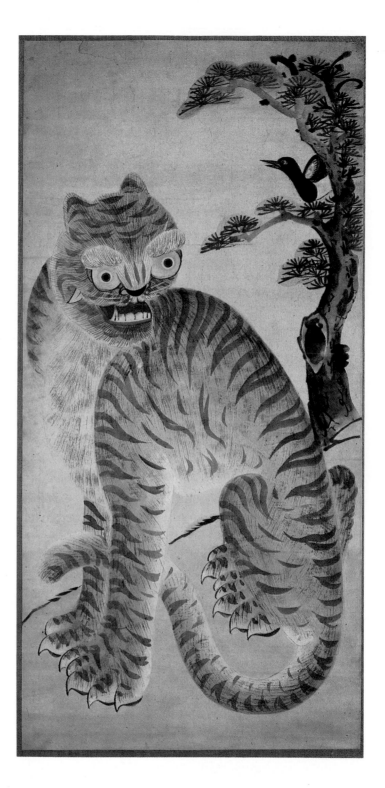

54. Tiger and Magpie
Hanging-scroll painting; ink and color on paper
H. 34¼″, W. 16½″ exclusive of mounting
Yi Dynasty, 19th century
Lent by Florence Selden   L81.18

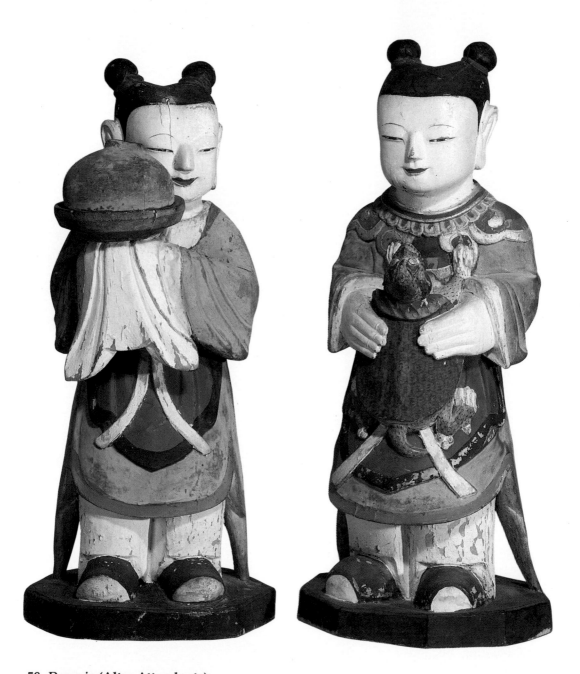

58. *Dong-ja* **(Altar Attendants)**
Pair of polychromed wood figures
H. 19" (.1), 20" (.2), W. 3½" each
Yi Dynasty, 18th century
Gift of Dr. & Mrs. Stanley Wallace   83.174.1 & .2

59. *Kirogi* **(Wedding Duck)**
Wood with traces of ink
H. 9½″, L. 13½″
Yi Dynasty, 19th century
Gift of the Guennol Collection   86.140

Clear Corneal Lens Surgery

Edited by
I. Howard Fine, MD
Oregon Health Sciences University
Portland, Oregon
Oregon Eye Associates
Eugene, Oregon

SLACK Incorporated, 6900 Grove Road, Thorofare, NJ 08086-9447

Publisher: John H. Bond
Editorial Director: Amy E. Drummond
Senior Associate Editor: Jennifer J. Cahill

The procedures and practices described in this book should be implemented in a manner consistent with the professional standards set for the circumstances that apply in each specific situation. Every effort has been made to confirm the accuracy of the information presented and to correctly relate generally accepted practices. The author, editor, and publisher cannot accept responsibility for errors or exclusions or for the outcome of the application of the material presented herein. There is no expressed or implied warranty of this book or information imparted by it.

Care has been taken to ensure that drug selection and dosages are in accordance with currently accepted/recommended practice. Due to continuing research, changes in government policy and regulations, and various effects of drug reactions and interactions, it is recommended that the reader carefully review all materials and literature provided for each drug, especially those that are new or not frequently used.

Printed in the United States of America
Published by: SLACK Incorporated
                   6900 Grove Road
                   Thorofare, NJ 08086 USA
                   Telephone: 609-848-1000
                   Fax: 609-853-5991
                   Website: www.slackinc.com

Clear corneal lens surgery/[edited by] I. Howard Fine.
     p. cm.
   Includes bibliographical references and index.
   ISBN 1-55642-381-0
   1. Cataract--Surgery. I. Fine, I. Howard.
   [DNLM: 1. Cornea--surgery. 2. Cataract Extraction--methods. WW 220C623 1999]
RE451.C636 1999
617.7'42059--dc21
DNLM/DLC
for Library of Congress   98-37810

Dedication

This book is dedicated to Dr. Charles Kelman, the innovator, and Drs. Richard Kratz, Robert Sinskey, James Little, and Jared Emery, the early converts. The insights and teachings of these men enhanced the lives of millions of people throughout the world and fostered satisfying careers for many who followed.

Contents

Dedication iii

Acknowledgments vi

Contributors vii

Foreword ix
Charles D. Kelman, MD

Chapter 1: **Introduction to Clear Corneal Lens Surgery** 1
I. Howard Fine, MD

Chapter 2: **Controversies Regarding Clear Corneal Incisions** 7
I. Howard Fine, MD, Richard S. Hoffman, MD

Chapter 3: **Clear Corneal Incisions and Astigmatism** 21
Emanuel Rosen, MD, FRCS, FRCOphth

Chapter 4: **Making the Transition to Temporal Clear** 43
Corneal Cataract Surgery Under Topical Anesthesia
Richard S. Hoffman, MD

Chapter 5: **Intraocular Anesthesia in Clear Corneal Cataract Surgery** . . 59
James P. Gills, MD, Myra Cherchio, COMT

Chapter 6: **The Choo-Choo Chop and Flip Phacoemulsification** 71
Technique
I. Howard Fine, MD

Chapter 7: **Deep Groove Corneal Incision** 85
David W. Langerman, MD, FACS

Chapter 8: **Personal Clear Corneal Cataract Technique** 95
John D. Hunkeler, MD

Chapter 9: **Tilt and Tumble Phacoemulsification** **99**
Richard L. Lindstrom, MD

Chapter 10: **Clear Corneal Incision: A Personal Method** **121**
Samuel Masket, MD

Chapter 11: **Techniques, Thoughts, Challenges** **131**
David M. Dillman, MD

Chapter 12: **Personal Techniques** **157**
James A. Davison, MD, FACS

Chapter 13: **Sub 3.0-mm Phaco** **185**
Harry B. Grabow, MD

Chapter 14: **Clear Corneal Micro Incision Surgery for Cataract** **211**
 and Refractive Implants
Charles H. Williamson, MD, FACS

Chapter 15: **Current Personal Phaco Procedure** **239**
Richard J. Mackool, MD

Chapter 16: **Clear Corneal Implant Surgical Techniques** **251**
Kenneth J. Hoffer, MD

Chapter 17: **Complications of Clear Corneal and Posterior** **263**
 Limbal Lens Surgery
Thomas Kohnen, MD

Chapter 18: **Clear Lensectomy** **281**
Robert H. Osher, MD

Chapter 19: **Implantable Contact Lens** **287**
Roberto Zaldivar, MD, Susana Oscherow, MD, Giselle Ricur, MD

Chapter 20: **Phakic Refractive Intraocular Lenses** **325**
Paul S. Koch, MD

Chapter 21: **Phakic Intraocular Lenses** **349**
George O. Waring III, MD, FACS, FRCOphth

Index **371**

Acknowledgments

I would like to acknowledge, with gratitude, the efforts and contributions of each of the authors of this book, all of whom are superb physicians, surgical technicians, and teachers. I would also like to thank those members of industry with whom I have worked in the development of knives and other concepts, facilitating the development of clear corneal lens surgery. These include Alan Huber, Doug Mastel, Ravi Nallakrishnan, Ron Dikes, Mary Christie, and especially John Bee. I would be remiss not to once again offer my gratitude to my wonderful editors at SLACK Incorporated: Amy Drummond and Jennifer Cahill. Their help is a pleasure to experience. Finally, as always, I want to acknowledge the help of my wife, Vicky, through whom all things have become possible for me.

Contributors

Myra Cherchio, COMT
St. Luke's Cataract and Laser Institute
Tarpon Springs, Florida

James A. Davison, MD, FACS
University of Utah
Salt Lake City, Utah
Marshalltown Medical Surgical Center
Marshalltown, Iowa
Iowa Methodist Medical Center
Des Moines, Iowa

David M. Dillman, MD
Dillman Eye Care Associates
Danville, Illinois

I. Howard Fine, MD
Oregon Health Sciences University
Portland, Oregon
Oregon Eye Associates
Eugene, Oregon

James P. Gills, MD
St. Luke's Cataract and Laser Institute
Tarpon Springs, Florida

Harry B. Grabow, MD
International Cataract Institute
Sarasota, Florida

Kenneth J. Hoffer, MD
University of California—Los Angeles
Los Angeles, California

Richard S. Hoffman, MD
Oregon Eye Associates
Eugene, Oregon

John D. Hunkeler, MD
Hunkeler Eye Center
Kansas City, Missouri

Paul S. Koch, MD
Koch Eye Associates
Warwick, Rhode Island

Thomas Kohnen, MD
Johann Wolfgang Goethe University
Frankfurt, Germany

David W. Langerman, MD, FACS
Langerman Eye Institute
Orangeburg, New York

Richard L. Lindstrom, MD
University of Minnesota
Phillips Eye Institute
Minneapolis, Minnesota

Richard J. Mackool, MD
The Mackool Eye Institute
Astoria, New York
New York Eye and Ear Infirmary
New York, New York

Samuel Masket, MD
Jules Stein Eye Institute
University of California—Los Angeles
Los Angeles, California

Susana Oscherow, MD
Instituto Zaldivar
Mendoza, Argentina

Robert H. Osher, MD
Cincinnati Eye Institute
Cincinnati, Ohio

Giselle Ricur, MD
Instituto Zaldivar
Mendoza, Argentina

Emanuel Rosen, MD, FRCS, FRCOphth
Consultant Ophthalmic Surgeon
Manchester, England

George O. Waring III, MD, FACS, FRCOphth
Emory University
Atlanta, Georgia

Charles H. Williamson, MD, FACS
The Williamson Eye Center
Baton Rouge, Louisiana

Roberto Zaldivar, MD
Instituto Zaldivar
Mendoza, Argentina

Foreword

It has been most gratifying for me to see other physicians involved in expanding and refining the art and science of phacoemulsification. It is especially rewarding when physicians of the caliber of Dr. I. Howard Fine and his contributors to *Clear Corneal Lens Surgery* are actively involved in the continuing advancement of the art.

I consider myself extremely fortunate to be able to witness this flowering of knowledge and skill, all directed to the patient's benefit. When I began work on phacoemulsification in the 1960s, the intracapsular cataract extraction was followed by 7 to 10 days in the hospital and 1 month's recuperation at home. At that time it was impossible to predict all the developments that would be made over the ensuing years in the evolution of cataract surgery.

My congratulations to all who have made contributions to phacoemulsification, and especially to those most dedicated physicians, such as Dr. Fine, who have spent considerable time and energy passing their skills on to others.

Charles D. Kelman, MD
The Eye Center
New York, New York

Chapter 1

Introduction to Clear Corneal Lens Surgery

I. Howard Fine, MD

The cornea as a location for cataract surgery goes all the way back to couching of the lens with a flat needle inserted through the cornea near the limbus. Jacques Daviel in 1745 utilized clear corneal incisions in his cataract surgery technique as did Albrecht von Graefe, who in the 1750s developed a clear corneal knife and a technique known as the Graefe section. His technique persists to the present day in some third world areas where intracapsular cataract extraction remains the dominant cataract extraction technique. With the utilization of operating microscopes and sutures in the latter half of the 20th century, ophthalmic surgeons fashioned a variety of incision construction techniques, architectures, and suturing methods favoring the limbus as the incision location.

Kratz is generally credited as the first phacoemulsification surgeon to move from the limbus posteriorly to the sclera in order to increase appositional surfaces, thus enhancing wound healing and reducing surgically induced astigmatism.[1,2] Girard and Hoffman were the first to name the posterior incision a "scleral tunnel incision" and were, along with Kratz, the first to make a point of entering the anterior chamber through the cornea creating a corneal shelf.[3] This corneal shelf was designed to prevent iris prolapse and was popularized by Maloney, Kratz's fellow, who described that architecture as both strong and waterproof (Figure 1-1).[4] In 1989, McFarland used this incision architecture and recognized that these incisions sized for phacoemulsification and implantation of foldable lenses were self-sealing.[5] Ernest recognized that McFarland's long scleral tunnel incision with a corneal shelf acted as a one-way valve, thus explaining the mechanism for self-sealability. Ernest

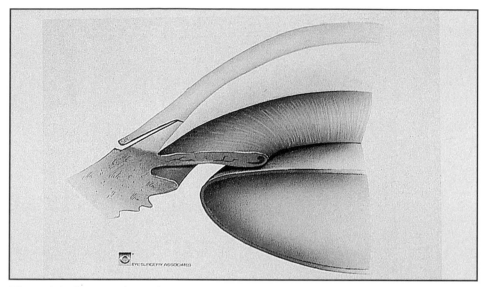

Figure 1-1. Cross-sectional view of the corneal shelf incision. Incision begins in sclera, is beveled into the clear cornea, and enters the anterior chamber producing a corneal shelf, which is watertight and prevents iris prolapse. Reprinted with permission from *Textbook of Phacoemulsification* by Dr. William F. Maloney.

changed the name from corneal shelf to posterior corneal lip.[6] In April 1992, I presented my self-sealing temporal corneal tunnel incision at the annual meeting of the American Society of Cataract and Refractive Surgery.[7] Finally, in May 1992, at the Island Ophthalmology Seminar, Kellan demonstrated on video a posterior limbal incision that he called the scleral-less incision. It was essentially a limbal stab incision through conjunctiva and the limbus, entering the anterior chamber through clear cornea, leaving a corneal shelf or lip (Figures 1-2 and 1-3).

There have been many surgeons who have favored corneal incisions for cataract surgery prior to their recent popularization. In 1968, Charles Kelman stated that the best approach for performing cataract surgery was with phacoemulsification through a clear corneal incision utilizing a triangular-tear capsulotomy and a grooving and cracking technique in the posterior chamber.[8] Harms and Mackensen in Germany published an intracapsular technique using a corneal incision in 1967 in an atlas of *Ocular Surgery Under the Microscope*.[9] Troutman was an early advocate of controlling surgically induced astigmatism at the time of cataract surgery by means of the corneal incision approach.[10] Arnott in England utilized clear corneal incisions and a diamond keratome for phacoemulsification, although he had to enlarge the incision for introducing an IOL.[11] Galand in Belgium utilized clear corneal incisions for extracapsular cataract extraction in his envelope technique,[12] and Stegmann of South Africa has a long history of having utilized the cornea as the site for incisions for extracapsular cataract extraction.[13] Finally, perhaps the leading proponent of clear corneal incisions for modern era phacoemulsification was Kimiya Shimizu of Japan.[14]

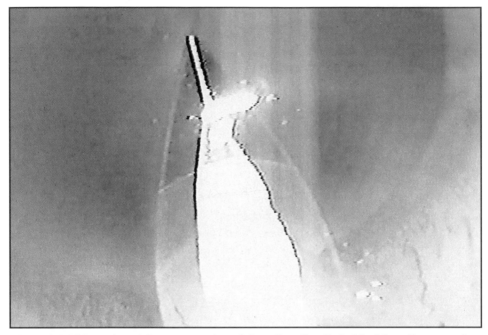

Figure 1-2. Video print of the construction of the self-sealing limbal incision. Courtesy of Dr. Robert Kellan.

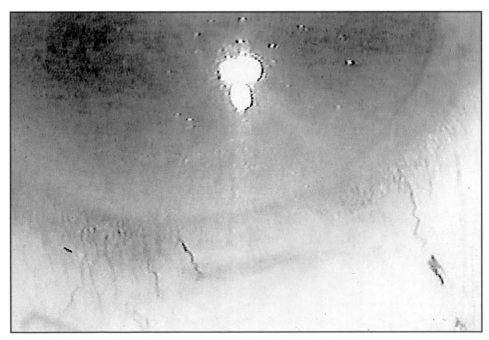

Figure 1-3. Video print of the appearance of the self-sealing limbal incision. Courtesy of Dr. Robert Kellan.

My personal experience with corneal incisions began in 1979 when the temporal clear cornea was utilized as the site for secondary anterior chamber IOL implantation. The temporal approach was preferred because of the vagaries and disturbed anatomy present at the superior limbus in eyes which had previous intracapsular cataract extraction. As soon as foldable lenses were available in 1986, I utilized sutured clear corneal incisions for phacoemulsification and foldable IOL implantation in patients who had pre-existing filtering blebs. After these procedures, a marked reduction in surgically induced astigmatism was noted despite the fact that these incisions were corneal rather than scleral. In 1992, I began routinely utilizing clear corneal cataract incisions for phacoemulsification and foldable IOL implantation with incision closure using a tangential suture modeled after John Shepherd's technique.[15] Within a very short period, the suture was abandoned in favor of self-sealing corneal incisions.[16]

In a recent survey in *Eye World* magazine,[17] 60% of the American surgeons surveyed were utilizing self-sealing clear corneal cataract incisions for phacoemulsification and foldable IOL implantation, which was nearly double compared to the year before. Internationally, the percentage of phacoemulsification surgeons may be even larger at this time. We anticipate that these incisions will also be increasingly utilized for refractive lens surgery, including clear lensectomy with IOL implantation and IOL implantation into phakic eyes.

REFERENCES

1. Colvard DM, Kratz RP, Mazzocco TR, Davidson B. Clinical evaluation of the Terry surgical keratometer. *Am Intraocular Implant Soc J*. 1980;6:249-251.
2. Masket S. Origin of scleral tunnel methods. [Letter to the editor.] *J Cataract Refract Surg*. 1993;19:812-813.
3. Girard LJ, Hoffman RF. Scleral tunnel to prevent induced astigmatism. *Am J Ophthalmol*. 1984;97:450-456.
4. Maloney WF, Grindle L. *Textbook of Phacoemulsification*. Fallbrook, Calif: Lasenda Publishers; 1988:31-39.
5. McFarland MS. Surgeon undertakes phaco, foldable IOL series sans sutures. *Ocular Surgery News*. 1990;8.
6. Ernest PH. Presentation at the Department of Ophthalmology, Wayne State University School of Medicine, Detroit, MI, February 28, 1990.
7. Brown DC, Fine IH, Gills JP, et al. The future of foldables. *Ocular Surgery News*. 1992;Aug15(suppl). Panel discussion held at the 1992 annual meeting of the American Society of Cataract and Refractive Surgery.
8. Kelman CD. Phacoemulsification and aspiration: a new technique of cataract removal: a preliminary report. *Am J Ophthalmol*. 1967;64:23.
9. Harms H, Mackensen G. Intracapsular extraction with a corneal incision using the Graefe knife. In: *Ocular Surgery Under the Microscope*. Stuttgart, Germany: Georg Thieme Verlag; 1967:144-153.
10. Paton D, Troutman R, Ryan S. Present trends in incision and closure of the cataract wound. *Highlights of Ophthalmology*. 1973;14:3,176.
11. Arnott EJ. Intraocular implants. *Transactions of the Ophthalmological Society of the United Kingdom*. 1981;101:58-60.
12. Galand A. *La Technique de L'Enveloppe*. Liege, Belgium: Pierre Mardaga; 1988.
13. Stegmann R. Personal communication, December 3, 1992.
14. Shimizu K. Pure corneal incision. *Phaco & Foldables*. 1992;5:5-8.

15. Shepherd JR. Induced astigmatism in small incision cataract surgery. *J Cataract Refract Surg*. 1989;15:85-88.
16. Fine IH. Corneal tunnel incision with a temporal approach. In: Fine IH, Fichman RA, Grabow HB, eds. *Clear-Corneal Cataract Surgery & Topical Anesthesia*. Thorofare, NJ: SLACK Incorporated; 1993:5-26.
17. Snapshot. *Eye World*. 1998;3:70.

Controversies Regarding Clear Corneal Incisions

I. Howard Fine, MD, Richard S. Hoffman, MD

Initially, the utilization of clear corneal incisions was limited to those patients with pre-existing filtering blebs, patients on anti-coagulants or with blood dyscrasias, or patients with cicatrizing disease, such as ocular pemphigoid or Stevens-Johnson syndrome. Subsequently, because of the natural fit of clear corneal cataract incisions with topical anesthesia, the indications for clear corneal cataract surgery have expanded. With the ability to avoid any injections into the orbit and utilization of IV medications, those patients who had cardiovascular, pulmonary, and other systemic diseases that might have contraindicated cataract surgery became surgical candidates. Subsequently, through the safety and increasing utilization of these incisions by some pioneers in the United States, including Williamson, Shepherd, Martin, and Grabow,[1] these incisions became increasingly popular and utilized on an international basis.

Studies utilizing topographical analyses of these incisions by Rosen have demonstrated that clear corneal incisions 3 mm in width or less were topographically astigmatism-neutral.[2] This led to an increasing interest in these incisions and an increasing utilization of techniques including T-cuts, arcuate cuts, and limbal relaxing incisions for managing pre-existing astigmatism at the time of cataract surgery. Without astigmatism neutrality in the cataract incision, the predictability of adjunctive astigmatism-reducing procedures would be decreased, making it more difficult to achieve the desired result. In the initial studies and ultimate utilization of multifocal IOLs, the need for astigmatism neutrality was again a factor for stimulating interest in clear corneal incisions. Finally, the availability of phakic IOLs and the

need for control of astigmatism at the time of implantation of these lenses has driven many surgeons to consider clear corneal incisions as the route for phakic IOL implantation.

Other advantages of the temporal clear corneal incision include better preservation of pre-existing filtering blebs,[3] preservation of options for future filtering surgery, increased stability in the refractive results because of the neutralization of the forces from lid blink and gravity, the ease of approach to the incision site, the lack of need for bridle sutures and resultant iatrogenic ptosis, and finally the location of the lateral canthal angle under the incision which facilitates drainage.

Soon after my (IHF) presentation and later publication[4] on self-sealing corneal tunnel incisions, there was criticism surrounding the use of what later became named "self-sealing clear corneal incisions." The major concern was a fear of a possible increased incidence of endophthalmitis secondary to poor wound sealing and delayed wound healing. This controversy stimulated many studies into the strength and safety of clear corneal incisions compared to limbal and scleral tunnel incisions. Unfortunately, because of a lack of standardization in the definition of what constitutes a limbal vs clear corneal incision, considerable confusion has been generated in this area, making it difficult for surgeons to communicate and compare the relative claims of their individual techniques. Based on Hogan's *Histology of the Human Eye: An Atlas and Textbook* ("The external surface of the limbus is covered by the conjunctiva which ends at the periphery of Bowman's membrane. The conjunctival vessels are seen with the slit lamp as fine arcades that extend into clear cornea for about 0.5 mm beyond the limbal edge.")[5] and topographical studies of incisions done by Menapace[6] in Vienna, I categorized these incisions using the parameters of location and architecture.[7] An incision is termed "clear corneal" when the external edge is anterior to the conjunctival insertion, "limbal corneal" when the external edge is through conjunctiva and limbus, and "scleral corneal" when it is posterior to the limbus (Figure 2-1). In addition to the anatomic designation of the external incision, these incisions are also classified by their architecture as being either "single plane" when there is no groove at the external edge of the incision, "shallow groove" when the initial groove is less than 400 microns, and "deeply grooved" when it is deeper than 400 microns (Figure 2-2). In order to reduce the confusion and facilitate communication regarding these incisions, we believe they should be classified as either clear corneal, limbal corneal, or scleral corneal incisions and either single plane, shallow groove, or deep groove (Figure 2-3).

One of the most controversial criticisms of clear corneal incisions has been their relative strength compared to limbal or scleral incisions. Paul Ernest demonstrated that rectangular clear corneal incisions in cadaver eye models were less resistant to external deformation utilizing pinpoint pressure than square limbal or scleral tunnel incisions.[8,9] Subsequently, Mackool demonstrated that once the incision width was 3.5 mm or less and the length 2 mm or greater, there was an equal resistance to external deformation in clear corneal incisions as compared to scleral tunnel incisions.[10] In Ernest's work as well, as incision sizes got increasingly smaller, the force required to cause failure of these incisions became very similar for limbal and clear corneal incisions, and thus this could be used to further document the safety of incisions 3 mm or less.

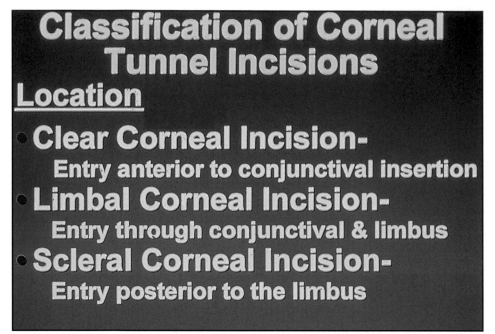

Figure 2-1. Classification of corneal tunnel incisions by external incision location.

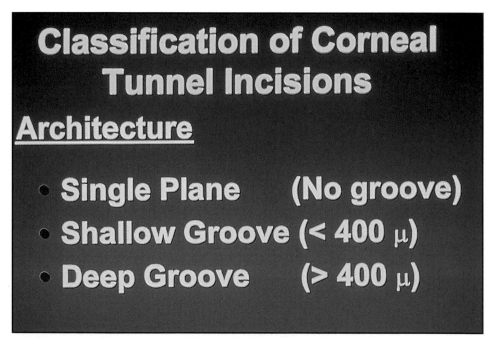

Figure 2-2. Classification of corneal tunnel incisions by wound architecture.

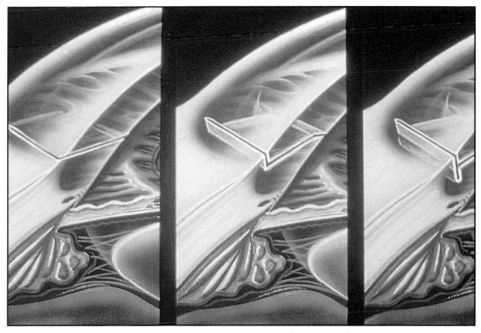

Figure 2-3. Architecture of clear corneal incisions. Single plane (left), shallow groove (center), and deep groove (right).

A major criticism of these cadaver studies is that there is a lack of functioning endothelium contributing to wound sealing. Others have also indicated that cadaver eye incision strength cannot be compared to incisions in vivo.[2] Ernest has compared in vivo posterior limbal incisions with clear corneal incisions and found that deep grooved clear corneal incisions performed better than shallow grooved or single-plane clear corneal incisions when challenged by pinpoint pressure. He also found that posterior limbal incisions performed better than clear corneal incisions when challenged by pinpoint pressure.[11]

Many surgeons have called into question the validity of pinpoint pressure as a clinically relevant test for cataract wound strength since the likelihood that anyone would challenge his or her own incision by pressing on it with something as fine as the instruments utilized to apply pinpoint pressure in these studies is highly unlikely. Regardless of whether more posteriorly placed incisions demonstrate increased strength compared to clear corneal incisions, the real question is whether that added strength is clinically significant or relevant. Surgeons, including myself (IHF), have demonstrated the stability of clear corneal incisions when a knuckle or a fingertip, the most likely way patients would challenge these incisions, was utilized (Figures 2-4a and 2-4b).[12,13] In addition, it is a well-known fact that a 1-mm "hypersquare" paracentesis will leak the day after surgery if pinpoint pressure is applied to its posterior lip; however, the likelihood of any paracentesis incision leaking spontaneously or with blunt pressure the day following surgery is extremely unlikely.

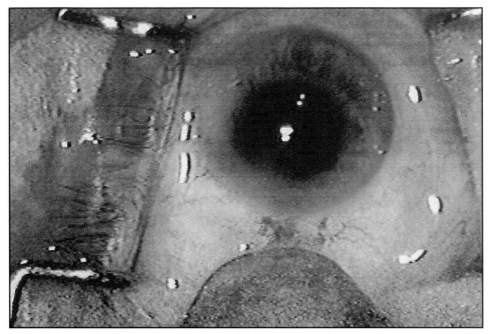

Figure 2-4a. Demonstration of self-sealability of clear corneal incision to the challenge of a blunt "knuckle" prior to application of pressure.

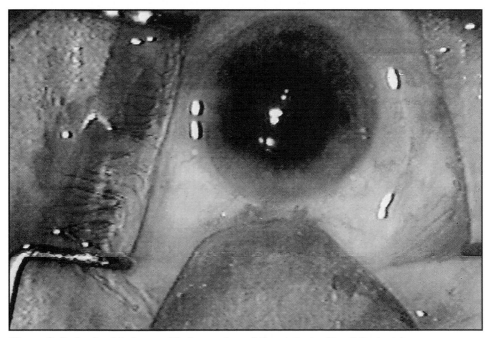

Figure 2-4b. Lack of leakage with depression of the posterior lip of the incision.

One final point of controversy regards the studies in cat eyes performed by Ernest et al.[14] These studies revealed a fibrovascular response in incisions placed in the limbus with extensive wound healing in 6 days compared to a lack of fibrovascular healing in clear corneal incisions. This study has been used to propose an increased safety for limbal incisions as compared to clear corneal incisions. Fortunately, the real issue for these various incisions is not healing but sealing. We feel that as long as an incision is sealed at the conclusion of surgery and remains sealed, the time before complete healing of the incision is accomplished is almost irrelevant, especially since there is still a 6-day period in which limbal incisions are not healed. An analogy can be drawn to the sealing that takes place during LASIK, in which there is no fibrovascular healing of the clear corneal interface, which has little effect on the strength, effectiveness, or safety of the wound, and in fact is an advantage by limiting scarring and an inflammatory healing response. Ultimately, the relative safety of one incision over another in the clinical setting will only be determined with the findings of a difference in the rate of incision-related complications which to date have not been demonstrated for incisions 4.0-mm wide or smaller.

One of the clear disadvantages of limbal corneal incisions is the greater likelihood of ballooning of conjunctiva, which can make visualization of anterior chamber structures during the surgical procedure more difficult. In addition, studies by Park[3] demonstrated that violation of the conjunctiva threatens the integrity not only of pre-existing filtering blebs but of the conjunctiva which would participate in filtering surgery at some future date. Finally, the presence of subconjunctival hemorrhage, although not important with respect to the ultimate function of the eye, may be of importance from a cosmetic perspective to the patient as well as to the survival of filtering blebs.

Controversy has led to an evolution of techniques and blade technology, and many surgeons have personal preferences for the architecture and construction of clear corneal cataract incisions. Single-plane incisions, as I (IHF) first described,[4] utilized a 3.0-mm diamond knife. After pressurization of the eye with placement of viscoelastic through a paracentesis, the eye was atraumatically fixated by the Fine-Thornton ring (Figure 2-5). The blade was placed on the eye in such a way that it completely applanated the eye with the point placed at the leading edge of the anterior vascular arcade. The knife was moved in the plane of the cornea until the shoulders, which are 2 mm posterior to the point of the knife, touch the external edge of the incision and then a dimple down technique is utilized to initiate the cut through Descemet's membrane. After the tip enters the anterior chamber, the initial plane of the knife is re-established to cut through Descemet's in a straight line configuration (Figure 2-6).

Williamson was the first to utilize a shallow 300- to 400-micron grooved clear corneal incision.[15] The rationale for the Williamson incision was that it led to a thicker external edge to the roof of the tunnel and less likelihood of tearing. Langerman later described the single-hinge incision in which requirements for the initial groove were 90% of the depth of the cornea anterior to the edge of the conjunctiva.[16] Initially, he utilized a depth of 600 microns and subsequently made the

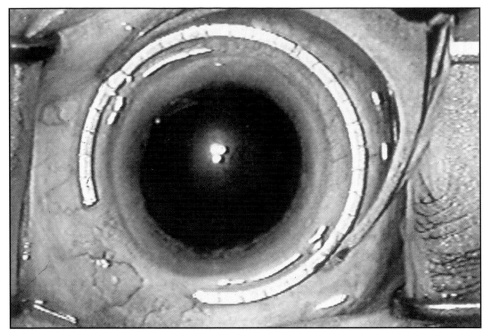

Figure 2-5. Application of the Fine-Thornton ring for side-port incision construction to the left.

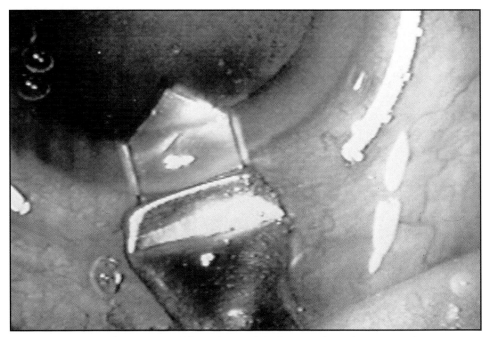

Figure 2-6. Completion of the incision with straight line cut through Descemet's membrane.

tunnel itself superficially in that groove, believing that this led to enhanced resistance of the incision to external deformation.

New blade technologies have been developed which have helped perfect incision architecture. The Fine Triamond knife (Figure 2-7) was developed in conjunction with Mastel Precision Instruments so that the incision could be made with an extremely sharp, thin, and narrow knife without a necessity for either dimpling down or cutting in a sawing motion, both of which resulted in some tendency for tearing of tissue or scrolling of Descemet's membrane. Subsequently, in conjunction with Rhein Medical, the 3-D blade (Figure 2-8) was developed which had differential slope angles to the bevels on the anterior vs the posterior surface (Figures 2-9a through 2-9d), resulting in an ability to just touch the eye at the site of the external incision location and advance the blade **in the plane of the cornea**. The differential slopes on the anterior vs posterior aspects of the blade allowed the forces of tissue resistance to create an incision that was characterized by a linear external incision, a 2.0-mm tunnel, and a linear internal incision without the need to dimple down or distort tissues to create the proper incision architecture (Figures 2-10a and 2-10b).[17,18] As one advances the knife, the blade automatically perforates Descemet's membrane 2.0 mm central to the external incision. The Rhein 3-D trapezoidal blade (Figure 2-11) also allows enlargement of the incision from 2.5 to 3.5 mm for IOL insertion without altering incision architecture as would occur by cutting to the side within the incision. With the trapezoidal 3-D blade, the surgeon merely replaces the knife in the incision and advances it forward as far as necessary.

The seal of the incision may be tested by covering the incision with fluorescein and depressing the posterior lip of the incision with a fingertip to demonstrate the presence of aqueous streaming through the pooled fluorescein on the surface of the eye. If necessary, one may enhance the seal by hydrating the stroma at the sides of the incision (Figure 2-12).

Clear corneal cataract incisions are becoming a more popular option for cataract extraction and IOL implantation throughout the world. Through the use of clear corneal incisions and topical and intracameral anesthesia, we have achieved surgery that is the least invasive of any kind in the history of cataract surgery with visual rehabilitation that is almost immediate. Clear corneal incisions have had a proven record of safety with relative astigmatic neutrality utilizing the smaller incision sizes. In addition, corneal incisions result in an excellent cosmetic outcome and should increase in popularity, especially as newer modalities such as phakic IOLs increase in popularity.

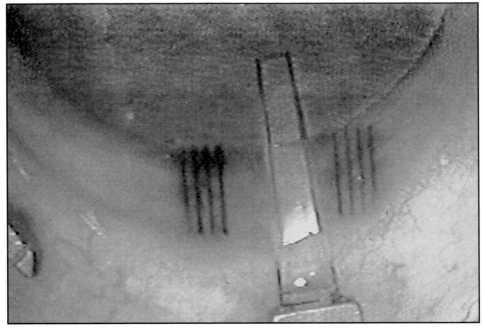

Figure 2-7. The Fine Triamond knife (Mastel Precision Instruments) cutting to the right in a cornea marked by the Fine cornea marker (Mastel Precision Instruments).

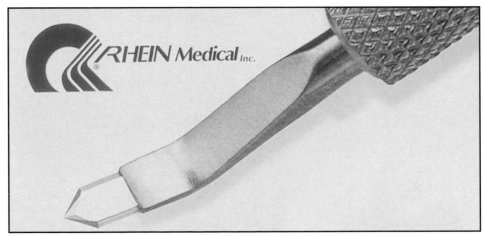

Figure 2-8. The Rhein 3-D diamond blade.

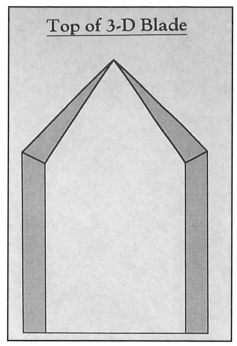

Figure 2-9a. Schematic representation of top view of the 3.0-mm Rhein 3-D diamond keratome.

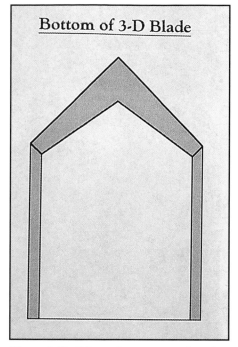

Figure 2-9b. Schematic representation of bottom view of the 3.0-mm Rhein 3-D diamond keratome.

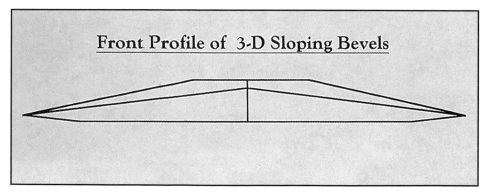

Figure 2-9c. The front profile of the keratome demonstrates the differential slopes on the anterior vs posterior aspects of the blade which allow the forces of tissue resistance to create the proper incision architecture.

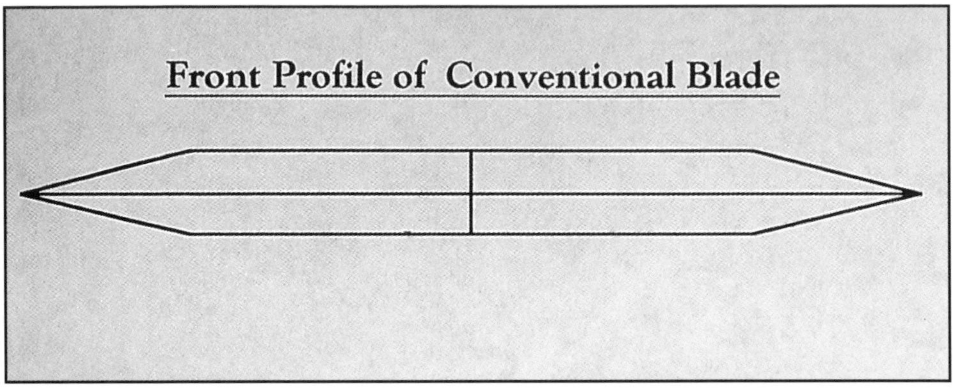

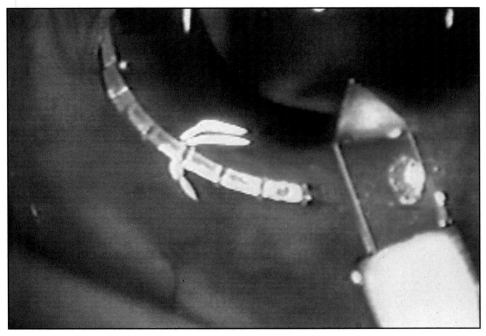

Figure 2-9d. Front profile of a conventional blade for comparison purposes.

Figure 2-10a. Entrance into Descemet's membrane 2 mm central to straight line external incision without dimple down maneuver.

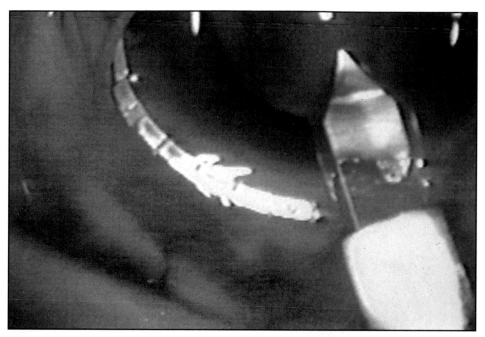

Figure 2-10b. Straight line internal construction with advancement of the blade.

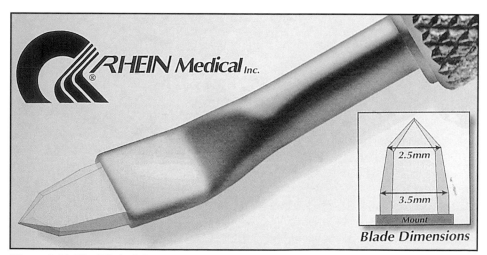

Figure 2-11. The Rhein 3-D trapezoidal blade with 2.5- to 3.5-mm blade dimensions.

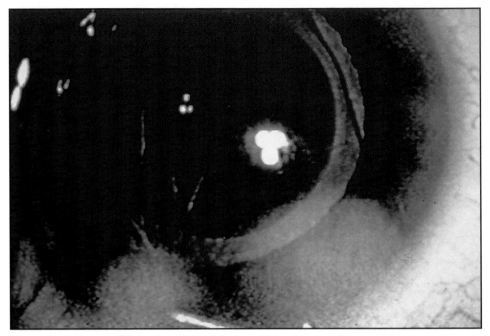

Figure 2-12. Stromal hydration with a 26-gauge blunt tip cannula.

REFERENCES

1. Fine IH, Fichman RA, Grabow HB, eds. *Clear-Corneal Cataract Surgery & Topical Anesthesia.* Thorofare, NJ: SLACK Incorporated; 1993.
2. Rosen ES. Clear corneal incisions: a good option for cataract patients. A roundtable discussion. *Ocular Surgery News.* 1998;Feb 1.
3. Park HJ, Kwon YH, Weitzman M, Caprioli J. Temporal corneal phacoemulsification in patients with filtered glaucoma. *Arch Ophthalmol.* 1997;115:1375-1380.
4. Fine IH. Self-sealing corneal tunnel incision for small-incision cataract surgery. *Ocular Surgery News.* 1992;May 1.
5. Hogan MJ, Alvarado JA, Weddell JE, eds. *Histology of the Human Eye: An Atlas and Textbook.* Philadelphia, Pa: WB Saunders Co; 1971:118-119.
6. Menapace RM. Preferred incisions for current foldable lenses and their impact on corneal topography. Abstract. Cataract Workshop on the Nile, Luxor-Aswan, Egypt, November 20, 1996.
7. Fine IH. Descriptions can improve communication. *Ophthalmology Times.* 1996;Dec 15.
8. Ernest PH, Lavery KT, Kiessling LA. Relative strength of scleral corneal and clear corneal incisions constructed in cadaver eyes. *J Cataract Refract Surg.* 1994;20:626-629.
9. Ernest PH, Fenzel R, Lavery KT, Sensoli A. Relative stability of clear corneal incisions in a cadaver eye model. *J Cataract Refract Surg.* 1995;21:39-42.
10. Mackool RJ, Russell RS. Strength of clear corneal incisions in cadaver eyes. *J Cataract Refract Surg.* 1996;22:721-725.
11. Ernest PH, Neuhann T. Posterior limbal incision. *J Cataract Refract Surg.* 1996;22:78-84.
12. Fine IH. New thoughts on self-sealing clear corneal cataract incisions. In: *Phaco Today— The Latest Developments in Phacoemulsification and Small Incision Cataract Surgery CD-ROM.* Ophthalmology Interactive Inc; 1995.
13. Fine IH. New thoughts on self-sealing clear corneal cataract incisions. *Eye Care*

Technology. 1995;5:67-68.

14. Ernest PH, Tipperman R, Eagle R, et al. Is there a difference in incision healing based on location? *J Cataract Refract Surg.* 1998;24:482-486.

15. Williamson CH. Cataract keratotomy surgery. In: Fine IH, Fichman RA, Grabow HB, eds. *Clear-Corneal Cataract Surgery & Topical Anesthesia.* Thorofare, NJ: SLACK Incorporated; 1993:87-93.

16. Langerman DW. Architectural design of a self-sealing corneal tunnel, single-hinge incision. *J Cataract Refract Surg.* 1994;20:84-88.

17. Fine IH. New blade enhances cataract surgery. Techniques spotlight. *Ophthalmology Times.* 1996;Sept 1.

18. Jacobi FK, Dick HB, Bohle RM. Histological and ultrastructional study of corneal tunnel incisions using diamond and steel keratomes. *J Cataract Refract Surg.* 1998;24:498-502.

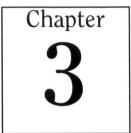

Chapter

3

Clear Corneal Incisions and Astigmatism

Emanuel Rosen, MD, FRCS, FRCOphth

CORNEAL INCISIONS AND CATARACT SURGERY: A HISTORICAL NOTE

Intracapsular cataract extraction, popular until the late 1970s, generally utilized a large corneal incision performed superiorly with against-the-rule astigmatism as a general consequence (Figure 3-1). The switch to extracapsular cataract extraction as IOL implantation became popular did little to resolve the post cataract astigmatic errors which prevailed because the large incision was necessary to incorporate a large IOL (Figure 3-2). As phacoemulsification extraction of the cataract was eventually followed by IOL designs capable of insertion through a small incision, the refractive aspects of cataract surgery assumed much greater relevance, particularly with reference to astigmatism. Initially, the concept of clear corneal incisions was rejected as the fear of induced astigmatism persisted. However, clear corneal incisions will not induce refractive change in the cornea if correctly managed. The utilization of corneal mapping has been an invaluable aid in our understanding of the effects of clear corneal incisions and graphically illustrates the issues considered herein.

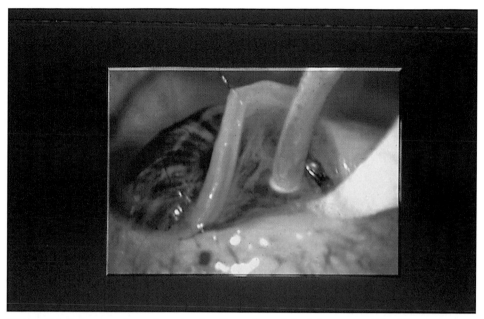

Figure 3-1. Intracapsular cataract extraction—the original clear corneal incision.

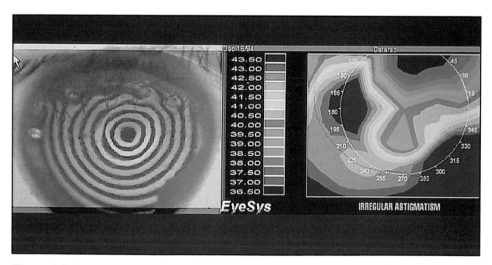

Figure 3-2. Large extracapsular cataract extraction clear corneal incision much too central with continuous suture resulting in gross corneal irregularity. Videokeratoscope view and tangential corneal topographic map.

RATIONALE OF CLEAR CORNEAL INCISIONS FOR CATARACT EXTRACTION AND IOL IMPLANTATION

- Excellent access to cataract/lens (Figures 3-3 through 3-7)
- Bloodless incision
- Quick and easy to perform
- Self-sealing/sutureless
- Variable incision architecture to reduce/eliminate pre-existing astigmatism
- Small incisions, <3 mm, will not induce astigmatism

REQUIREMENTS

- Phaco probe <3 mm preferred (Figure 3-8)
- Rigid irrigation sleeve to prevent corneal burns preferred (see Figure 3-8)
- Suitable knife for incision construction (eg, Mastel triamond, diamond keratome [various designs], steel keratomes [various designs]); see Figure 3-4

PRINCIPLE: THE SMALLER, THE BETTER

It is well understood that the larger a corneal incision is, the greater its effect on corneal refraction will be. Further, the closer the incision to the optical zone of the cornea, the greater its effect. Clear corneal incisions for cataract extraction and lens implantation are governed by two factors:

1. The size of the incision necessary to extract the cataract
2. The size of the incision necessary to enable IOL implantation

In fact, cataracts can be removed with exceptionally small phacoemulsification probes (1-mm Surgical Design Corp, Figure 3-9), but usually with a 2.5-mm standard probe from the same source. Other manufacturers of phacoemulsification equipment are increasingly making a 2.5-mm probe available. However, even in this era of foldable IOL implantation, 2.5 mm is too small to accommodate the injector or forceps used to deliver the IOL; 2.8 mm to 3.0 mm is the necessary minimum dimension. The question therefore arises: what is the largest clear corneal incision for cataract extraction and IOL implantation that will not have any effect on corneal refraction? The answer seems to be <3.0 mm in general but possibly <3.5 mm. There are individual eye/corneal factors as well as the precise nature of the corneal incision architecture. Another consideration is the protection of the clear corneal incision from the heat of the phacoemulsification needle probe, for if an incisional "burn" were to occur, then the corneal architecture would be grossly varied with dramatic refractive effects. Hence the preference for a rigid irrigation sleeve to preclude the possibility of a corneal burn with attendant permanent tissue shrinkage when utilizing a "tight" incision.

CLEAR CORNEAL INCISION DEFINITIONS

- Single-plane incision (Figure 3-10)—2.5- x 1.5-mm rectangular tunnel
- Two-plane incision (Figure 3-11)—2.5- x 1.5-mm rectangular tunnel
- Three-plane incision (Figure 3-12)—2.5- x 1.5-mm rectangular tunnel plus a perpendicular arcuate component

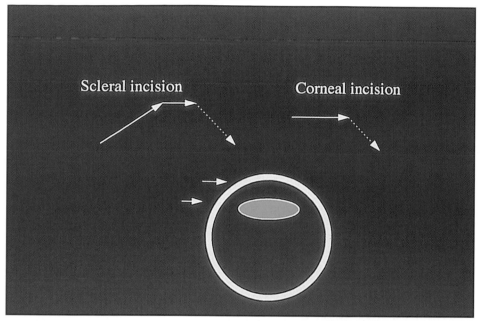

Figure 3-3. Phaco probe access to cataract. Scleral approach—uphill and downhill. Corneal access much easier.

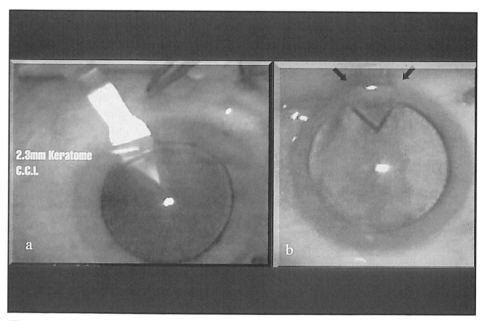

Figure 3-4. Clear corneal incisions (single plane) performed by a) 2.3-mm steel keratome and b) 2.5-mm diamond keratome. Approximate tunnel length: 1.5 mm.

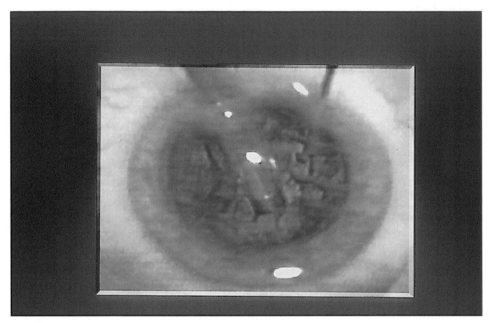

Figure 3-5. 2.5-mm Cobra Surgical Design phaco probe through a 2.4-mm clear corneal incision. Note polysulfone "rigid" irrigation sleeve to preclude the possibility of a corneal burn by inserting the probe through a tight incision.

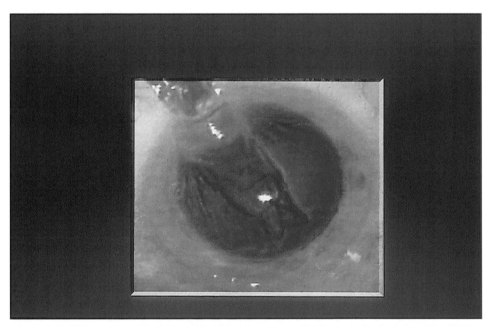

Figure 3-6. Clear corneal incision with IOL injector nozzle through the incision. The IOL is emerging from the injector (Staar AA plate haptic IOL).

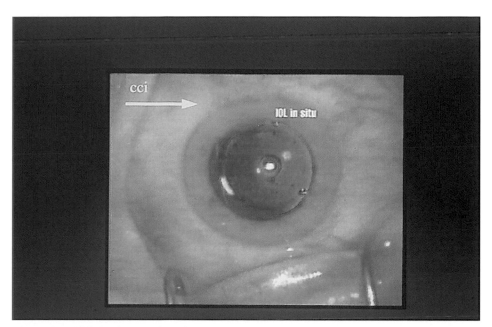

Figure 3-7. IOL in situ—self-sealing clear corneal incision.

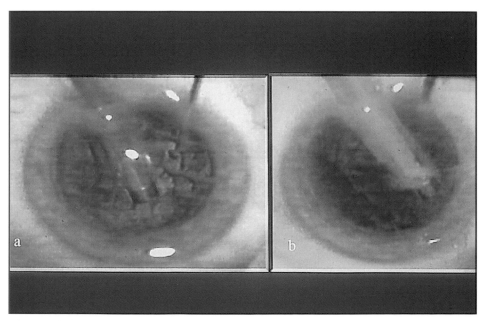

Figure 3-8. 2.5-mm phaco probe and 3.2-mm phaco probe and a clear corneal incision. The smaller probe has obvious advantages in limiting the size of the incision.

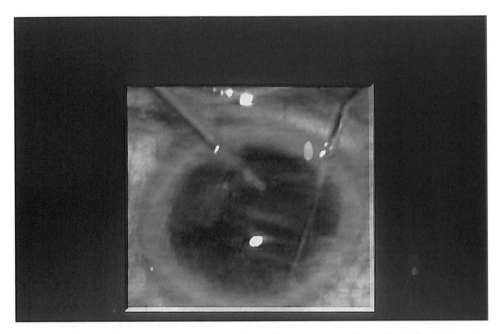

Figure 3-9. 1-mm Cobra phaco probe removing a dense cataract through a 1.1-mm clear corneal incision.

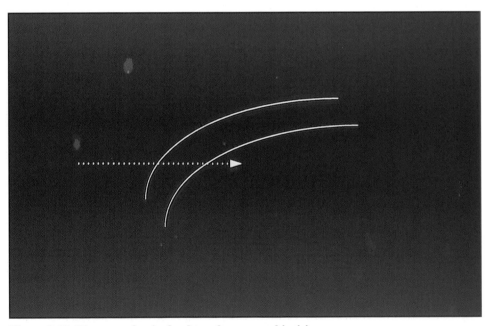

Figure 3-10. Diagram of a single-plane clear corneal incision.

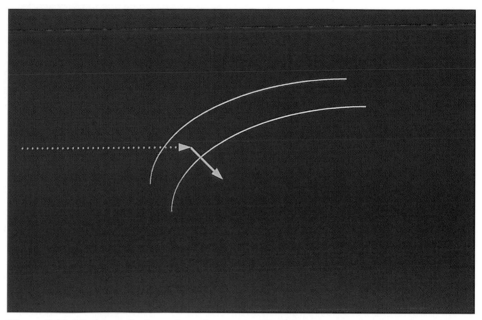

Figure 3-11. Diagram of a two-plane clear corneal incision.

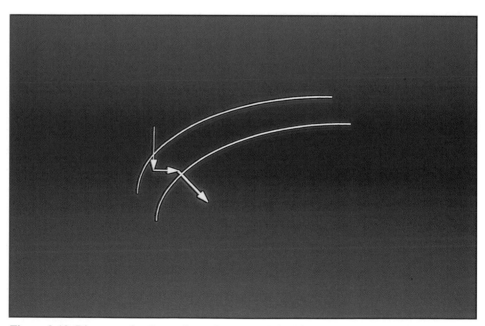

Figure 3-12. Diagram of a three-plane clear corneal incision wherein the first plane is a 50% perpendicular arc at the base of the clear corneal incision tunnel.

The difference between the single- and two-plane and the three-plane is the capacity of the three-plane to modify pre-existing astigmatism by its placement with centration on the steep corneal meridian.

As is well understood, the larger incision formerly employed in planned extra-capsular cataract extraction yielded an against-the-rule shift (Figure 3-13), ie, the radius of curvature of the cornea of the meridian on which the corneal incision was based would be increased, the reason being that the incision heals with a quantum of scar/fibrous tissue throughout its length. Tight sutures may reduce the effect, loose sutures would exacerbate the effect. By incorporating an arcuate component into the small clear corneal incision used for phacoemulsification cataract surgery, a planned increase in the radius of curvature (flattening) of the corneal meridian upon which it is based will occur. The longer the perpendicular arcuate component and the deeper the incision, the greater the effect (Table 3-1). Thus if an eye has preopera-tive astigmatism of sufficient degree (eg, >1.5 DC), then the three-plane incision can be based on the steep meridian to allow for its reduction while anticipating the 1:1 coupling effect which is usual but not invariable in this situation (Figure 3-14).

INDIVIDUAL VARIATION

Clear corneal incisions have an individual nature both from the surgeon's and the operated eye's perspective. No two incisions are really identical, but the general principle of the effect does hold well. If the effect is inadequate or exaggerated in an individual eye, then, using incisional corneal refractive methods, later adjustments are possible. Thus, clear corneal cataract and lens implant surgery should be viewed as a process in which a convenient (ie, a simple procedure such as arcuate keratoto-my and/or radial keratotomy) can improve the refractive outcome if either party so wishes. This point is emphasized because no surgical process is so precise that a 100% guarantee can be given. Accordingly, the algorithm for the length and depth of the arcuate component of a three-plane clear corneal incision has to be individu-ally compiled, yet Table 3-1 may be useful as a starting point.

It is strongly recommended that all surgeons performing clear corneal incisions for cataract surgery study the effect of their incisions on the cornea through the medium of corneal topography, particularly utilizing the local radius of curvature (tangential) algorithm which allows both peripheral corneal and central corneal shape effects to be evaluated (Figure 3-15).

RULES FOR CONTROL OF CORNEAL SHAPE

The usual refractive aim of lens extraction/IOL surgery is emmetropia, low degree of myopia, or in order to improve the depth of focus of an eye implanted with a monofocal IOL, a small degree of myopic astigmatism (Sturm's conoid). To achieve these ends from a purely astigmatic viewpoint, the following rules should apply.

Rule 1

Perform corneal topography preoperatively so that the pre-existing corneal astigmatism may be recognized and recorded. Astigmatism at the corneal plane is different than the spectacle astigmatic correction.

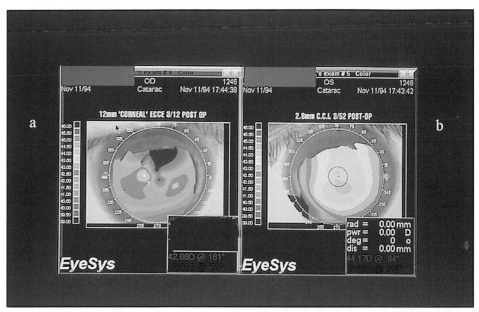

Figure 3-13. a) Large incision clear corneal incision with resultant against-the-rule astigmatism and b) 2.8-mm clear corneal incision, no astigmatism.

Table 3-1 Potential Algorithms		
Astigmatism Magnitude (Plus Cylinder)	**Arcuate Incision Degrees**	**Arcuate Incision Depth**
1 D	30	50%
1 to 2 D	45	50%
2 to 3 D	60	50%
3 to 4 D	90	50%

- S = C/1+VS where
- S = Spectacle correction in diopters
- C = Corneal plane refraction
- V = Vertex distance in meters

(The greater the vertex distance, the more effective is a plus lens and the less effective a minus lens, ie, a plus cylinder astigmatic component of a spectacle lens will be greater than the cylindrical component at the corneal plane as revealed by topography.) It is the corneal plane element that is to be reduced or eliminated by surgical adjustment.

Rule 2

If no change in corneal shape is required (ie, no significant preoperative astigmatism), then an astigmatically neutral clear corneal incision should be performed (ie, <3 mm). See Figure 3-16.

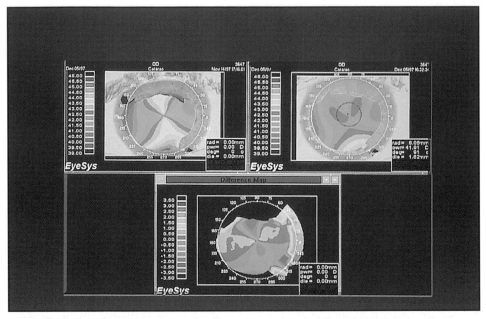

Figure 3-14. Preoperative with-the-rule three-dimensional astigmatism offset by three-plane clear corneal incision incorporating perpendicular arc based on the 100 degree meridian. Corneal topographic difference map. Note coupling effect.

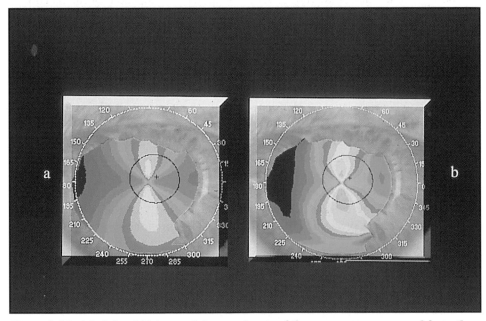

Figure 3-15. a) Axial and b) tangential corneal map of the same cornea prepared from the same data to illustrate some subtle differences in appearance. The tangential map gives a more accurate representation of true corneal shape.

Rule 3

If preoperative corneal astigmatism is identified, then note the location of the steep corneal meridian and base the clear corneal incision thereupon utilizing a three-plane clear corneal incision, wherein the initial component is a perpendicular arc of 50% depth and an extent commensurate with the degree of astigmatism bearing in mind the probability of a 1:1 coupling effect (see Table 3-1 and Figure 3-17).

EVOLUTION OF INCISIONS

Cataract surgery in evolving from larger incision extractions to small incisions has naturally coincided with an increasing awareness of the refractive aspects of visual rehabilitation. The early answer to reduction of incision size was to place the incision as far back as possible into the so-called "funnel of astigmatic neutrality"— the scleral tunnel incisions. Frowns, smiles, and many variations were explored as were one-suture and sutureless incisions as IOL design allowed their implantation through smaller incisions, though still larger than that strictly necessary for cataract extraction. The limitations of scleral incisions were overcome by the recognition that clear corneal sutureless incisions were not only possible but advantageous for modern cataract/lens IOL surgery by Dr. I. Howard Fine in particular. Most surgeons accepted that clear corneal sutureless incisions for lens surgery were simpler and desirable, but in the main they were and still are opposed to the concept, for fear of not being able to control the refractive (ie, astigmatic) component of the incision.

THE EFFECTS OF CLEAR CORNEAL INCISIONS

Of course, clear corneal tunnel sutureless incisions for lens extraction and IOL implantation require a sufficient bore ideally to allow the IOL to be inserted through the same incision without enlargement. The question therefore arises: What is the effect on corneal refraction of such incisions and how important are their construction and dimensions?

In order to understand the effects of clear corneal sutureless incisions, it is necessary to consider the design and optical characteristics of the cornea and its lamellar structure. The shape of the corneal dome derived in part from its coherent lamellar collagen bundles is altered locally or generally by incisions into its substance. Traumatic corneal lesions affect the regularity of the corneal surface, their local refractive properties, through their effect upon the optical zone as well as its transparency.

Comprehending the refractive outcome of some corneal trauma led to the emergence of surgical techniques to effect a controlled change in the refractive properties of the cornea by planned incisions. Clear corneal incisions for lens surgery are merely an extension of that process. As long as they are controlled (ie, planned) and their outcome understood, they can be used to significant advantage as part of the process of lens refractive surgery, the cornea as it were providing the opportunity for fine tuning that process. The cornea is a toroidal asphere, ie, it is steeper centrally than peripherally with degrees of toricity varying from minor to major. Its intrinsic design is calculated in the natural sense to offset optical aberrations, spherical aberrations in particular.

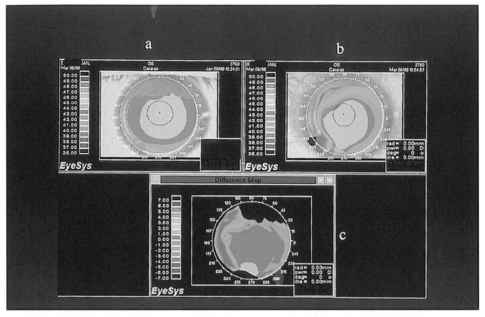

Figure 3-16. Corneal topography difference map (EyeSys) showing a) the preoperative corneal map, b) the postoperative corneal map, and c) the difference between the two. Note there is no difference for the clear corneal incision was <3 mm.

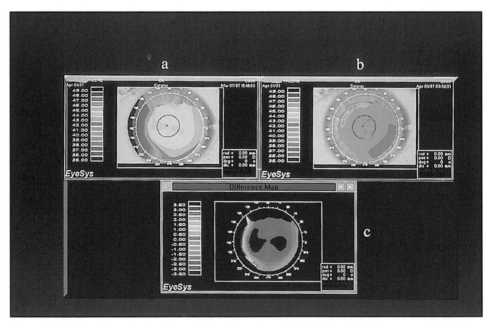

Figure 3-17. An example of a three-plane clear corneal incision on 180 degree meridian to control pre-existing astigmatism, flattening of the steep meridian is the main effect. a) Preoperation corneal map, b) postoperative corneal map, and c) difference = effect of three-plane incision.

The optical zone of the cornea is approximately central and overlies the "entrance pupil," ie, the image of the actual pupil which appears 14% larger to the observer as a consequence of corneal magnification. The central portion of the optical zone of the cornea through the Stiles Crawford effect handles about 80% of the light rays which form the retinal image. Accordingly, more peripheral light rays passing through the periphery of the optical zone are less relevant to the patient's image perception. Thus the effects of clear corneal tunnel sutureless incisions have to be weighed from the refractive viewpoint against their actual impingement upon the optical zone. To take two extremes: a 1-mm clear corneal incision at the edge of the cornea will have no effect whatsoever upon the shape of the optical zone or its optical properties (Figure 3-18). At the other extreme, a large extracapsular cataract extraction incision into clear cornea extending through an arc of 150 to 180 degrees even if sutured will have a profound effect on central corneal refraction with the well-understood against-the-rule astigmatic effect (see Figure 3-13a). The large incision with edges not firmly bound together by the healing process incorporates a microgape, albeit infilled with fibrous scar tissue. The net result is a lengthening of the radius of curvature of the meridian upon which the incision is centrally based (ie, the meridian is flatter than it was originally). In eyes with no preoperative astigmatism, change must not be induced. But this is an effect that can be utilized to advantage in the neutralization of a pre-existing astigmatic component. However, the temptation to combine the cataract surgical incision which embraces an element to correct pre-existing astigmatism with independent arcuate keratotomy incisions is best resisted until the cornea has stabilized postoperatively when the residual astigmatism, if any, can be properly assessed. A secondary intervention is then appropriate (see below).

KERATOMETRY STUDY ON CLEAR CORNEAL INCISIONS AND MORE

It is frequently argued that temporal placement of clear corneal incisions has less refractive effect than incisions placed elsewhere. Further, it is argued that if an element of astigmatism were induced it would be with-the-rule rather than against-the-rule resulting from superior incisions. Though there is some justification in these beliefs (Figures 3-19 and 3-20),[1] it is the size of the incision and its juxtaposition to the optical zone of the cornea that is more important. Once again, surgeons are advised to evaluate the effects of their incisions based upon a consistent architecture and location. Figures 3-21 and 3-22 illustrate the refractive effects of clear corneal sutureless incisions <3 mm and >5 mm. Corneal topography provides an immediate recorded graphic expression of the corneal refractive status following clear corneal incision. Sequential studies also illustrate the temporal effects of the healing incisions. Keratometric studies will provide data on the outcome of a series of cases (see Figures 3-19 and 3-20). We all imprint our own art onto the science of incisions, and therefore must recognize that even for the individual surgeon, no two incisions are exactly identical. Thus the scope for variation needs to be assimilated by surgeons in order to achieve a consistent outcome.

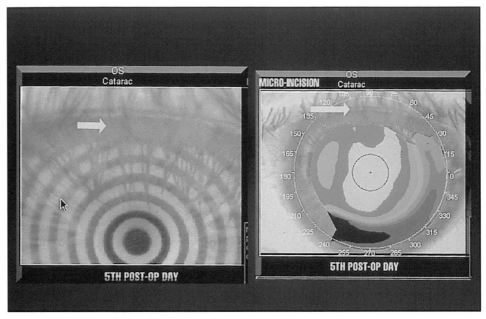

Figure 3-18. 1.1-mm clear corneal incision for cataract extraction in high myopia where no IOL was required to achieve a low myopic postoperative refraction. Note no refractive effect of the small incision <3 mm.

SUTURES AND CLEAR CORNEAL INCISIONS

It may be necessary on occasion to place an interrupted 10-0 nylon suture even in a small clear corneal incision as a temporary measure or to initiate stability of a three-plane clear corneal incision incorporating the longer perpendicular arcuate component (Figure 3-23). By so doing and studying the topography of the cornea, valuable information can be gleaned regarding clear corneal incision management. As the suture is removed 10 days postoperatively (Figures 3-24 and 3-25), there is an immediate localized flattening of the peripheral cornea through the arcuate component of the incision. This change is transmitted to the steep meridian causing an immediate flattening of 1 D at the corneal plane. The actual difference is clearly revealed on the topographic difference map.

In summary, clear corneal incision has many attributes generally and rather than creating refractive problems, it provides the means for a satisfactory solution to pre-existing astigmatic errors of refraction.

POST CATARACT SURGERY ASTIGMATISM ADJUSTMENT

The management of residual refractive errors after cataract and IOL surgery is part of the process, for however hard we try, there will be eyes that have not responded as expected and troublesome astigmatism lingers or is induced. Therefore, post surgical adjustment of residual refractive errors is part and parcel of both cataract and IOL surgery as well as lens refractive surgery. The principle of post surgical adjustment is that it should be convenient (ie, rapid, inexpensive, and comfortable).

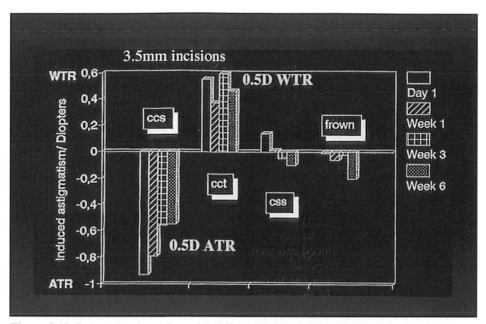

Figure 3-19. Induced astigmatism with different 3.5-mm self-sealing incisions. ccs = clear corneal superior, cct = clear corneal temporal, css = cornea scleral superior, frown = scleral frown superior. Autokeratometer evaluation of 3.5-mm incisions at 1 day, 1 week, 3 weeks, and 6 weeks postoperatively. 3.5-mm incisions ccs = 0.5 D against-the-rule and cct = 0.5 D with-the-rule incisions. Reprinted with permission from Nielsen J. *J Cataract Refract Surg.* **1995;21(1):43.**

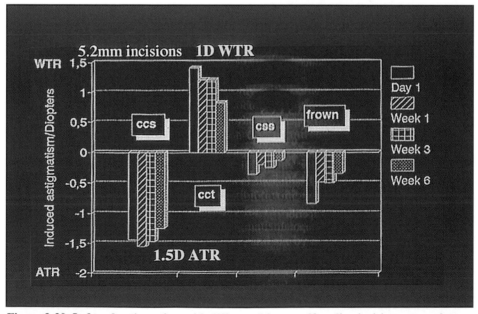

Figure 3-20. Induced astigmatism with different 5.2-mm self-sealing incisions. ccs = clear corneal superior, cct = clear corneal temporal, css = cornea scleral superior, frown = scleral frown superior. Autokeratometer evaluation of 5.2-mm incisions at 1 day, 1 week, 3 weeks, and 6 weeks postoperatively. 5.2-mm incisions ccs = 1.5 D against-the-rule and cct = 1.0 D with-the-rule incisions. Reprinted with permission from Nielsen J. *J Cataract Refract Surg.* **1995;21(1):43.**

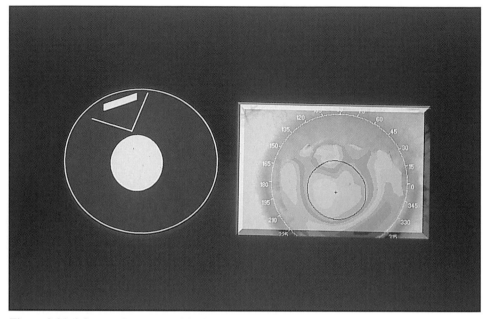

Figure 3-21. 2.8-mm clear corneal incision causes local effect only. Optical zone spherical.

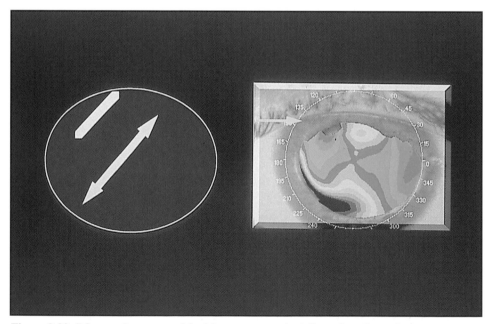

Figure 3-22. 5.5-mm clear corneal incision causes against-the-rule astigmatism.

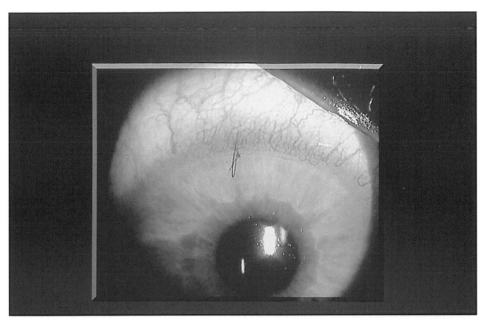

Figure 3-23. Three-plane clear corneal incision incorporating 60 degree arcuate component plus one tight suture.

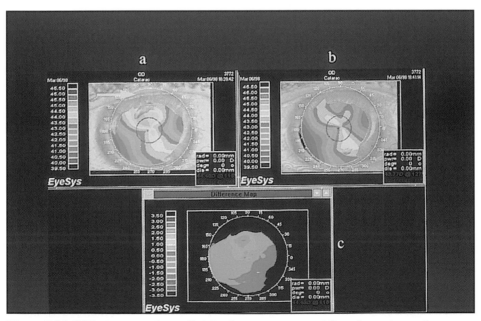

Figure 3-24. Difference map immediately after suture removal 2 weeks postoperative demonstrating localized peripheral corneal flattening, reduction of optical zone astigmatism to 1 D, and good visual acuity in spite of symmetrical three-arm steeper hemi-meridians. a) Suture in place (arrow), b) suture removed, and c) demonstrates the difference (ie, flattening effect of released suture tension).

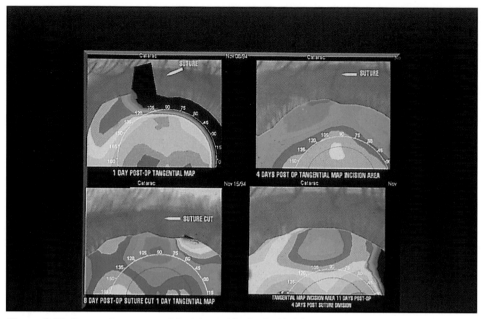

Figure 3-25. 3-mm clear corneal incision with single 10-0 interrupted nylon suture removed at 8 days postoperative. a) Suture in place 1 day postoperative, b) corneal map 4 days postoperative, c) suture cut 8 days postoperative with immediate localized corneal flattening invading the optical zone, and d) 11 days postoperative regression of flattening effect a process which continued so that the optical zone remained anastigmatic.

This implies that a simple arcuate keratotomy (Figures 3-26 and 3-27) or non-contact laser thermal keratoplasty (LTK) may be applied for the fine tuning of the refractive result. Figure 3-28 illustrates an eye with post cataract against-the-rule treated by LTK to complete the refractive process of lens extraction and IOL implantation (see Figures 3-29 and 3-30 for difference maps).

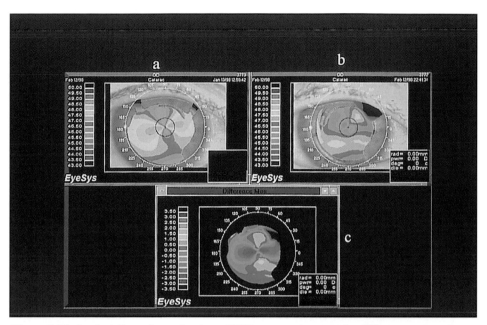

Figure 3-26. Against-the-rule post cataract/IOL surgery topography difference map. a) Before arcuate keratotomy -2.0/+4.0 x 10 = 20/20, b) after arcuate keratotomy -0.50/+0.75 x 50 = 20/20, and c) with resultant difference correction of astigmatism. Uncorrected visual acuity = 20/25.

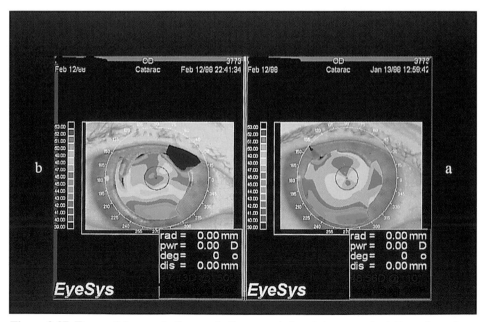

Figure 3-27. Tangential maps before and after arcuate keratotomy, against-the-rule post cataract/IOL surgery. a) Before arcuate keratotomy -2.0/+4.0 x 10 = 20/20 and b) after arcuate keratotomy -0.50/+0.75 x 50 = 20/20. Uncorrected visual acuity = 20/25.

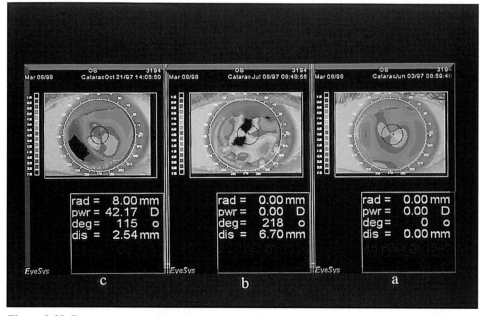

Figure 3-28. Post cataract astigmatism treated by astigmatic non-contact holmium (Sunrise 1000) LTK. Tangential maps. a) Pretreatment, b) immediately after LTK, and c) 4 months later stable spherical central cornea (ie, large incision extracapsular corneal cataract extraction against-the-rule astigmatism eliminated).

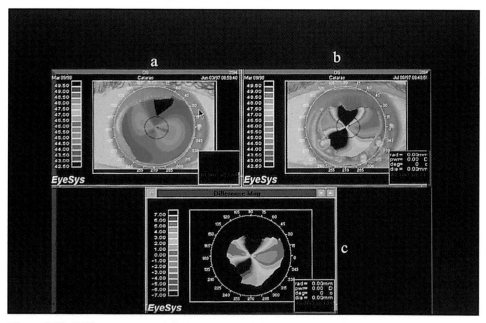

Figure 3-29. Difference map. a) Post cataract against-the-rule astigmatism, b) immediate effect of LTK, steepening of flat meridian alone, and c) difference to show steepening effect with no coupling.

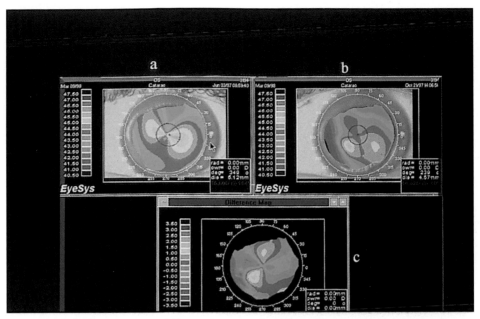

Figure 3-30. Difference map. a) Post cataract against-the-rule astigmatism, b) 4 months later stable spherical optical zone of the cornea, and c) difference to show steepening permanent effect now with coupling (ie, flat meridian steepened and steep meridian flattened).

REFERENCES

1. Prospective evaluation of surgically induced astigmatism and astigmatic keratotomy effects of various self-sealing small incisions per Julius Nielsen. *J Cataract Refract Surg.* 1995;21(1):43.

Making the Transition to Temporal Clear Corneal Cataract Surgery Under Topical Anesthesia

Richard S. Hoffman, MD

INTRODUCTION

There are essentially two methods one can undertake to transition from a superior scleral tunnel cataract extraction technique under local anesthesia to temporal clear corneal surgery under topical and intracameral anesthesia. The first method involves a complete shift from the former technique to the latter—analogous to jumping into a pool of refreshing yet very cold water. Although in retrospect this seems a simple and straightforward change in approach, prior to beginning clear corneal surgery the notion of undertaking this change can be extremely intimidating to many surgeons. The second method involves a slow methodical transition in incremental steps, changing one aspect of the surgical procedure at a time, in order to reduce the anxiety that can occur with making any transition to a new surgical procedure or technique. This slow, incremental wading into the pool of clear corneal surgery allows the surgeon to master each new aspect of the new surgical procedure and confront the potential complexities and complications of each step prior to adding additional changes to his or her technique.

When making this slow transition to clear corneal surgery, it is best to first become familiar with the various foldable lenses and insertion devices available for small incision surgery. Once use of these devices is mastered, shifting the surgical location to the temporal location and introduction of the clear corneal incision should then follow. If the surgoen is unfamiliar with surgery under topical anesthesia, comfort with the clear corneal incision and all of its nuances should occur prior to undertaking the apprehensive but simple transition to topical anesthesia. It is by

means of these progressive changes that each surgeon can make a safe, composed, and confident transition to this rewarding and satisfying technique.

FOLDABLES

As the first step in making the transition to clear corneal surgery, one should become familiar with the use of foldable IOLs inserted through a superior scleral tunnel incision. Foldable IOLs come in essentially two varieties: plate haptic lenses and three-piece lenses. The instruments used to insert these lenses are numerous but can also be divided into two varieties: cartridge injectors and folding and inserting forceps.

Plate lenses offer some advantages over three-piece lenses in that they are perhaps easier to insert and fit better into the smaller lens capsules of hyperopic eyes. Although older style plate lenses were reported to have an increased tendency for lens decentration,[1,2] alterations in the lens positioning holes have been shown to allow for better fixation within the capsular bag.[3] Although easier to insert, complications that may arise during the phacoemulsification procedure, such as a torn anterior capsulorrhexis or torn posterior capsule, may prohibit their use requiring the insertion of a three-piece foldable lens within the capsular bag or ciliary sulcus. In addition, the recently released multifocal AMO Array is a three-piece foldable lens which should become increasingly popular for insertion in appropriate patients requesting useful acuity at both distance and near. Thus, familiarity with both lens styles is suggested, especially if plate lenses are used as the primary lens for insertion.

Some of the newest advances in lens insertion technology surrounds the use of cartridge injector systems. There are many perceived advantages of implanting foldable IOLs with injector systems as compared to folding forceps. These advantages include the possibility of greater sterility, ease of folding and insertion, and implantation through smaller incisions.[4-6]

AMO has designed a new cartridge injector system called the Unfolder AMO Phacoflex II Implantation System for second-generation silicone three-piece foldable lenses with PMMA haptics (Figure 4-1). It has a cartridge with a 45 degree bevel-down configuration which can implant the SI40 and Array IOLs through a 2.8- to 3.0-mm clear corneal incision. The tip of the insertion rod has a Teflon cap so that tearing of the lens is avoided. After the viscoelastic-lined cartridge has been loaded and the lens folded, the cartridge tip is inserted through the incision into the anterior chamber with the bevel down. The bevel is then rotated slightly to the surgeon's left so that the leading haptic is pointing to the surgeon's left as the optic is advanced with the handpiece rod. The leading loop of the IOL should always point to the surgeon's left throughout the entire procedure. As the optic is advanced, the bevel will need to be rotated down and then to the surgeon's right in order to keep the lens in proper orientation (Figure 4-2). The leading haptic is placed into the bag as the IOL is released. Once the optic is completely out of the cartridge, the handpiece rod is retracted proximal to the end of the trailing haptic and then advanced with the bevel down in order to place the trailing haptic within the bag. Placing the bevel completely within the capsulorrhexis at this stage of insertion will keep the optic in place and ensure placement of the trailing loop.

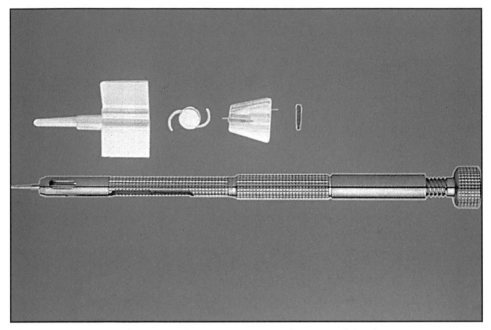

Figure 4-1. AMO Unfolder cartridge injector system. Courtesy of AMO.

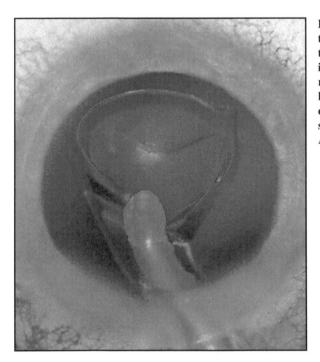

Figure 4-2. Implantation of a three-piece foldable IOL using the AMO Unfolder cartridge injector. The cartridge bevel is rotated to the right in order to keep the lens in the proper orientation as it is ejected by the soft blue Teflon tip. Courtesy of AMO.

Although cartridge injector systems have become the preferred method for lens insertion, familiarity with folders and forceps is important especially in those instances when lenses will need to be inserted into the ciliary sulcus because of bag compromise. Newer forceps for foldable lens implantation include the Fine Universal III forceps (Rhein #05-2339R) (Figure 4-3), the Nichamin II loader and inserter (Rhein #05-2346 and #05-2348) (Figure 4-4), the Buratto insertion forceps (Asico AE-4275), and the Lehner II loader and inserter (Rhein #05-2376 and #05-2377) (Figure 4-5). Although these folders can insert both silicone and acrylic IOLs, the Buratto and Lehner II forceps have been specifically designed for acrylic lens insertion.

All three-piece foldable lenses are being manufactured with PMMA haptics in order to increase haptic stability and decrease the rate of lens decentration. Older lens insertion techniques for use with prolene haptics utilized tucking the haptics between the folded halves of the lens prior to insertion through the incision. This technique does not work well with PMMA haptics, which may snap permanently or kink when being tucked. In general, the technique for folding and implanting three-piece lenses with PMMA haptics is as follows.

The lens is grasped with the insertion forceps held in the dominant hand and then placed into the folder or on the surface from which it can be purchased by the folder in the non-dominant hand. The lens is folded and then the insertion device, in the dominant hand, holds the folded lens which is ready for insertion. When lenses are folded across the 12 and 6 o'clock axis, they are oriented in the holding or insertion instrument with a leading and trailing haptic. This is the preferred orientation for inserting and unfolding a lens in the anterior chamber for dialing into the ciliary sulcus. In contrast, folding across the 10 and 4 o'clock axis (oblique axis) or across the 9 and 3 o'clock axis will yield a folded configuration with both haptics pointed inferiorly with the fold superiorly. For placement into the capsular bag, after insertion through the incision, the hand is brought into a proper position so that the fold is superior. After the leading haptic has been delivered under the distal capsulorrhexis, the forceps are slowly opened (direct-acting forceps) or closed (reverse-acting forceps), allowing the lens to unfold. The trailing haptic is then usually dialed into the capsular bag to the left. Using the folded orientation with both haptics directed inferiorly will negate the need for dialing in the trailing haptic since both haptics will unfold into the capsular bag pulling the optic through the capsulorrhexis.[7-9]

TEMPORAL SURGERY

Perhaps one of the most challenging aspects of making the transition to clear corneal surgery is the change from the superior to the temporal location. The temporal location offers many advantages including better access to the lens without brow obstruction and improved visualization with a better red reflex. Other advantages include better preservation of pre-existing filtering blebs,[10] preservation of options for future filtering surgery, the lack of need for bridle sutures with resultant iatrogenic ptosis, increased stability in the refractive results because of the neutral-

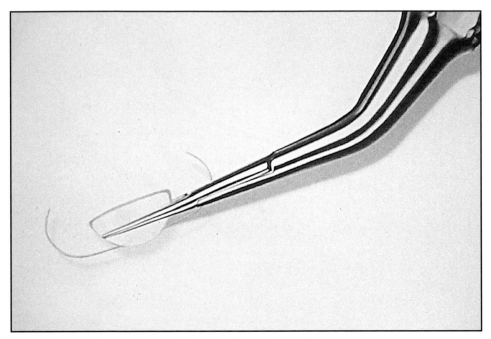

Figure 4-3. The Fine Universal III forceps (Rhein #05-2339R).

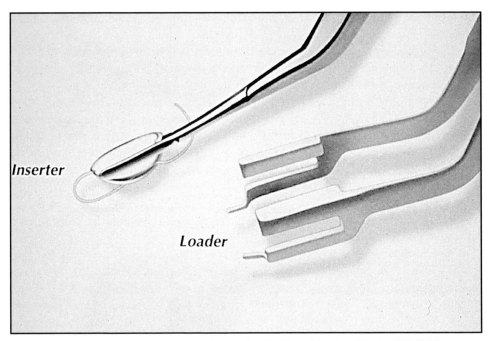

Figure 4-4. The Nichamin II inserter (Rhein #05-2348) and loader (Rhein #05-2346).

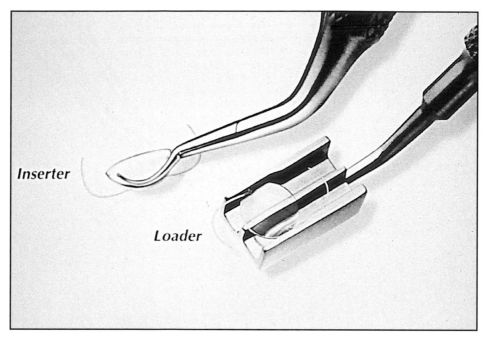

Figure 4-5. The Lehner II inserter (Rhein #05-2377) and loader (Rhein #05-2376).

ization of the forces from lid blink and gravity, and finally the location of the lateral canthal angle under the incision which facilitates drainage.

Two of the obstacles to overcome when rotating to the temporal location include loss of wrist support by the patient's forehead and the difficulty with leg placement under and around the head of the operating table.

Although not necessary, if available, a Chan wrist rest (Figure 4-6) can allow the surgeon to operate temporally with similar hand support as is present when operating superiorly. The wrist rest should be set at a level so that a hand resting on the support arm, and parallel to the floor, does not rise above the level of the lateral canthus (Figure 4-7). If the wrist rest is set too high, access to the patient's eye becomes awkward; thus it is better to err on setting the support too low rather than too high. Eventually, the Chan wrist rest can be abandoned, although it does allow for a nice pocket to be created between the patient's head and the support arm for drainage collection.

One of the most awkward aspects of temporal clear corneal surgery is the difficulty with leg and pedal placement under the operating table. Even with the best of operating tables, it is difficult, if not impossible, to operate temporally with the surgeon's legs under the table. An operating stretcher with a tapered head (Figure 4-8) allows the surgeon easier access to the head of the bed by allowing him or her to straddle the table with his or her legs (Figure 4-9). Depending on which foot is used to perform phacoemulsification, the pedals are positioned with the phaco pedal adjacent to and to the outside of the stretcher wheel with the focusing pedal at the head of the bed when operating on the right eye (Figure 4-10). If surgery is performed on

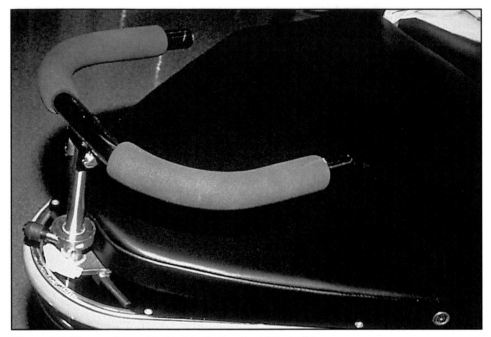

Figure 4-6. Chan wrist rest bolted to the head of OR stretcher.

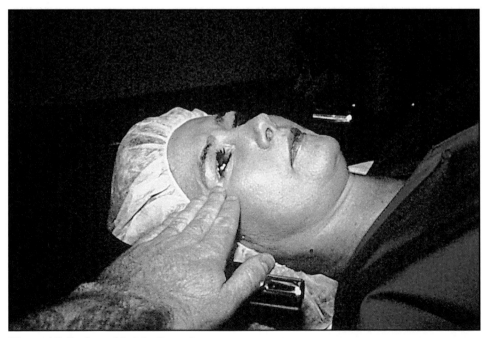

Figure 4-7. Preferred height for wrist rest arm.

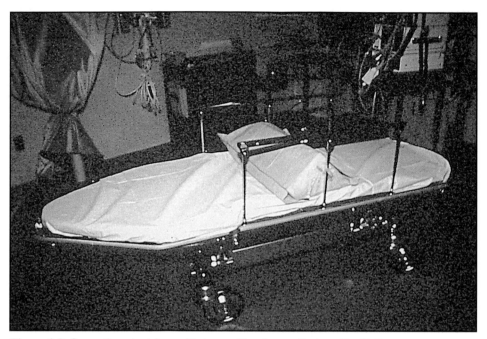

Figure 4-8. Operating stretcher with tapered head manufactured by Reliance.

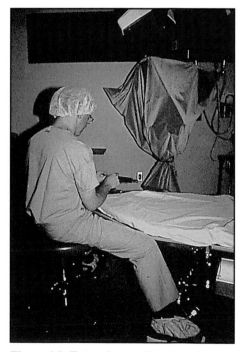

Figure 4-9. Tapered operating stretcher allows the surgeon to straddle the head of the bed with his or her legs.

a square hospital OR table, there is usually more leg room under the foot of the bed than at the head; thus, placing the patient's head at the foot of the bed will permit more leg room. In addition, using a thinner mattress allows the bed to be raised a few inches which can many times make a significant difference in leg positioning.

Prior to proceeding with clear corneal surgery, the surgeon may wish to perform scleral tunnel phacoemulsification from the temporal location in order to become accustomed to the temporal location before adding the additional change in technique of a clear corneal incision. Since the vascular arcade is located more posteriorly at the temporal limbus than the superior limbus, using this landmark as the site for anterior chamber entry (as is customary for superior scleral tunnel incisions) will usually result in premature entry and difficulty

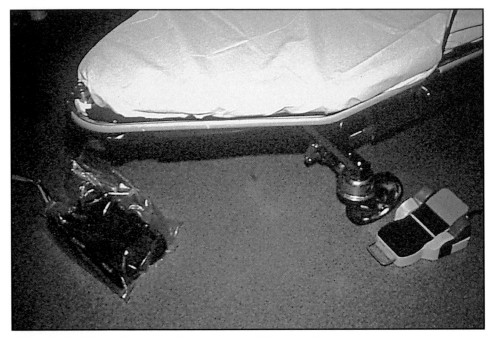

Figure 4-10. Pedal orientation of operating on right eye using temporal approach.

with potential iris prolapse. Thus, it is important to ensure that the internal incision entry into the anterior chamber is at least 2 mm from the temporal limbus when a temporal scleral tunnel incision is used. Usually, after one or two temporal scleral tunnel cases, familiarity with the temporal position is adequate to proceed with the clear corneal incision.

CLEAR CORNEA

The ideal patient for your first clear corneal cataract extraction is one with a small amount of against-the-rule astigmatism and a moderate nuclear sclerotic cataract—not too hard and not too soft. Essentially, the grade of cataract with which the surgeon is most comfortable removing from a scleral tunnel approach is the best candidate for initial clear corneal surgery. When beginning this technique, avoid patients with extremely dense nuclei, corneal endothelial dystrophy, and miotic pupils or floppy irides. As familiarity with this incision grows, these more challenging cases can be added with ease.

When making the incision, a decision must be made as to whether to groove or not groove the external aspect of the incision. Non-grooved single-plane incisions[11] utilize a 2.5- to 3.0-mm diamond knife. After pressurization of the eye with placement of viscoelastic through a paracentesis, the blade is placed on the eye so that it completely applanates the limbus with the point placed at the leading edge of the anterior vascular arcade. Using a Fine-Thornton ring for fixation, the knife is moved in the plane of the cornea until the shoulders, which are 2 mm posterior to the point of the knife, touch the external edge of the incision. A dimple down technique is then

used to initiate the cut through Descemet's membrane. After the tip enters the anterior chamber, the initial plane of the knife is re-established to cut through Descemet's in a straight line configuration. If the blade is allowed to fully enter the anterior chamber in the dimple down position, the edges of the internal incision will many times tear similar to the effect of opening a can with a triangular can opener.

A grooved clear corneal incision[12] is created in the same fashion differing only in that a 300- to 400-micron deep groove is placed just anterior to the temporal limbus first (with either a guarded diamond step knife or a diamond RK knife if a step knife is not available) prior to creating the corneal tunnel incision (Figure 4-11a). The tunnel incision is formed by placing the tip of the diamond keratome in the base of the groove, applanating the posterior lip of the incision, and entering the anterior chamber in the same orientation as is used for the single-plane incision (Figure 4-11b). The rationale for a grooved incision is that it produces a thicker external edge to the roof of the tunnel with less likelihood of tearing. One disadvantage of a grooved incision is that instruments may occasionally get caught in the floor of the incision when entry into the anterior chamber is attempted.

For a transitioning surgeon's first cases, a grooved incision approximates the technique previously used for scleral tunnel incision construction and thus seems a natural and less intimidating step to clear corneal surgery conversion. Although diamond knives offer the advantages of more precise wound construction, steel keratomes can be used successfully for a surgeon's first cases until the investment in diamond keratomes is made.

One of the newer advances in diamond keratome design is Rhein Medical's 3-D blade. The 3-D knife was developed with differential slope angles to the bevels on the anterior and the posterior surfaces resulting in an ability to create a perfect incision just by advancing the blade in the plane of the cornea in a manner similar to placing a paracentesis site. The differential slopes on the anterior and posterior aspects of the blade allow the forces of tissue resistance to create a single-plane incision that is characterized by a linear external incision, a 2-mm tunnel, and a linear internal incision without the need to dimple down or distort tissues to create the proper incision architecture.[13] The trapezoidal 3-D blade also allows enlargement of the incision to 3.5 mm for IOL insertion without altering incision architecture (Figure 4-12). When using the 3-D knife it is important to angle the blade up into the plane of the cornea and not the plane of the iris since the latter will result in a shortened corneal tunnel with an increased incidence of iris prolapse and loss of incision self-sealability.

Once the clear corneal incision is constructed, cataract surgery can then proceed using the surgeon's preferred technique. Performing cortical cleaving hydrodissection[14] prior to hydrodelineation allows for easier cortical clean-up by breaking the cortical-capsular connections at the lens equator. Frequently, cortex can be completely removed during trimming and flipping maneuvers of the lens epinucleus without the need for the I/A handpiece.[15]

Following phacoemulsification, lens implantation, and removal of residual viscoelastic, stromal hydration of the clear corneal incision can be performed in order to help seal the incision.[16] This is performed by placing the tip of a 26- or 27-gauge

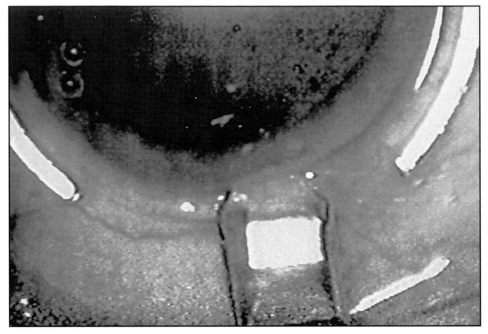

Figure 4-11a. Guarded diamond knife produces grooved incision in temporal clear cornea.

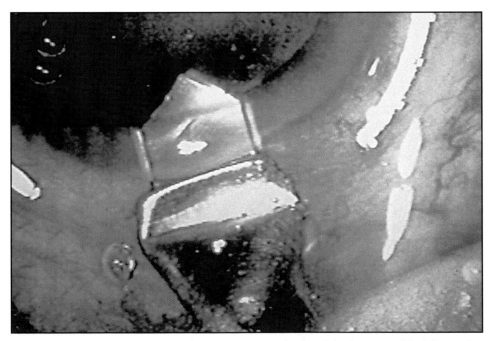

Figure 4-11b. After the tip of the diamond keratome is placed in the grooved incision and the posterior lip of the incision is depressed, the keratome is advanced in order to produce a shallow and deep grooved incision.

cannula in the side walls of the incision and gently irrigating balanced salt solution into the stroma (Figure 4-13). This is performed at both edges of the incision in order to help appose the roof and floor of the incision. Once apposition takes place, the hydrostatic forces of the endothelial pump will help seal the incision. In those rare instances of questionable wound integrity, a single radial 10-0 nylon suture should be placed to ensure a tight seal.

TOPICAL ANESTHESIA

One of the most profound changes in the evolution of cataract surgery has been the transition from local anesthesia to topical and intracameral anesthesia. This transition is perhaps the most intimidating step for the average cataract surgeon because of a perceived loss of control of the operating field. In reality, this change from local to topical anesthesia is an easy transition with many rewards for the patient and surgeon.

If the surgeon is already familiar with topical anesthesia through a scleral tunnel approach, switching to clear corneal surgery under topical anesthesia is really no different and can be made easily once the surgeon becomes familiar with the temporal approach. For the novice topical surgeon, certain precautions for the initial cases will make this transition simple and less stressful.

The ideal patient for one's first topical cataract removal are similar for the ideal patient for one's first clear corneal case. The surgeon's "Goldilocks" lens (not too hard and not too soft) in a cooperative patient with a small amount of against-the-rule astigmatism is ideal. Although most anyone can undergo cataract surgery under topical anesthesia, certain personality types and observations have been found to be indicators for the appropriateness for topical anesthesia. Dementia, mental retardation, hysteria, language barrier, and deafness are obviously not good patient traits for a surgeon's early topical anesthesia cases.[17] In general, how well a patient performs during tonometry, A-scan biometry,[18] and indirect ophthalmoscopy is a good predictor of patient suitability for topical anesthesia.

Topical anesthesia can be performed with almost any topical anesthetic including tetracaine,[19] Marcaine, and lidocaine.[20] Although adjusting the pH of topical lidocaine has been found to result in higher aqueous concentrations,[21] more complete analgesia can result from placing 0.3 to 0.5 cc of nonpreserved lidocaine 1% directly into the anterior chamber as an adjunct to topical anesthesia.[21-23] Intracameral lidocaine has been demonstrated to be safe and well tolerated by both the corneal endothelium and the retina.[24-26] In addition, it allows for a more profound anesthetic effect which allows for increased intraocular manipulations such as iris stretching and scleral fixation of IOLs.

One of the major advantages of topical and intracameral anesthesia, other than the added safety from the elimination of orbital injections and immediate visual recovery, is the ability to have the patient assist with the surgical procedure. Since full ocular motility is maintained, the patient can improve exposure by looking up or down during placement of the paracentesis and during insertion of secondary instruments through the paracentesis. During lens insertion, the patient can assist by

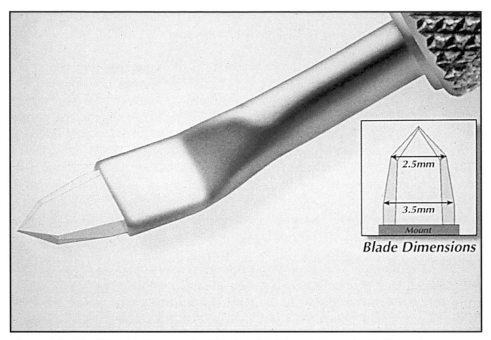

Figure 4-12. The Rhein 3-D trapezoidal blade with 2.5- to 3.5-mm blade dimensions.

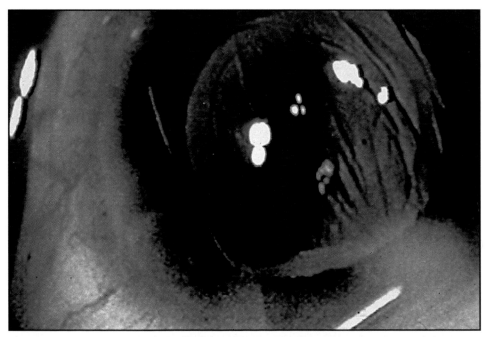

Figure 4-13. Stromal hydration of the incision is created by placing the tip of a 26-gauge cannula in the side walls of the incision and gently irrigating balanced salt solution into the stroma. This is performed at both edges of the incision in order to help appose the roof and floor of the incision.

looking slightly temporal while the lens injector or folding forceps is inserted. This allows for added resistance to the forces directed nasally by the injector or forceps being placed through a small incision.

During the majority of the procedure, the patient can maintain relative ocular immobility by looking straight into the light of the operating microscope. The light should be turned down prior to beginning the case in order to help the patient adapt to the intense brightness. After viscoelastic is placed in the eye and the clear corneal incision is constructed, the light intensity can slowly be increased to maximize visualization during capsulorrhexis formation and phacoemulsification. If the patient is unable to find the light during the procedure and increased ocular motility and wandering develop, asking the patient to look straight ahead usually stops the movement. Warning the patient about sensations of pressure (during fixation ring placement and lens insertion) and loss of vision (during hydrodelineation and phacoemulsification) helps keep both the patient and surgeon calm during the procedure.

Perhaps the most amazing aspect of clear corneal surgery under topical and intracameral anesthesia is the lack of patient discomfort even during significant ocular manipulation. As comfort with this technique increases and anxiety abates, the novice surgeon can rapidly address more challenging cases under topical anesthesia such as hard nuclei and small pupils. Topical anesthesia should eventually become the preferred method for cataract extraction in most patients, except perhaps the intractable lid squeezers, patients with dementia, and small children. It is safe, effective, and well tolerated by patients, without the need for systemic sedation.[27]

ADJUNCTIVE ASTIGMATIC REDUCTION TECHNIQUES

The final step in the transition to clear corneal lens surgery under topical anesthesia is the addition of astigmatic reduction techniques. With small amounts of against-the-rule astigmatism, a 3.0-mm temporal clear corneal incision can reduce up to 0.5 D of astigmatism. Numerous studies have been performed documenting the safety and low magnitudes of astigmatism induced by these incisions depending on their size. Masket has documented by vector analysis 0.50 D of induced cylinder and <0.25 D of cylinder change in the surgical meridian using 3.0- x 2.5-mm self-sealing temporal clear corneal incisions. He was also able to demonstrate the refractive stability of these incisions 2 weeks following surgery.[28] Kohnen compared the surgically induced astigmatism of 3.5-, 4.0-, and 5.0-mm grooved temporal clear corneal incisions and found a mean induced astigmatism of 0.37 D, 0.56 D, and 0.70 D, respectively, after 6 months.[29]

When reduction of larger amounts of astigmatism is desired, various means are available to reduce pre-existing astigmatism. Fine continues to utilize a temporal location for the cataract incisions and adds one or two T-cuts made by the Feaster knife with a 7-mm ocular zone and a 640-micron blade setting. Others, including Lindstrom and Rosen, rotate the location of the incision to the steep axis in order to achieve some increased flattening at the steepest axis to address pre-existing astigmatism. Arcuate keratotomies, using a standard arcuate keratotomy nomogram, can

be placed at a 7.0-mm optical zone in the steep axis prior to constructing a temporal clear corneal incision for those accustomed to this technique. Kershner utilizes the corneal incision in the temporal half of the eye by starting with a nearly full thickness T-cut through which he then makes his corneal tunnel incision. For large amounts of astigmatism he uses a paired T-cut in the opposite side of the same meridian.[30] Finally, the popularization of limbal relaxing incisions by Nichamin[31] and Gills and Gayton[32] adds an additional means of reducing large amounts of pre-existing astigmatism by utilizing the groove for the limbal relaxing incision as the site of entry for the clear corneal cataract incision. Paired limbal relaxing incisions can be used to reduce large amounts of pre-existing astigmatism.

CONCLUSION

From a personal perspective, the transition from a scleral tunnel cataract incision under local anesthesia to a temporal clear corneal incision under topical anesthesia seems to have been unnecessarily prolonged. Although a change to this rewarding technique can be made in one single jump, a slow methodical transition can reduce the stress and anxiety that many surgeons experience when making any alterations in their surgical technique and approach. By changing one aspect of the surgical procedure at a time, the aspiring surgeon should be less intimidated by this transition and able to make a safe and atraumatic passage into the soothing waters of advanced clear corneal surgery.

REFERENCES

1. Mackool RJ. Decentration of plate-haptic lenses. [Letter.] *J Cataract Refract Surg.* 1996;22:396.
2. Gonzalez GA, Irvine AR. Posterior dislocation of plate haptic silicone lenses [Letter.] *Arch Ophthalmol.* 1996;114:775-776.
3. Kent DG, Peng Q, Isaacs RT, Whiteside SB, Barker DL, Apple DJ. Security of capsular fixation: small- versus large-hole plate-haptic lenses. *J Cataract Refract Surg.* 1997;23:1371-1375.
4. Steinert RF, Deacon J. Enlargement of incision width during phacoemulsification and folded intraocular lens surgery. *Ophthalmology.* 1996;103:220-225.
5. Mackool RJ, Russell RS. Effect of foldable intraocular lens insertion on incision width. *J Cataract Refract Surg.* 1996;22:571-574.
6. Olson R, Cameron R, Hovis T, Hunkeler J, Lindstrom R, Steinert R. Clinical evaluation of the Unfolder. *J Cataract Refract Surg.* 1997;23:1384-1389.
7. Fine IH. Response. In: Masket S, ed. Consultation section. *J Cataract Refract Surg.* 1992;18:207-208.
8. Oh KT, Oh KT. Optimal folding axis for acrylic intraocular lenses. *J Cataract Refract Surg.* 1996;22:667-670.
9. Shugar JK. Implantation of AcrySof acrylic intraocular lenses. *J Cataract Refract Surg.* 1996;22:1355-1359.
10. Park HJ, Kwon YH, Weitzman M, Caprioli J. Temporal corneal phacoemulsification in patients with filtered glaucoma. *Arch Ophthalmol.* 1997;115:1375-1380.
11. Fine IH. Self-sealing corneal tunnel incision for small-incision cataract surgery. *Ocular Surgery News.* 1992;May 1.
12. Williamson CH. Cataract keratotomy surgery. In: Fine IH, Fichman RA, Grabow HB, eds. *Clear-Corneal Cataract Surgery & Topical Anesthesia.* Thorofare, NJ: SLACK Incorporated; 1993:87-93.

13. Fine IH. New blade enhances cataract surgery. Techniques spotlight. *Ophthalmology Times*. 1996;Sept 1.

14. Fine IH. Cortical cleaving hydrodissection. *J Cataract Refract Surg*. 1992;18:508-512.

15. Fine IH. The chip and flip phacoemulsification technique. *J Cataract Refract Surg*. 1991;17:366-371.

16. Fine IH. Corneal tunnel incision with a temporal approach. In: Fine IH, Fichman RA, Grabow HB, eds. *Clear-Corneal Cataract Surgery & Topical Anesthesia*. Thorofare, NJ: SLACK Incorporated; 1993:5-26.

17. Fichman RA. Topical anesthesia. In: Fine IH, Fichman RA, Grabow HB, eds. *Clear-Corneal Cataract Surgery & Topical Anesthesia*. Thorofare, NJ: SLACK Incorporated; 1993:101-103.

18. Fraser SG, Siriwadena D, Jamieson H, Girault J, Bryan SJ. Indicators of patient suitability for topical anesthesia. *J Cataract Refract Surg*. 1997;23:781-783.

19. Fichman RA. Phacoemulsification with topical anesthesia. In: Fine IH, Fichman RA, Grabow HB, eds. *Clear-Corneal Cataract Surgery & Topical Anesthesia*. Thorofare, NJ: SLACK Incorporated; 1993:114-118.

20. Williamson CH. Topical anesthesia using lidocaine. In: Fine IH, Fichman RA, Grabow HB, eds. *Clear-Corneal Cataract Surgery & Topical Anesthesia*. Thorofare, NJ: SLACK Incorporated; 1993:122-128.

21. Zehetmayer M, Rainer G, Turnheim K, Skorpik C, Menapace R. Topical anesthesia with pH-adjusted versus standard lidocaine 4% for clear corneal cataract surgery. *J Cataract Refract Surg*. 1997;23:1390-1393.

22. Gills JP, Cherchio M, Raanan MG. Unpreserved lidocaine to control discomfort during cataract surgery using topical anesthesia. *J Cataract Refract Surg*. 1997;23:545-550.

23. Koch PS. Anterior chamber irrigation with unpreserved lidocaine 1% for anesthesia during cataract surgery. *J Cataract Refract Surg*. 1997;23:551-554.

24. Garcia A, Loureiro F, Limao A, Sampaio A, Ilharco J. Preservative-free lidocaine 1% anterior chamber irrigation as an adjunct to topical anesthesia. *J Cataract Refract Surg*. 1998;24:403-406.

25. Fry LL. Intracameral preserved lidocaine. [Letter to the editor.] *J Cataract Refract Surg*. 1997;23:10.

26. Hoffman RS, Fine IH. Transient no light perception visual acuity after intracameral lidocaine injection. *J Cataract Refract Surg*. 1997;23:957-958.

27. Johnston RL, Whitefield LA, Giralt J, et al. Topical versus peribulbar anesthesia, without sedation, for clear corneal phacoemulsification. *J Cataract Refract Surg*. 1998;24:407-410.

28. Masket S, Tennen DG. Astigmatic stabilization of 3.0 mm temporal clear corneal cataract incisions. *J Cataract Refract Surg*. 1996;22:1451-1455.

29. Kohnen T, Dick B, Jacobi KW. Comparison of the induced astigmatism after temporal clear corneal tunnel incisions of different sizes. *J Cataract Refract Surg*. 1995;21:417-424.

30. Kershner RM. Clear corneal cataract surgery and the correction of myopia, hyperopia, and astigmatism. *Ophthalmology*. 1997;104:381-389.

31. Nichamin L. Refining astigmatic keratotomy during cataract surgery. *Ocular Surgery News*. 1993;Apr 15.

32. Gills JP, Gayton JL. Reducing pre-existing astigmatism. In: Gills JP, et al, eds. *Cataract Surgery: The State of the Art*. Thorofare, NJ: SLACK Incorporated; 1998:53-66.

Intraocular Anesthesia in Clear Corneal Cataract Surgery

James P. Gills, MD, Myra Cherchio, COMT

ANESTHESIA IN CLEAR CORNEAL CATARACT SURGERY

The development of clear corneal surgery spurred a concurrent interest in topical anesthesia.[1] The less invasive nature of the temporal clear corneal wound and the quicker procedure made topical anesthesia more feasible. Topical anesthesia provides a number of advantages over regional blocks, including cost, safety, and quicker visual rehabilitation. However, forgoing a regional block requires calm and cooperation from the patient. Many patients, due to anxiety, were not considered suitable candidates for topical anesthesia without supplemental IV sedation, which presents its own set of risks. Moreover, some patients complained of sensations from intraocular manipulations.

We have found intraocular anesthesia with unpreserved lidocaine a safe and effective method of addressing the limitations of topical anesthesia.[2] Intraocular anesthesia reduces or eliminates the sensations caused by intraocular manipulations that occur during phacoemulsification, thus reducing anxiety. Most patients have no need for supplemental IV, eliminating problems such as bruising or anxiety over the needle.

INTRAOCULAR ANESTHESIA

Anecdotal reports[3] of inadvertent intracameral injection of lidocaine indicated no complications and a normal postoperative course. These case reports led us to hypothesize that intracameral injection of an appropriate solution of this drug could

safely eliminate discomfort that patients may experience with topical anesthesia alone. In fact, Fichman had already described the use of preservative-free tetracaine for intracameral injection to reduce intraoperative discomfort in select patients undergoing surgery under topical anesthesia,[1] in instances where patient anxiety mounted during phacoemulsification.

The rationale for use of intraocular lidocaine is summarized in Table 5-1. We began using small doses of intracameral lidocaine for select cases with limited visual potential and found no adverse effects. The solution used was 1% unpreserved and epinephrine-free. Lidocaine is potent and has a very fast onset. The duration, though relatively short, is adequate. These features, combined with low toxicity, make it a good choice for intraocular anesthesia. Impressed with the efficacy observed in these cases and assured that there was no endothelial damage, we increased the dose to 0.1 cc.

CLINICAL STUDIES OF INTRAOCULAR LIDOCAINE

We designed a masked, randomized, prospective, parallel group study to evaluate the safety and efficacy of intraocular lidocaine. Patients were eligible for the randomized study if they were to undergo uncomplicated cataract extraction by phacoemulsification with insertion of a folded silicone IOL through an incision size of 3.2 mm or less and there were no contraindications for topical anesthesia. Contraindications included known allergic response to the topical anesthetics or lidocaine and any corneal or ocular conditions precluding the use of topical anesthesia. Patients scheduled for triple procedures (IOL + trabeculectomy) were also excluded. However, patients with small pupils were not excluded as long as they were eligible for the phacoemulsification procedure. Patients scheduled for either corneal and/or limbal relaxing incisions to correct astigmatism were also eligible for the study.

All study patients received topical anesthesia under the following regimen: proparacaine 0.5%, 1 drop administered twice, and Marcaine 0.75%, 1 drop instilled four times. Patients who expressed anxiety were given Versed just prior to surgery regardless of study treatment.

The study treatments were as follows: 0.10 cc unpreserved, epinephrine-free lidocaine at 1.0%, or 0.10 cc unpreserved BSS. Study medication for the day was dispensed by preloading the syringes ready for intracameral injection and was administered after entry into the anterior chamber. After intracameral injection, an interval of 1 minute passed before starting phacoemulsification. At specified intervals (1, 3, and 5 minutes after administration), the patient's discomfort/pain level was measured using a predefined uniform scale administered by the nurse anesthetist. In addition, the patient was asked if there was discomfort or pain midway during phacoemulsification and midway during lens insertion. The patient had also been instructed to utilize a predetermined hand motion to spontaneously signal any pain or discomfort if necessary, including both mild pressure and increased pressure. The goal was to evaluate all sensations the patient might feel, although mild pressure was not uncomfortable to the patient.

Table 5-1
Use of Intraocular Lidocaine
• Documentation of inadvertent injection into anterior chamber with no adverse effects • Selected clinical use in patients with limited vision potential • Gradual dosage increase • Randomized study • Routine use of 0.5 cc 1% lidocaine

The surgeon would then determine, based on patient response, if an additional dose of lidocaine was needed. The level of pain or discomfort was quantified with a five-point scale:

0 = No sensation

1+ = Mild pressure (no discomfort)

2+ = Increased pressure (uncomfortable)

3+ = Moderate pain

4+ = Sharp pain

5+ = Severe pain

Efficacy of treatment was assessed by comparing pain or discomfort level as determined using the scale. The pain/discomfort scores were assessed during phacoemulsification and during lens insertion. In addition, patients were classified according to the highest expressed pain/discomfort score occurring at any time during the procedure. The need for additional medication (added lidocaine for the lidocaine group or a first dose of lidocaine for the BSS group) and/or the need for sedation were also used to monitor efficacy. The safety of intraoperative lidocaine was assessed by IOP, visual acuity, anterior chamber cell and flare measurements, and endothelial cell counts.

Mean age and the means of the pain scores for each group (range: 0 to 5+) were compared using two-tailed t-tests. The distributions of gender, pain/discomfort scores, visual acuities, and scores for aqueous flare and cells were compared between groups using a chi-square test with continuity correction. All statistical analyses were carried out using SAS[4] or Statmost.[5]

Results

Placebo-Controlled Study

A total of 303 procedures were performed under topical anesthesia: 183 received intraoperative lidocaine and 120 received BSS and constituted the control group. A pain/discomfort score was not obtainable from one of the lidocaine patients. The groups were comparable with respect to age and sex distribution, the use of Versed administered for anxiety, and the use of astigmatic keratotomy.

Discomfort or pain was assessed at several predetermined times during the operative procedure. The distribution of pain/discomfort scale scores is shown in Table 5-2 and in Figure 5-1 for each treatment group. First, we evaluated the highest score experienced at any point intraoperatively. The distribution of pain scale scores was

shifted in the direction of increased discomfort among the BSS cases compared with lidocaine cases. Mild sensation, expressed as pressure, was reported by 26% of BSS patients and 23% of lidocaine patients. Increased pressure was reported in 19% of BSS procedures compared with 8% of procedures performed with lidocaine. Moderate pain (score = 3+) was reported in 7% of BSS procedures vs 1% of lidocaine procedures. Thus, 26% of patients with no lidocaine treatment experienced increased pressure or moderate pain vs 9% of lidocaine-treated cases. This finding was statistically significant (p<0.0001).

When the scores were examined according to when the discomfort occurred (during phacoemulsification or during lens insertion), it was found that pain/discomfort scores of 2 (increased pressure) or 3 (moderate pain) occurred more frequently during lens insertion than during phacoemulsification (see Table 5-2 and Figure 5-2). This result suggested that patients were describing, to some extent, sensation resulting from the wound manipulation as the IOL was introduced. During phacoemulsification, only four lidocaine patients (2%) had reported increased pressure (score = 2). None of the lidocaine patients reported pain (score ≥3) during phacoemulsification. Two of the 15 lidocaine patients expressing increased pressure during surgery did so before phaco began. In the BSS group, nine (8%) reported increased pressure (score = 2) during phacoemulsification and three (2%) reported moderate pain (score = 3). No patient in the study reported sharp or severe pain (score = 4 or 5, respectively) at any time during surgery.

The two treatment groups were comparable with respect to the need for intraoperative Versed for anxiety. Nineteen percent of BSS patients and 18% of lidocaine patients required Versed to control anxiety.

There was no difference in pain score distribution between patients receiving astigmatic keratotomy and those with no relaxing incisions regardless of whether the patient was given lidocaine or BSS. However, patients receiving limbal relaxing incisions had more discomfort postoperatively.

There were no significant differences between the groups with respect to mean IOP at 1 day postoperatively or in anterior chamber flare/cells measurements. Visual acuity (pinhole) at 1 day postoperatively was comparable between the groups, with 80% of BSS eyes and 83% of lidocaine eyes seeing 20/40 or better with pinhole.

Postoperative endothelial cell counts were collected for a 20% sub-sample of cases. No significant differences between treatment groups were found in cell counts or percent cell loss from baseline. Mean postoperative cell count for the sample was 1602 (SD = 279) for lidocaine patients and 1588 (SD = 285) for BSS patients. Mean central pachymetry measurements were also equivalent.

Blood pressures were compared between the groups just prior to surgery, intraoperatively, and in the recovery room. If multiple measurements were charted at an interval, the highest was used for analysis. There were no group differences in the means of systolic or diastolic pressure at any time point. There were no adverse events among the study participants.

Secondary Studies

The statistically significant results of the controlled study documented the overall efficacy of intracameral lidocaine in optimizing patient comfort during surgery.

Table 5-2
Distribution of Discomfort/Pain Scale Scores
by Treatment Group and Intraoperative Interval

Intraoperative Interval	Treatment	(0) None	(+1) Mild	(+2) Increased	(+3) Moderate	Total
Phaco-emulsification	Lidocaine	152 (83.0%)	26 (14.3%)	4 (2.2%)	0 (0%)	182
	BSS	89 (74.2%)	19 (15.8%)	9 (7.5%)	3 (2.5%)	120
Lens Insertion	Lidocaine	140 (76.9%)	31 (17.0%)	9 (4.9%)	2 (1.1%)	182
	BSS	78 (65.0%)	23 (19.2%)	14 (11.7%)	5 (4.2%)	120
Highest Reported Level	Lidocaine	123 (67.6%)	42 (23.1%)	15 (8.2%)	2 (1.1%)	182
	BSS	58 (48.3%)	31 (25.8%)	23 (19.2%)	8 (6.7%)	120

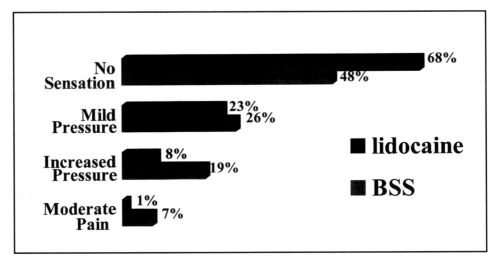

Figure 5-1. Histogram illustrating the distribution of pain scores among patients treated with intraocular lidocaine (dark bars) and control patients treated with balanced saline solution (light bars).

After data analysis, it was felt necessary to suspend the controlled study to avoid placebo treatment. Nevertheless, there were remaining questions:
1. The optimal dose of lidocaine to eliminate any discomfort, and indeed, any sensation at all
2. Whether a larger dose of lidocaine would impact on safety

To answer these questions, a consecutive series of 300 patients were enrolled under the same general protocol but all patients were given 0.5 cc 1% unpreserved lidocaine. The pain scale was administered in the same way except that additional questions were asked to determine if the patient could distinguish between intraocular discomfort or pain and discomfort or pain felt extraocularly (ie, in the wound area or lids). This additional information was collected because of the finding that scores were much lower during phacoemulsification than for lens insertion, which

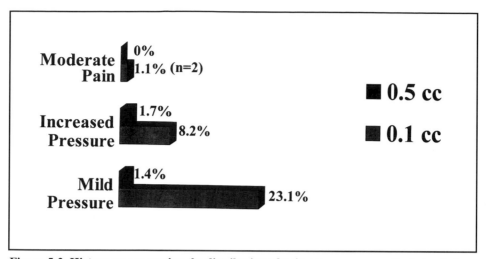

Figure 5-2. Histogram comparing the distribution of pain scores among patients treated with 0.5 cc of 1% unpreserved lidocaine (dark bars) with patients treated with 0.1 cc unpreserved lidocaine (light bars).

led the surgeon to believe that in some cases the source of discomfort to the patient came from manipulation of the wound during lens insertion and was not intraocular.

In this series, 286 of the 300 patients met study criteria and had complete data for analysis. Intraocular increased pressure (score = 2+) was experienced by 0.7% of cases (two patients) during phacoemulsification and by 1% (three patients) during lens insertion. Two patients experienced external discomfort from wound manipulation which they rated as 2 or 3+. When the results of the 0.5 cc study were compared to the 0.1 cc lidocaine group from the randomized study (see Figure 5-2), it was found that the rate of discomfort (any increased pressure or pain as defined by a score ≥2) was reduced to 1.7%. None of the 0.5 cc cases had 3+ scores. The presence of any intraocular sensation was reduced to 3.1%. At the 0.1 cc dose, 23.1% had felt mild pressure and 9.3% had increased pressure or moderate intraocular pain during either phaco or lens insertion.

Postoperative endothelial cell counts and pachymetry measurements were collected at 2 weeks from 109 patients who received 0.5 cc intraoperative lidocaine (Table 5-3). There were no differences in mean preoperative vs postoperative endothelial cell count and the mean percent change in cell count (preop to postop) was not significant. There were no adverse events among the 286 patients.

The results of the study documented a statistically significant decrease in pain or discomfort scores among patients receiving intraoperative lidocaine vs placebo. In the controlled study using a 0.1 cc dose, lidocaine patients mainly felt no sensation or mild pressure with no discomfort, while placebo patients experienced increased pressure and moderate pain in many instances. In the subsequent study of 286 patients given 0.5 cc doses, no intraocular pain was experienced by lidocaine patients, and increased pressure was felt by only 1.7%. Furthermore, 97% felt no sensation at all, including mild pressure. Thus, increasing the dose to 0.5 cc dramatically reduced even mild pressure.

Table 5-3
Evaluation of Changes in Endothelial Cell Count
and Corneal Thickness at 2 Weeks Postoperative
Among 109 Eyes Receiving 0.5 cc 1% Lidocaine

	Mean	Standard Deviation	10th	50th	90th
Preop ECC	1895	231	1500	1900	2200
Postop ECC	1884	244	1600	1900	2200
% Cell Loss	3.2%	1.86	11% (loss)	0%	10% (gain)*
Preop Pachymetry	0.57	0.028	0.54	0.58	0.60
Postop Pachymetry	0.56	0.096	0.54	0.58	0.60

Recorded "gain" due to normal measurement error.

There were no adverse events. Patients did not experience any untoward effects or significant endothelial cell loss at either the 0.1 cc dose or the 0.5 cc dose. The average 3% endothelial cell loss was less than that recently reported by Dick et al for clear corneal cases.[6] Two-week endothelial cell count data are not generally considered stable. However, microscopy was done at this routine visit to check for any acute toxicity effects. The decision not to alter the routine visit schedule was based on repeated observation of clear, healthy corneas. A long-term follow-up of these patients is underway to monitor endothelial health.

Currently, all patients receive 0.5 cc unpreserved lidocaine intraoperatively. There is less need for supplemental anesthesia during phacoemulsification or lens insertion and fewer problems due to squeezing lids when lidocaine is administered. The effectiveness of lidocaine lasts for approximately 10 minutes and works best when administered prophylactically.

Since the study was performed, we have altered our regimen for topical anesthesia, because we observed that the repeated administration of proparacaine and Marcaine tended to increase the rate of keratitis. Currently we use 1 drop of Alcaine and 1 drop of lidocaine, administered just prior to the procedure. We also use lidocaine in a 2% jelly, administered through a sterile dropper, 1 drop preoperatively, 1 drop in the OR, and 1 drop in the recovery room. We find the jelly formulation to provide a longer duration and reduce dryness and the incidence of keratitis.

SIDE EFFECTS WITH TOPICAL ANESTHESIA AND INTRAOCULAR LIDOCAINE

In rare instances, there could be a need to convert to regional anesthesia in the event of an intraocular complication requiring substantially more operating time.

One interesting effect we have observed is that lidocaine seems to have an effect on pupil size during surgery.[2] In the controlled study, almost three times as many lidocaine cases (24% vs 9%) maintained pupil sizes of 9 mm or more. This effect was modest due to the overwhelming effect of the epinephrine we routinely use in our irrigating solution.

Our studies have indicated that intraocular lidocaine causes no endothelial cell damage; there is no cell loss and the corneas are clear and healthy.

We have found that in rare instances (four cases among over 15,000 performed to date), intracameral irrigation with lidocaine can, in fact, result in a limited regional block with associated transient visual loss such as that which commonly occurs during retrobulbar block. In the four cases we have observed, the posterior capsule has not been intact. We have hypothesized that the preservative-free lidocaine migrated posteriorly into the vitreous where it bathed the ganglion cells. There was a complete visual recovery within hours, just as when retrobulbar blocks are used. The patients were given thorough retinal exams and no damage was found. In essence, these few patients, due to the non-intact posterior capsule, simply received a regional block along with the concomitant transient visual loss. Nevertheless, it is important not to assume that any visual loss occurring under topical anesthesia is related to lidocaine use. The patient must have a thorough evaluation to rule out vascular occlusion and any other complications.

EFFECTIVE APPROACHES TO CATARACT SURGERY

Intraocular lidocaine has greatly broadened our inclusion criteria for topical anesthesia. However, a select number of patients remain who still require regional anesthesia. Each patient is carefully evaluated to determine which anesthesia is best for him or her. Patients receive regional anesthesia for the following reasons: hearing problems, language barrier and no interpreter, extreme anxiety, senility, and nystagmus. Currently, about 95% of our patients are given topical anesthesia with intraocular lidocaine.

The use of intraocular lidocaine has completely changed our approach to cataract surgery. Our patient preparation and care has become more personalized. Topical anesthesia, even when supplemented by intraocular lidocaine, is most effective when there is a good rapport between surgeon and patient. Preoperative patient counseling and education are especially important. We make a point to establish communication preoperatively and earn the patient's trust. It is important that patients view the doctor not only as their surgeon, but as their caregiver. The patient thus feels a partnership with the surgeon, and they are completely dependent on each other.

It is also important to give patients a detailed explanation of what they will see and feel during surgery. The clinical and surgical staff join me (JPG) in reassuring the patients that they will feel no discomfort whatsoever. I do explain that there may possibly be some sensation of my fingers around the eye. Patients are encouraged to alert me if they feel any sensation other than the light pressure of my fingers. I also explain that if they are aware of any pressure whatsoever during the procedure, I can irrigate the eye with "special solutions" to eliminate it. In these occasional instances, the additional dose of lidocaine brings rapid relief from the increased pressure. I have found that most patients are very cooperative and less likely to move at inopportune moments when they are thoroughly educated, allowing patients to enter the OR in a totally relaxed, cooperative state of mind.

The OR staff is able to be more relaxed and focus their energy on the patient's needs, rather than worrying about the patient's next jump. I encourage the staff to focus all conversation on the patient. The nurse anesthetist holds the patient's hand during the entire procedure.

SPECIFIC PREOPERATIVE AND SURGICAL PROCEDURES

The intraocular lidocaine is administered prophylactically during hydrodissection. Phacoemulsification is started after a 1-minute interval. The duration of effect of the lidocaine is approximately 15 to 20 minutes. Rarely, irrigation with additional lidocaine is required later in the case if the patient has discomfort.

We have noted that excessive drops increase the incidence of keratitis. Thus, we have reduced our topical anesthesia drops to a single drop each of lidocaine and Alcaine, with most of the topical anesthesia provided by a lidocaine jelly preparation. The ointment formulation provides an extended duration and protects the cornea from drying during surgery. As a result, the patients are more comfortable postoperatively. The jelly can easily be transferred into a sterile dropper bottle and administered as a drop. We administer 1 drop preoperatively, 1 drop in the OR, and 1 drop in the recovery room.

CHANGING SURGICAL PRACTICE PATTERNS

As ophthalmologists, we are always looking for ways to improve cataract surgery, to make it safer and more effective, while at the same time making it easier for our patients to experience. Topical anesthesia with intraocular lidocaine had an enormous impact on the roles played by patients, surgeons, and surgical staff during surgery. The patient retains more control both during and after surgery and is better able to communicate and assist the surgeon and staff concerning his or her own comfort and well-being. The need for sedation is very low and can generally be predicted using good patient screening procedures. While routine IV access has traditionally been a standard part of cataract surgery, we have begun to reassess its usefulness. The purpose of IV access is to allow for easy administration of medications which may be used during surgery, such as those used in blood pressure control and sedation. It has been shown, however, that receiving an IV creates almost as much apprehension as receiving a retrobulbar block.

We have found that there is less need for IV access during cataract surgery with the routine use of intracameral lidocaine and with thorough preoperative patient education. Avoiding the use of an IV line decreases patient anxiety and apprehension without the use of medications, making the procedure even easier for our patients and increasing the safety.

We have been able to eliminate the use of IVs in 90% of our cataract surgical cases. Some indications do remain for the use of IVs during cataract surgery. These include the very nervous patient, those with poorly controlled hypertension or diabetes, and the non-communicative patient. An IV is also valuable for patients with a cardiac condition who may become bradycardic with the use of sedatives. We may never totally eliminate the need for IV access during cataract surgery. However, lim-

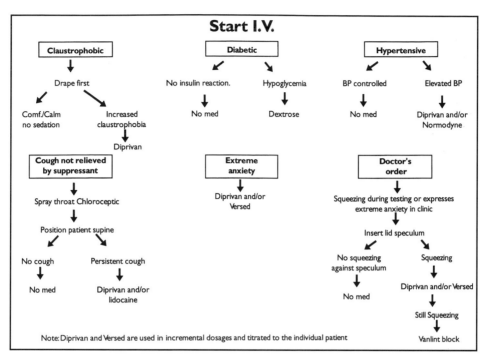

Figure 5-3. Decision tree diagram with suggested indications for IV and initiation of added anesthesia.

iting its use to only when it is indicated will make our patients more comfortable and ultimately more satisfied (Figure 5-3).

Without the use of regional blocks, sedation, and routine IV access, the role of the nurse anesthetist in cataract surgery at our facility has changed dramatically. At this time, the need for the nurse anesthetist to be involved throughout the procedure is greatly changed. In this environment, the skills of the nurse anesthetist are better used for the infrequent complicated cases and for other intraocular procedures requiring blocks or general anesthesia.

SUMMARY

Since our introducing the use of intracameral lidocaine as an adjunct to topical anesthesia, the use of this technique has increased rapidly. In the 1996 Leaming American Society of Cataract and Refractive Surgery survey, 52% of large-volume surgeons (>50 cases per month) were using intraocular lidocaine.[7] We believe that this technique is effective and safe and has had a great impact on postoperative outcome and patient satisfaction.

REFERENCES

1. Fichman RA. Topical anesthesia. In: Fine IH, Fichman RA, Grabow HB, eds. *Clear-Corneal Cataract Surgery & Topical Anesthesia*. Thorofare, NJ: SLACK Incorporated; 1993:97-162.
2. Gills JP, Cherchio M, Raanan MG. The use of intraoperative unpreserved lidocaine to control discomfort during IOL surgery under topical anesthesia. *J Cataract Refract Surg*. 1997;23:527-535.
3. Gills JP, Hustead RF, Sanders DR, eds. *Ophthalmic Anesthesia*. Thorofare, NJ: SLACK Incorporated; 1993.
4. SAS System for Windows, Release 6.11. SAS Institute Inc, Cary, NC.
5. StatMost Version 2.5 for Windows, DataMost Corp, Salt Lake City, Utah.
6. Dick HB, Kohnen T, Jacobi FK, Jacobi KW. Long-term endothelial cell loss following phacoemulsification through a temporal clear corneal incision. *J Cataract Refract Surg*. 1996;22:63-70.
7. Leaming DV. Practice styles and preferences of ASCRS members—1996 survey. *J Cataract Refract Surg*. 1997;23:527-535.

Chapter

6

The Choo-Choo Chop and Flip Phacoemulsification Technique

I. Howard Fine, MD

This technique is designed to take maximum advantage of various new technologies available through the Alcon 20,000 Legacy,[1] the AMO Diplomax,[2] the Mentor SIStem, and the Storz Millennium phacoemulsification systems. These technologies include high vacuum cassettes and tubing, multiple programmable features on all systems, as well as the Mackool MicroTip with the Legacy and burst mode and occlusion mode capabilities with the Diplomax (Tables 6-1 through 6-4). The result is enhanced efficiency, control, and safety. The procedure is done as follows.

After stabilizing the globe with a Fine-Thornton ring, a side-port incision is made to the left with a 1-mm trifaceted diamond knife (Figure 6-1), after which the anterior chamber is irrigated with 0.5 cc preservative-free Xylocaine. Utilizing the soft-shell technique described by Dr. Steve Arshinoff, Viscoat is placed into the anterior chamber angle distal to the side port through the side-port incision. It fills the anterior chamber but allows the eye to remain relatively soft. Provisc is instilled on top of the center of the lens capsule under the Viscoat. Provisc forces the Viscoat up against the cornea, creating a soft shell which helps stabilize the anterior chamber and protect the endothelium. Additionally, Provisc, which is a cohesive viscoelastic, decreases any tendency for iris prolapse during the hydro steps. The globe is again stabilized with the Fine-Thornton ring and the trapezoidal 3-D blade is positioned without applanating the globe so that the point touches the desired edge of the external incision (Figure 6-2). The blade is simply pushed in the plane of the cornea. Due to the differential bevels on the edges of the blade, the force of tissue resistance will result in three accurate and reproducible architectural characteristics during incision

Table 6-1 Fine Phacoemulsification Parameters Alcon Legacy, January 1998					
Mackool System Hi-Vac Choo-Choo Chop and Flip					**I&A**
Memory Mode	**Chop Mem 1 Pulse**	**Trim Mem 2 Pulse**	**Flip Mem 3 Pulse**	**Cortical Mem 1-3**	**Viscoat Mem 4**
Power	50	35	35	Surg vac.	Surg asp.
Asp.	28/33 cc/min	20/18 cc/min	22 cc/min	38	60
Vacuum	350 mmHg	180 mmHg	180 mmHg	500+	500+
Mode	Pulse 2/sec	Pulse 7/sec	Pulse 7/sec	Cont. irrig.	Cont. irrig.
Bt. Ht.	78 cm	72 cm	72 cm	70 cm	70 cm

Hi-vac tubing with gold handpiece and gold tips. Put expand-a-pole on (extends IV pole by 32 cm).

Table 6-2 Fine Phacoemulsification Parameters AMO Diplomax, 1998					
Hi-Vac/Chop and Flip				**I&A Control Surg Vac Control**	
	Chop Phaco 1	**Trim Phaco 2**	**Flip Phaco 3**	**Cortical Clean-Up**	**Viscoat Removal**
Power	60	60	60		
Asp. Cont. Flow	26/30 cc/min	32/26 cc/min	32/16 cc/min	10 cc/min	30 cc/min
Vacuum	50/250 mmHg	40/90 mmHg	70/150 mmHg	500 mmHg	500 mmHg
Mode	Cont. burst	Cont. burst	Cont. burst	Cont. irrig.	Cont. irrig.
Bt. Ht.	32 inches	32 inches	32 inches	28 inches	28 inches

construction: the external incision will be linear, the point of the blade will perforate Descemet's membrane 2 mm central to the external incision without beveling down, and the internal incision will be linear. Advancing the blade to the shoulders makes an internal incision 2.5 mm (Figure 6-3). Advancing the blade all the way in enlarges the internal incision to 3.5 mm, without altering the architecture. Therefore, enlarging the phaco incision for IOL implantation can be achieved without side-cutting of the incision which **does** alter the architecture and may compromise self-sealability. Alternatively, incision construction may be accomplished by touching the point of the 3-D blade at the desired site of the internal incision after fixating the globe with the Fine-Thornton ring. With the blade aligned at the plane of the cornea, one may simply use the Fine-Thornton ring to rotate the globe on to the blade, reproducibly creating the same incision architecture.

Following clear corneal incision, cortical cleaving hydrodissection is performed in the two distal quadrants followed by hydrodelineation. After the two hydro steps, the nucleus should rotate easily within the capsular bag. The Mackool/Kelman MicroTip on the Legacy is introduced bevel down to aspirate the epinucleus uncovered by the capsulorrhexis, and is then turned bevel up. With the other systems, a 30

Table 6-3
Fine Phacoemulsification Parameters
MENTOR SIStem, February 1998

	Bt. Ht.	Aspiration	Vacuum	Power/Pulse
Chop & Quadrant Removal	98	22	225	60%/2 sec
Epinuclear Trimming	98	20	135	50%/2 sec
Epinuclear Flipping	98	24	180	50%/2 sec
Cortex Removal	98	24	500	NA
Viscoat Removal	98	40	500	NA

Table 6-4
Fine Phacoemulsification Parameters
Storz Millennium, March 1998

	Bt. Ht.	Vacuum	Power/Pulse
Chop & Quadrant Removal	70	300	20%/2 sec
Epinuclear Management	70	300	5%/2 sec
Cortex/Viscoat Removal	70	550	

degree standard tip, bevel down, is used throughout endonuclear removal. The Fine/Nagahara chopper (Rhein Medical) is placed in the golden ring and is used to stabilize the nucleus by lifting and pulling toward the incision slightly (Figure 6-4), after which the phaco tip lollipops the nucleus in either pulse mode at 2 pulses/second or 80 millisecond burst mode (see Tables 6-1 through 6-4). With the energy set in this way, we minimize ultrasound energy into the eye and maximize our hold on the nucleus as the vacuum builds between pulses or bursts. Because of the decrease in cavitational energy around the tip at this low pulse rate or in burst mode, the tunnel in the nucleus in which the tip is embedded fits the needle very tightly and gives us an excellent hold on the nucleus, thus maximizing control of the nucleus as we score and chop it (Figure 6-5) in foot position 2.

The Fine/Nagahara chop instrument is grooved on the horizontal arm close to the vertical "chop" element with the groove parallel to the direction of the sharp edge of the vertical element. In scoring the nucleus, the instrument is always moved in the direction the sharp edge of the wedge-shaped vertical element is facing (as indicated by the groove on the instrument), thus facilitating scoring. The nucleus is scored by bringing the chop instrument to the side of the phaco needle. It is chopped in half by pulling the chopper to the left and slightly down while moving the phaco needle, still in foot position 2, to the right and slightly up. Then the nuclear complex is rotated. The chop instrument is again brought into the golden ring (Figure 6-6), the nucleus is again lollipopped, scored, and chopped with the resulting pie-shaped segment now lollipopped on the phaco tip (Figure 6-7). The segment is then evacuated utilizing high vacuum and short bursts or pulse mode phaco at 2 pulses/second (Figure 6-8). The nucleus is continually rotated so that pie-shaped segments can be scored, chopped, and removed essentially by the high vacuum assisted by short bursts or pulses of phaco. The short bursts or pulses of ultrasound energy continu-

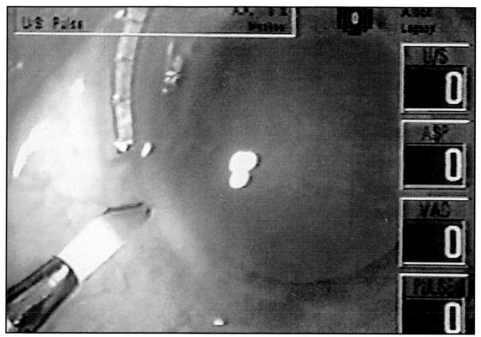

Figure 6-1. Initiating side-port incision.

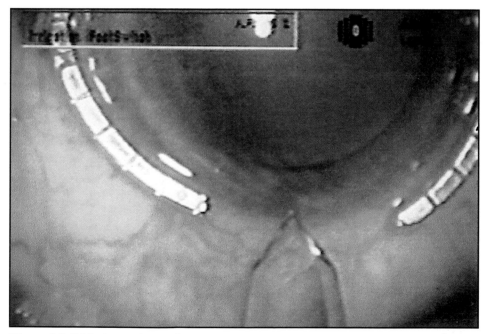

Figure 6-2. Initiating main incision by touching cornea at site of external incision and aiming the knife in the plane of the cornea.

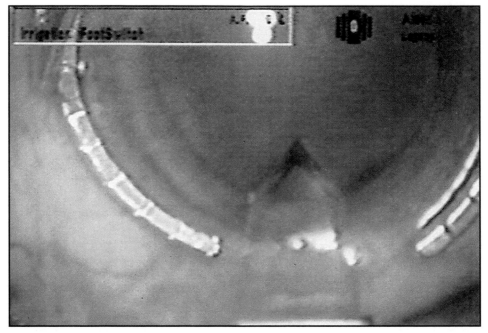

Figure 6-3. Completion of 2.5-mm incision by stopping 3-D trapezoidal knife as shoulders reach Descemet's membrane.

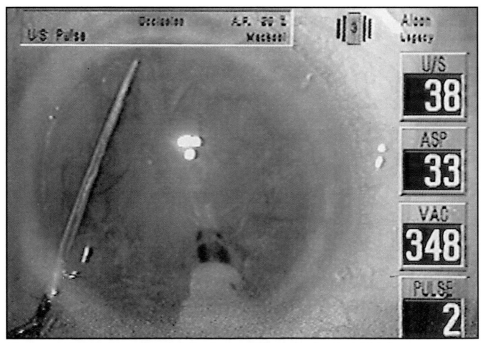

Figure 6-4. Stabilization of the nucleus during lollipopping for the initial chop.

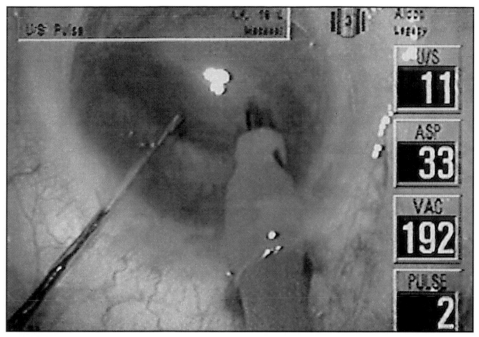

Figure 6-5. Completion of the initial chop.

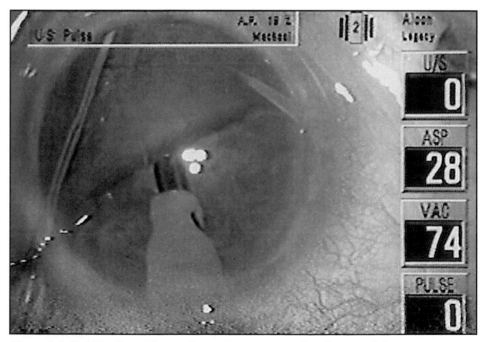

Figure 6-6. Stabilization of the nucleus prior to commencing the second chop.

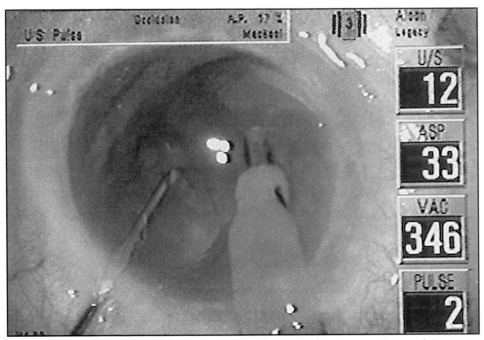

Figure 6-7. Pie-shaped segment adherent to the phaco tip following completion of the second chop.

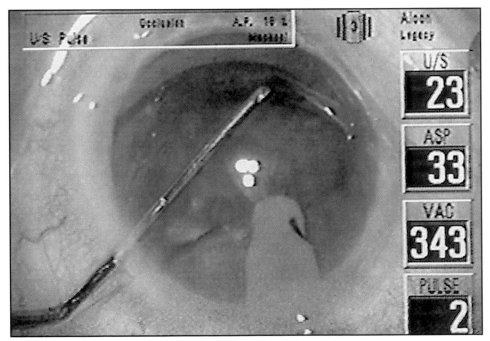

Figure 6-8. Mobilization of the first pie-shaped segment.

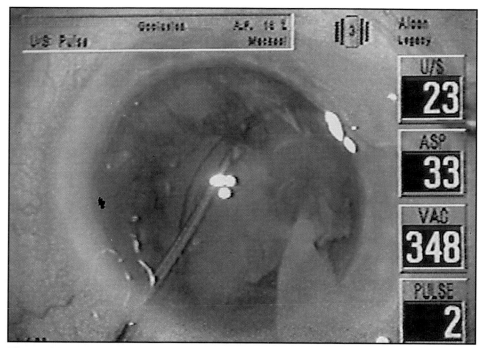

Figure 6-9. Scoring of the second heminucleus.

ously reshape the pie-shaped segments which are kept at the tip, allowing for occlusion and extraction by the vacuum. The size of the pie-shaped segments is customized to the density of the nucleus with smaller segments for denser nuclei. Phaco in burst mode or at this low pulse rate sounds like "choo-choo-choo-choo"; ergo the name of this technique. With burst mode or the low pulse rate, the nuclear material tends to stay at the tip rather than chatter as vacuum holds between pulses. The chop instrument is utilized to stuff the segment into the tip or keep it down in the nuclear shell.

After evacuation of the first hemi-nucleus, the second hemi-nucleus is rotated to the distal portion of the bag and the chop instrument stabilizes it while it is lollipopped. It is then scored (Figure 6-9) and chopped. The pie-shaped segments can be chopped a second time to reduce their size (Figure 6-10) if they appear too large to easily evacuate.

There is little tendency for nuclear material to come up into the anterior chamber with this technique. Usually it stays down within the epinuclear shell, but the position of the endonuclear material can be controlled by the chop instrument. Following evacuation of all endonuclear material (the Diplomax tip is turned bevel up) (Figure 6-11), the epinuclear rim is trimmed in each of the three quadrants, mobilizing cortex as well in the following way. As each quadrant of the epinuclear rim is trimmed, the cortex in the adjacent capsular fornix flows over the floor of the epinucleus and into the phaco tip. Then the floor is pushed back to keep the bag on stretch until three of the four quadrants of epinuclear rim and forniceal cortex have

been evacuated. It is important not to allow the epinucleus to flip too early, thus avoiding a large amount of residual cortex remaining after evacuation of the epinucleus.

The epinuclear rim of the fourth quadrant is then utilized as a handle to flip the epinucleus (Figure 6-12). As the remaining portion of the epinuclear floor and rim is evacuated from the eye, 80% to 90% of the time all of the cortex is evacuated with it (Figure 6-13). Continuing with the soft-shell technique, the capsular bag is filled with Provisc and Viscoat is injected into the center of the capsular bag to help stabilize the anterior chamber and to blunt the movement of the foldable IOL as it is implanted into the eye. If the cortex was incompletely mobilized during epinuclear removal, Viscoat (rather than Provisc) is instilled first to viscodissect the cortex into the capsular fornix and drape some of it on top of the capsulorrhexis. Provisc is then injected into the bottom of the bag, forcing the Viscoat anteriorly. The foldable IOL is then implanted (Figure 6-14).

The lens we use most frequently is the Staar Surgical AA4207VF plate haptic foldable silicone IOL, which is injected into the eye using a shooter and microcartridge through the unenlarged 2.5-mm incision (Figure 6-15). This does not stretch the incision. Alternatively, we inject into the eye an AMO SA40NB multifocal silicone foldable IOL utilizing the AMO Unfolder, without enlarging the 2.5-mm incision. This stretches the incision at least 0.3 mm.

Residual cortex is evacuated with residual viscoelastic, the posterior capsule being protected by the optic of the IOL. Mobilization of Viscoat is greatly facilitated as it is encased within the much more highly cohesive Provisc and less time is necessary to evacuate residual viscoelastic. At the completion of the case, the wound is tested for leakage with fluorescein dye. If necessary, the seal can be enhanced with stromal hydration.

The choo-choo chop and flip technique utilizes the same hydro forces to disassemble the nucleus as in cracking techniques, but substitutes mechanical forces (chopping) for ultrasound energy (grooving) to further disassemble the nucleus. High vacuum is utilized as an extractive technique to remove nuclear material rather than utilizing ultrasound energy to convert the nucleus to an emulsate that is evacuated by aspiration. This technique maximizes safety and control as well as efficiency in all cases, and allows for phaco of harder nuclei in the presence of a compromised endothelium. This technique facilitates the achievement of two goals: minimally invasive cataract surgery and maximally rapid visual rehabilitation with foldable IOLs.

This is an updated version of a previous publication. Reprinted with permission.[3]

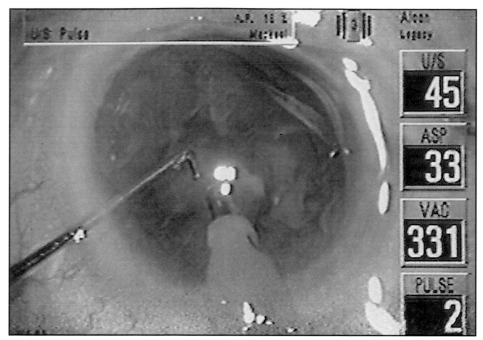

Figure 6-10. Mobilizing the final quadrant.

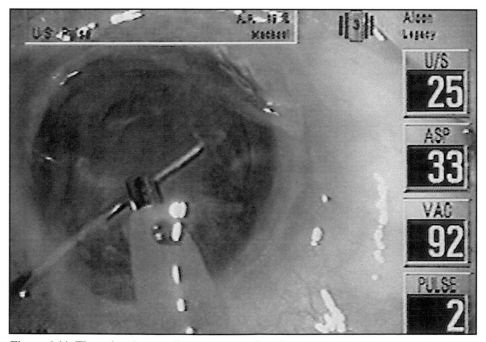

Figure 6-11. The epinuclear shell being rotated for trimming.

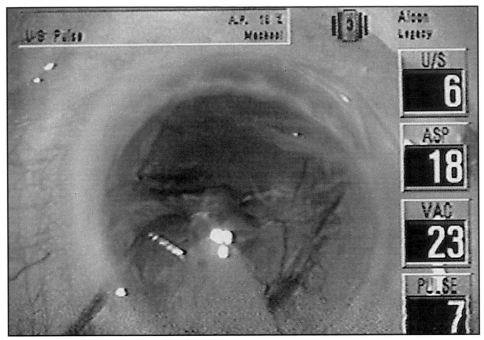

Figure 6-12. Flipping of the epinucleus.

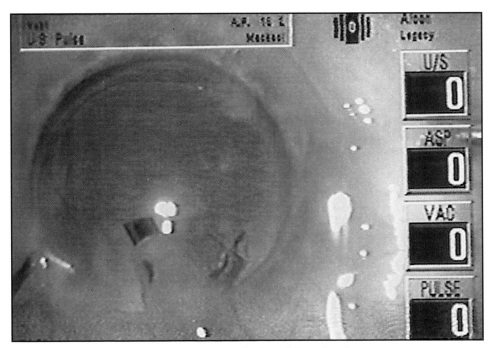

Figure 6-13. Empty capsular bag following flipping of the epinucleus.

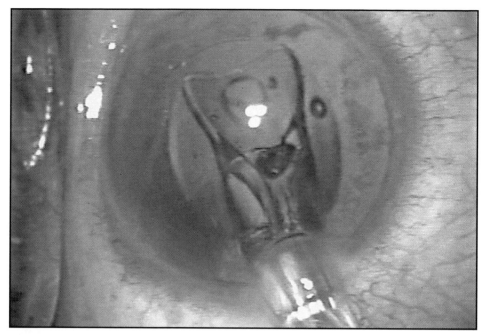

Figure 6-14. Plate haptic IOL opening.

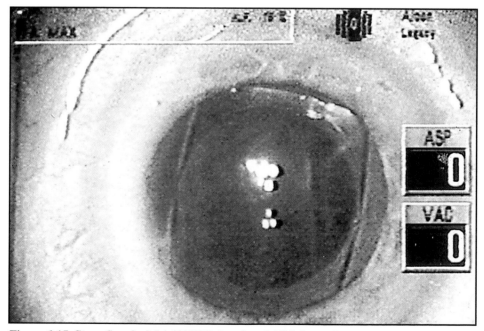

Figure 6-15. Staar Surgical AA4207VF plate haptic IOL immediately following implantation.

REFERENCES

1. Fine IH. Choo-choo chop and flip phacoemulsification. *Phaco & Foldables*. In press.
2. Masket S, Thorlakson R. The OMS Diplomax in endolenticular phacoemulsification. In: Fine IH, ed. *Phacoemulsification: New Technology and Clinical Application*. Thorofare, NJ: SLACK Incorporated; 1996:67-80.
3. Fine IH. The choo choo chop and flip phacoemulsification technique. *Operative Techniques in Cataract and Refractive Surgery*. 1998;1(2):61-65.

Chapter

7

Deep Groove
Corneal Incision

David W. Langerman, MD, FACS

INTRODUCTION

A discussion of the hinge incision would not be complete without a historical perspective of corneal tunnel incisions. Corneal tunnel incisions have been popular since they were first described by Dr. I. Howard Fine in Spring 1992 (Figure 7-1).[1]

The procedure was called clear corneal because the incision originated anterior to the termination of the conjunctival vascular arcade. Shortly thereafter, Kellan, also in Spring 1992, described his sclera-less corneal tunnel approach which began by making a small conjunctival peritomy.[2] His paracentesis-styled incision began at the limbus and entered the anterior chamber through a 1.5-mm corneal tunnel. He felt that the limbal area added stability to his wound construction and was less tissue traumatic. At about the same time, Williamson described a trapezoidal corneal tunnel in which he made a clear corneal groove 300-microns deep and a 1.5-mm tunnel length (Figure 7-2).[3] The external incision measured 3.5 mm and the internal 3.2 mm. He felt that a thicker roof would add wound stability and the smaller internal opening would help in preventing leakage. The larger external opening would accommodate the IOL.

After these innovative procedures were introduced, reports of wound leakage and infection appeared, as well as the need to suture these wounds.[4-7] Stromal hydration was then advocated by Dr. Fine to help create a better sealing effect.[8] We now realize that those incidents probably occurred because a great deal of force was used to push a foldable IOL through the corneal tunnel, thereby stretching the wound and increasing the circumference of the corneal tunnel.[9-11] The result was poor apposi-

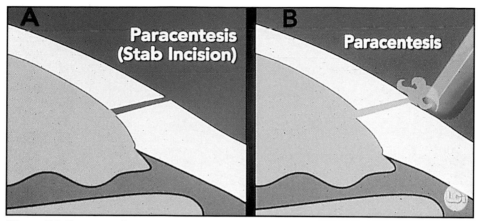

Figure 7-1. Paracentesis.

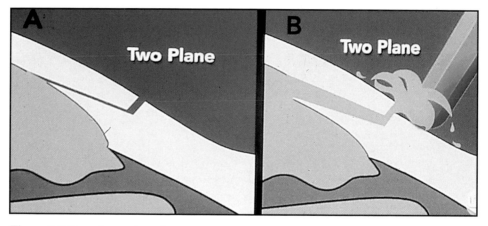

Figure 7-2. Two step or two plane.

tion of the tissues leading to a loss of self-sealing and the appearance of spontaneous leakage.

After visiting Dr. Fine in June 1992, I began performing clear corneal tunnels, but did not experience the above problems. However, the reports were disturbing and I tried to find a better way to increase the sealability of the clear corneal tunnel. The hinge technique was therefore developed in 1993 and was reported in Spring 1994 at the American Society of Cataract and Refractive Surgery meeting (Figure 7-3).[12] It came into being to alleviate the concern expressed in the above publications, and I frankly thought that the clear corneal tunnel was an elegant, tissue-friendly procedure.

An understanding of changes in tunnel circumference during the surgical procedure came later.

The hinge incision was designed to have two components:
1.   A self-sealing feature
2.   A no-leak feature

Self-sealing means that the wound does not leak spontaneously. The no-leak feature means that leakage does not occur when pressure is applied to the posterior lip.

PHYSIOLOGY

To create a hinge incision that has the two components, the guiding principle is that the base of the groove should be maximally separated from the plane of the tunnel (Figures 7-3 and 7-4). This permits both tunnel and groove to act independently of one another. The deep groove disrupts the contiguity of the tissues in the same manner as a relaxing incision. The deep groove permits the thin rim of tissue at the base of the groove to function as a movable hinge, so that when pressure is applied to the posterior lip the hinge enables the groove to separate and widen, but the tunnel is able to remain independently sealed (see Figure 7-3).

If the groove is too shallow as in a two-plane or step incision, a hinge effect cannot be achieved, since the tissues of the tunnel and the base of the groove are too close and contiguous to one another (see Figure 7-2). This close proximity of the tunnel to the base of the groove unites the tissues functionally into a block of tissue. Pressure on the posterior lip causes the entire unit or block of tissue to open up and leakage occurs.

With a paracentesis incision, the floor of the tunnel and the tissue of the posterior lip are contiguous and function as a block of tissue (see Figure 7-1). Pressure on the posterior lip can cause a 2.0-mm tunnel to open and leakage will occur. As a general rule, corneal tunnels longer than 2.5 mm will not leak even with pressure. However, visibility during phacoemulsification becomes difficult due to folds in the cornea that are created during the phaco portion of the procedure.

There are a number of factors that are most important in order to create an effective hinge incision.

PROCEDURE

For accuracy, a template is my preference to outline the dimensions of the hinge incision, but it is not absolutely necessary (Figure 7-5).

The groove is made with a diamond set at 600 microns, and must be perpendicular to the corneal curvature (Figure 7-6). The width of the groove can be 2.6, 3.0, 3.2, or 3.5 mm, but this is optional.

The tunnel begins at one third stromal depth and must be perpendicular to the groove. The tunnel follows the corneal curvature for 2.0 mm and then enters the anterior chamber (Figure 7-7). The diamond, if the sides are sharp, must be depressed to enter the anterior chamber, otherwise, the heel of the diamond may tear the roof of the corneal tunnel. The width of the tunnel can be 2.6, 3.0, 3.2, or 3.5 mm, but this is optional.

Another important factor in maintaining the effect of the hinge incision is not to change the circumference of the corneal tunnel. This can occur if one uses a great deal of force to push a lens through the corneal tunnel. This excessive force stretch-

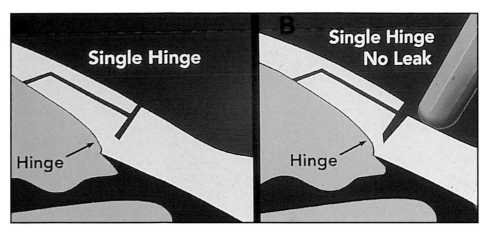

Figure 7-3. Hinge incision.

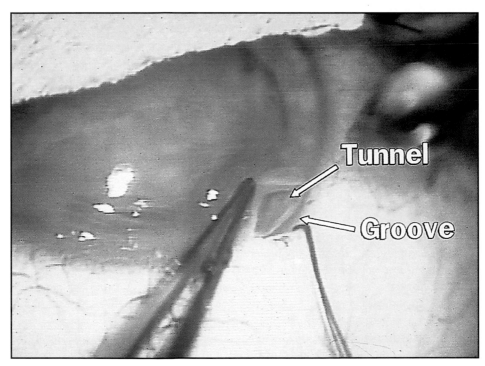

Figure 7-4. Hinge incision with no-leak feature.

es and dilates the tunnel, thereby increasing its circumference. This increased circumference can cause a loss of one or both components leading to a dysfunctional hinge. The way to avoid changing the circumference or stretching the tunnel is to cut the distal half of the tunnel (Figure 7-8). This permits the lens to be guided through the tunnel without counterpressure (Figure 7-9), and both the self-sealing and no-leak components can be preserved (Figure 7-10).

Mackool demonstrated that the external opening of a 3.0-mm clear corneal tunnel can stretch anywhere between 0.10 to 0.65 mm and internally by 0.50 to 0.75 mm depending on a variety of insertional devices and foldable IOLs.[10] Dr. Steinert and I also demonstrated that the circumference of the corneal tunnel can increase during various stages of the operation.[9,13] For example, IOL insertion may widen the incision by 0.3 mm, and phaco can widen the wound by about 0.1 mm.[11]

With the growth in popularity of inserting foldable IOLs with shooters, inserters, and lens unfolders, the chance of losing the self-seal with all three incision types increases. Most inserters are cone shaped and increase in diameter from the tip upward. Pushing the inserter beyond the 2.0-mm tunnel into the anterior chamber may stretch and increase the diameter of the wound, thereby increasing its circumference. Therefore, one should not push the tip of inserters beyond the 2.0-mm tunnel length. Alternatively, manufacturers might reduce the diameter of inserters to accommodate smaller and smaller wounds.

Using the corneal approach, and with the introduction of topical anesthesia by Fichman,[14] and thanks to the revolutionary idea by Gills[15] that one can safely instill 1% nonpreserved Xylocaine into the anterior chamber, we can now perform what I call "cosmetic cataract surgery."[16] This simply means that a patient should look as natural after the procedure as before the procedure. Therefore, subconjunctival hemorrhage and redness should be avoided. This can be achieved by not using needle anesthesia and by touching the surface of the eye with instruments as little as possible. If an instrument is necessary for counterpressure I strongly recommend the Fine-Thornton ring, since the ring is a benign instrument due to its broad-based teeth, which has no negative effect on the surface of the eye. I do not use sharp instruments such as the 0.12 forceps for counterpressure because of the likelihood of causing subconjunctival hemorrhage, which is something that I want to avoid. These new modalities permit patients to leave the OR without patching. With the trend toward cosmesis in cataract surgery, it could appear on the managed care outcomes list one day.

Recent cadaver and feline studies have demonstrated that square wounds are stronger than rectangular wounds.[11] However, from a practical point of view it is very difficult to employ square wounds in corneal tunnel surgery. Corneal tunnels longer than 2.0 to 2.5 mm create optical difficulties during phacoemulsification and may possibly encroach upon the visual axis. Therefore, most corneal tunnels are rectangular in shape. Adding a hinge component to a rectangular wound provides increased sealability and resistance to leakage when pressure is applied to the posterior lip, thereby making square wounds less critical. Animal studies have also demonstrated that limbal incisions seal in 7 days whereas clear corneal wounds take a little longer.[17-20] This makes sense, considering that it takes months for a corneal transplant to fully heal and surgeons can still peel back the corneal cap months after the original surgery.

SURGICAL TECHNIQUE

In my personal phacoemulsification technique, I use a variety of modalities to debulk the lens. I prefer using topical and intracameral anesthesia on all patients, reserving a parabulbar block on the few patients who are unable to cooperate. The

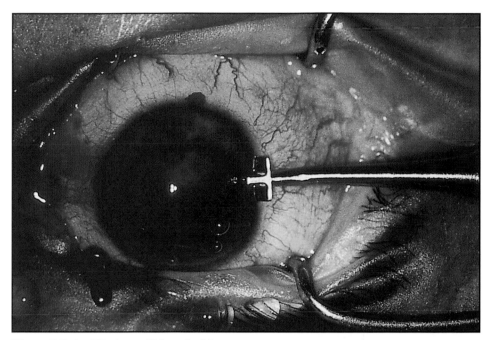

Figure 7-5. Architecture of hinge incision.

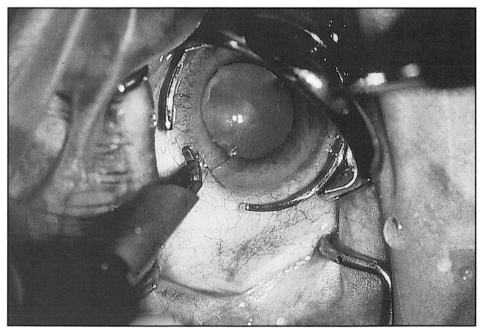

Figure 7-6. Hinge template.

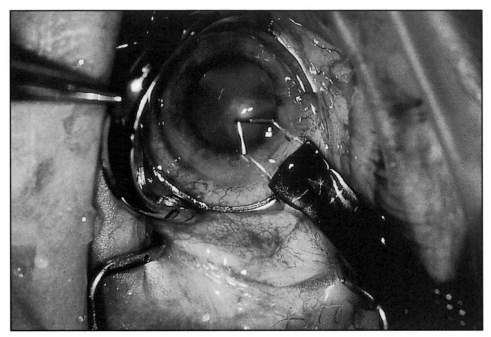

Figure 7-7. Diamond set at 600 microns.

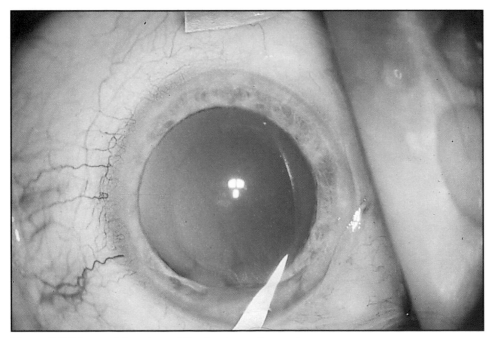

Figure 7-8. Diamond keratome following corneal curvature.

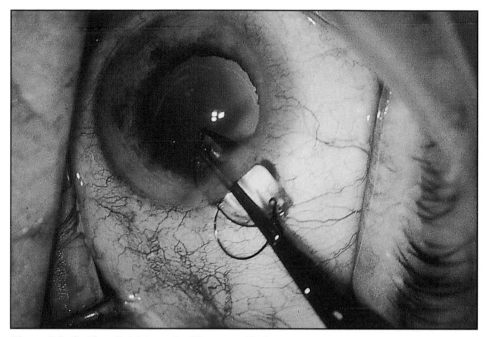

Figure 7-9. Cutting distal tunnel with a superblade.

Figure 7-10. Insertion of IOL with no counterforce.

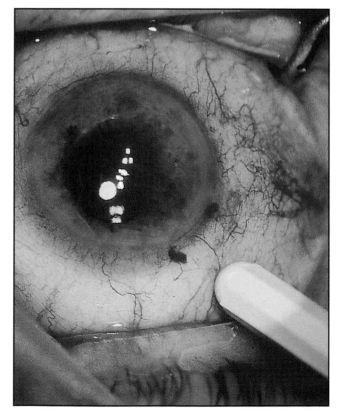

phaco machine that I currently use is the Diplomax from Allergan. One of the most important factors that enables me to determine my phaco technique is the size of the capsulorrhexis. A 6.0- to 7.0-mm capsulorrhexis or larger will permit the edge of the lens to rise above the capsular bag and will lend itself to debulking. Most of the lens is in the capsular bag and about one fourth to one third of the lens is in the anterior chamber, covered with viscoelastic, and away from the corneal endothelium. A Kugelin spatula through the side-port guides and rotates the lens toward the phaco tip, and also prevents the lens from touching the endothelium. To start the debulking process, I prefer position 1 with settings of power 70, aspiration 16, vacuum 30. After 50% of the lens has been debulked I switch to position 2 with higher vacuum. The settings in position 2 are power 70, aspiration 30, vacuum 350. In position 2, I prefer a burst mode of 8 pulses.

If the lens does not elevate itself spontaneously, my preference is to sculpt the nucleus into four quadrants, fracture, and emulsify. Sculpting is performed in position 1 with settings of power 70, aspiration 16, vacuum 30. Emulsification takes place in position 2 with burst mode of 8 pulses, power 70, aspiration 30, vacuum 350. If the quadrants are large, I will chop the lens into smaller pieces using the Kugelin hook and vacuum levels of 350 to 400.

In performing the hinge incision, my goal is to achieve the two components—the self-sealing and no-leak features. To achieve the no-leak feature, which is that leakage is not observed when pressure is applied to the posterior lip of the wound, construction of the wound as outlined is critical. If the no-leak feature has not been achieved, and the self-sealing effect is still present, nothing further is done. If there is spontaneous leakage, then stromal hydration with balanced salt solution is performed, and this generally will cause the leakage to cease.

REFERENCES

1. Fine IH. Introduces clear corneal incision. American Society of Cataract and Refractive Surgery meeting, April 1992.
2. Kellan R. Introduces sclera-less corneal tunnel. *Ocular Surgery News*. 1992;10:12.
3. Williamson C. Williamson Eye Surgery Center. Cataract keratotomy course. Baton Rouge, La, August 1992.
4. Gills J. Evaluation of early post-operative intraocular pressure in IOL patients with cornea and scleral tunnel incisions. American Society of Cataract and Refractive Surgery meeting, April 1994.
5. Grabow H. Complications of clear corneal cataract incisions. *Ocular Surgery News*. 1993:II;8.
6. Koch P. Why I stopped doing clear corneal incisions. *New England Ophthalmological Society*. 1992;Dec.
7. McFarland M. Not so clear cornea. *Ocular Surgery News*. 1993:II;8.
8. Fine IH. Enhancing the seal in clear corneal incisions. *Ocular Surgery News*. 1992;March:40.
9. Langerman DW. Circumference changes in corneal tunnels following IOL insertion. Royal Hawaii meeting, January 1995.
10. Mackool R. Insertion of foldable IOLs can increase incision length. *Ophthalmology Times*. 1994;May.
11. Steinert R. Enlargement of incision width during phaco and foldable intraocular lens implant surgery. American Society of Cataract and Refractive Surgery meeting, April 1995.

12. Langerman DW. Architectural design of a self-sealing corneal tunnel, single hinge incision. American Society of Cataract and Refractive Surgery meeting, April 1994.
13. Langerman DW. Architectural design of a self-sealing corneal tunnel, single hinge incision. *J Cataract Refract Surg*. 1994;20:84-88.
14. Fichman R. Topical eye drops replace injection for anesthesia. *Ocular Surgery News*. 1992;March:10:5.
15. Gills J. Intracameral injection of Lidocaine. Ocular Surgery News symposium, New York City, September 1995.
16. Langerman DW. Cosmetic cataract surgery. Royal Hawaii meeting, Maui, Hawaii, January 1997.
17. Ernest PH. Relative strength of scleral corneal and clear corneal incisions constructed in cadaver eyes. *J Cataract Refract Surg*. 1994;20:626-629.
18. Ernest PH. Relative stability of clear corneal incisions in a cadaver eye model. *J Cataract Refract Surg*. 1995;21:39-42.
19. Ernest PH. Wound stability determined by incision shape, construction and location. *Ocular Surgery News*. 1996;14:28-29.
20. Ernest PH. Incisional healing, based on location in the feline model. American Society of Cataract and Refractive Surgery meeting, June 1996.

Personal Clear Corneal Cataract Technique

John D. Hunkeler, MD

Following the development of foldable IOLs, the evolution of cataract surgical technique led to smaller and more simply constructed cataract incisions. Utilizing phacoemulsification techniques, it became possible that the cataract extraction can be accomplished through a 3.0-mm incision. Depending on variables, the incision could be slightly larger or smaller than 3.0 mm.

Previously, with planned extracapsular techniques and phacoemulsification techniques, when combined with PMMA lens implants, scleral incisions were needed to minimize astigmatic refractive changes after cataract surgery. Often, the incisions were over 2 mm posterior to the limbus and required meticulous dissection from the sclera into the clear cornea.

With the advent of foldable technology, the implant incision has migrated anteriorly, become smaller, and moved closer to the limbus. Because of the reduction in incision size, the anterior migration of the incision was not accompanied by any significant change in astigmatism. The reduction of induced astigmatism resulted directly from the reduced size of the incision.

Clear corneal cataract surgery was popularized by Dr. I. Howard Fine in the 1990s. His technique involved a beveled clear corneal incision temporally with the insertion of a foldable IOL and self-sealing closure. Occasionally, a suture was necessary to enhance wound integrity. Variations in technique and modifications have occurred over the years with the creation of rhomboidal incisions, grooving prior to keratome incision, and movement of the incision away from the temporal location to oblique superior or nasal entry point. Irregardless, the procedure has led to overall success with clear corneal cataract surgery.

The procedure can be combined with additional techniques to facilitate the cataract procedure, such as iris hooks for small pupils, chamber maintainers, or astigmatic surgery. In order to reduce pre-existing corneal astigmatism, clear corneal relaxing incisions in the form of arcuate keratotomy offer one option. An alternative is the limbal relaxing incision.

My current cataract surgical technique has evolved over the past several years from the initial phase of creating a clear corneal temporal groove and then utilizing a stainless steel rounded bevel-up blade to dissect further into clear cornea and make a stainless steel keratome through this lamellar corneal dissection. This technique was successful, but often led to dissection too far into clear cornea and a difficulty in cutting through the lamellar sheets of cornea. It was soon replaced with a diamond blade trapezoidal technique to create a more consistent, uniform, and easily reproducible incision into the anterior chamber. The 3.5-mm, 400-micron deep groove was created temporally and the keratome passed through the groove, corneal stroma, and through Descemet's membrane. The technique resulted in a 3.2-mm internal incision compared to a 3.5-mm external incision. The cataract procedure could be performed with a standard phaco tip and insertion of a first-generation silicone easily through the self-sealing incision. Wound hydration was necessary to close the incision satisfactorily. The incision worked very nicely for clear temporal incision resulting in a mean 0.38 D flattening in the meridian of the incision.

My technique has evolved over a period of time to the use of stainless steel disposable blades again, which are actually used as "re-sposable." Although the blades were originally designed for a single use, it has been my experience that they can be used multiple times until usually, as is the case, the leading tip of the disposable keratome is damaged and easy penetration of the anterior chamber is made more difficult by the damage to the tip. No longer do I feel it is necessary that a groove be created, and I prefer to make the beveled keratome incision directly into the cornea through the stroma and into the anterior chamber. The usual approach is temporal clear corneal although, occasionally, a limbal incision may be made. The drawback to the limbal incision is the ballooning of the conjunctiva that occurs intraoperatively and persists postoperatively, which has a temporary cosmetically bothersome appearance, but resolves very quickly over the first 24 hours after surgery. Also, in patients with 0.5 D or greater of with-the-rule astigmatism, a superior clear corneal incision is used. With the presence of 1.5 D or more of keratometric with-the-rule astigmatism, I prefer to perform refractive keratotomy at the time of cataract surgery. Previously, paired linear astigmatic keratotomies were performed for astigmatism up to 3.00 D. The paired incisions were placed at the 6.5-mm optical zone with a depth of 110% of the central corneal pachymetry. The incisions were placed with the paired incisions at 1.0 mm per diopter.

The most recent change is to limbal relaxing incisions which are placed just in front of the vascular arcade with a diamond blade setting of 600 microns, and the arcuate incision is placed at 5 mm for 1.5 D, at 6 mm for 2 D, at 7 for 2.5 D, and 8 mm for 3 D. Should there be residual astigmatism postoperatively, additional linear or arcuate keratotomy can be added to enhance the outcome postoperatively.

With the limbal relaxing incision, the clear corneal incision is placed in the center of the incision utilizing the inner corneal wall of the 600-micron groove as the entry point for the beveled incision through the clear cornea. It is wise to reduce the keratome incision by about 0.2 micron to reduce wound gaping during the cataract procedure. Should the astigmatism be with-the-rule or oblique, the clear corneal incision will be centered in the steep meridian very much in the center of the limbal relaxing incision.

I prefer to use a stainless steel blade, having gone through many diamond blades over the years that the economic reality offers a compelling argument for the use of stainless steel. With each procedure, the stainless steel blade is inspected for the integrity of the tip. I select a tapered bevel-up keratome which puts the blade with the lateral cutting edge posteriorly giving a linear incision into the clear cornea. The incision is initially made with the tip and a forward thrust of the blade with a right-and-left rocking motion as needed to facilitate the advance of the tip while lifting gently on the blade rather than depressing it, which guides the blade through the corneal stroma before engaging Descemet's membrane. Once Descemet's membrane has been penetrated, the blade is advanced directly into the anterior chamber. Previously, a stainless steel blade was used to create a side-port incision 1 to 1½ clock hours temporal to the anticipated entry point into the anterior chamber. A side-port incision facilitates with the two-handed surgical techniques that I use for cataract extraction. The side-port incision remains self-sealing, as will the primary incision. The incision width is measured at 3.0 mm, which allows for phacoemulsification with a standard phaco tip and insertion of the folded silicone lens implant with the currently available insertion systems. The superthin stainless steel keratomes that are used create a consistent rectangular, rather than trapezoidal, incision into the anterior chamber, but with enough relaxing of the incision to allow movement of the phaco tip for phacoemulsification or I/A tip in the anterior chamber.

After the cataract extraction and lens implantation, the incision may require some hydration and verification of wound integrity. Should there be leakage from the incision, the wound can be sutured with one simple radial 10-0 Mersilene, which ususally can be removed within 1 week following the cataract procedure.

Although I am very comfortable with this current surgical technique, I would anticipate that further modifications may be forthcoming, but none are anticipated in the immediate future. The current technique and instrumentation provide easily reproducible results with minimal postoperative complications other than transient localized corneal swelling and minimal induced astigmatism.

Tilt and Tumble Phacoemulsification

Richard L. Lindstrom, MD

I was fortunate to be introduced to phacoemulsification in 1977 during a fellowship with Dr. William S. Harris in Dallas, Texas. At that time, phacoemulsification techniques were generally divided into anterior chamber phaco as championed by Dr. Charles Kelman, iris plane phaco as championed by Dr. Richard Kratz, and posterior chamber phaco as championed by Drs. John Sheets and Robert Sinskey. Under the tutelage of Dr. Harris, I had the opportunity to try all of these techniques, and over a period of time I selected the iris plane phacoemulsification technique of Dr. Kratz as my procedure of choice.

In this era prior to capsulorrhexis and hydrodissection, I would perform a relatively large can-opener anterior capsulectomy just inside the zonules. Following this, a portion of the central core nucleus was emulsified leaving an inferior shelf of tissue. Then, utilizing a bimanual technique, the superior pole of the nucleus was tilted above the capsule and engaged by a beveled phacoemulsification tip. The nucleus was then supported in the iris plane with a nucleus rotator and emulsified (Figure 9-1).

I still found occasions to subluxate the nucleus into the anterior chamber, particularly when I was in trouble or concerned about a capsular tear. I also had indications for posterior chamber phacoemulsification, particularly in very soft nuclei in younger patients. Yet, Kratz's iris plane phacoemulsification remained my procedure of choice for many years, and I taught this technique successfully to hundreds of residents, fellows, and fellow ophthalmologists.

Like others in the 1980s, I experimented with and eventually adopted the tech-

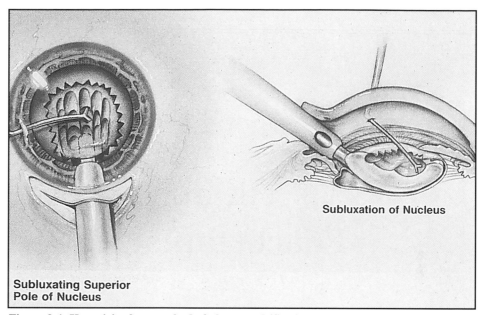

Subluxation of Nucleus

**Subluxating Superior
Pole of Nucleus**

Figure 9-1. Kratz iris plane method of phacoemulsification.

nique of continuous tear anterior capsulectomy (capsulorrhexis). Initially, I utilized a relatively small diameter capsulorrhexis in the range of 4.0 to 5.0 mm, especially when utilizing 5.5-mm round optic PMMA IOLs. This small continuous tear anterior capsulectomy made it impossible to subluxate the nucleus safely into the iris plane or anterior chamber, and I, therefore, converted to posterior chamber, endocapsular phaco techniques. In most nuclei I would utilize a nuclear cracking technique, but still found a technique where I would emulsify the core nucleus and then infracture the peripheral bowl of retained nuclear material and nuclear plate in a so-called one-handed technique useful for soft nuclei in younger patients. Soon thereafter, hydrodissection and hydrodelineation became a standard part of my technique in order to loosen the nucleus and allow it to be rotated more easily, and with a small continuous tear anterior capsulectomy, the nucleus always remained localized in the posterior chamber. While there are many positive features to the endocapsular cracking techniques, I did find they were more difficult to teach with a longer learning curve. In addition, I found my procedure times to be somewhat longer than they had been with the iris plane technique. I also noted a mild increase in my capsular tear rate from approximately 1% to 1.8%. On the positive side, visual recovery was very rapid, especially when I adopted foldable IOLs, and most patients had a crystal clear cornea on the first postoperative day. In time I was able to reduce my capsular tear rate to 1.3%, but I continued to have an operative procedure that required 10 to 15 minutes to complete. In addition, in some instances when my capsulorrhexis was somewhat smaller, in the 4-mm range, particularly in patients with loose zonules, such as patients with pseudoexfoliation, I noted other undesirable side effects such as the capsular-contraction syndrome.

After being influenced by several Japanese investigators who suggested that retained subcapsular epithelium might play a role in postoperative inflammation and capsular opacity, I began to investigate using larger diameter continuous tear anterior capsulectomies. Utilizing a continuous tear anterior capsulectomy of 5.5 to 6.5 mm, I returned to the size of anterior capsulectomy that I had utilized in my early phacoemulsification years when utilizing iris plane and anterior chamber phacoemulsification. During hydrodissection I would, in many cases, partially or totally subluxate the nucleus anterior to the capsular rim inadvertently. In those cases I would simply push the nucleus back into the capsular bag and complete the procedure utilizing a nuclear fracture technique. Over a period of time I learned to take advantage of this capability to subluxate the nucleus into the anterior chamber in high risk cases. When there was a large anterior segment, as in a myopic patient, a healthy cornea, and a relatively soft nucleus, I would often subluxate the nucleus to a position anterior to the capsular bag and complete a deep anterior chamber phacoemulsification supporting the nucleus with a nucleus rotator. I found the larger anterior capsulectomy allowed an easier phacoemulsification, and I did not appear to be sacrificing anything in regards to IOL centration. Fundus visibility was good, and my occasional case of capsular-contraction syndrome disappeared. Capsular opacity rates appeared low, and a small randomized study suggested that they were somewhat lower than with the smaller anterior capsulectomy that I had utilized in the past. The impact of capsulorrhexis size on capsular opacity rate and postoperative inflammation remains controversial with studies supporting both sides of the equation. I remain impressed that my incidence of capsular opacity and inflammation is somewhat lower with a larger anterior capsulectomy.

I was next influenced by Drs. David Brown and Bill Maloney, who have championed the concept of supracapsular phacoemulsification where the nucleus is hydrodissected and tumbled and then pushed back into the posterior chamber anterior to the capsule. After evaluating this technique for a period of time, I found it technically somewhat difficult to tumble the nucleus safely in all eyes. I also found that my first-day postoperative corneas were not as clear as I had been accustomed to seeing them when utilizing an endocapsular approach. I did, however, become quite adept at hydrodissecting until the nucleus tilted, which was the first step prior to tumbling the nucleus in a supracapsular approach. One day while working on my supracapsular and tumbling technique, I realized that the first step of this procedure tilted the nucleus to a position very similar to that which I had utilized for years in the Kratz iris plane phacoemulsification approach. Rather than completing the tumbling of the entire nucleus, I simply supported the nucleus in the plane of the iris and anterior capsular leaflet and then emulsified half of it. At that time, with a much smaller nuclear remnant, I tumbled the remaining one half upside down and completed the emulsification as I would have in the classical supracapsular approach. To my delight, the surgical technique was fast, simple, and safe. The following day the corneas of the patients upon whom I utilized this technique were similarly clear to those with my endocapsular nuclear fracture approach. I chose to call the technique "tilt and tumble" and began to refine it so that I could teach it effectively to residents, fellows, and other ophthalmologists with confidence. It is basically "back to Kratz"

with help from Brown and Maloney, in the capsulorrhexis, hydrodissection, viscoelastic, and modern phaco machine era. In the following paragraphs I will attempt to describe this technique in enough detail to allow an ophthalmologist to evaluate it for his or her own patients.

INDICATIONS

The indications for the tilt and tumble phacoemulsification technique are quite broad. It can be utilized in either a large or small pupil situation. I am aware of surgeons who favor it in small pupil settings where the nucleus can be tilted up such that the equator is resting in the center of a small pupil and is then carefully emulsified away. It does require a larger continuous tear anterior capsulectomy of at least 5.5 mm. If a small anterior capsulectomy is achieved, I believe that the hydrodissection step where the nucleus is tilted can be dangerous, and it would be possible to rupture the posterior capsule during the hydrodissection step. If inadvertently a small anterior capsulectomy is created, I favor converting to an endocapsular phacoemulsification technique or enlarging the capsulorrhexis. If I am unable to tilt the nucleus with either hydrodissection or manual technique, I will also convert to an endocapsular approach. Occasionally the entire nucleus will subluxate into the anterior chamber. In this setting, if the cornea is healthy, the anterior chamber roomy, and the nucleus soft, I will often complete the phacoemulsification in the anterior chamber supporting the nucleus away from the corneal endothelium. The nucleus can also be pushed back inferiorly over the capsular bag to allow the iris plane tilt and tumble technique to be completed. In patients with severely compromised endothelium, such as Fuchs' dystrophy or previous keratoplasty patients with a low endothelial cell count, I will often utilize endocapsular phacoemulsification to reduce endothelial trauma to the minimum possible. In a normal eye I am unable to differentiate my first-day postoperative corneal clarity in my endocapsular eyes vs my nuclear tilt and tumble eyes, but the tilting and tumbling maneuvers do increase the chance of endothelial cell contact of lens material vs an endocapsular phacoemulsification. I, therefore, favor the latter in eyes with borderline corneas. The technique is a very good transition technique for teaching residents, fellows, and surgeons who are transitioning to phacoemulsification because it is easy to convert to a planned extracapsular cataract extraction with the nucleus partially subluxated above the anterior capsular flap at the iris plane.

PREOPERATIVE PREPARATION

The patient enters the anesthesia induction or preoperative area and tetracaine drops are placed in both eyes. The placement of these drops increases the patient's comfort during the placement of the multiple dilating and preoperative medications, decreases blepharospasm, and also increases the corneal penetration of the drops to follow. I dilate the patient with 2.5% Neo-Synephrine and 1% cyclopentolate every 5 minutes for 3 doses. I also treat the patient preoperatively with topical antibiotic and anti-inflammatory drops at the same time as dilation. I favor preoperative topical antibiotic, topical steroid, and topical non-steroidal. The rationale for this is to

preload the eye with antibiotic and non-steroidal prior to surgery. The pharmacology of these drugs and the pathophysiology of postoperative infection and inflammation support this approach. An eye that is preloaded with anti-inflammatories prior to the surgical insult is likely to demonstrate a much reduced postoperative inflammatory response. Both topical steroids and non-steroidals have been confirmed to be synergistic in the reduction of postoperative inflammation. In addition, the use of perioperative antibiotics appears to be supported by the literature as helpful in reducing the small chance of postoperative endophthalmitis. Since the patient will be sent home on the same drops utilized preoperatively, there is no additional cost.

My usual anesthesia is topical tetracaine reinforced with intraoperative intracameral 1% nonpreserved (methylparaben-free) Xylocaine. For patients with blepharospasm a "mini-block" Obrien facial nerve anesthesia, utilizing 2% Xylocaine with 150 units of hyaluronidase per 5 cc of Xylocaine, can be quite helpful in reducing squeezing. This block lasts 30 to 45 minutes and makes surgery easier for the patient and the surgeon. Patients are sedated prior to the block to eliminate any memory of discomfort. One way to screen for patients where this facial nerve block might be useful is to ask the technicians to make a note in the chart when they have difficulty performing applanation pressures or A-scan because of blepharospasm. In these patients a mini facial nerve block can be quite helpful.

In younger anxious patients and in those where I am quite concerned about cooperation, I continue to perform a peribulbar block. This is basically a clinical impression type decision. Naturally general anesthesia is used for very uncooperative patients and children. While this is controversial in some patients where general anesthesia is chosen and a significant bilateral cataract is present, I will perform consecutive bilateral surgery completely re-prepping and starting with fresh instruments for the second eye. Again, this is a risk-benefit clinical decision weighing the risk-benefit ratio of operating both eyes on the same day vs the risk of two general anesthetics.

In summary, in the induction area the patient is dilated maximally and the eye is preloaded with antibiotic, steroid, and non-steroidal anti-inflammatory drops. Appropriate anesthesia is obtained. Oculopression can be utilized at the surgeon's discretion, and I still favor this in most patients, even when utilizing topical anesthesia. The patient is visited by the anesthetist, if utilized, as well as the circulating nurse and the surgeon. Any questions are answered. The patient is then brought into the surgical suite.

Upon entering the surgical suite, the patient table is centered on preplaced marks so that it is appropriately placed for microscope, surgeon, scrub nurse, and anesthetist access. I favor a wrist rest, and the patient's head is adjusted such that a ruler placed on the forehead and cheek will be parallel to the floor. The patient's head is stabilized with tape to the wrist rest to reduce unexpected movements, particularly when the patient may fall asleep during the procedure and suddenly awaken. A second drop of tetracaine is placed in each eye. I find that if the tetracaine is placed in each eye, blepharospasm is reduced. A periocular prep with 5% povidone-iodine solution is completed. I do not personally irrigate the ocular surface and fornices with povidone-iodine, as under topical anesthesia I find that the patients note

a significant burning. If a few drops leak into the eye this is certainly acceptable.

I have found an aperture drape helpful to increase comfort for topical anesthesia patients, as I have noted that when I tuck the drape under the lids this often irritates the patient's eye and also reduces the malleability of the lids, decreasing exposure. Since it is important to isolate the meibomian glands and lashes, if an aperture drape is utilized I recommend a reversible, solid-bladed speculum (Lindstrom/Chu speculum, Rhein Medical). Utilizing temporal and nasal approaches to the eye, the solid blades of the speculum are not in the way. In those cases where a superior approach is planned, I will utilize a drape where the drape is tucked under the lids, and, in those cases, I favor a Kratz modified Barraquer wire, as this enhances access to the globe. I do, however, find that I am using a superior approach incision less and less. I currently utilize balanced salt solution in all cases. I have not found for the short duration of a phacoemulsification case that BSS Plus provides any clinically meaningful benefit. I place 0.5 cc of the intracardiac nonpreserved (sodium bisulfate-free) epinephrine in the bottle for assistance in dilation and perhaps hemostasis. I also place 1 mL (1000 units) of heparin sulfate to reduce the possibility of postoperative fibrin. This is also a good anti-inflammatory and coating agent. At this dose there is no risk of enhancing bleeding or reducing hemostasis. I personally also favor 10 mg of vancomycin in the 500 cc of balanced salt solution, although this remains controversial. I personally consider an IOL a high-risk prosthetic case in that the risk of significant loss of vision is clearly high, even though the incidence of infection is relatively low. While there are currently no studies to fully document the risk-benefit ratio to the individual patient and to society in general utilizing this approach, my own personal incidence of endophthalmitis has been reduced from approximately 1/1000 to 0 in approximately 6000 consecutive cases since utilizing vancomycin in the bottle intraoperatively. Dr. Manus Kraff of Illinois and Dr. James Gills of Florida have reported similar experiences (personal communication, 1998).

The lids are separated with a solid-blade speculum. A solid-blade Barraquer speculum is satisfactory, but my associate, Dr. Y. Ralph Chu and I have recently designed an aspirating speculum called the Lindstrom/Chu speculum available from Rhein Medical. This instrument, which can be placed temporally or nasally, isolates the lashes and also can be hooked up to aspiration to remove any pooling of fluid. A final drop of tetracaine is placed in the operative eye or the surface is irrigated with the nonpreserved Xylocaine. I am now ready to begin the surgical procedure. I do not like to utilize more than 3 drops of tetracaine or other topical anesthetic as excess softening of the epithelium can occur, resulting in punctate epithelial keratitis, corneal erosion, and delayed postoperative rehabilitation.

OPERATIVE PROCEDURE

The patient is asked to look down. The globe is supported with a dry Merocel sponge, and a counterpuncture is performed superiorly at 12 o'clock with a diamond stab knife (Osher, Storz). I favor approximately a 1-mm stab incision (Figure 9-2). Approximately 0.25 mL of 1% nonpreserved methylparaben-free Xylocaine is injected into the eye (Figure 9-3). I advise the patient that he or she will feel a "tin-

gling" or "burning" for a second, and then "the eye will go numb." This provides psychological support for the patient that he or she will now have a totally anesthetized eye and should not anticipate any discomfort. I tell the patient that while he or she will feel some touch and fluid on the eye, "you will not feel anything sharp," and if he or she does, should advise me, and I will supplement the anesthesia. This injection also firms up the eye for the clear corneal incision. I do not find it necessary to inject viscoelastic.

I prefer a temporal or nasal anterior limbal or posterior clear corneal incision. I define my incision as a modified Langerman incision. A groove is made 400 to 500 microns deep into the perilimbal capillary plexus just anterior to the insertion of the conjunctival (Figure 9-4). Care is taken not to incise the conjunctivae as this can result in ballooning during phacoemulsification and irrigation/aspiration. Some surgeons define this as being a posterior clear corneal incision and others as an anterior limbal incision. The anatomical landmark for me is the perilimbal capillary plexus and the insertion of the conjunctivae. When the groove is made there will be a small amount of capillary bleeding. Since the incision is into a vascular area, long-term wound healing can be expected to be stronger than it is with a true clear corneal incision. True clear corneal incisions, such as performed in radial keratotomy, clearly do not have the wound healing capabilities that a limbal incision demonstrates where there are functioning blood vessels present. The anterior chamber is then entered parallel to the iris at a depth of approximately 300 microns or above the deepest portion of the groove. This creates a hinge type or Langerman type of incision (Figure 9-5). I like the width of the incision to be 1.75 to 2.0 mm and have designed a keratome with Storz with two small black lines which can serve as a guide to the surgeon in creating an appropriate width incision (Lindstrom keratome, Storz).

In right eyes, my favorite incision is temporal, and in left eyes, nasal. I have found a nasal clear corneal incision for left eyes to be excellent, allowing the surgeon to sit in the same position for right and left eyes. I simply need to move over approximately 2 to 3 inches in my sitting position, and I can continue with my phacoemulsifier, scrub nurse, and instruments to my right sitting comfortably oblique at an approximately 45 degree angle at the patient's head. The nasal cornea is thicker, has a higher endothelial cell count, and allows very good access for phacoemulsification. The nasal limbus is approximately 0.3 mm closer to the center of the cornea than the temporal limbus, and this can, in some cases where there is excess edema, reduce first-day postoperative vision more than one might anticipate with a temporal incision. There also can, in some patients, be pooling. For this reason, I do favor an aspirating speculum. It is also helpful to tip the head slightly to the left side. Nonetheless, I have found in my left eyes a nasal clear corneal approach to be excellent, and offer this as an alternative for surgeons who find the left temporal position uncomfortable. While I personally create my groove by simply taking the keratome and tipping it up and utilizing the tip of the keratome, many surgeons will utilize a guarded knife to create a consistently deep incision. I find that an astigmatic keratotomy blade can be quite useful in this regard. This blade can also be helpful when patients present with high astigmatism and an intraoperative astigmatic keratotomy

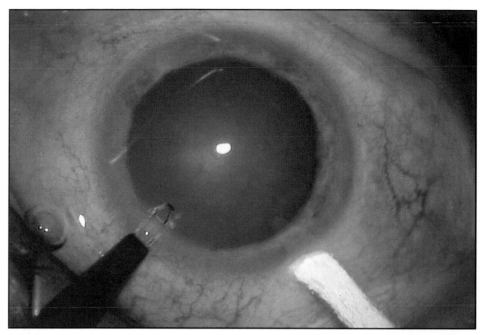

Figure 9-2. A clear corneal counterpuncture is made at 12 o'clock with a l-mm diamond blade.

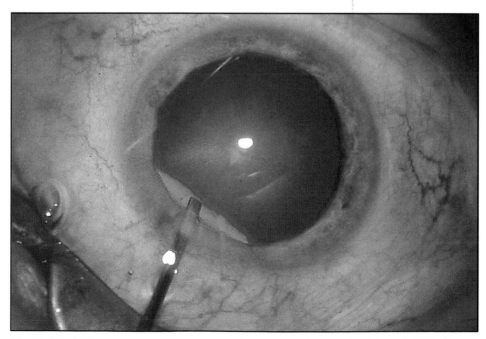

Figure 9-3. 0.25 mL of nonpreserved (methylparaben-free) Xylocaine is injected into the anterior chamber.

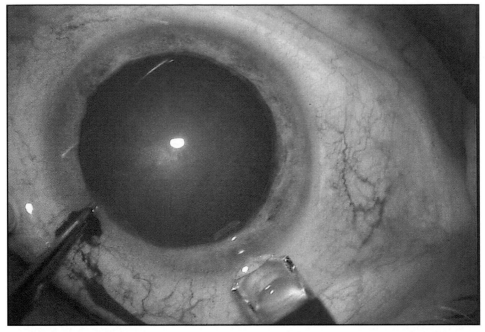

Figure 9-4. A "modified Langerman"—anterior limbal incision is created with a 2.5- to 3.2-mm diamond keratome.

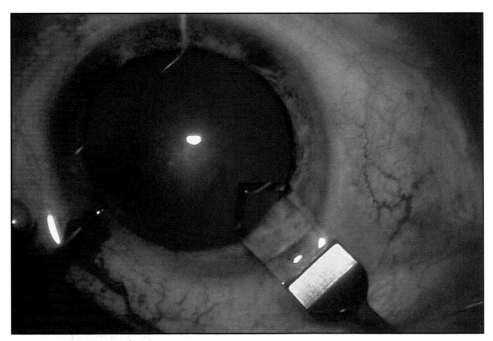

Figure 9-5. A "modified Langerman"—anterior limbal incision is created with a 2.5- to 3.2-mm diamond keratome.

is felt to be appropriate.

In some patients I will select a corneal scleral incision, eg, those who have had a previous radial keratotomy or demonstrate findings of peripheral corneal ulcerative keratitis, in some patients with very low endothelial cell counts, and any case where there was any significant peripheral pathology or thinning. I do find that my type of anterior limbal or posterior corneal incision can be made temporally, nasally, in the oblique meridian, or even superiorly without induction of significant corneal edema or endothelial cell loss.

When I select a corneal scleral incision I will raise a small conjunctival flap with a Westcott scissors. Prior to this I will hold a Merocel sponge in the area of the limbus where the conjunctival flap will be raised, soaked in tetracaine or nonpreserved Xylocaine, for 30 to 60 seconds to enhance anesthesia. Mild cautery can be applied or one can utilize a Merocel soaked in thrombin 1/1000 in BSS to effect hemostasis. If there is minimal capillary oozing the mild bleeding can also simply be ignored. Thrombin solution is also very useful in anterior segment reconstruction cases where excess bleeding is noted and may be safely injected into the anterior chamber if diluted in BSS.

I personally close all clear corneal incisions larger than 4 mm with a horizontal mattress, X, or single radial suture. I have found that the least early astigmatism is induced with the horizontal mattress suture, and I personally favor this. A corneal scleral incision greater than 5.5 mm is also closed with one horizontal mattress suture. I find that my incision, if 3 mm in length, tends to cause an induction of 0.25 $\pm$ 0.25 D of astigmatism. If it is placed on the steeper meridian, it can therefore be expected to reduce the astigmatism somewhere between 0 and 0.50 D. If the incision is 4 mm in length, I find a reduction in astigmatism of 0.50 $\pm$ 0.50 D or 0 to 1.00 D if the incision is placed on the steeper meridian. In routine cataract surgery I do not utilize incisions larger than 4 mm, and I do favor an incision in the 3-mm range as I am very secure that these will be self-sealing. I find that with modern injector systems most foldable IOLs can be implanted through a 3-mm anterior limbal incision.

In select patients I will perform an intraoperative astigmatic keratotomy at the 7- to 8-mm optical zone. I personally will do this at the beginning of the operation. The patient's astigmatism axis is marked carefully using an intraoperative surgical keratometer which allows one to delineate the steeper and flatter meridian and not be concerned about globe rotation. I find that one 2-mm incision at a 7- to 8-mm optical zone will correct 1 D of astigmatism and two 2-mm incisions will correct 2 D of astigmatism in a cataract age patient. One 3-mm incision will correct 2 D, and two 3-mm incisions 4 D. One can combine a 3 mm and 2 mm correcting 3 D. Larger amounts of astigmatism can also be corrected utilizing the Arc-T nomogram.

Depending on the age of the patient one can correct up to 8 D of astigmatism with two 90 degree arcs. Many surgeons have moved to a more peripheral corneal limbal arcuate incision, but I continue to favor the 7- to 8-mm optical zone because of my years of experience with this approach. There certainly is a variation in response, but I have not found any significant induced complications with this approach. My outcome goal is 1 D or less of astigmatism in the preoperative axis. I would prefer to undercorrect rather than overcorrect. The key in astigmatism surgery

is "axis, axis, axis." If one is not careful in preoperative planning and the incisions are placed more than 15 degrees off axis, one is better avoiding this approach.

The anterior chamber is constituted with a viscoelastic. My studies have not found any significant difference between one viscoelastic or another in regards to postoperative endothelial cell counts. I have found Ocucoat to be an excellent viscoelastic which can also be utilized to coat the epithelial surface during surgery. This eliminates the need for continuous irrigation with BSS. It gives a very clear view. It is also economically a good choice in most settings. I have also been very happy with the Amvisc Plus, as we can obtain 0.8 cc of it at a very fair price.

I then fashion a relatively large diameter continuous tear anterior capsulectomy (Figures 9-6 and 9-7). This can be made with a cystotome or forceps. I personally prefer a cystotome. I would like it to be 5.5 to 6.5 mm in diameter and inside the insertion of the zonules (usually at 7 mm). In my opinion, larger is better than smaller, as there is less subcapsular epithelium and an easier cataract operation. I still believe that less subcapsular epithelium leaves one with a lower inflammation postoperatively and less capsular opacity. I have not seen any change in the incidence of IOL decentration. With some IOLs, the capsule will seal down to the posterior capsule around the loops rather than be symmetrically placed over the anterior surface of the IOL. These eyes, in my opinion, do extremely well, and I am beginning to wonder if this is not preferred to having the capsule anterior to the optic. This is also certainly a controversial position.

I then perform hydrodissection utilizing a Pearce hydrodissection cannula on a 3-cc syringe filled with BSS. Slow continuous hydrodissection is performed gently lifting the anterior capsular rim until a fluid wave is seen. At this point irrigation is continued until the nucleus tilts on one side, up and out of the capsular bag (Figure 9-8). If one retracts the capsule at approximately the 7:30 o'clock position with the hydrodissection cannula, usually the nucleus will tilt superiorly. If it tilts in another position, it is simply rotated until it is facing the incision (Figure 9-9).

Once the nucleus is tilted, some additional viscoelastic can be injected under the nucleus pushing the iris and capsule back. Also, additional viscoelastic can be placed over the nuclear edge to protect the endothelium. The nucleus is emulsified outside-in while supporting the nucleus in the iris plane with a second instrument, in my case, a Rhein Medical or Storz Lindstrom Star or Lindstrom Trident nucleus rotator (Figure 9-10).

Once half the nucleus is removed, the remaining one half is tumbled upside-down and attacked from the opposite pole (Figure 9-11). Again it is supported in the iris plane until the emulsification is completed (Figures 9-12 and 9-13). Alternatively, the nucleus can be rotated and emulsified from the outside edge in, in a carousel or cartwheel type of technique. Finally, in some cases, the nucleus can be continuously emulsified in the iris plane if there is good followability until the entire nucleus is gone.

I have found this to be a very fast and very safe technique, and as mentioned before, it is a modification of the iris plane technique taught by Kratz in the late 1970s and 1980s. It is basically "back to Kratz" with help from Brown and Maloney in the modern phacoemulsification, capsulorrhexis, hydrodissection, and viscoelas-

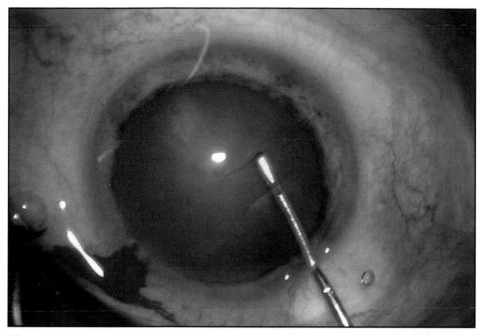

Figure 9-6. A large (5.5- to 6.5-mm) continuous tear anterior capsulectomy is performed.

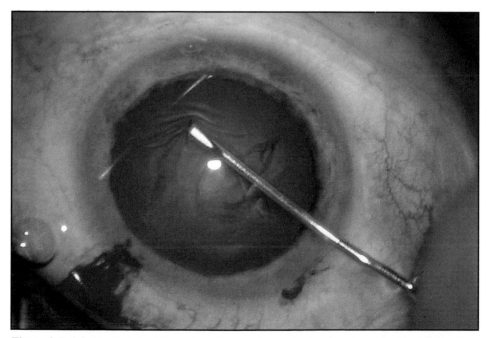

Figure 9-7. A large (5.5- to 6.5-mm) continuous tear anterior capsulectomy is performed.

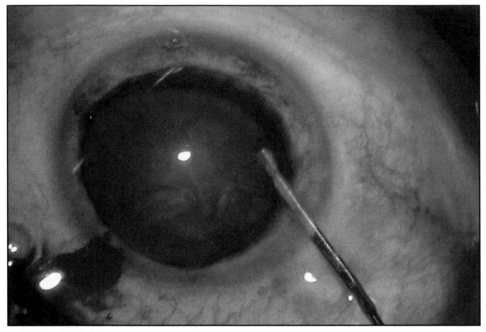

Figure 9-8. Hydrodissection is continued until the nucleus tilts out of the capsular bag. If necessary, the nucleus is rotated to face the incision.

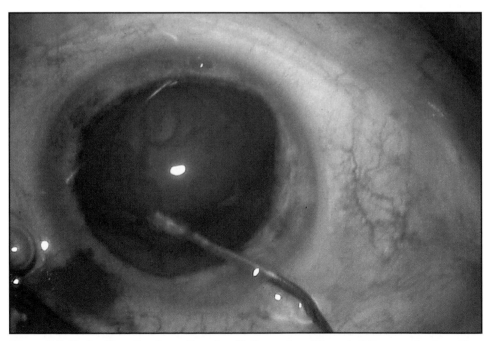

Figure 9-9. Hydrodissection is continued until the nucleus tilts out of the capsular bag. If necessary, the nucleus is rotated to face the incision.

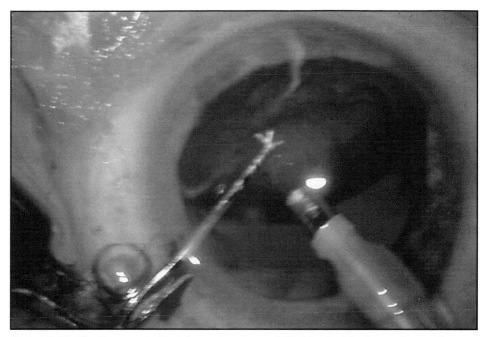

Figure 9-10. The first one half of the nucleus is emulsified in the iris plane using an "outside in" phacoemulsification approach. I prefer a 30 degree bevel MicroFlow Plus needle and Storz Millennium machine.

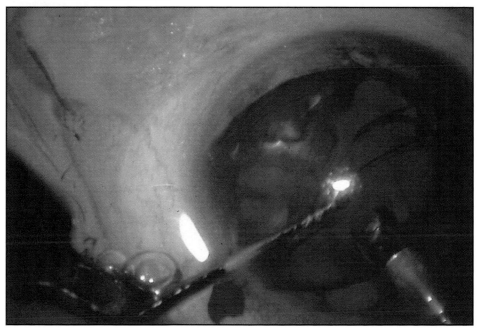

Figure 9-11. The remaining one half of the nucleus is tumbled upside down with a nucleus rotator.

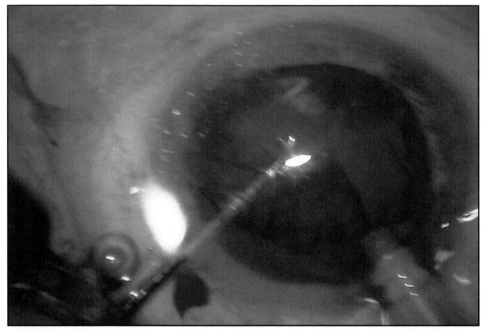

Figure 9-12. The remaining one half of the nucleus is supported in the iris plane with a nucleus rotator and emulsified outside in.

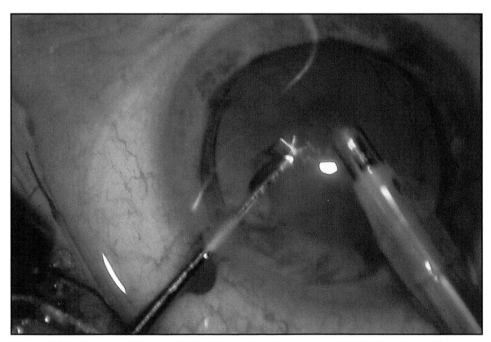

Figure 9-13. The remaining one half of the nucleus is supported in the iris plane with a nucleus rotator and emulsified outside in.

tic era. My surgery times now range between 5 and 10 minutes with this approach rather than 10 to 15 minutes for endocapsular phacoemulsification. In addition, my capsular tear rate has now gone under 1%. I have, therefore, found it to be a technique that is easier, faster, and safer. It is true that in this technique the phacoemulsification tip is closer to the iris margin and also somewhat closer to the corneal endothelium. There is, however, a significantly greater margin of error in regards to the posterior capsule. Care needs to be taken to position the nucleus away from the corneal endothelium and away from the iris margin when utilizing this approach.

If the nucleus does not tilt with simple hydrodissection, it can be tilted with a second instrument such as a nuclear rotator, Graether collar button, or hydrodissection cannula.

When utilizing this approach of phacoemulsification with the Storz Premier instrument, I utilize a vacuum of 60 mmHg and an anterior chamber maintainer pressure of 60 mmHg. I personally favor the Storz MicroFlow Plus needle with a 30 degree bevel.

When utilizing a peristaltic machine, I will utilize a slightly higher vacuum in the range of 80 to 100 mmHg. I favor a relatively high bottle with some overflow of fluid. Again, I find for me a 30 degree bevel needle is appropriate for this approach. When utilizing tilt and tumble, very high vacuum settings are not necessary and may be inappropriate. The reason being is that the iris margin is in the vicinity of the phacoemulsification tip, and it is possible to core through the nucleus and aspirate the iris margin if very high vacuums are utilized.

More recently I have had an opportunity to work with the dual function Storz Millennium, and I find this machine to be excellent for all cataract techniques including tilt and tumble. I will set my vacuum with a range of 60 to 100 mmHg and my ultrasound power from 10% to 50% with the Storz Millennium. I will arrange the foot pedal such that I have surgeon control over ultrasound on the vertical or pitch motion of the foot pedal, and then on the yaw or right motion foot pedal, I will have vacuum control. I, therefore, can engage the tissue, emulsify it, and, as needed, apply additional ultrasound with a downward movement and additional vacuum with a right movement of the foot pedal. This allows very efficient emulsification, and the Millennium is my current preferred machine. Again, I favor the MicroFlow Plus needle with a 30 degree angle tip with the Millennium.

Following completion of nuclear removal, the cortex is removed with the I/A handpiece. I favor a 0.3-mm tip and utilize the universal handpiece with interchangeable tips. I will use a curve-linear tip for most cortex removal and then remove the cortex under the incision with a Lindstrom right angle sandblasted tip currently manufactured by Rhein and Storz (Figure 9-14). If there is significant debris or plaque on the posterior capsule, I will attempt some polishing and vacuum cleaning, but I do not favor extensive polishing or vacuum cleaning as I have found many of my capsular tears with this technique occur during capsular polishing and vacuuming. Many times there is an unexpected small burr or sharp defect on the I/A tip which results in a capsular tear after a case that was otherwise well done.

The anterior chamber is reconstituted with viscoelastic, and I will insert an IOL utilizing an injector system (Figures 9-15 and 9-16). My current lenses of choice

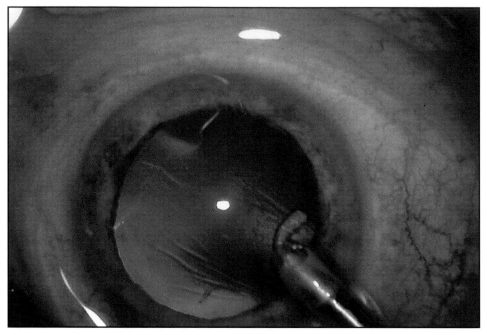

Figure 9-14. The cortex under the incision is removed with a Lindstrom sandblasted right angle tip.

include the plate haptic silicone IOL and the three-piece silicone lenses which are injectable through a 3-mm incision. In select cases I will utilize an acrylic implant, although with a cross-action folder this requires enlargement of the incision. I have found that one can inject the acrylic lens with care through a Bartelt injector, but proper technique is necessary or the loops can be damaged.

Excess viscoelastic is removed with irrigation/aspiration. I simply push back on the IOL and slowly turn the irrigation/aspiration to the right and left two or three times allowing a fairly complete removal of viscoelastic under the IOL.

I favor injection of a miotic and personally prefer carbachol over Miochol at this time, as it is more effective in reducing postoperative intraocular tension spikes and has a longer duration of action. I find it is necessary to dilute the carbachol 5 to 1, or one can obtain an excessively small pupil which results in dark vision for the patient at night for 1 to 2 days. I firm up the eye through the counterpuncture and evaluate the incision. If the chamber remains well constituted and there is no spontaneous leak from the incision, I do not feel that wound hydration is necessary. If there is some shallowing in the anterior chamber and a spontaneous leak, I will then perform wound hydration injecting BSS peripherally into the incision and hydrating it to push the edges together. I believe that within a few minutes these clear corneal or posterior limbal incisions seal, much as a LASIK flap will stick down, through the negative swelling pressure of the cornea and capillary attraction. It is important to leave the eye slightly firm at 20 mmHg or so to reduce the side effects of hypotony and also help the internal valve incision to appropriately seal (Figure 9-17).

At completion of the procedure I place another drop of antibiotic, steroid, and non-steroidal on the eye. I also use 1 drop of an anti-hypertensive such as Betagan or Alphagan to reduce postoperative intraocular tension spikes.

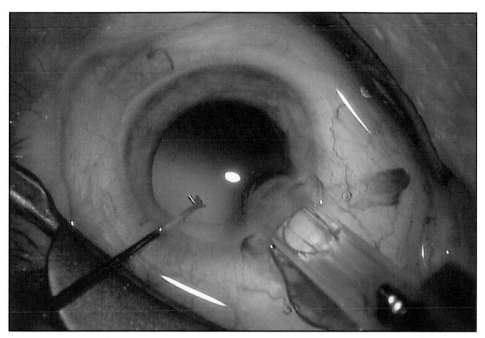

Figure 9-15. A foldable IOL is implanted with the capsular bag using an injector system.

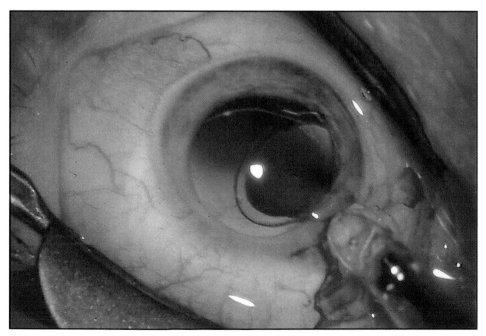

Figure 9-16. A foldable IOL is implanted with the capsular bag using an injector system.

POSTOPERATIVE CARE

No patch is routinely utilized for the topical and intracameral approach. If a mini-block of the lids has been performed, this will wear off in 30 to 45 minutes, and there is usually adequate lid function for a normal blink at the completion of the procedure. Patients are advised that they will have some erythropsia, meaning they will see a pink after-image for the rest of the day, but usually this will resolve by the next morning. They are also told that their vision may be a little dark at night from the miotic, and not to be concerned if they wake up at night and their vision seems dark.

The patient is seen on the first-day postoperative and then at approximately 2 to 3 weeks postoperative. At this time a refraction and complete examination with the slit lamp and fundus evaluation are performed. If there is no inflammation, patients are seen again 1-year postoperative. If at 3 weeks there is still persistent inflammation, additional postoperative anti-inflammatory medications are recommended, and the patient is asked to return again at 2 to 3 months postoperative.

Topical antibiotic, steroid, and non-steroidal are utilized twice a day, usually requiring a 5-cc bottle and 3 to 4 weeks of therapy. Occasionally a second bottle of steroid and non-steroidal are necessary if flare and cell persist at the 3-week examination. There are minimal restrictions, including a request that there be no swimming and no very heavy lifting for 2 weeks. Many patients are given half-glasses the first postoperative day allowing functional vision at distance and near. I personally consider the ideal postoperative refractive spherical equivalent for a monofocal lens to be -0.62 D with less than 0.50 D of astigmatism in the same axis as preoperative. Most patients can see 20/30+ and J3+ with this type of correction. I will utilize monovision in the appropriate settings. More recently I am finding good results with the Allergan Array multifocal IOL. In this setting I target +0.25 to -0.25 D with minimal astigmatism.

The second eye is done at 1 month or greater postoperative, except in rare situations. I prefer to defer any YAG lasers for 90 days in order to allow the blood aqueous barrier to become intact and capsular fixation to be firm, especially in plate haptic IOLs. In my experience, the lowest YAG laser capsulotomy rates have been with the plate haptic silicone IOL and the Acrysoft IOL.

CONCLUSION

In summary, the key points are listed in Figures 9-18 through 9-20. I hope other surgeons will find this approach to cataract surgery useful. These techniques must be personalized, and all surgeons will find that slight variations in technique are required to achieve optimum results for their own individual patients in their own individual environment. Continuous efforts at incremental improvement result in meaningful advances in our ability to help the cataract patient obtain rapid, safe, visual recovery following surgery.

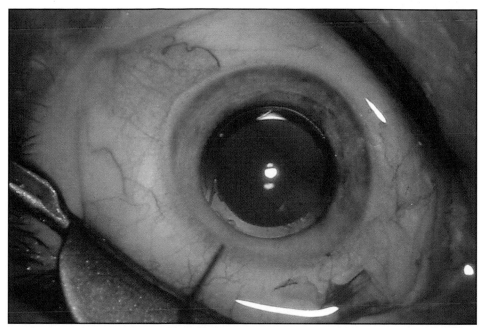

Figure 9-17. The eye at completion of the procedure. Note the left nasal clear corneal incision.

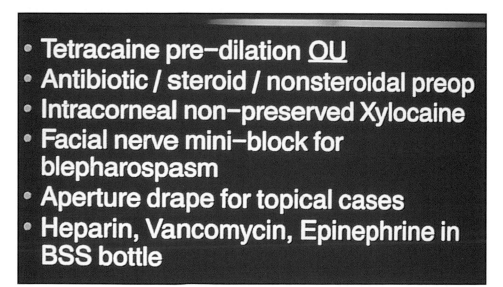

Figure 9-18. Summary of key steps in tilt and tumble phacoemulsification procedure.

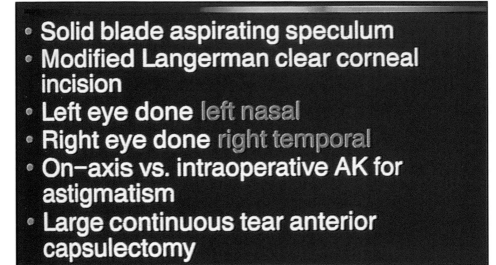

Figure 9-19. Summary of key steps in tilt and tumble phacoemulsification procedure.

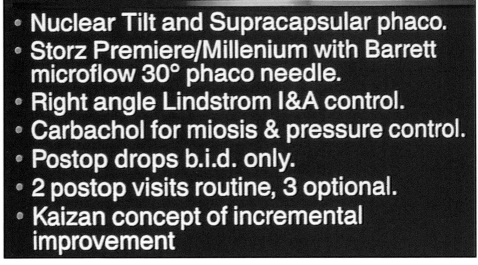

Figure 9-20. Summary of key steps in tilt and tumble phacoemulsification procedure.

Clear Corneal Incision: A Personal Method

Samuel Masket, MD

Clear corneal incision has become the technique of choice for many cataract surgeons. When compared with sclerocorneal incisions, advantages include reduced surgical time, reduced surgical trauma, and improved cosmesis. There are limitations, however, in that corneal incisions are less forgiving than are sclerocorneal tunnels, require exacting surgical precision in order to be self-sealing, and should be limited to incision sizes no greater than 3.8 mm in order to safely avoid the need for sutures. Furthermore, many believe, as do I, that clear corneal incisions should be limited to the temporal aspect of the globe. Temporally oriented incisions are further from the visual axis than are those placed superiorly or superonasally, owing to external limbal anatomy. As a result, temporally placed corneal incisions exhibit less astigmatic consequence and are further from the endothelial surface than are clear corneal incisions placed superiorly. While some surgeons prefer to operate in the astigmatically steepest axis and use the incision to reduce overall corneal astigmatism, I prefer to employ an incision system that induces little-to-no change in corneal curvature in order to provide early stability of the keratorefractive results of surgery. In those cases where reduction of pre-existing astigmatism is desirable, I combine astigmatic keratotomy with a stable temporal clear corneal incision. Incisional stability, with respect to induced astigmatism, is achieved in less than 2 weeks after surgery.

In a study of 45 eyes having unsutured pre-grooved (350-micron depth) temporally oriented clear corneal incisions, induced astigmatism, as noted in Figures 10-1 and 10-2, was approximately 0.5 D by vector analysis and 0.21 D in the incisional meridian when using simulated keratometry determined from computerized video-

keratography.[1] Most importantly, the data noted in Figures 10-1 and 10-2 suggest that the 2- and 6-week postoperative changes are identical, indicating that the corneal shape change is stable within 2 weeks after surgery.

I began temporal clear corneal cataract surgery routinely in mid-1993. Prior to that, I employed a superiorly oriented sclerocorneal tunnel with a frown-shaped external configuration for implantation of either foldable IOLs or one-piece rigid PMMA 5.5-mm lenses. Because corneal incisions are not protected with conjunctival closure, I used suture closure for all clear corneal cases for approximately 1 year, during which time I employed both 3.5-mm incisions for foldable lenses and 5.5-mm incisions for rigid lenses (Figure 10-3). The data as noted in Figures 10-4 and 10-5 compared the surgically induced astigmatism with 5.5-mm superior frown incisions (N = 50) to temporally placed 5.5-mm (N = 20) and 3.5-mm (N = 30) clear corneal incisions. The results indicated that the 3.5-mm temporally oriented incision exhibited the narrowest range of astigmatic change after surgery. Additionally, the temporal incisions, as expected, induced a small amount of with-the-rule astigmatic change while the superiorly oriented incision altered the cornea in an against-the-rule manner. I concluded from the data that small temporally oriented incisions were likely the most stable. Additionally, in short order it became evident that operating temporally offered many advantages with respect to exposure of the globe and for access to the anterior chamber. Furthermore, small clear corneal incisions mated very well with topical anesthesia which became part of my routine early in 1994. It became evident that the most efficient method for cataract surgery would provide rapid and stable surgical results, would include the use of topical anesthesia, would employ clear corneal incisions placed temporally, and would utilize foldable lenses which could be implanted through unenlarged phacoemulsification incisions. Subsequently, all cases, where possible, have been performed in that manner.

As mentioned above, during the initial year of my experiences with clear corneal surgery, I sutured virtually all incisions. Irrespective of a self-sealing corneal tunnel, I theorized that the absence of the conjunctival protection barrier (with which I was accustomed) mandated the need for suture closure. However, I began to experience suture-related complications. Corneal neovascularization was noted along suture tracts, I observed an induced pterygium in two patients (Figure 10-6), and, commonly, sutures would erode and induce a foreign body sensation. One patient with an eroded suture experienced a suture abscess. A growing body of personal experience and literature evidence suggested that small clear corneal temporal incisions did not require sutures. And, with the observed complications associated with sutures, I abandoned the use of routine suturing early in 1994.

Based upon the studies and theories of Langerman,[2] and the laboratory investigations of Ernest,[3] I employed a grooved clear corneal incision for more than 2 years. The Langerman theory suggests that a deep (600-micron) pre-cut groove creates an internal hinge that stabilizes the incision against force applied directly to the globe posterior to the incision. In fact, in laboratory cadaveric studies performed by Ernest et al, the Langerman-type incision tolerated greater point pressure applied

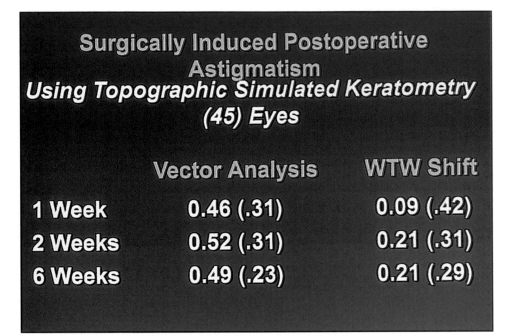

Figure 10-1. Mean induced astigmatic change for 45 eyes with 3-mm temporal clear corneal incision. The left column is by vector analysis and the right column by with-the-wound shift using a Cravy-Holladay-Koch software. Numbers in parentheses represent standard deviation.

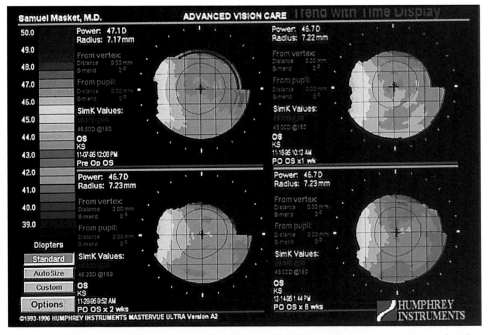

Figure 10-2. Representative patient with serial topographic analysis preoperative and 1, 2, and 6 weeks postoperatively.

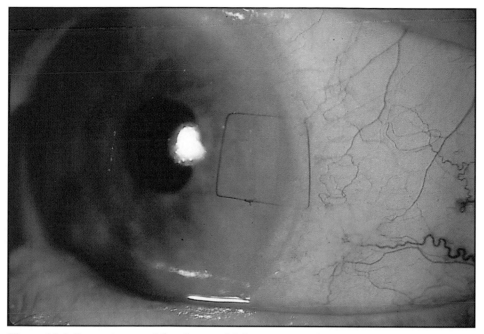

Figure 10-3. Box suture used for closure of 3.5-mm temporally oriented clear corneal incision.

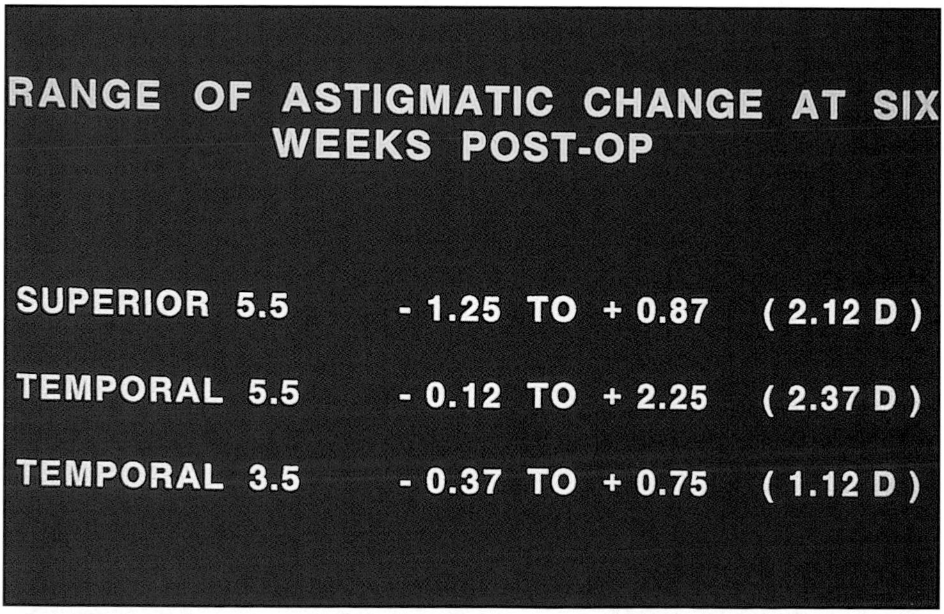

RANGE OF ASTIGMATIC CHANGE AT SIX WEEKS POST-OP		
SUPERIOR 5.5	- 1.25 TO + 0.87	(2.12 D)
TEMPORAL 5.5	- 0.12 TO + 2.25	(2.37 D)
TEMPORAL 3.5	- 0.37 TO + 0.75	(1.12 D)

Figure 10-4. Tabular form of range of induced astigmatism at 6 weeks after surgery using algebraic analysis. Superior orientation (50 eyes), temporal 5.5-mm incision group (20 eyes), and temporal 3.5-mm incision group (30 eyes). The numbers in parentheses represent the algebraic sum of the range of induced astigmatism for each group.

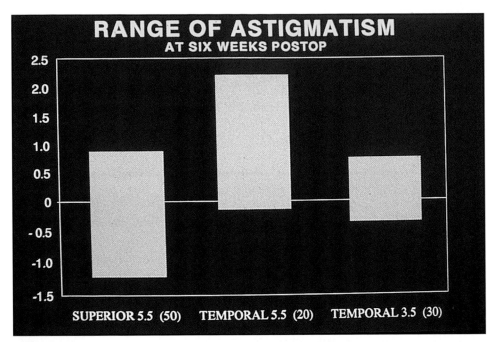

Figure 10-5. Bar graph presentation for same data in Figure 10-4.

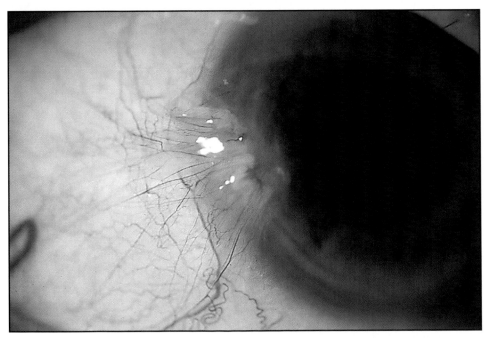

Figure 10-6. Pterygium induced by temporal clear corneal incision with 10-0 nylon suture closure. The patient, a 70-year-old male, had no sign of pterygium formation prior to surgery.

posterior to the incision without wound leakage when compared to other incision styles. Nevertheless, the very deep groove risks accidental perforation, physical instability, and, perhaps, additional induced astigmatism. Therefore, it was my preference to use no deeper than a 350-micron pre-cut groove for sutureless clear corneal cataract surgery. The incision system provided stability and in no case did I experience postoperative wound leaks or ocular hypotony.

However, a number of patients with grooved incisions complained of chronic foreign body sensation after surgery. In an attempt to reduce surgical time and eliminate postoperative sensation, I investigated a paracentesis-type clear corneal incision. Previous personal experience with this method often resulted in incisions that were triangulated or irregular on their external surface as a result of the thickness and configuration of the diamond keratome. However, with the advent of the 3-D blade (Rhein Medical) designed in part by Dr. I. Howard Fine, I was able to achieve a reliable method for non-grooved straight cut (paracentesis-type) 3-mm clear corneal incisions without the need for suture closure.

Currently, I employ a surgical method that I believe is safe, efficient, and reproducible. Virtually all cases are performed under topical and intracameral anesthetic. After appropriate asepsis and draping, a single side-port incision is fashioned with my non-dominant hand. The self-sealing side-port incision is made with a 15 degree blade using counterforce with a closed forceps at the opposite limbus (Figure 10-7). Care is taken to avoid vascular tissue. The Bores forceps provide stability owing to two-point fixation. Through the side-port, intracameral 1% nonpreserved lidocaine is added after which I **partially** fill the chamber with viscoelastic. If the eye is over-inflated or very firm, the incision tract tends to be too short and may not self-seal at the close of surgery. On the other hand, if the eye is too soft, the incision tract may be too long, creating the potential for an incision that is too central; incisions of this nature induce striae with poor visibility during surgery and promote corneal edema after surgery. Working with an eye at near physiologic pressure seems best. I fixate the globe with a closed MacPherson forceps placed through the side-port incision for counterpressure and control of eye movement. I use a 3-mm 3-D diamond blade and initiate the incision just central to the limbal vascular arcade. Using both tactile and visual clues, the blade is advanced through corneal tissue to create a 2-mm long tunnel (Figure 10-8). In this manner, the surface geometry of the incision is 3 x 2 mm. Following capsulorrhexis and cataract removal, a foldable lens is secured in the capsular bag. Given current technology and my methodology, I insert either silicone or acrylic lenses through the unenlarged 3.0-mm incision. In the case of looped silicone lenses (Allergan SI 40 or SA 40), I use the Unfolder device. While this system will deliver lenses through smaller incisions, I found a tendency for incision stretch and incompetent sealing with 2.8-mm incisions. However, with the 3.0-mm incision it is very rare that the incision will not self-seal. Regarding acrylic lenses (Alcon MA 30BA), the 5.5-mm optic of any dioptric power can fit through the unenlarged incision if the lenses are warmed, folded properly, and grasped with a Spaleck implanting forceps (Katena). Just prior to placing the lens through the incision, I use the broad portion of the shaft of a MacPherson forcep to "squeeze" the implanting forceps in order to further reduce

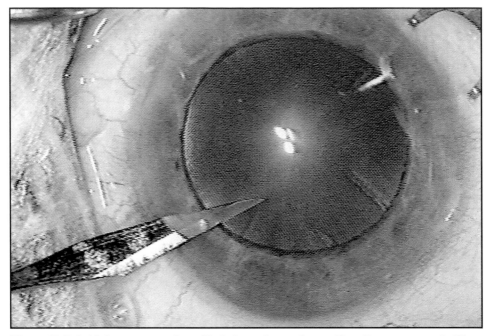

Figure 10-7. A 15 degree supersharp blade is used to make a self-sealing paracentesis. The globe is fixated with a Bores forceps held 180 degrees away from the paracentesis incision.

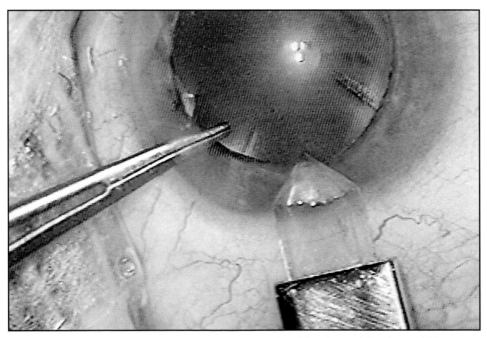

Figure 10-8. The clear corneal tunnel incision is made with a 3-mm 3-D diamond blade (Rhein Medical) while maintaining countertraction through the paracentesis incision with a closed MacPherson forceps. Note the straight edge of the external aspect of the corneal incision.

its diameter. With all of these steps I have experienced no difficulty implanting the lens without undue incision stretch or need for enlargement.

Following lens implantation, it is my routine to perform stromal hydration of the 3.0-mm incision as well as the side-port incision **prior** to removal of the viscoagent (Figure 10-9). While it may not be necessary to use stromal hydration in every case, I prefer to perform it while the viscoagent is still in the eye. In this manner, once the viscoagent is removed from the chamber, it is no longer necessary to place a cannula or any instrument into the corneal tunnel; such maneuvers could allow the chamber to shallow. Since the surgery is nearly completed, the patient might be anxious and tend to squeeze against the lid speculum. Chamber shallowing could, therefore, be significant enough to bring the implant in contact with the cornea. To preclude this complication I perform hydration before removal of the viscoagent and do not further manipulate the corneal tunnel. After the viscoagent is removed, the eye is pressurized with balanced salt solution through the side port and a surgical tonometer, much like the one used for LASIK, is used to establish IOP at approximately 20 mmHg (Figure 10-10). Following this, a fluorescein strip is wiped across both incisions. Gross leakage is evidenced by a positive Seidel test, which is very rare. I challenge the competence of the incision with point pressure applied by a Weck-cel sponge posterior to the incision. With rare exception, the incision is noted to be watertight and surgery is completed without additional manipulation (Figure 10-11). In the unusual circumstance where an obvious leak is observed, one radial suture of 10-0 nylon is placed and the knot buried. I estimate that a suture is required in one of 40 to 50 cases.

Following surgery, no ocular hypotensive agents are used unless the patient has a history for glaucoma or significant ocular hypertension. While employing clear corneal incision surgery for nearly 5 years, I have not experienced one case of postoperative wound leak or ocular hypotension on the first postoperative day or thereafter.

Cataract surgery continues to evolve as a procedure that brings rapid recovery with stable optical results to a very high proportion of patients. The clear corneal temporal incision popularized by Fine[4] has been a major component of the modernization of cataract surgery.

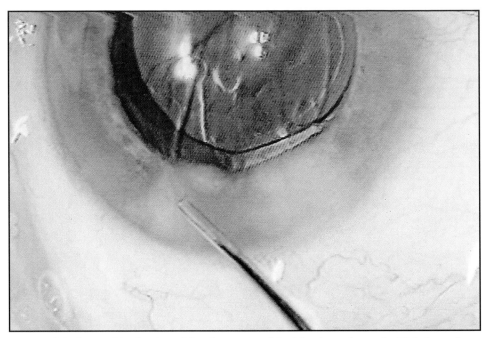

Figure 10-9. Stromal hydration of the clear corneal incision is performed with balanced salt solution following lens implantation but prior to removal of the viscoelastic agent.

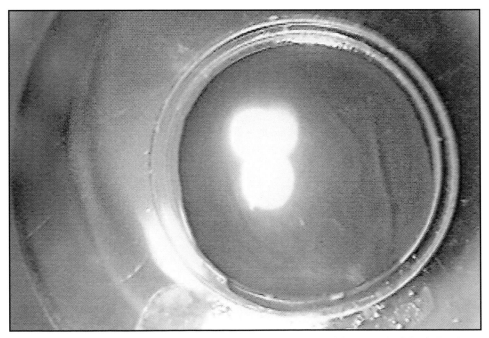

Figure 10-10. After removal of the viscoelastic, IOP is re-established at physiologic levels by adding balanced salt solution through the paracentesis. IOP is measure with a modified Barraquer-Kratz tonometer (Ocular Instruments). The outer ring corresponds to an IOP of 15 mmHg while the inner ring is equivalent to 21 mmHg. Note that the applanation mire falls just inside the inner ring, indicating that IOP is slightly above 21 mmHg.

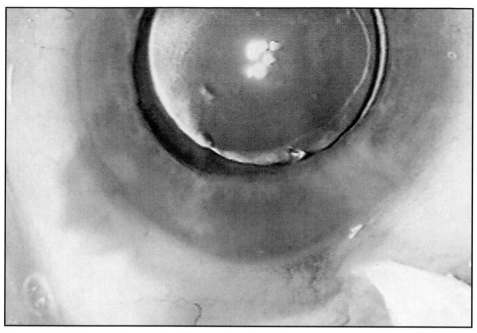

Figure 10-11. Surgery is completed by performing an intraoperative Seidel test while placing point pressure posterior to the incision with a Weck-cel cellulose sponge. Note that neither the tunnel incision nor the paracentesis demonstrates leakage.

REFERENCES

1.   Masket S, Tennen DG. Astigmatic stabilization of 3.0 mm temporal clear corneal cataract incisions. *J Cataract Refract Surg.* 1996;22:1451-1455.
2.   Langerman DW. Architectural design of self-sealing corneal tunnel, single-hinge incision. *J Cataract Refract Surg.* 1994;20:84-88.
3.   Ernest PH, Fenzel R, Lavery KT, Sensoli AM. Relative stability of clear corneal incisions in a cadaver eye mode. *J Cataract Refract Surg.* 1995;21:39-42.
4.   Fine IH. Clear corneal cataract incision with a temporal approach. In: Fine IH, Fichman RA, Grabow HB, eds. *Clear-Corneal Cataract Surgery & Topical Anesthesia.* Thorofare, NJ: SLACK Incorporated; 1993.

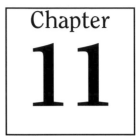

Chapter

11

Techniques, Thoughts, Challenges

David M. Dillman, MD

INCISION

July 18, 1992 was a momentous day in my professional life. It was on that day that I attended a (perhaps the first ever conducted) topical anesthesia/clear corneal incision seminar. It was hosted by Dr. Charles Williamson at his ambulatory surgery center in Baton Rouge, Louisiana. The guest of honor was my dear friend, Dr. I. Howard Fine. Both topics were so well taught and so beautifully demonstrated (via Chuck's live surgery session) that I was able to return to Danville, Illinois, and immediately employ them.

There are only a very few aspects of my surgical armamentarium that I use essentially 100% of the time. The clear corneal incision is one of them. Thus, let me share some thoughts about my particular approach to the clear corneal incision by placing them into three categories:
1. Equipment
2. Technique
3. Location

Equipment

First of all, I would like to argue in favor of the use of specific-sized (eg, 2.5-mm, 2.8-mm, 3.0-mm, etc) keratomes. Granted, a clear corneal incision can be made by "free-handing" it with more of an all-purpose type of knife. However, by so doing, the surgeon runs the very real risk of creating a mismatch between the incision size and his or her particular phaco needle/sleeve configuration. The negative

consequences of such a mismatch could run the spectrum of being bothersome, all the way to disastrous (with a corneal burn if the incision is too narrow and excessive incisional leakage if the incision is too wide). The worse the leakage, the worse the fluidics, and the surgeon might well have a very difficult time controlling the operation.

Okay, so I am going to use a specific-sized keratome. Now is a good time for you to ask me two questions:

1.   Metal or diamond keratome?
2.   What size?

There is absolutely no doubt about it, a good clear corneal incision can be constructed with both metal and diamond keratomes. Thus, you need to be cognizant of the advantages and disadvantages of both.

Metal keratomes are disposable, relatively inexpensive, do not require any special care, and are easier to "control" since their cutting edges are not quite as sharp as their diamond counterparts. Thus, if you want a 2.8-mm wide incision, you are likely to get just that with a 2.8-mm metal keratome. On the other hand, since they are more dull, they do require better fixation (ie, countertraction) in order to appropriately incise. And, since there is more tissue drag, they tend to create an "envelope-patterned" external incision rather than the straight incision created by a good diamond keratome (Figures 11-1a and 11-1b). This has the potential to negatively affect the self-sealability.

A good diamond keratome is exquisitely sharp and is capable of creating clear corneal incisions with the ease of "a hot knife through warm butter." The flip side, however, is that they are relatively expensive, are not disposable, require special care, and, because of their sharpness, are more difficult to control. That is to say, they are so sharp that if the entering and exiting paths of the diamond keratome are not exactly the same, it is quite possible to create an incision wider than intended. For example, imagine that we desire a 2.8-mm clear corneal incision for which we choose a 2.8-mm wide diamond keratome. If we impart any lateral movements during the entering path and/or the exiting path, we might well inadvertently widen the incision and end up with a 3.0-mm (or larger) incision instead of the intended 2.8 mm. In that scenario, we have that dreaded incision/phaco needle mismatch with resultant excessive incisional leakage and compromised phaco fluidics.

With all that as a backdrop, I will share with you that I have a strong preference for diamond keratomes. I am blessed to work in an environment where they are respected and well cared for and they can work and last for a long, long time. Now, any particular manufacturer or design that I recommend? No, at least at the time of this writing. I have tried all the heavily advertised (and not so heavily advertised) designs by the various manufacturers, and I have found that they all work quite well...and, in my opinion, equally well.

Also, let's not forget that the creation of the corneal tunnel is a two-handed technique. A second instrument is needed to both stabilize the eye (since so many of these are done with topical anesthesia and, hence, an eye capable of sudden movement) as well as provide for countertraction (more important when utilizing metal keratomes). The Fine/Thornton fixation ring has truly been a mainstay for many

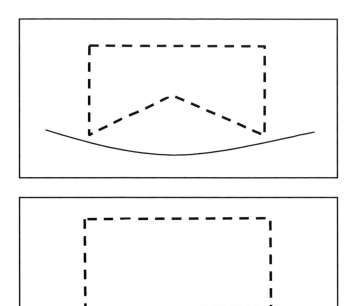

Figure 11-1a. Good clear corneal incisions can be made with both metal and diamond keratomes. Because there is more tissue drag with the metal blades, they have a tendency to create what I call an "envelope-patterned" incision.

Figure 11-1b. Contrast that to the more linear incision made by a diamond keratome.

clear corneal surgeons. I myself have designed a blunt, two-point fixation device called the Dillman fixation hook. But, to be honest, something as simple as a cotton swab or even a finger from the opposite hand placed at the limbus 180 degrees away from the corneal tunnel also works well.

Some surgeons are fond of using their side-port incision for the purpose of stabilization and countertraction. By using something such as a cyclodialysis spatula, a thin pair of forceps, or even the dull, backside of the blade used to create the side-port incision, the mission can certainly be well accomplished.

Okay, so what size? Most assuredly, this is an extremely important fluidics question, because it is imperative to good phaco fluidics to have the phaco incision properly match the phaco needle/silicone sleeve configuration. For me, it is 2.8 mm. For you, it might be 2.9 mm, 2.7 mm, 2.6 mm, or 2.5 mm. Notice I did not list 3.0 mm and certainly not 3.2 mm. For standard-sized phaco needles (internal lumen diameter approximately 0.9 mm) with a standard outer silicone sleeve, I believe an incision of 2.8 or 2.9 mm results in the optimum fluidics. For the downsized systems (internal lumen 0.8 to 0.6 mm) with, perhaps, specialized outer sleeves (eg, the Mackool System, Alcon Surgical Co), an incision of, perhaps, 2.5 mm would be more appropriate. The take-home point is simply this. Just because you have used (likely for years now) a 3.0- or 3.2-mm incision for your scleral-based phaco incision, please do not just assume that it will automatically convert into your clear corneal incision. I challenge you to really be persnickety about this and to consciously arrive at the correct amount of phaco incisional leakage that is appropriate for your phaco needle/sleeve configuration that will properly balance phaco fluidics with adequate cooling of the handpiece.

Technique

I am aware of three primary techniques for creating a clear corneal incision, and then multiple variations on each of the three. To my knowledge, and I apologize to any surgeon I might inadvertently and innocently not recognize, the three primary techniques and their (modern) originators are as follows:

1. The single-plane, paracentesis-type incision—Dr. I. Howard Fine
2. A 300- to 400-micron corneal groove followed by a two-plane corneal tunnel—Dr. Charles Williamson
3. The Langerman hinge—Dr. David Langerman

Williamson and Langerman describe their techniques elsewhere in this book. So as not to be redundant, and since I prefer the single-plane, paracentesis-type incision, that is the one I will describe.

What I do is embarrassingly simple. Using a 2.8-mm, parallel-sided, diamond keratome, I place the tip of the blade just anterior to the limbal arcade of vessels, thereby starting the incision in avascular tissue. Basically, the plane of the incision is parallel to the plane of the iris. Occasionally, I might slightly (10 degrees or so) drop the butt of the blade downward, imparting an ever-so-slight upward angle to the tip. Then, using the now-famous Dillman hook in my left hand, I simply advance the blade straight forward to its full width and back it straight out. I make no attempt at making bi- or tri-planed incisions. It truly is nothing more than a giant-sized, paracentesis incision. Hopefully, the width of the resultant tunnel is 2.8 mm. The length is approximately 1.5 to 2.0 mm.

I do alter this technique slightly when using a metal keratome. In an effort to avoid the envelope-configuration external incision (see Figures 11-1a and 11-1b), I intentionally drop the butt of the blade 15 to 20 degrees, thereby definitely pointing the tip somewhat up toward the dome of the cornea. This usually does necessitate a wee bit of a dimple down maneuver to break through Descemet's and complete the incision.

Location

When Dr. Mike McFarland shattered the incision paradigm in 1990 and presented to us the concept of self-sealing incision architecture, the term "astigmatically neutral" appeared on the scene. Its meaning is self-explanatory. During that fateful summer of 1992, I coined the term "astigmatically beneficial." The thought behind it was perhaps it would be possible to create an incision that would go beyond neutral to beneficial, ie, one that might actually improve the patient's astigmatic status, not only early on, but for his or her lifetime. It seemed to me that the clear corneal incision had a better chance of doing that than scleral-based incisions. And that for patients with either pre-existing against-the-rule astigmatism or spherical corneas, the temporal location made the most sense. Thus, in very short fashion, I found myself doing the vast majority of my procedures via a temporal, clear corneal incision.

But not all, not 100%. That is to say, not all temporal. I continue to do 100% clear corneal incisions, but not all temporally. And this might well be a point of con-

tention between myself and other contributing authors to this text. There are those who advocate (some fervently) that clear corneal incisions should only be temporal, and never superior. I believe, however, that if the clear corneal incision is a good incision then, doggone it, it is a good incision everywhere. Therefore, in the unusual situation in which I have a cataract patient with greater than about 1.5 D of with-the-rule astigmatism, I will usually attempt to be astigmatically beneficial by employing a superior clear corneal incision. I will openly admit that I do not necessarily appreciate or welcome the ergonomic awkwardness of working over the brow again. But, from an astigmatic management perspective, it just makes the most sense to me. Certainly, there is the argument that for these with-the-rule patients, one could use a temporal clear corneal incision for the phaco/IOL components and then couple them with some form of corneal relaxing incisions on the vertical meridian. With all due respect, I call that the Steven Wright approach. Steven Wright is a comedian who has a very dry sense of humor delivered in a distinctive, characteristic monotone manner. One of his routines is about his dog which he named "Stay." He talks about how difficult it was for him to train the dog when he would give the command "Come, Stay!" It seems to me that giving out that type of mixed statement can occur when combining a temporal clear corneal incision with vertical relaxing incisions. The cornea might get confused as to what you are asking it to do.

Therefore, I continue to use superior clear corneal incisions. I create them in an identical fashion to that which I use for temporal clear corneal incisions. But, be aware that, in general, there is more astigmatic bang for the buck with a superior clear corneal incision. The natural shape of the human cornea will usually place a superior clear corneal incision closer to the central cornea than a temporal clear corneal incision, thereby giving it more potential to affect central corneal shape (Figure 11-2). That is why my personal criteria for the superior clear corneal incision is at least 1.5 D of vertically oriented steep axis.

CAPSULORRHEXIS

Just prior to a recent American Academy of Ophthalmology meeting, I had the real pleasure of participating in a focus group regarding cataract surgery. The list of invitees included many surgeons I had long admired and respected. As you might imagine, it was quite the learning experience. The very first question posed to the group was something like this, "If you could isolate and improve only one part of cataract surgery, what would it be?" I knew exactly what my choice would be, but I was almost ashamed to admit it. I mean, what would this group of stalwarts think of the Danville hick who picked the capsulorrhexis procedure? Well, you might also imagine my sheer delight when I learned that was precisely the very part chosen by the majority of the group!

For sake of this discussion, I am going to classify the capsulorrhexis procedure into two categories:
1. The easy, routine capsulorrhexis
2. The difficult capsulorrhexis

The easy, routine capsulorrhexis is, well…easy and routine. You know the scenario: big pupil, good red reflex, little-to-no tension underneath the anterior capsule, low anterior capsular elasticity, good visualization, etc. Truly, the clinical setting just described is absolutely wonderful when taking on the task of performing a capsulorrhexis. However, we all know that the reality of life is that we often encounter clinical settings that can make the capsulorrhexis extraordinarily challenging. It would be beyond the intended scope of this particular chapter to delineate each and every clinical setting that makes doing the capsulorrhexis anything but easy and routine. Therefore, for the sake of simplicity, I am going to lump them all together into the category I am calling "the difficult capsulorrhexis."

In dealing with the difficult capsulorrhexis, I believe there are two principles that deserve serious consideration:

1. The maintenance of a closed system
2. The use of non-coaxial light sources

Two of the many objectives in the successful completion of the capsulorrhexis are to exert total control over the intraocular contents and to keep the anterior surface of the anterior capsule as flat as possible, thereby relieving stress forces that tend to direct the shearing forces laterally. In order to best accomplish these two objectives in the difficult capsulorrhexis, I feel it is mandatory to maintain the most closed system physically possible that will still allow you to perform the capsulorrhexis. To me, that translates to utilizing the smallest possible incision. Let me be even more blunt. To utilize the phaco incision, even if as small as 2.0 mm, for the capsulorrhexis in the difficult capsulorrhexis setting is absolutely counterproductive! Even if you are using a viscoelastic material with very low cohesion, it can still be very difficult to maintain the control and pressurization needed in a difficult setting. As such, I have long advocated, and I continue to advocate, the use of an incision that is somewhere in the area of 0.5 to 1.0 mm.

This specialized capsulorrhexis incision can be created in one of two simple ways. The one I most commonly employ is to use the same 2.8-mm diamond keratome that I routinely use for the creation of the clear corneal phaco incision. The big difference is that I proceed extremely slowly and pay extra careful attention to the tip of the diamond microkeratome. Once I have seen that it has incised Descemet's membrane, I advance it ever so slightly until I feel an internal incision of 0.5 to 1.0 mm has been made (Figure 11-3). I then quickly back the diamond keratome out of the eye. It is through this very small internal clear corneal incision that I then attempt to do the capsulorrhexis and hydrodissection. Once they are completed, and in order to admit the phacoemulsification handpiece, I then enlarge that incision to 2.8 mm. Although that could be done with the same 2.8-mm diamond keratome, I strongly prefer to do so with a more blunt metal blade. The reason is simply that the diamond is so very sharp, it would be possible to inadvertently create a whole new incision, rendering a "sandwiching" effect to the corneal tunnel that could become problematic. Therefore, I routinely use a 2.8-mm metal keratome and, ideally, one that has a blunted tip with sharp sides. That gives the highest probability of locating the original incision via the blunted tip and then expanding it laterally via the sharp sides. The second way of creating this tiny capsulorrhexis incision

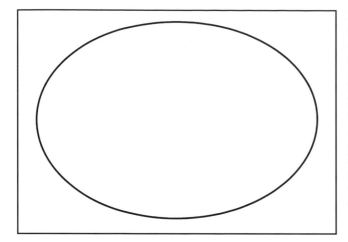

Figure 11-2. For sake of illustration, I purposely exaggerated the dimensions of this cornea. The reminder here is that the horizontal diameter of the human cornea is greater than the vertical diameter. As such, full thickness corneal incisions have a higher tendency to influence central corneal shape when placed in the vertical meridian.

is to go slightly to the side of the intended clear corneal phaco incision (to the right if you are right-handed and to the left if you are left-handed) and simply to create a second side-port incision with a width of 0.5 to 1.0 mm (Figure 11-4). It is through this ancillary side-port incision that you can attempt the closed system capsulorrhexis.

You might very well have already posed the question "How am I possibly going to work with my capsulorrhexis forceps through such a tiny opening?" The answer is, you can't. Or, at least, you can't with any of the capsulorrhexis forceps with which I am familiar. Indeed, the ophthalmic community is wonderfully global and, although I try to keep abreast of instrumentation, techniques, etc, worldwide, I know enough to know that I don't know everything. Thus, I admit that there might very well be a very good capsulorrhexis forceps design that will work well through a 0.5 to 1.0 mm incision…I simply am not aware of it. Therefore, in my hands, I am forced to use a capsulorrhexis cystotome for the difficult capsulorrhexis. My personal preference is a 25-gauge pre-bent cystotome. A little pearl I can offer you with the cystotome is to place it on the cannula of the viscoelastic material of your preference. The cannula then becomes the "handle" for the cystotome. The advantage of this, I hope, is obvious. If, at any time, you need to add viscoelastic material in order to flatten the dome of the anterior capsule, move cut anterior capsule around, enlarge the pupil, etc, you can do so instantaneously without having to remove one set of instruments and inserting another. If this notion of a tiny incision, cystotome driven, using the viscoelastic cannula as the cystotome handle makes sense to you and you are currently unfamiliar with it, I would suggest that you start using it in the easy, routine scenarios. This is a great way to become familiar and comfortable with it so that when the day comes along to employ it in the difficult capsulorrhexis situation, it will be a technique in which you have confidence.

The second principle that I like to advocate in attempting to perform the difficult capsulorrhexis is the use of non-coaxial light sources. This is a little trick that I learned from Dr. Richard Mackool several years ago. The application for non-coaxial lighting is during the clinical situation in which surgeon visualization is significantly compromised. Indeed, we have all been there, done that. A significantly

Figure 11-3. My preferred method for creating the closed system capsulorrhexis incision is simply to initiate the phaco clear corneal incision. I carefully observe the advancing tip of the keratome and stop when I feel the internal incision is 0.5 to 1.0 mm.

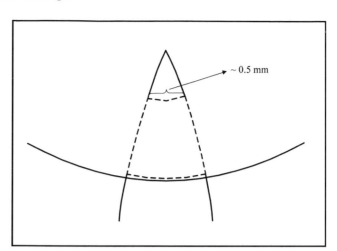

Figure 11-4. Another good way of creating a useful incision for the closed system capsulorrhexis approach is to simply create a second side-port incision to the immediate right (or left for you southpaws) of the intended phaco incision.

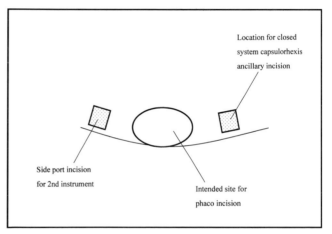

blunted or absent red reflex, a very white solid cataract, anterior capsular plaques, etc, all wreak havoc on our ability to visualize the progression of a capsulorrhexis, often causing us to abandon the rhexis altogether and convert to a can-opener type of a capsulotomy. Now, I want to be very careful not to put on airs here. I am not saying that using non-coaxial light sources in any way makes it easy to do these low visual circumstance capsulorrhexes. All I am saying is that in many instances, it does makes them at least doable.

Here's how it works. If you have not already done so, have all of the room lights turned off, then turn off the coaxial light of the operating microscope. That's right, I said turn off the light of the operating microscope. Now, bring in from the side an oblique light source. Probably the easiest and most convenient to use is an endoscopic retinal light probe. This small light pipe is very easy to manipulate and maneuver. The objective here is to create different angles of lighting and shadows within the anterior chamber. This is accomplished by directing the external light source with varying angles, positions, and levels of intensity. So doing will often greatly assist you in identifying the leading edge of the capsulorrhexis and moving

it along. Please know that it is sometimes, in fact often, necessary to continuously alternate between the coaxial light source and the external oblique light source. It can truly be a painstaking and tedious process. I can honestly tell you that I have spent as long as 40 minutes in an effort to complete a good continuous tear anterior capsulotomy under very trying circumstances. However, it is often under these very difficult circumstances that we most need the advantages that a good capsulorrhexis brings to bear on the remainder of the procedure. Therefore, it is my personal belief that I owe it to the patient to do everything I possibly can to say that I gave it my absolute best shot at completing a capsulorrhexis.

CATARACT REMOVAL
Hydrodissection

Good mobility of the lens within the capsular bag is a function of hydrodissection. The vast majority of the phacoemulsification techniques that I am aware of for either endocapsular or supracapsular phacoemulsification are predicated upon good mobility of the lens within the capsular bag and, therefore, are predicated on good hydrodissection. And, certainly, my phaco technique is no exception.

So, how do you know when you have accomplished good hydrodissection? Well, it's that beautiful posterior fluid wave I can see, isn't it? No! Emphatically, no. The only way you can prove to yourself, beyond a shadow of a doubt, that you have accomplished thorough hydrodissection is by demonstrating the ability of being able to easily spin the cataract inside the contents of the capsular bag. For most of us, this is simply done by utilizing the same cannula and syringe apparatus that we use to create the hydrodissection.

Now, hang onto to your scrub caps for this one! In the presence of a good capsulorrhexis and normal anterior segment anatomy, you should be able to perform good hydrodissection 100% of the time. That's right, I said 100% of the time. I will accept no excuses…none…nada! I can hear some of you now, "Come on, Dave, I have had cases where I tried and tried and tried and I just couldn't make it happen. I tried one quadrant, and then another quadrant, and then another quadrant, and then another quadrant. I tried straight cannulae, u-shaped cannulae, flat cannulae, and round cannulae. I squirted and I squirted and I squirted and I squirted…and all I got for my efforts was a fluffy mess through which I couldn't see, and no hydrodissection." Well, friends, I hear you. I have been down that road more than once. And then, about 4 years ago, Dr. Michael Colvard showed me salvation, although he did so in a wonderfully indirect way.

Mike developed an ingenious little device to help surgeons transitioning into phacoemulsification either from planned extracapsular cataract extraction or residents who had no surgical experience at all. He called this device the Phaco Shield. It is a very thin piece of silicone that is shaped very much in the shape of a plate style IOL. The objective of the Phaco Shield is to place it under the inferior anterior capsule and then advance it all the way around the inferior equator until it rests centrally in a position between the posterior capsule and the cataract. Therefore, when properly placed, it would be a virtual impossibility to break the posterior capsule by

phacoing through the cataract. And, here is where Dr. Colvard indirectly taught me the secret to the "no excuse hydrodissection." As you might imagine, in an effort to place his Phaco Shield, a fair amount of space needs to be created. Therefore, the first step in the placement of the Phaco Shield is to take the I/A handpiece and to rather aggressively remove as much cortex and epinuclear material as one possibly can. The neat thing Dr. Colvard taught me was that this can be safely accomplished not only centrally, but also under the anterior capsule and out into the periphery as well. And, that's the key to the no excuse hydrodissection. When you are in that situation in which no matter what you try, you just cannot get good hydrodissection, and cortical and epinuclear material are starting to fluff up, simply refrain from further efforts at that time and ask the scrub nurse to take the I/A lines off the phaco handpiece and transfer them to the I/A handpiece. Employing the same high vacuum, high flow settings that you would normally use for cortical removal, aggressively remove as much cortex and epinucleus as you possibly can. Again, not only from the very center, but also under the anterior capsule and as far into the periphery as you feel comfortable with (Figure 11-5). In order to be successful with this, it will be necessary for you to constantly turn the opening so that it faces all directions, including port down. Once done, you will likely want to at least partially refill the anterior chamber with the viscoelastic agent of your choice. Now, get out that hydrodissection cannula again, put in under the anterior capsule, slide it out into the periphery a bit, and try it again. To date, I have never had this fail. On my honor. In fact, how much do I believe in this maneuver? I used it on my own mother's first eye. I tried and tried and tried to hydrodissect, and the cataract apparently didn't care that I was sweating blood. Her doggone lens would not spin for anything. Therefore, I did the "Colvard maneuver" and, lo and behold, the next attempt at hydrodissection resulted in wonderfully comforting mobilization.

Phaco Quick Chop

My fastball phaco technique is one that I call "phaco quick chop." I learned it by repeatedly watching an instructional videotape made by Dr. Vladimir Pfeifer from Slovenia. He calls his technique "phaco crack." Phaco quick chop is essentially Dr. Pfeifer's technique with some simple variations and an American marketing department. It has all the marvelous efficiency of traditional phaco chop, but with what I feel to be considerably greater safety.

The main difference between traditional phaco chop and phaco quick chop is so subtle and, yet, makes all the difference in the world. It simply deals with the placement of the chopper itself. With traditional phaco chop, once the phaco tip is buried into the center of the lens, the chopper is placed under the inferior capsule and then advanced peripherally until it reaches the equator of the lens (Figures 11-6 and 11-7). The chopper is then pulled toward the buried phaco tip in a near horizontal movement (Figure 11-8). Well, at least that's the theory. Unfortunately, sometimes with traditional phaco chop I just can't see the position of the chopper. On at least two occasions that I recall, I thought I had the chopper under the anterior capsule when, in fact, I was on top of the anterior capsule. When I attempted the actual chop, I suc-

ceeded only in creating a huge rent in the anterior capsule which quickly wrapped around to include the posterior capsule early in the case.

You can imagine how happy I was to see Dr. Pfeifer ignore the anterior capsule altogether. He simply placed the chopper basically on top of the buried phaco tip, pretty much at the center of the lens (well away from the anterior capsule) and initiated the chop with a near vertical movement (Figure 11-9)...Voilà! The efficiency of phaco chop, but with what I perceived to be considerably greater safety.

Following capsulorrhexis and hydrodissection, the phaco needle is introduced into the eye through the phaco incision and then the chopper is introduced into the eye through the side-port incision. It is important to get the chopper into the eye before burying the phaco tip. There is a strong natural tendency to retract the phaco tip if it is buried with the chopper external to the eye and then the chopper introduced secondarily. The phaco needle is placed on the surface of the lens just in front of the edge of the capsulorrhexis nearest you (Figure 11-10). The phaco needle is then buried, aiming it toward the dead center of the lens (Figure 11-11). Since this means you will be very quickly working with a totally occluded phaco needle, and since a totally occluded phaco needle is a prime set-up for a corneal/scleral burn, I would strongly suggest this burying process be done with 3 to 4 short (foot-pulsed) bursts of phaco (foot position 3) as opposed to a single continuous, uninterrupted one. Once buried, remain in foot position 2 (aspiration).

The chopper is now lightly placed on the surface of the lens either directly above the end of the buried phaco needle or it can be as much as a millimeter in front of it (Figure 11-12). You are now ready to make the first chop. Simultaneously, the chopper is moved downward while the buried phaco needle is moved upward (Figure 11-13). For a long time, I thought this was an "equal opportunity" type of a maneuver with 50% of the effort devoted to the downward movement of the chopper and 50% of the effort devoted to the upward movement of the buried phaco needle. More recently, I have convinced myself that it is really the chopper that is doing most of the work...probably a more accurate ratio would be 90% chopper to 10% buried phaco tip.

The downward movement with the chopper is an aggressive movement. "Whoa, now," you're thinking, "orthopedic surgeons have aggressive moves, not ophthalmologists!" We do now. But, it is controlled aggression. Please remember three things have preceded this:
1. A good capsulorrhexis
2. Excellent hydrodissection
3. A securely buried phaco tip

To put a phaco chopper on the middle of the lens in the absence of any of those three prerequisites and to aggressively chop down wouldn't be aggressive...it would be downright stupid! However, if you are confident that all three have been successfully completed, then chop away. Mentally, aim that chopper toward the optic nerve and go for it.

This "vertical" maneuver initiates the division of the lens centrally. However, the peripheral propagation of the division is accomplished by yet a third maneuver that virtually follows on the heels of the first two. Once the chopper and buried

Figure 11-5. I think you will be pleasantly surprised by how much cortex and epinucleus you can remove, not only within the boundaries of the capsulorrhexis, but under the anterior capsule as well.

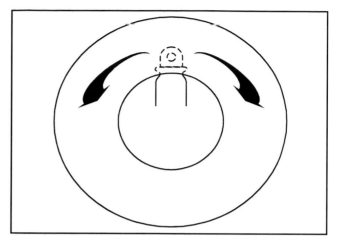

phaco needle have come into very near contact (or they can even come into contact), they are laterally separated (Figure 11-14). This triad of maneuvers—chopper down, buried phaco needle up, and lateral separation—when properly done, smoothly flow into what might well be perceived to be a single movement by a first time observer.

Because excellent hydrodissection precedes this initial chop (and, therefore, good mobility of the lens within the capsular bag is an unquestionable given), the lateral separation maneuver might well be accompanied by a spinning of the lens within the bag. If so, fine! Because the next intended maneuver is to spin it anyway. Rotate the lens (clockwise or counterclockwise, it's your call) so that the split in the lens is in the horizontal position from your perspective (Figure 11-15). (Another way of couching that would be so that the split in the lens is parallel to the phaco incision.)

It is prudent at this point to take a moment to ensure that this first chop is truly complete (ie, both the posterior and peripheral nuclear plates are completely severed). This is easily accomplished by placing both the phaco needle (you are now in foot position 1, irrigation only) and chopper within the split, and then pushing the inferior one half of the lens away from you with the phaco needle while simultaneously pulling the superior one half toward you with the chopper (Figure 11-16).

Now that you have two completely separated halves, there are a variety of ways in which to proceed but, for the sake of simplicity, here I am going to follow the quartering approach. The phaco needle is now buried into the center of the inferior one half (foot position 3). Once again, I would recommend doing this in 2 or 3 short bursts of ultrasound as opposed to 1 continuous burst. The chopping of this half into quarters is accomplished in exactly the same fashion as the initial chop. The chopper is lightly placed on the surface of the lens, essentially on top of the end of the buried phaco needle (which is now in foot position 2) and in front of the edge of the capsulorrhexis. The aforementioned triad of maneuvers is then carried out:
1.   Chopper down (90% of the effort)
2.   Buried phaco tip up (10% of the effort)
3.   Lateral separation (Figures 11-17a and 11-17b)

Prudence, again, enters the picture and, before advancing, I would strongly recommend ensuring that this second chop is also complete both posteriorly and peripherally.

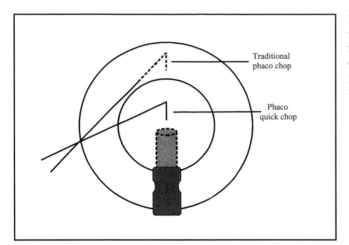

Figure 11-6. Top view of the contrasting locations for the placement of the chopping instrument for phaco quick chop vs traditional phaco chop.

Traditional phaco chop

Phaco quick chop

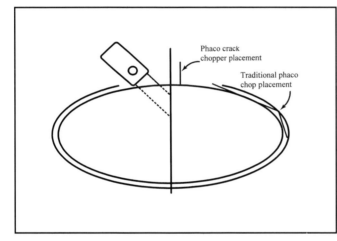

Figure 11-7. Side view of the contrasting locations for the placement of the chopping instrument for phaco quick chop vs traditional phaco chop.

Phaco crack chopper placement

Traditional phaco chop placement

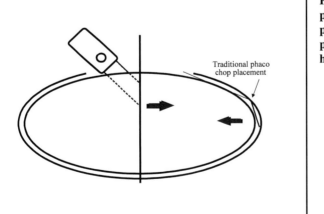

Figure 11-8. In traditional phaco chop, the chopper is pulled toward the buried phaco needle in a near horizontal fashion.

Traditional phaco chop placement

With the first half nicely quartered, a whole myriad of options now present themselves. The density of the lens, plus your surgical personality, will likely dictate how you decide to proceed. But, by way of example, here would be a few roads you might choose to travel:

- Remove both quarters
- Chop one quarter into eighths, remove each eighth, chop the second quarter into eighths, and remove them
- Leave both quarters alone, spin the lens 180 degrees so as to bring the other half into the inferior capsular bag, and chop it into quarters

As you read this, I'm sure you're already thinking of other options as well.

Pearls

It would be unfair and inappropriate to deny the fact that there is definitely a learning curve to phaco quick chop. That's the bad news. The good news is that it should be a fairly painless one. Hopefully, in an effort to smooth out some potential bumps along the way, let me now share with you a few observations regarding phaco quick chop that are not readily obvious at first.

The first two deal with the initial chop. The strong tendency is to be way too tentative both with burying the tip and using the chopper. Let's start with the phaco needle. You definitely want it buried into the substance of the lens. In order to facilitate this, I retract the silicone sleeve approximately double the amount I would normally do for a divide and conquer technique (Figure 11-18). I can hear you now, so I'll go ahead and reply…no, I'm not concerned about breaking the posterior capsule with this extra exposure. Let's do the math. The center thickness of the human lens is some 3.5 to 4.0 mm. We have exposed 2 mm of the titanium tip. The silicone sleeve will act as a physical barrier to further advancement of the tip. If we approached the center of the lens at a 90 degree angle and went straight down, we would only reach the middle of the lens, well away from the central posterior capsule. But, in real phaco quick chop life, we're not going to approach the lens at a 90 degree angle, we're going to be much more at a 45 degree angle (see Figure 11-10). As such, the actual penetration of the centrally buried tip will actually be less than 50%.

Once the phaco needle is well buried, keep in mind that it is the action of the chopper that most determines the success or failure of the initial chop. I know I'm beating this to death, but "be one with the chopper!" Use it with controlled aggression. Sink that baby into the substance of the lens and push down with authority.

Now, ready for some really good news? Let's say that, for whatever reason, that initial chop just doesn't happen successfully with the first effort. Fine, no harm done. You can either immediately abort phaco quick chop and convert to your divide and conquer technique, or you can spin the lens 90 degrees or so and try it again. Just be sure to pick a new place to bury the phaco needle. This time a little more peripherally than the first attempt. What if it doesn't work the second time? Fine, again, no harm done. At that point, you could choose to convert to your fastball technique or if you're feeling particularly spunky that day, you could spin it another 90 degrees

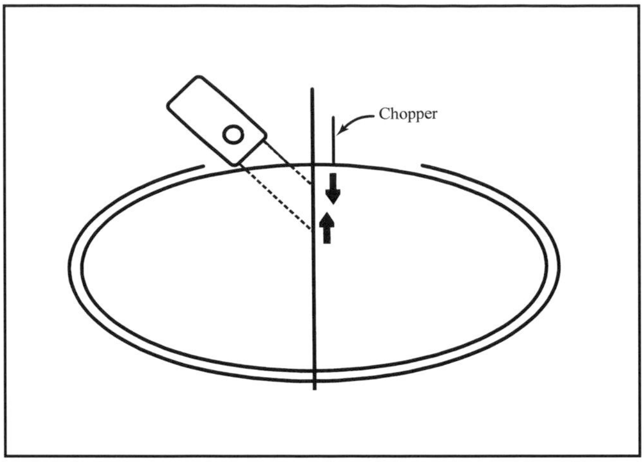

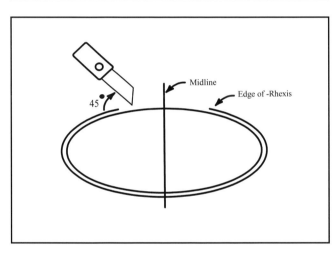

Figure 11-9. In phaco quick chop, the chopper is moved straight downward and the buried phaco tip is moved straight upward, resulting in a "vertical" chopping maneuver. Contrast this to the "horizontal" chopping maneuver of traditional phaco chop (see Figure 11-8).

Figure 11-10. The angle with which the phaco needle contacts the surface of the lens is determined by the size of the capsulorrhexis. A smaller capsulorrhexis will demand a steeper angle whereas a larger capsulorrhexis will allow for a flatter angle. In general, aim for approximately a 45 degree angle.

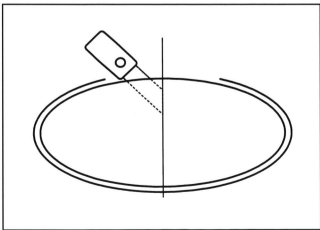

Figure 11-11. Using short, interrupted bursts of ultrasound, the phaco needle is buried into the center of the lens. Please note that the buried tip does not come anywhere close to the posterior capsule.

Figure 11-12. The chopper is placed anywhere from right on top of the end of the buried phaco needle to a millimeter in front of it.

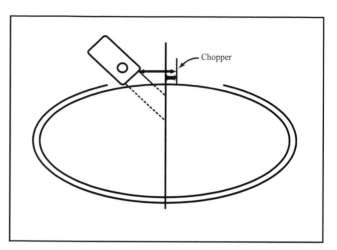

Figure 11-13. The first chop is initiated by vigorously moving the chopper in a downward fashion while gently moving the buried phaco tip in an upward fashion.

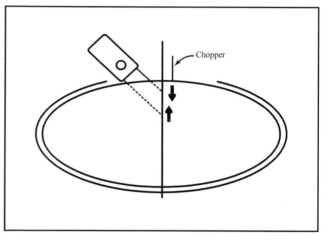

Figure 11-14. The central chop is propagated out to the periphery by laterally separating the buried chopper and buried phaco needle.

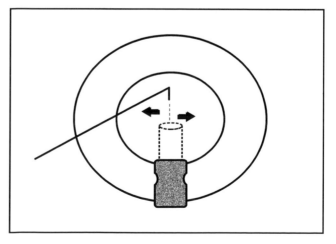

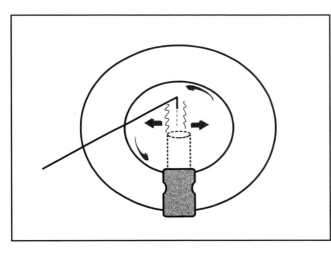

Figure 11-15. Because excellent hydrodissection is a quick chop prerequisite, it will be easy to rotate the lens into a position that puts the two halves in a "horizontal" position.

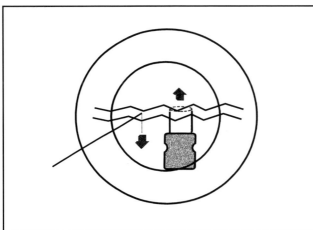

Figure 11-16. As with any chopping or cracking technique, it is crucial to ensure complete separation of individual pieces. Therefore, before proceeding beyond the initial chop, use the phaco needle and chopper to "work the split" until you are convinced of a through and through chop.

or so and try it again. But let common sense prevail. Granted, persistence is a virtue in many cases, but not always inside the eye.

Also, please don't be frightened or concerned if your initial chop does not result in a lens split perfectly right down the middle. It might well be that you won't have two absolutely equal-sized halves. You might end up with a one third – two thirds type split. Again, no harm done. The bigger piece will simply need more further chopping than the smaller piece.

This next little variation was taught to me by Dr. Bruce Wallace from Alexandria, Louisiana, and it is well worth sticking in your bag of quick chop tricks. After the initial chop if, for some reason (eg, the size of the pupil and/or capsulorrhexis is smallish) there is little-to-no room in front of the buried phaco needle to place the chopper...fine, simply place the chopper to the side (left side if you control the phaco handpiece with your right hand) of the buried phaco needle and carry on exactly as if it were right on top of it. Remember, one of the aims of phaco quick chop is to avoid unintentional contact with the anterior capsule. This "side chop-

Figure 11-17a. Further chops are made in a near identical fashion to the initial chop. The phaco needle is buried into the lens, the chopper placed on top, and a vertical chopping maneuver is carried out.

Figure 11-17b. The vertical chopping maneuver is followed by lateral separation.

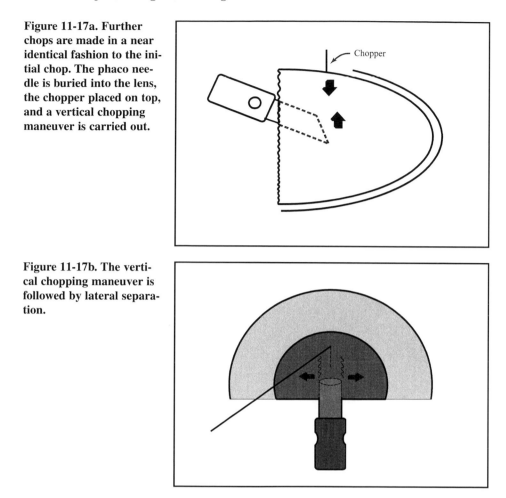

ping" is great for that endeavor. And, in fact, I have since learned that "opposite side" chopping is, perhaps, the easiest way of all to create all the chops after the first one. By opposite side chopping I mean that I place the chopper over the buried phaco tip (I hold the phaco handpiece with my right hand, therefore, I bury the tip with my right hand and, with my left hand, I bring the chopper over the buried tip, place it on top of the cataract immediately to the right of the tip), chop down (with authority), and push the newly chopped piece away from the buried tip with a cross-handed maneuver (Figures 11-19a and 11-19b). I do this a lot.

Here's a truly important pearl. I've actually already discussed it once, but it's worth re-emphasizing. Just because you see a chop, do not assume that it's a through and through chop. Be very active with both the chopper and the phaco needle. Use them to poke and pry, push and pull, rock and roll. Separation is a whole lot better than desperation.

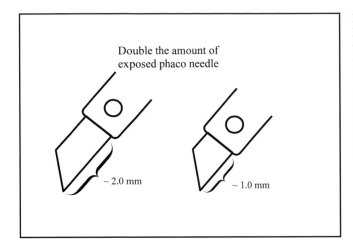

Double the amount of
exposed phaco needle

~ 2.0 mm

~ 1.0 mm

Figure 11-18. If you are like me, you will be too tentative when burying the phaco tip at first. Exposing more of the titanium needle facilitates burying. Just be careful not to overdo it and have the irrigating sleeve out of the eye…bad form!

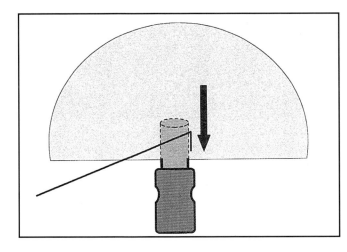

Figure 11-19a. Opposite side chopping has become my preferred method for making all of the chops following the initial central chop. With the phaco needle buried into the substance of the lens, the chopper is placed directly to the right side (as opposed to the top or left side) and that same "aggressive" downward chop is made, followed by a cross-action separation of the two pieces.

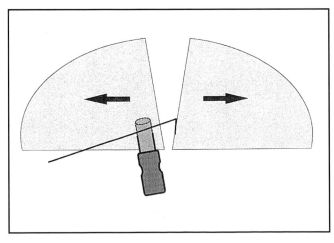

Figure 11-19b. A cross-action separation of the two pieces.

Lens Implantation

Several hundred years ago, the country of Italy prided itself in the art of designing and manufacturing exquisite violins. Interestingly enough, in one small village in northern Italy, there were three families who all lived on the same block and whose family business was the production of such violins. And, apparently, marketing was popular even back then. The first family, the Alberto family, had a large sign outside of their business which stated "The Best Violins in All of Italy." Next to them, the Giaroni family had a sign outside of their business which said "The Best Violins in All the World." Lastly, the sign of the third family, the Stradivarius family, read "The Best Violins on the Block." And, thus, the question begs, is there a "best" IOL/insertion system combination? Certainly, at the time of this writing, my answer would be a fairly emphatic "No!" As I presently put pen to paper, I am using three different materials: silicone, acrylic, and a hybrid hydrogel. I am using three different designs:

1. Single-piece plate design
2. The three-piece design with polypropylene haptics
3. The three-piece design with extruded PMMA haptics

I am using both monofocal and multifocal optics. To implant these various lenses, I employ a wide variety of folders, unfolders, forceps, spatulas, and kitchen sinks.

Therefore, in an effort to keep the length of this chapter somewhat less than that of *War and Peace*, rather than talk about each of the individual IOLs, insertion devices, and their multiple combinations, I am going to direct my thoughts and observations to three topics:

1. Quality of vision
2. Biocompatibility
3. Required incision size/ease of insertion

And, before going any further, you need to be fully cognizant of the fact that the majority of what I am about to say is based upon personal experience and perceptions as compared to rigorous prospective, double blind, highly regimented and regulated studies that I have conducted.

Quality of Vision

I hope it goes without saying that I feel all of the lenses that I implant will provide good quality of vision. There are, however, some differences as should be expected from the design of the optics. Multifocal IOLs provide simultaneous multiple images to the macula. Therefore, by their very nature, they will have a slightly adverse effect on contrast sensitivity. Thus, while both the monofocal and multifocal patients may test equally well under the conditions of high contrast, Snellen acuity, my experience has been that the monofocal people appreciate a little more sharpness and crispness to their functional vision. On the other hand, the multifocal optics, again by their very design, create an expanded depth of field that their monofocal counterparts are not capable of producing. As such, my experience has been that my multifocal patients (when implanted bilaterally) are able to function overall without glasses better than their monofocal counterparts. Therefore, much as in the world of refractive surgery, patient selection is absolutely crucial in determining the recommended optic design for any one individual.

Biocompatibility

To me, biocompatibility is something that I cannot define, but I know it when I see it. Should we define biocompatibility by formalized flare and cell measurements? By posterior capsule opacification rates? By the presence or absence of precipitates on the surface of the implanted IOL? By the presence or absence of adhesions between the iris and the anterior capsule? The incidence of cystoid macular edema? Or, all of the above? Well, probably all of the above plus other criteria that you have already identified that I did not mention. Those are things that we can definitely reach out and touch if you will.

Let me share with you a couple of thoughts regarding biocompatibility and how it is influenced by materials and designs. I am not aware of any indisputable scientific study that has proven beyond a shadow of a doubt that one material is more biocompatible than another. Certainly, PMMA, the various silicones, the acrylics, and the hydrogels all appear to be within a very acceptable range of biocompatibility. Indeed, there is anecdotal evidence to support one or more over the others and, indeed, we all have our own personal biases. Here's mine…placing materials in descending order of biocompatibility starting with the most biocompatible: hydrogel and hydrogel hybrids, acrylics and PMMAs, and the silicones.

While I do not feel that the material itself makes a huge difference, I do believe that the design characteristics do influence biocompatibility. In 1994, I did a small study on my patients by doing a retrospective chart review. The intent of the study was to compare the incidence of "unusual" postoperative inflammation in one-piece, plate style silicone lenses vs three-piece silicone lenses. I defined "unusual" inflammation in a very loose and subjective manner. All of us have what we call our "routine" postoperative regimen in terms of topical medications. These would likely contain topical steroids, non-steroidals, antibiotics, and perhaps other agents. My point simply is that each one of us has identified a routine regimen that we feel will nicely keep in check both inflammation and infection. Any time we see a clinical situation that we think is beyond the norm, we will then do something to either intensify or prolong our therapy. And, that is quite simply how I defined "unusual" inflammation. Any time I saw a clinical situation that I felt warranted intensifying or prolonging my routine anti-inflammation regimen, I labeled it as an unusual inflammation case.

Details of Study

The study involved some 500 eyes. Seven percent of the eyes exhibited "unusual" inflammation with the plate design vs 1% with the three-piece design. The number jumped dramatically to almost double (13% vs 1%) when considering diabetic eyes only. With intensified therapy, virtually all of the non-diabetic eyes eventually ended with their preop projected result. Unfortunately, essentially one third of the diabetic eyes developed cystoid macular edema that did not respond to intensified therapy.

Based upon that experience, I was led to believe, at least in my hands, that my patients tended to experience more inflammation with the plate style silicone lens vs

the three-piece style silicone lens. However, it also led me to believe that at least the non-diabetic eyes could handle the added inflammation with intensified therapy. The diabetic eyes, however, did not fare nearly as well. Based upon that experience, I discontinued using the plate style silicone lenses in anyone who I felt would be predisposed to unusual inflammation postoperatively. Certainly, for my practice, the biggest group to be put in that category would be persons with diabetes. However, I also added blacks, those with previous glaucoma surgery, and the move obvious cases, such as those with a previous history of uveitis of any etiology.

So, what would be the possible mechanism of a tendency toward more postoperative inflammation with a plate style lens vs a three-piece lens? The theory that I have heard the most often and the one that is most plausible to me is really quite simple. If you simply envision the physical design of the plate style IOL, you will realize that there is a significant amount of cross-sectional area in which the anterior and posterior capsules do not come into contact. This leaves a significant population of the anterior subcapsular epithelial cells to have free reign, if you will. It is at least conceivable that the combination of the population and freedom of these cells can result in some type of metabolic activity that enhances the normal postoperative inflammatory stimuli. It is for that very reason that we sometimes hear proponents of the plate style lens recommending a large capsulorrhexis and/or a concerted effort to remove as many of the subcapsular epithelial cells as possible, especially in those areas occupied by the plate haptics.

Size of Incision and Ease of Insertion

There have been and continue to be a whole slew of insertion systems for foldable IOLs. Therefore, once again, in order to stay within the intended parameters of this chapter, rather than engage in a dissertation on each of them individually, I am going to basically lump them together and discuss insertion systems vs the incision size necessary to employ them.

I think, in general, it is safe to say that the concept that "smaller is better" still holds true. The more difficult question is how small is "good small?" And, obviously, there are many issues that demand attention in answering that question. At least a few that would be included are as follows:

• Effect upon astigmatism (both in the short-term and for the long-term)
• Effect upon sealability without requiring the use of sutures
• Ease of wound construction

And, while certainly there is not unanimous agreement, I am going to throw out the number of 3.0 mm as being "good small." Now, you or anyone else might pose the question, "Does 0.5 mm (500 microns) really make that much clinical difference?" Well, probably not. "If not, then does 1.0 mm really make that much clinical difference?" Well, probably. At least in terms of the ability to seal an incision without requiring sutures.

That said, please allow me to share with you my personal incision sizes for the various insertion systems that are available at the time of this writing for the implants that are available at the time of this writing. My phaco incision size for the standard sized phaco tips and their standard accompanying silicone sleeves for the

longest time has been 2.8 mm. In the ideal clinical setting, I would like an IOL/insertion system that I can easily employ through a 2.8-mm incision. And, let's step back just a moment here to put a huge emphasis on the word easily. To my way of thinking, a really good IOL/insertion system is one that is essentially effortless. Effortless in assembling and effortless in inserting. And, when I say effortless, I mean without effort! In my humble opinion, that combination does not yet exist. They all require, in my mind, what I would classify as too much effort in their assembly and/or too much effort in their insertion. Keep in mind, I'm talking about a desired incision of approximately 3.0 mm here.

Okay, here are my general sizes. For the single-piece plate style silicone lenses, I feel that I can repeatedly and without undo effort insert them through an un-enlarged 2.8-mm incision. (However, loading the delivery system is more involved than I would like to see.) For the three-piece silicone lenses, depending upon the insertion system, I use anywhere from a 3.2- to a 3.5-mm incision. For both the three-piece acrylic lens and three-piece hydrogel hybrid lens, I need an incision that is very close to 4.0 mm.

Closure

At the conclusion of the surgery, it is our responsibility to make sure that the patient leaves the OR with an incision that is well-sealed. Please note, I said well-sealed and not well-healed. There is, indeed, a distinct difference that I think sometimes gets lost in the shuffle. I am aware of three modalities through which today's clear corneal incisions can be properly sealed.

The first would be a wound construction that beautifully self-seals itself upon proper re-pressurization of the globe. I have significant experience with all three of the primary techniques for creating these clear corneal incisions. In my hands, and I emphasize in my hands, none of these types of wound construction adequately self-seal when simply left to their own devices. I realize full well that that is a potentially inflammatory observation. There are numerous, highly talented, and extremely conscientious surgeons who feel, with great confidence, that in their hands their clear corneal incisions self-seal very nicely. I am sure their rebuttal to my statement would go something like, "Dave, poor fellow, please come to my operating suite and I will show you the proper way of making a truly self-sealing clear corneal incision." Until that day of reckoning comes, let me simply state that when I challenge my clear corneal incisions, again, regardless of the type of wound construction, they leak. As a result, I feel compelled to, therefore, resort to one of the other two alternatives.

The second way to deal with the business of sealing these clear corneal incisions is to revert to the old tried and true suturing process. Truth is, for the first 6 months or so of my clear corneal incision life, I was suturing essentially 100% of the cases. That's the bad news. The good news is that because the vast majority of these cases will involve an incision of 4 mm or less, there is not a lot of suturing required. I have tried horizontal sutures, one or two vertical interrupted sutures, and a single "x" suture. Of the three, I found that I preferred the single "x" suture. (Note: If I know

in advance that suturing is going to be required, eg, I know I will be using a 6.0- to 7.0-mm clear corneal incision for the implantation of a rigid PMMA IOL, I will be sure to employ a wound construction that utilizes a corneal groove of some 300 to 500 microns. It is, indeed, considerably easier to suture a clear corneal incision that has a "shelf" to hang on to. I will usually close such cases with a running 10-0 nylon, "baseball" type suture.)

It was right around that 6-month time period when I first learned about the process of stromal hydration. It was a true revelation for me. Virtually within a heartbeat, I went from essentially 100% suturing to essentially 0% suturing for the routine clear corneal incision cases. I always try to be exceedingly careful when giving particular individuals credit for innovations. Invariably, I overlook someone, not out of malice, but rather ignorance. That said, I believe it is Dr. Fine who deserves credit for bringing the phenomenon of stromal hydration to these present-day clear corneal incisions. However, I also wish to acknowledge Dr. Mackool. In the 1970s, he reported a form of stromal hydration that he developed for use in pediatric cataract surgery cases.

Stromal hydration is exactly what its name implies. I accomplish it by placing a 30-gauge cannula into the corners of my clear corneal incision and injecting, fairly aggressively, balanced salt solution (Figures 11-20a through 11-20c). The goal of stromal hydration is a simple one. By injecting fluid into the corneal stroma, we cause an outward expansion of the corneal lamellae. This causes the two cut surfaces to come into more firm apposition. It would be somewhat akin to injecting water into two sponges that were stacked one on top of the other. I am not aware of any study that actually verifies exactly how long the effect of the stromal hydration impacts the cornea. My personal guess would be no more than a few hours and, perhaps, even considerably shorter than that. My personal belief (and please keep in mind this is purely theoretical without any laboratory experimentation to substantiate it) is that the stromal hydration serves only to bring the cut surfaces into tight apposition for a short time period. Within a very short time, I believe that some combination of the action of the glycosaminoglycans and the endothelial pump then take over the business of further sealing and then healing the clear corneal incision. I am sure you have already recognized that my theory is far from original or unique. Indeed, it is much the same theory as that behind the incredible phenomenon of the re-adherence of the corneal cap in LASIK surgery. For the past many years, and still at the time of this writing, I stromal hydrate 100% of my routine clear corneal incisions.

PARTING THOUGHTS

We are so blessed to have such wonderful technology and techniques available to us today. And, just as important, so many wonderful ways in which to share them. It's okay, in fact, even appropriate, to be pleased with them, but let's not be satisfied with them. As wonderful as they are, every single one of them needs to be better. Now, true, outside regulatory interventions seem, at times, to be ruthless predators of innovation. And, true, the business of medicine is becoming more and more just that, hardcore, hardball business that is seemingly evaporating research and development dollars.

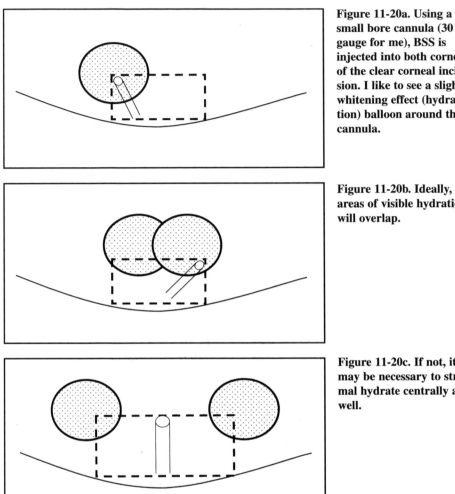

Figure 11-20a. Using a small bore cannula (30 gauge for me), BSS is injected into both corneas of the clear corneal incision. I like to see a slight whitening effect (hydration) balloon around the cannula.

Figure 11-20b. Ideally, the areas of visible hydration will overlap.

Figure 11-20c. If not, it may be necessary to stromal hydrate centrally as well.

But let's not allow ourselves to be either disillusioned or deluded. We must keep reaching, keep stretching. My greatest wish for this chapter is that it will be totally obsolete 5 years from now. Ophthalmology is truly a global family, and together, I hope we can make that happen.

Personal Techniques

James A. Davison, MD, FACS

INTRODUCTION

In 1992 I was inspired by my good friend, Dr. I. Howard Fine, to adopt clear corneal temporal incisions for cataract surgery. Dr. Fine's pioneering work and his scientific presentations convinced me that clear corneal temporal incisions would be superior to the corneoscleral incisions from the superior approach that I was making at the time. I adopted Dr. Fine's technique, but in 1993, I adopted a refinement that I learned from Dr. David Brown of Fort Myers, Florida. Dr. Brown employed a free-hand technique using a diamond blade made by Diamatrix, Inc (Brown Universal Cataract Knife [BUCK]). Having one blade that could accomplish everything was very appealing, especially in our setting of operating in multiple hospitals and multiple cities and towns in urban and rural Iowa. Hospitals, of course, were reluctant to purchase seemingly expensive diamond blades since steel blades had gotten the job done. To them, even though disposable steel could be proven to be cumulatively expensive, at least the cost per case was predictable and seemed small relative to the high expense of a single diamond blade. Since the BUCK knife was a universal diamond blade, I initially purchased three (two for use and one for backup) and took them to the various locations where I operated, where they were rented by the hospitals from me. I was soon able to convince each hospital to purchase their own as we were providing a superior technique more efficiently (faster and with ultimately less expense). Because of the availability of the knives, many of my partners adopted the technique, so that multiple surgeons were able to accomplish clear corneal temporal incisions at multiple locations using the same diamond blades without

extraordinary expense and unnecessary redundancy associated with various types and sizes of keratome-style diamond knives.

The advantage of clear corneal temporal surgery is that it not only creates the cleanest, most precise incision furthest away from the visual axis, but it also allows safer access to the intraocular contents (Figure 12-1). No longer did I have to struggle to get over the brow and endure the substantial corneal distortion and compromised visibility that accompanied superior corneoscleral incisions. The temporal pathway provided me with safer access, and it has improved my cataract surgery substantially.

My average induced keratometric astigmatism with clear corneal temporal incision freehand technique is 0.2 D of flattening at 6 to 8 weeks. Because of this small amount, I perform all cases, regardless of preoperative astigmatism, with a clear corneal temporal technique. I have been able to routinely prescribe a spectacle lens change at 2 weeks after the surgery. Because of the incision's safety and stability, I see my patients about 40 minutes after surgery. I find that their wounds are secure, their IOLs are in place, their chambers are formed, and I can discharge them with drops (antibiotic and prednisolone acetate 1% qid for 2 weeks, then prednisolone acetate 1% bid for 2 weeks) and an instruction package, and just recheck them in 2 weeks for their final lens prescription. I have found that it is not necessary to check them on the day after surgery. Again with our relatively rural environment, this saves travel, risks, hazards, and expense for our patients, and they have been uniformly very enthusiastic about this follow-up plan.

I have performed approximately 8000 clear corneal temporal incision cataract surgeries and have had only four wound leaks.

One was a patient who I thought about placing one suture (I suture about 1% because of poor wound sealing), I actually had the 10-0 nylon open at surgery but ultimately convinced myself that it wasn't going to be necessary to suture it at the time. I ended up suturing that wound later the same day because the patient demonstrated half depth anterior chamber and low IOP and was Seidel positive at the wound. Two were real nervous, squeezing, eye rubbing men who precipitated an iris prolapse 2 days and 3 days, respectively, after surgery. The fourth was a patient who was in automobile crash and had an air bag explode in her face prolapsing her iris (but leaving the IOL capsular bag, etc, intact) 2 weeks after surgery. I have had no cases of endophthalmitis.

In the earlier years of using this incision, I created a groove that was between 150- and 300-microns deep, depending on the blade stop calibration, and then completed my incision through the groove. Later, again at Dr. Fine's suggestion, I abandoned the groove but continued to freehand the incision. The epithelial entry of the diamond is almost invisible 1 day after surgery, whereas the groove continues to be obvious indefinitely. Less foreign body sensation has been reported by my patients since abandoning the initial groove. The non-groove technique actually makes the incision making process a little bit easier, rather than more difficult, since more tissue resistance is available without the weakening effect that the groove creates by disrupting the peripheral countertraction which is available with an intact cornea without the groove.

TECHNIQUE

The patient is prepped and draped in the usual fashion and an open-wire speculum is placed curling the edges of the 3M Model 1060 drape underneath the lash margin, draping the lashes away from the operative field. A caliper is set at 2.8 mm (Figure 12-2), and an indentation created on the corneal surface (Figure 12-3). If desired, a 150- to 300-micron deep groove can be created for approximately a length of 3.2 mm (the length that we will need for IOL insertion) (Figure 12-4). In our current technique, however, the initial step is to create a paracentesis opening (Figure 12-5), which is followed by incision creation without a groove. The blade is placed against the cornea at the corneal limbus and driven into the stroma in a uniplanar fashion not ever being parallel to the corneal surface. The Descemet's target entry point is 1.75 mm from epithelial penetration. The entry of the blade is ultimately accomplished with an oblique, right-to-left motion, rather than a direct straight-in penetration. This is done because the diamonds are sometimes a little dull or the cornea seems a little tougher and straight-in penetration generates a "pop" as the resistance gives way when the blade enters the anterior chamber, which can result in touching of the iris or lens or generate an actual patient movement reaction. If an oblique entry is utilized, there is more of a gradual entry slowly slicing into stroma and arriving through Descemet's level more slowly so that this sudden loss of resistance can be avoided. The initiation point is slightly to the right (Figure 12-6) and at approximately 1.75 mm into the cornea Descemet's membrane is encountered. If the blade is slightly dull, even a dimpling can be seen, especially in grooved cases (Figure 12-7), prior to entry. It is more obvious in the grooved example because corneal tissue tends to pile up in a distorted accumulation because of loss of peripheral corneal countertraction as the diamond blade pushes centrally. This is one of the reasons that grooving should be avoided, ie, the accuracy of wound width creation is more consistent and the sudden release of compressed central stroma is less with non-grooved, uniplanar incisions. The blade is simply swept then to the left (Figure 12-8) to the spot underlying the dimple that has been created with the caliper and then to the right (Figure 12-9). After the incision is created, the blade is carefully withdrawn, retracted, and placed in its case. If the diamond blade is dull or the cornea seems tough, a slight sawing motion needs to be employed This sawing motion should be of very low amplitude and with not much force, while alternating driving in and withdrawing the blade. If too much of the cut is made while driving in the blade, the incision tends to extend peripherally into the conjunctival limbus, making a broader peripheral flap. If the incision is extended as the blade is being withdrawn, the incision seems to shallow and centralize the external portion extending further into the cornea making a narrower flap, but interestingly, sometimes the opposite may seem to occur. So if a sawing motion is needed, small movements, ie, almost an micro-oscillation created by finger motion, are necessary.

Seen from a side view, the blade enters the cornea at the limbal junction (Figure 12-10), a slight dimpling can be seen just prior to Descemet's entry (Figure 12-11), followed by a sweeping motion to the left (Figure 12-12), and then a sweeping motion to the right (Figure 12-13).

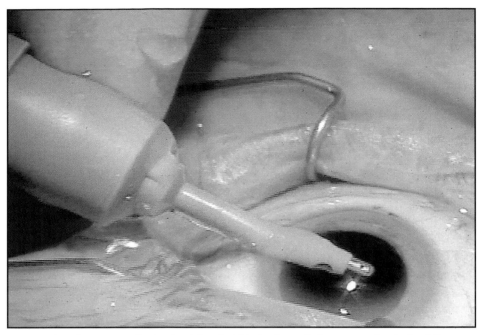

Figure 12-1. Easy access is obtained for the I/A tip through the temporal palpebral fissure. The surgeon has an opportunity to use his or her left index finger as a fulcrum to create finer control of the I/A tip.

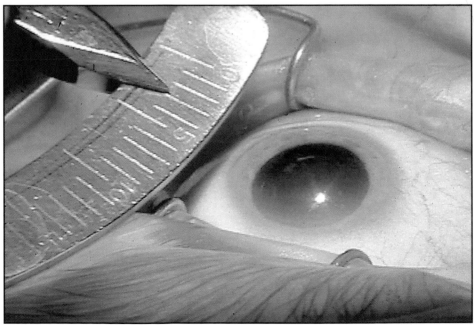

Figure 12-2. The caliper is set at 2.8 mm.

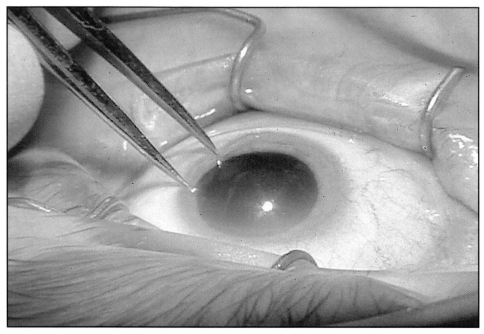

Figure 12-3. A slight indentation on the peripheral corneal surface is created with the pointed ends of the caliper.

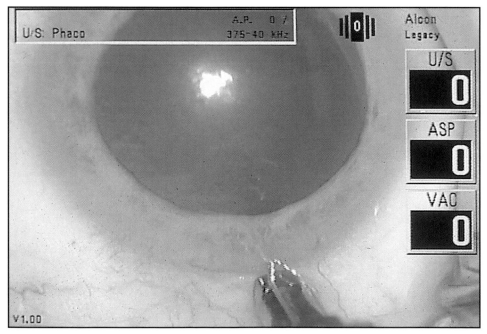

Figure 12-4. A 150- to 300-micron depth groove is created (older technique).

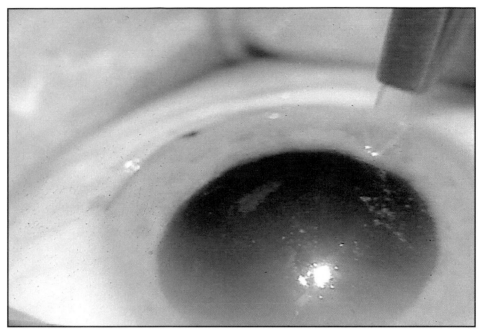

Figure 12-5. A paracentesis incision is created with the diamond blade fully extended.

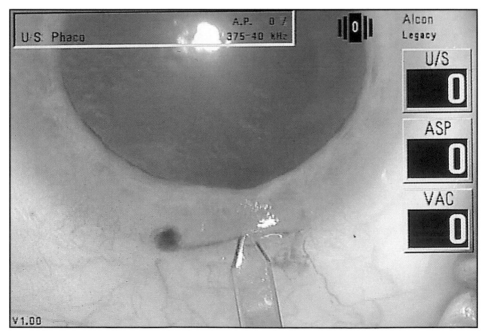

Figure 12-6. The initiation of the incision is created at the epithelial corneal level at the corneal portion of the limbus. The starting point is just to the right of center.

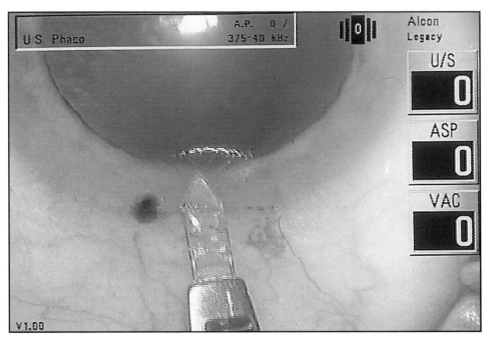

Figure 12-7. An oblique entry is created as the blade not only is driven through the corneal stroma to Descemet's level, but also slices to the surgeon's left. Notice the dimple being created because of the relatively dull blade and groove used in this case.

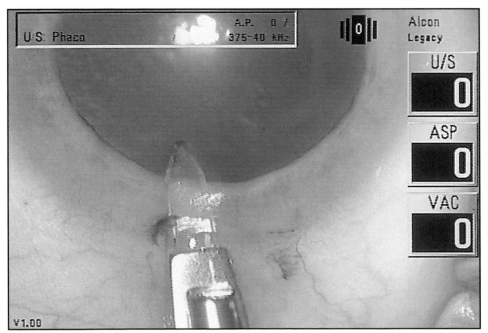

Figure 12-8. Descemet's level has been entered 1.75 mm from the epithelial level and the blade is swept to the left.

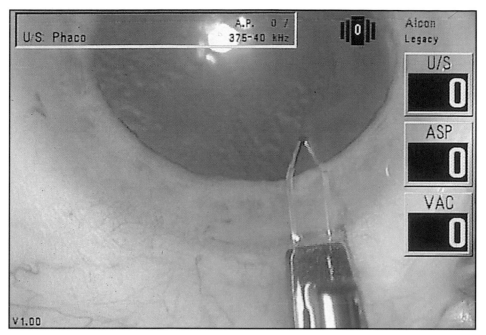

Figure 12-9. The blade is swept to the right so that its lateral aspect is just underneath the indentation created by the caliper.

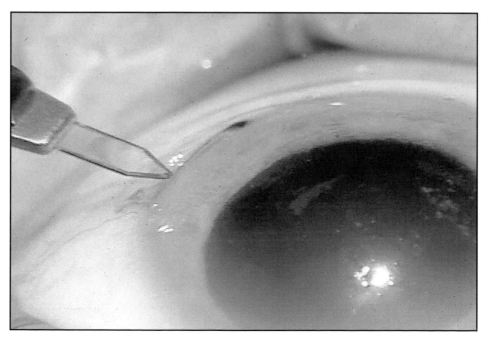

Figure 12-10. Side view. The diamond blade is on the corneal side of the epithelial limbus.

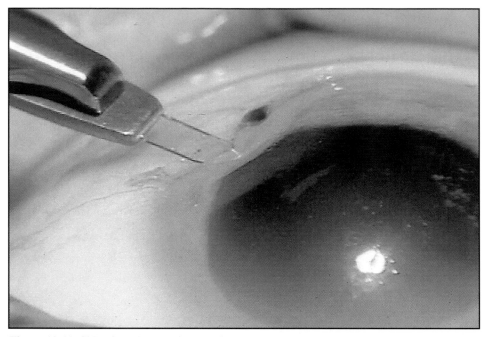

Figure 12-11. Side view. A slight indentation has been created as the blade is driven to the Descemet's level.

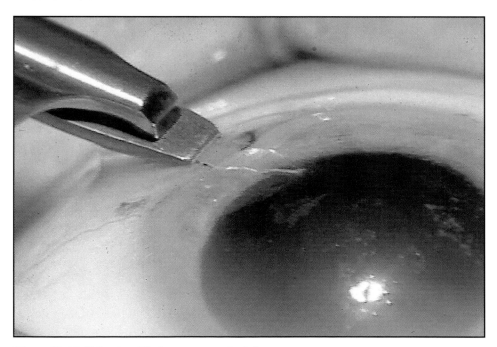

Figure 12-12. Side view. Blade sweeps to the left.

All subsequent steps in surgery are made with the important thought of keeping the incision tunnel intact and not disturbing any of the layers of the cornea involved around it. It is important for the incision not to be made any further peripheral than the one demonstrated; actually a totally clear corneal incision without limbal bleeding is preferable. If it is more peripheral, conjunctival ballooning or subconjunctival hemorrhage may make the operation more difficult and generate patient complaints.

A capsulorrhexis is created with a cystotome starting centrally and sweeping to the left (Figure 12-14). The rhexis continues toward the surgeon and by the time it sweeps past the 3 o'clock hour, the correct radius will have been achieved (Figure 12-15). It is nice to have this transition toward the surgeon as the important part of the intact capsular bag during the phacoemulsification and lens implantation process is the portion that is away from the surgeon, ie, the capsular bag that receives all the driving forces of phacoemulsification and lens implantation is 180 degrees away from the incision.

Hydrodissection is accomplished with a 30-gauge cannula (Figure 12-16). A 30-gauge cannula gives a fine directional quality to the dissecting fluid resulting in a safe, low volume, and well-controlled process.

PHACOEMULSIFICATION

I prefer the Alcon Legacy 20,000 phacoemulsification machine and the 0.9-mm MicroTip with aspiration bypass system (ABS) opening in the shaft (Figures 12-17 and 12-18). A 175-micron hole has been placed in the shaft of the ABS phacoemulsification tip approximately 3 mm from the end. During quadrant removal, as complete aperture occlusion is accomplished, the ABS will permit a substantial amount of fluid to be withdrawn into the phacoemulsification tip from the ABS hole. I use a setting of 30 cc/min in the quadrant removal phase, and with complete tip occlusion 11 cc/min can be withdrawn through the ABS opening.

Phacoemulsification—Non-Occluded Phase

Phacoemulsification is accomplished in Memory 1 (ultrasound 90% maximum, maximum vacuum potential 50 mmHg, aspiration flow rate 14 cc/min). A divide and conquer method variation is used employing a combination of capsular bag phacoemulsification and iris plane phacoemulsification of nuclear fragments. Deep grooves are possible because of the good visualization around and in front of the smaller tip and also the 45 degree configuration of the tip itself (Figure 12-19).

Using a specially modified 0.35-mm cyclodialysis spatula, a cross-handed cracking technique is used to tear the posterior nuclear plate from the periphery centrally (Figure 12-20).

As phacoemulsification proceeds, the tip is allowed to go deeper and grooves made. There is a tendency to "see" just the tips of the phacoemulsification unit and assisting cyclodialysis spatula, but careful attention needs to be paid so that the instruments, especially the phacoemulsification tip, stay well centered loosely within the very center of the incision, both from left and right and top to bottom. When the phacoemulsification tip (Figure 12-21) is involved in creating a deeper pass, the

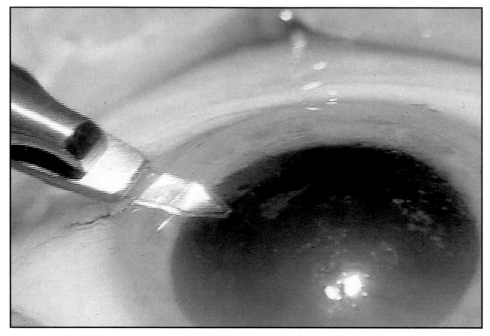

Figure 12-13. Side view. Blade then sweeps to the right. Notice that the angle of the blade has not changed from the epithelial entry in Figure 12-10.

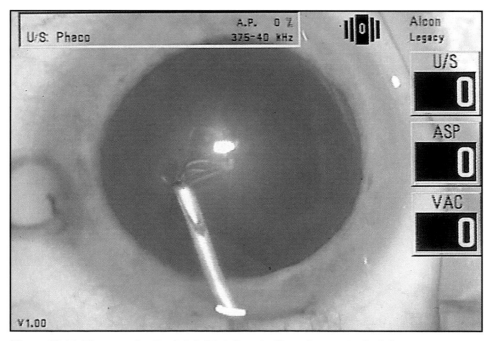

Figure 12-14. The capsulorrhexis is initiated centrally and swept to the left.

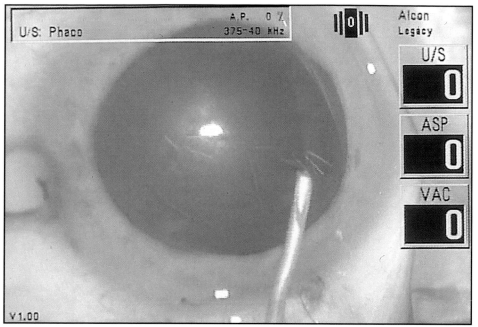

Figure 12-15. The rhexis has spiraled to an approximate 2.5-mm radius.

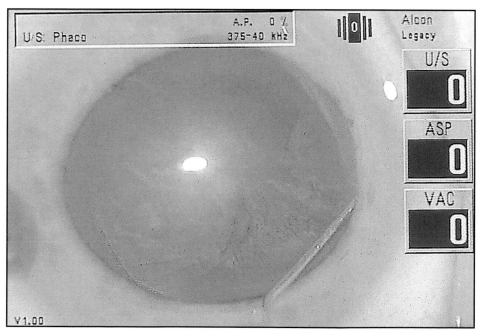

Figure 12-16. A 30-gauge cannula is placed underneath the anterior capsule and a fluid wave has progressed almost all the way across the posterior cortical interface.

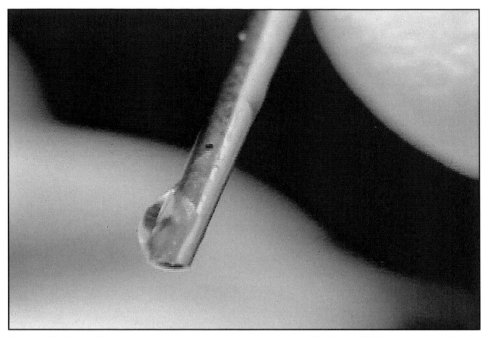

Figure 12-17. A 175-micron hole has been placed in the shaft of the ABS phacoemulsification tip approximately 3 mm from the end.

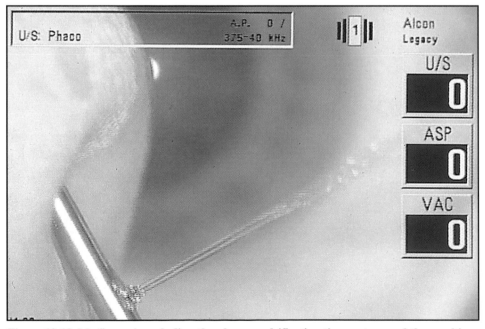

Figure 12-18. My finger is occluding the phacoemulsification tip aperture and the machine is in the reflux mode. Note the stream of BSS exiting the ABS aperture.

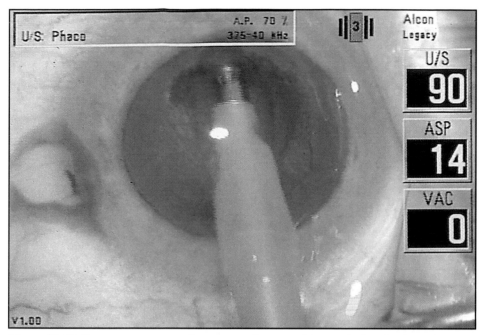

Figure 12-19. Deep grooves are easier to create because of the good visualization in front of and beside the 0.9-mm 45 degree phacoemulsification tip.

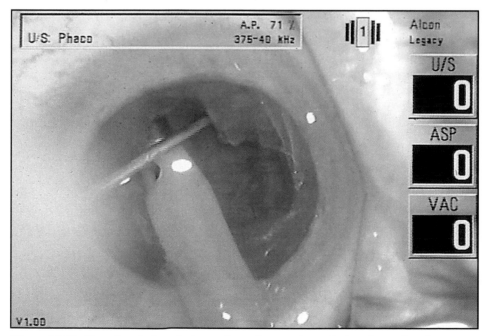

Figure 12-20. Cross-handed posterior nuclear plate tearing technique is employed.

tip is observed to be in appropriate position. But because of the shallower depth of focus and narrower field associated with higher magnification during this process, the surgeon may not see that the cornea is distorted because the shaft of the phacoemulsification tip may be pushing against one of the wound tunnel walls (right, left, top, or bottom). The friction generated can cause immediate heat absorption by any component of the elliptical corneal tunnel where contact has been made. Thermal absorption results in chemical collagen changes and ultimately wound shrinkage and poor wound sealing. Constant awareness of shaft centration within the elliptical tunnel helps prevent this problem (Figure 12-22).

Phacoemulsification—Occluded Phase

The phacoemulsification machine is now switched to Memory 3 for most normal quadrant removals (phacoemulsification maximum energy 70%, vacuum 400 mmHg, aspiration flow rate 30 cc/min); if very soft lenses are being aspirated, an intermediate setting (Memory 2) is used to slow down the operation (phacoemulsification maximum energy 50%, vacuum 300 mmHg, aspiration flow rate 25 cc/min).

The flat aperture of the 45 degree tip is placed sideways against the flat wall of the separated nuclear quadrant. Vacuum is allowed to build, with very little ultrasonic energy applied so that the tip can bore in and adhere to the quadrant (Figure 12-23). As vacuum builds, the nuclear fragment is held even more securely on the phacoemulsification tip aperture. The tip is drawn centrally and rolled over so that the fragment is rolled centrally and vertically in a simultaneous unlocking motion (Figure 12-24). The tip is rotated 90 degrees so that the previously side-facing aperture faces up. The nuclear fragment is rotated so that it is basically within the upper capsular bag or lower iris plane, well away from the posterior capsule and corneal endothelium with the tip aperture facing the corneal endothelium. The initial part of the nuclear fragment is aspirated with ultrasonic assistance while the rollover occurs. Vacuum is assisted with low levels of ultrasonic energy as needed so that the rest of the quadrant can be aspirated while it is in that location (Figure 12-25). A little more ultrasonic energy may be needed in the later phases of nucleus removal as the firmer portion of the deeper nucleus is ultimately the last to be acquired (Figure 12-26). As the very last of the firm nuclear fragments are removed, the cyclodialysis spatula is placed immediately underneath the phacoemulsification tip to prevent aspiration of capsule or involuntary presentation of the next nuclear quadrant (Figure 12-27).

Seen with side view, the nuclear wall is engaged with the face of the 45 degree tip. The quadrant is withdrawn and the tip rotated 90 degrees so it faces superior (Figures 12-28 through 12-30). The nuclear fragment is within the deeper iris plane and aspirated with the cyclodialysis spatula assisting in procurement and manipulation of nuclear material while protecting the posterior capsule from inadvertent aspiration (Figures 12-31 and 12-32).

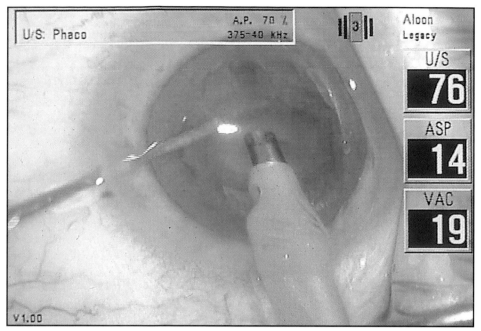

Figure 12-21. Note the striae in the superficial layer of the corneal wound from distortion due to the phacoemulsification tip pushing against the right-hand side of the wound. Notice the tip position within the sleeve.

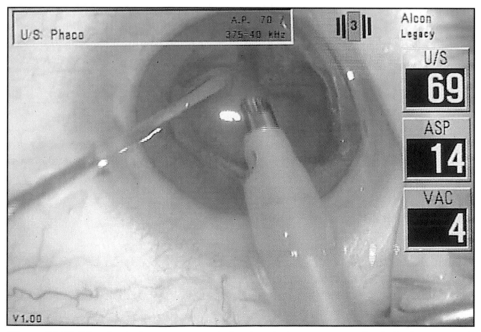

Figure 12-22. The shaft of the phacoemulsification tip is now appropriately in the center of the elliptical wound tunnel. No corneal distortion is seen.

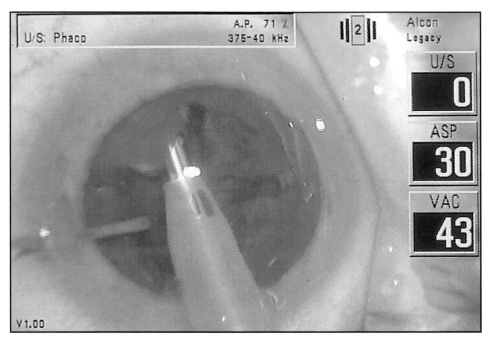

Figure 12-23. The 45 degree tip aperture is applied to the wall of nuclear fragment and vacuum allowed to build.

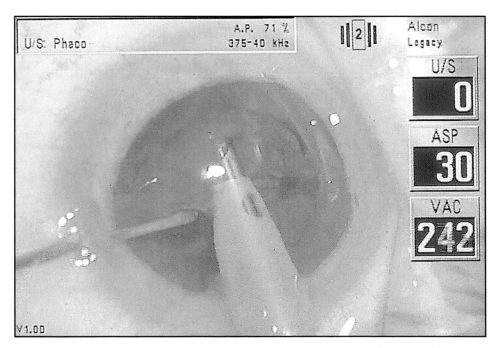

Figure 12-24. As vacuum is building, the fragment is drawn central but also rotated so that the peripheral portion will become the superficial portion and the deeper, firmer portion will be removed last.

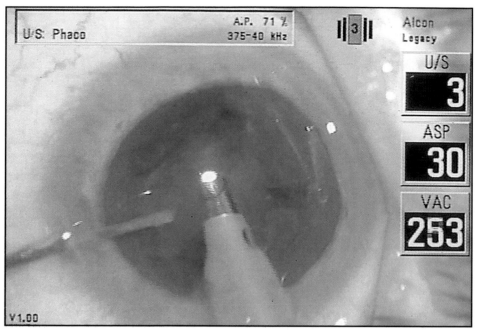

Figure 12-25. The nuclear fragment is being removed. The phacoemulsification tip is facing the corneal endothelial surface. The softer peripheral nuclear material is now the most central and drawn in easiest.

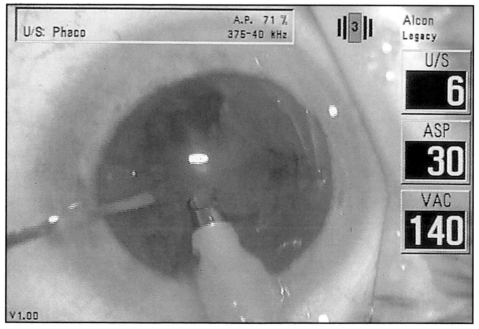

Figure 12-26. The firmer nuclear material is being aspirated with low levels of phacoemulsification energy.

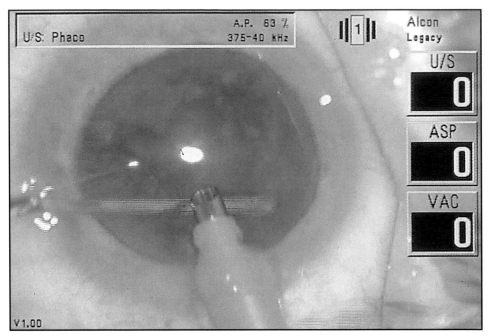

Figure 12-27. The cyclodialysis spatula is protecting the posterior capsule and additional peripheral nuclear pieces from being withdrawn.

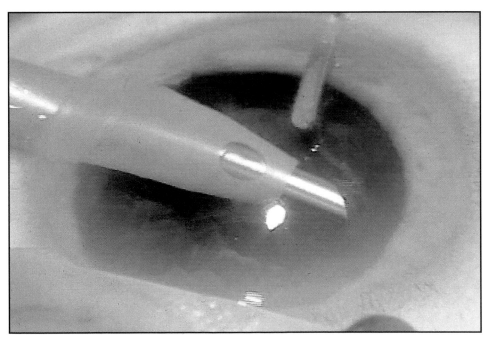

Figure 12-28. Side view. The aperture of the 45 degree tip has been applied to the wall of the nuclear fragment and vacuum is allowed to build.

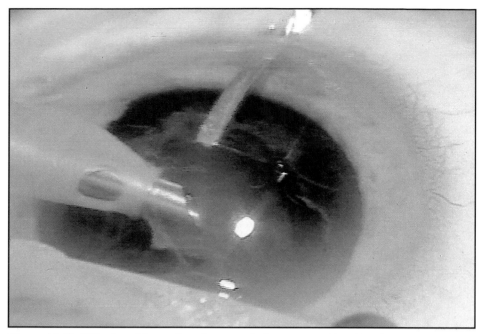

Figure 12-29. Side view. The nuclear fragment is drawn centrally while simultaneously rolling it over 90 degrees.

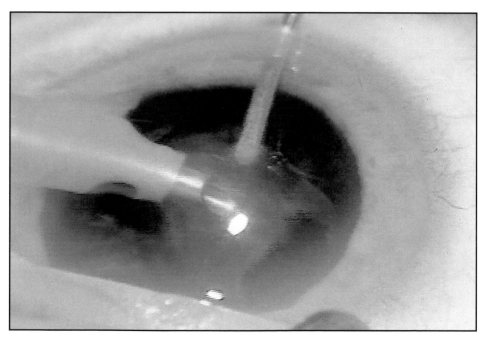

Figure 12-30. The phacoemulsification tip is facing the endothelium and the nuclear fragment is being withdrawn.

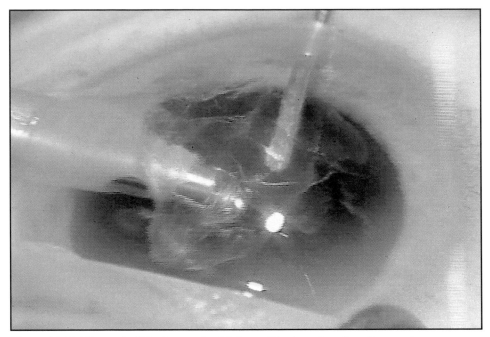

Figure 12-31. The cyclodialysis spatula aids in positioning of nuclear fragment.

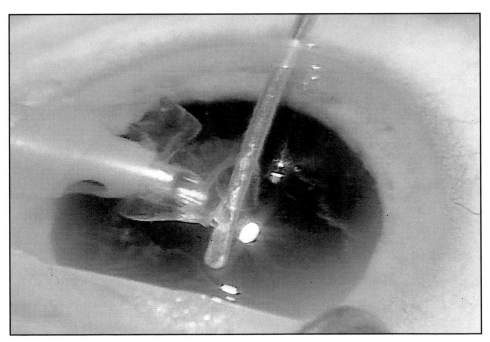

Figure 12-32. The cyclodialysis spatula protects the posterior capsule against inadvertent aspiration.

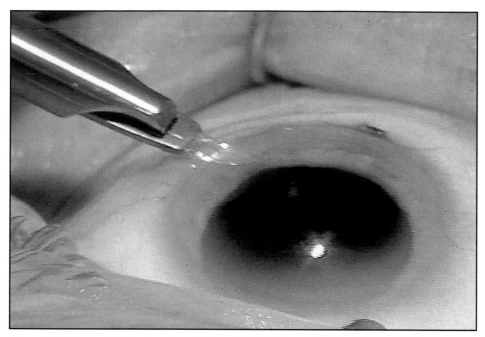

Figure 12-33. The incision is enlarged from 2.8 to 3.2 mm with the diamond blade.

INCISION ENLARGEMENT

After the phacoemulsification process and the aspiration of cortex are completed, the posterior capsule is polished with a 0.2-mm I/A tip (vacuum 11 mmHg, aspiration flow rate 11 cc/min). When vacuuming of the posterior capsule is completed, viscoelastic is placed in the anterior chamber. The diamond blade is extended fully and the incision lengthened from 2.8 mm to approximately 3.2 mm to accommodate IOL insertion (Figure 12-33).

IOL IMPLANTATION

I feel that the following implantation technique is the most gentle on the incision tunnel tissue and also creates the least acute distortion of the acrylic IOL PMMA haptics. I currently prefer to implant acrylic IOLs.

The folded lens is removed from the modified Acrypak compression device with insertion forceps (Figure 12-34). The surfaces of the forceps' paddles have been cleaned with an instrument wipe so that they do not harbor any foreign material that might be impressed on the optic surface. The leading haptic is extended with counterpressure by straightening so that it can go through the incision (Figures 12-35 and 12-36). The superficial portion of the incision is lifted gently so that the optic can slide between the superficial portion and the deeper tunnel walls. Care is taken not to mar the lens with the 0.12 forceps (Figure 12-37). Care is also taken not to disturb the stroma or epithelium which makes up the surface of the superficial tunnel flap. If the wound is tight, it should be extended. Globe stabilization through coun-

tertraction can be accomplished by placing a cyclodialysis spatula in the side-port incision. No substantial traction should be attempted with the 0.12 forceps on the wound edge as disruption of the epithelium or stroma or both may occur. The 0.12 forceps should be used only to lift slightly (see Figure 12-37). The lens is allowed to unfold, again being careful of the endothelial surface of the cornea, not only centrally but peripherally near the wound (Figure 12-38). The lens is dialed into position with a Lester manipulator (Figure 12-39). Viscoelastic is removed with the 0.3 I/A tip. Aspiration is not engaged until the tip has been placed under the IOL optic. If the tip is under the optic, the posterior capsule will not be encountered and all viscoelastic will be removed from the space between the posterior capsule and the optic of the IOL (Figure 12-40). The tip can then be brought into the anterior chamber to finish thorough viscoelastic removal.

WOUND CLOSURE

The side-port incision is irrigated with a 30-gauge cannula, not only to close the side-port incision with stromal hydration, but also to make sure that there is no nuclear fragment hiding there. The stroma is then hydrated with brief and minimal pressure from the 3-cc syringe on the 30-gauge cannula. Hydration of the stroma should be accomplished with the tip at mid-stroma, well away from the epithelial and endothelial edges (Figure 12-41). The eye is overinflated so that the tunnel interfaces become opposed. If the eye is left overinflated, the wound will seal but the IOP will be too high and the patient will be almost immediately uncomfortable. Normal pressure is obtained by expressing some of the fluid from the incision with gentle pressure using a Weck-cel sponge. If the wound is too well sealed and fluid will not express with this technique, it can be let out passively by placing the 30-gauge cannula within the side-port incision, but the appropriate pressure of the eye must be still be assessed by tactile sensation with the Weck-cel sponge over the incision. Pressure in the eye at the conclusion of this tamponade should be normal to low normal, ie, not hard or firm (Figure 12-42). When the IOP is normal to low normal, a final inspection is made. The external wound, internal wound, paracentesis, anterior chamber, capsulorrhexis border, IOL, and iris are all inspected to make sure that they are secure and their positions are appropriate and that no foreign bodies are present (Figure 12-43). The wound edges may moisten a bit, but no frank gross leakage should be apparent. The speculum is then carefully withdrawn while the patient is asked to keep his or her eyes open. The adhesive drape can then be slowly removed, while again asking the patient to keep his or her eyes open. The patient is then asked to just close his or her eyes gently, but not to squeeze. Any remaining fluid is gently dried with a towel so that the patient does not feel like he or she has to reach up and wipe the eye.

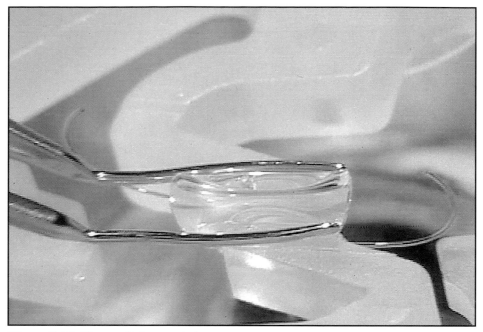

Figure 12-34. The acrylic lens optic is grasped with implantation forceps.

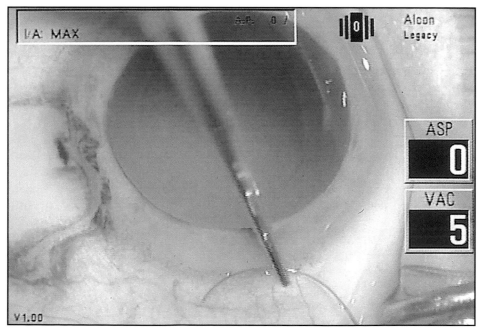

Figure 12-35. The leading haptic is in a position to be straightened as the optic is pulled slightly away from the 0.12 forceps.

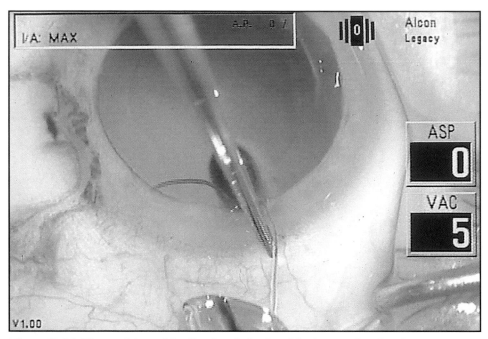

Figure 12-36. The straightened leading haptic is placed in the anterior chamber.

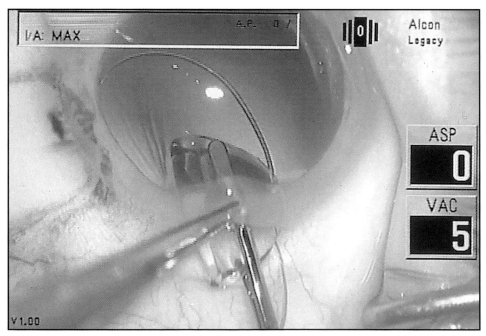

Figure 12-37. The 0.12 forceps lifts the superficial portion of the wound so that optic entry can be initiated.

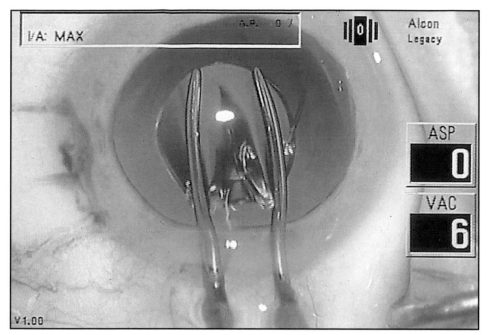

Figure 12-38. The IOL is unfolded, being careful of the corneal endothelium.

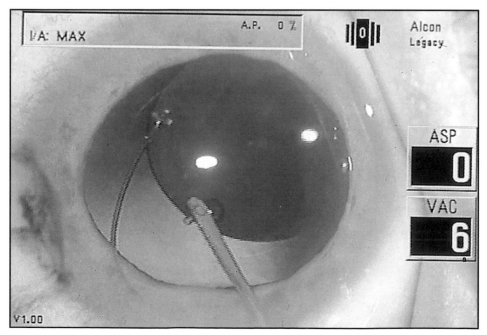

Figure 12-39. The trailing haptic is dialed into place within the capsule bag.

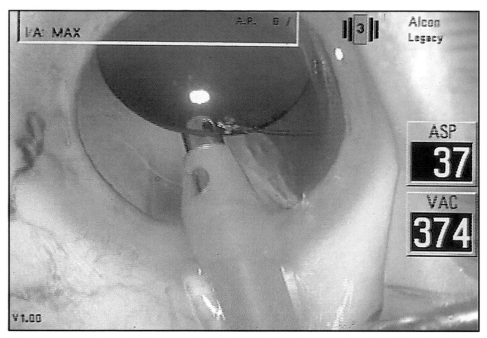

Figure 12-40. Viscoelastic is removed with a 0.3 tip first in a retrolental position, later in the anterior chamber.

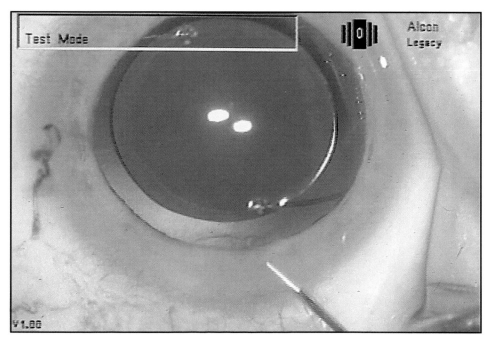

Figure 12-41. Stromal hydration is accomplished with a 30-gauge cannula.

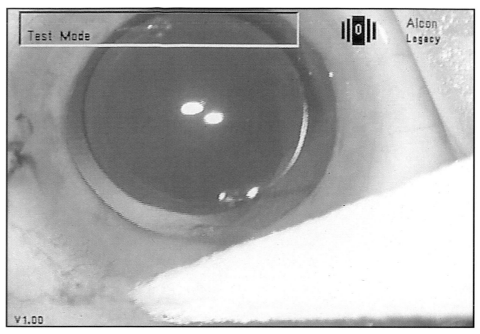

Figure 12-42. IOP is adjusted to normal by wound compression with a Weck-cel sponge.

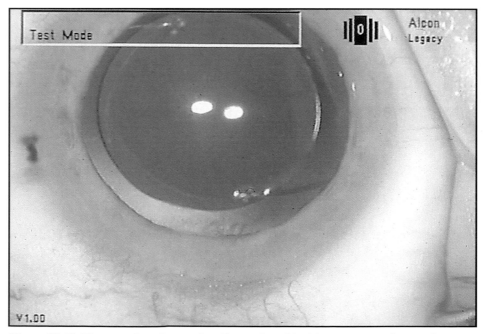

Figure 12-43. The procedure is complete. Inspection of incision, paracentesis, anterior chamber, iris, rhexis, capsule, and IOL is accomplished.

Sub 3.0-mm Phaco

Harry B. Grabow, MD

INCISION

For all cases of adult lens surgery, which includes cataract, refractive clear lensectomy, phakic foldable lens implantation, and secondary IOL implantation, I employ one form or another of a temporal clear corneal incision. For all cases of pediatric lens surgery, I employ a superior scleral tunnel incision. Because of its increased tunnel length, the scleral incision may function to resist external inadvertent pressure, as is more likely to occur in a child, with greater strength than shorter-tunnel-length clear corneal incisions.[1] In addition, the scleral component of the tunnel may theoretically heal more rapidly due to its increased vascularity.

I prefer the temporal location for adult lens procedures for four reasons. First, it is believed that the temporal clear corneal incision, in contrast to the superior clear corneal incision, is safer in regard to the incidence of postoperative infectious endophthalmitis. It is theoretically proposed that both lid-blink and gravity may contribute to an increased incidence of anterior chamber microbial inoculation with superior clear corneal incisions, particularly if they are longer than 4.0 mm and unsutured.

Second, the temporal location has been shown to result in less average corneal endothelial cell loss[2] than both the superior and the oblique locations (Figure 13-1), and, third, to also demonstrate less surgically induced astigmatism[3] (Figure 13-2). Finally, the temporal approach provides greater ergonomic access to the globe, eliminating the superior orbital rim, and simultaneously providing a more central position of the globe with maximized red reflex.

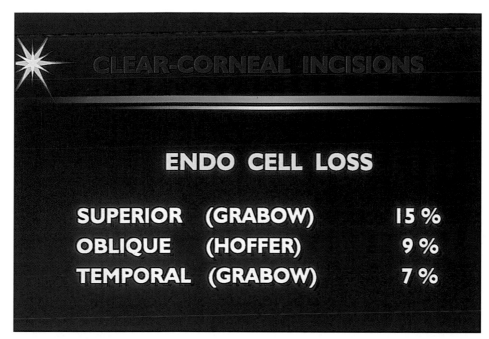

Figure 13-1. Clear corneal incision endothelial cell loss by location.

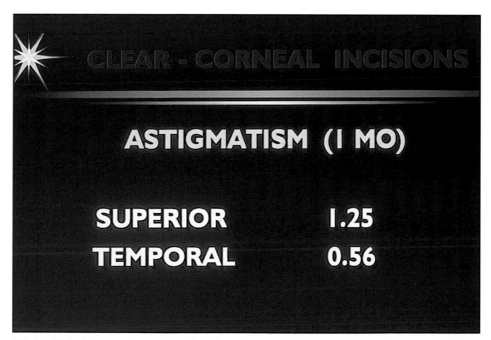

Figure 13-2. 3.0-mm clear corneal incision absolute (scalar) surgically induced astigmatism at 1 month by location.

Astigmatism Management

Like no other incision in cataract surgical history, the clear corneal incision offers a variety of construction variables that, for the first time, allow the cataract surgeon to truly be a refractive surgeon. When the incision is temporal and is less than 3.0 mm, as is used with most phacoemulsification and foldable IOL cases, the incision is usually astigmatically neutral. That is, it has no effect on altering the corneal curvature. However, if made longer than 3.0 mm or placed more centrally on the cornea, it can produce a major effect on corneal curvature, up to as much as 5.0 D of astigmatic change. With the advent of "sub 2-mm" surgery, with small ultrasonic emulsification tips[4] and laser phacolysis systems,[5] the use of longer and "on-axis" clear corneal incisions for cataract surgery may soon become undesirable. In addition, the development of foldable toric IOLs[6] may render all additional corneal incisional surgery for astigmatism virtually obsolete. Until such time, however, cataract surgeons are limited to currently available techniques for astigmatic reduction. These include on-axis incisions, one of three methods of astigmatic keratotomy, surface or stromal excimer laser astigmatic ablation, and toric IOLs.

While on-axis incisions are preferred by some surgeons, I prefer to use the temporal location exclusively for clear corneal incision cataract surgery, for reasons mentioned earlier in this chapter. Since beginning phacoemulsification and foldable lens implantation through 3.0-mm sutureless clear corneal incisions in 1992, and after a 6000-case experience, I became comfortable and familiar with the astigmatic effects of this cataract incision. Its predictability allowed the development of a systematic approach to pre-existing astigmatism. The system is called the "Six Steps to Sphericity," and involves six combinations of four variables:

1. Ungrooved uniplanar clear corneal incision (Figures 13-3 and 13-4)
2. Grooved biplanar clear corneal incisions (Figures 13-5 and 13-6)
3. Astigmatic keratotomy (Figures 13-7 and 13-8)
4. Toric IOLs (Figure 13-9)

The system is designed to be used with temporal clear corneal incisions only, and for the purposes of this system and its application to astigmatism reduction, "temporal" is defined as within 30 degrees of the horizontal axis.

Step 1

The first step to sphericity (Figure 13-10) is applied to **spherical eyes**. In these cases, we want the postop corneal curvature to match the preop curvature. Therefore, a simple single-plane, very peripheral temporal stab incision is used. This 2.5-mm incision is astigmatically neutral, usually resulting in either no change in astigmatism or no more than 0.37 D induction with-the-rule.

Step 2

For **mild astigmatism against-the-rule of 0.50 D to 1.25 D**, a two-step grooved incision is used. The groove depth used in this system is 300 microns. However, depths of 400 microns (Williamson) and 600 microns (Langerman) can be used. The deeper the groove, the greater the effect. In addition, as with all pure incisional ker-

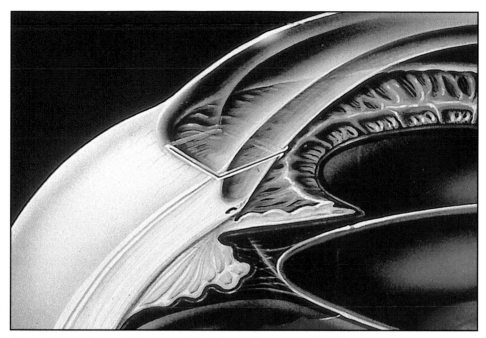

Figure 13-3. Diagram of ungrooved uniplanar clear corneal incision.

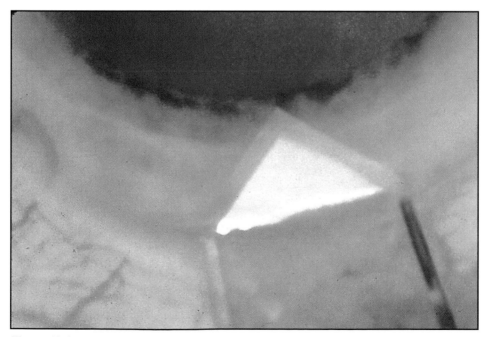

Figure 13-4. Ungrooved uniplanar clear corneal incision with trapezoid diamond blade.

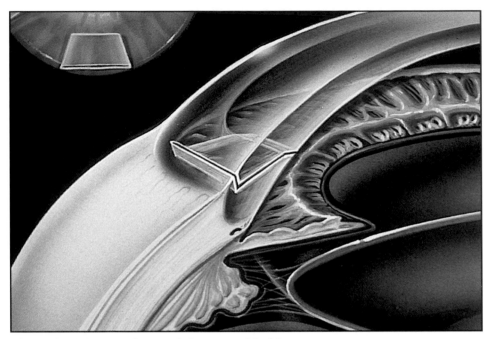

Figure 13-5. Diagram of grooved clear corneal incision.

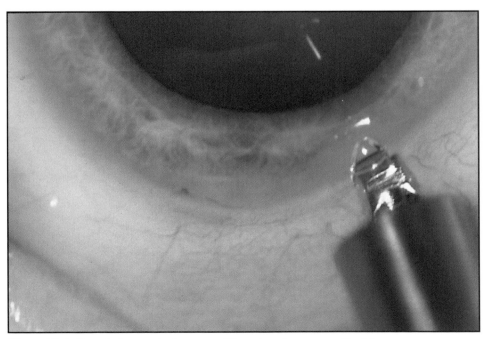

Figure 13-6. Completing vertical groove of two-step clear corneal incision.

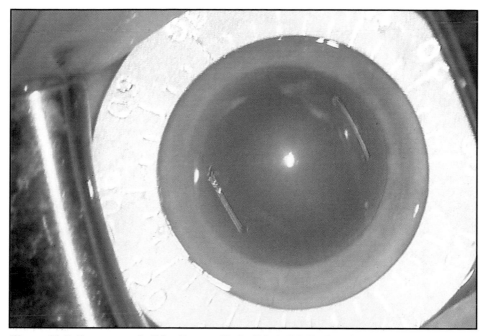

Figure 13-7. Cornea marked for Feaster blade (Rhein Medical) astigmatic keratotomy.

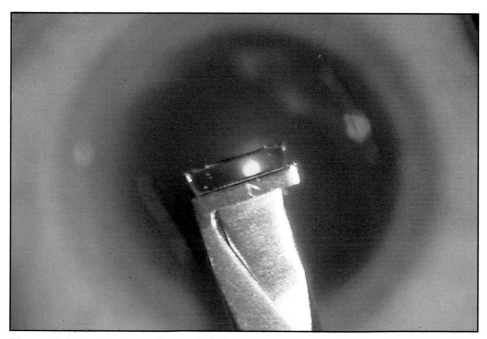

Figure 13-8. Feaster 3-mm diamond blade (Rhein Medical) ready for astigmatic kerato-tomy.

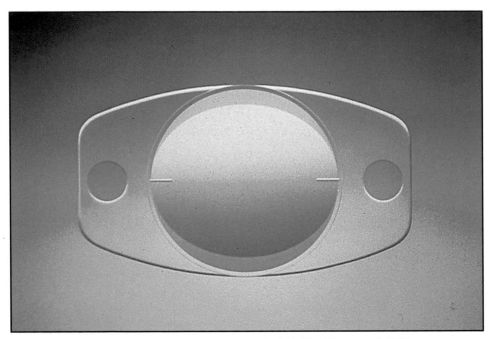

Figure 13-9. Staar AA4203T one-piece plate haptic foldable silicone toric IOL.

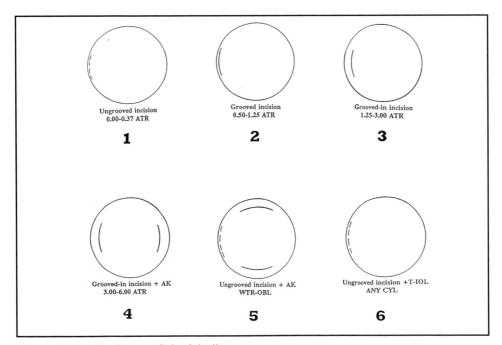

Figure 13-10. "Six Steps to Sphericity."

atorefractive procedures (RK and AK), age is a factor. The 60-year-old cataract patient might result in only a 0.50 D change in cylinder, whereas the 80-year-old would get a 1.25 D shift from the same incision.

Step 3

For **moderate against-the-rule astigmatism of 1.50 D to 3.0 D**, the same two-step grooved incision is used; however, it is moved 0.5 to 1.0 mm centrally on the corneal surface. Moving the vertical groove centrally effectively reduces the optical zone of the "AK portion" of the two-step phaco-foldable incision, thereby increasing its effect. Again, the effect is age-related.

Step 4

For **high degrees of against-the-rule astigmatism, 3.00 D to 6.00 D**, the two-step incision is used, as in Step 3. However, an AK incision is added across the cornea 180 degrees away, for more effect. For 4.00 D, the full-thickness phaco incision would be placed at an optical zone of 8.0 mm. An AK incision would then be added at the 8.0-mm optical zone (180 degrees away) and two additional AK incisions (a pair) at the 7.0-mm optical zone. For 6.00 D of astigmatism, a triple set of incisions may be desired, especially in a younger patient, at optical zones of 6.0, 7.0, and 8.0 mm. Beware: the full-thickness grooved phaco incision moved in on the cornea can be very powerful in the elderly, those over 80 years of age. The Feaster blade, not being translated through corneal tissue, must be set with greater exposure than previous 15 degree and square AK blades. From experience, the empiric blade setting for a 6.0-mm optical zone is 620 microns, for a 7.0-mm optical zone is 680 microns, and for an 8.0-mm optical zone is 720 microns. With-the-rule astigmatism is visually preferable to against-the-rule astigmatism. Therefore, overcorrection of against-the-rule and undercorrection of with-the-rule are recommended.

Step 5

For **oblique-axis or with-the-rule astigmatism**, the astigmatically neutral, single-plane, ungrooved temporal clear corneal incision is used and the appropriate AK incisions are placed on-axis. I prefer to make all of my AK incisions first, before entering the eye with the phaco-foldable incision, as the eye is more firm and the incision depths are more reliable.

Step 6

This is the ultimate step which will eventually add to and replace many of the previous steps in this system of astigmatism management: **the toric IOL.** In the United States, Staar will soon have available (pending the FDA's expected approval in 1998) 2.00 D and 3.50 D models for approximately 1.00 D to 1.25 D and 2.00 D to 2.50 D of cylinder, respectively. We will be able to use these alone or in combination with AK to ultimately have the simplest, safest, and most predictable method of reducing astigmatism in our cataract patients.

CAPSULORRHEXIS

The continuous circular capsulorrhexis (CCC), as developed by Neuhann and Gimbel,[7] is the capsular opening I prefer, whether for routine anterior openings for emulsification and implantation; for posterior openings, to stabilize an inadvertent opening created during cortical aspiration; or for vitrectomy in pediatric cases or in adults with asteroid hyalosis. With newer lens removal instrumentation being developed, such as laser phacolysis, impeller extraction,[8] hot water, and focused electromagnetic field[9] technologies, the possibility of evacuation of the capsular contents through 1.0-mm CCC openings is once again emerging. This then re-opens the door for expanded research in the area of liquid or expandable lens replacement materials for virtually intact capsular bag surgery with the potential for accommodation.

A-CCC Technique

The current technique I currently employ involves injecting viscoelastic, currently regular Healon, through a pre-bent 25-gauge needle into the anterior chamber through the 2.5-mm phacoemulsification incision. Once the chamber is full, with all aqueous replaced, as evidenced by expression of viscoelastic around the needle through the incision, injection is stopped and the 25-gauge needle is used to create an initial C-shaped central capsulotomy. A puncture is performed in the estimated geometric center of the intended resultant circle, and the needle tip is moved to the surgeon's left for 0.5 to 1.0 mm, using the sharp side-cutting edge of the down-turned portion of the 25-gauge needle. The tip is then drawn toward the entry incision, using the blunt cylindrical shaft of the down-turned portion of the tip, making this excursion long enough to be 0.5 mm shorter than the radius of the intended circle. The tip of the needle is then drawn to the surgeon's right, beginning the actual arc of the circle to be created. At this point, the needle capsulotomy is complete and viscoelastic is injected as the needle is withdrawn from the eye.

The second step in the A-CCC involves completion of the capsulectomy with Utrata or Brown-Grabow forceps (Figure 13-11). Arshinoff has explained two methods of tearing the capsule with forceps. The first involves stretching the capsule, pulling it apart by directing the force vector centrally with the flap not inverted. The central flap is then in contest with the zonule and peripheral elastic capsule. This technique is less controllable and often results in openings larger than intended or radial tears to the equator of the capsule. The second technique is shearing. With this method, the flap is inverted with its posterior surface facing anteriorly and the vector of the tear is directed circumferentially. This technique does not engage the elastic forces of the zonule or capsule and, therefore, becomes ultimately controllable.

To achieve the desired result, the first circular tear with the forceps usually is continued for approximately 5 clock hours (Figure 13-12). The flap then becomes long and unmanageable and is released. It is regrasped nearer to the tear and rhexis is continued for another 3 clock hours (Figure 13-13). The flap is released and regrasped a third and final time, continuing the tear 4 more clock hours until the starting point is approached. In order to create a smooth and strong transition zone, the tear is directed slightly more peripherally at the junction of the beginning and

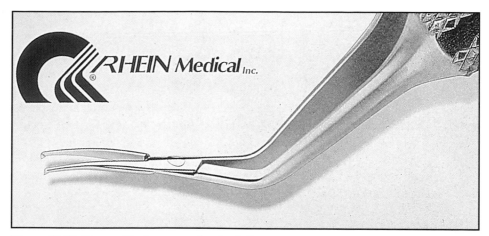

Figure 13-11. Brown-Grabow capsulorrhexis forceps.

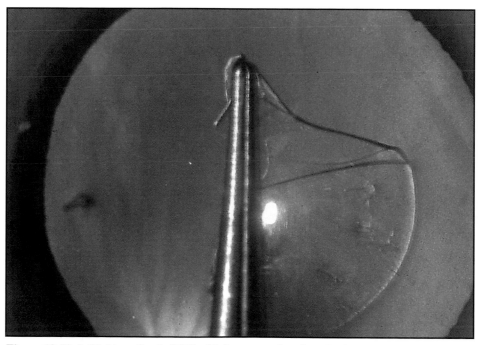

Figure 13-12. Initial tear for A-CCC with forceps under viscoelastic.

ending points. Each time the flap is released, it is deposited in the center of the rhexis so as to provide visibility of the tear line and to avoid inadvertent radial extension.

The diameter of the completed A-CCC is intended to be 0.5 mm less than the IOL optic to be implanted. Therefore, for a 6.0-mm optic, a 5.5-mm A-CCC is desirable.

HYDRODISSECTION

Following capsulorrhexis, Fine cortical-cleaving hydrodissection[10] is performed. A 30-gauge cannula on a 3-cc syringe with BSS is employed, the cannula being angled near the hub and straight at its intraocular portion. The tip is placed through the CCC, out near the equator of the capsule, and is elevated so as to appose the inner surface of the anterior capsule. Smooth injection of the BSS, hopefully, in a potential cleavage plane between the capsule and the cortex is then undertaken, watching for the dissecting fluid wave to traverse the posterior capsule (Figure 13-14). If the phaco is to be performed inside the capsular bag, as it is for all 2+, 3+, and 4+ nuclei, in eyes with guttata, and in eyes with shallow or short anterior segments (short anterior chamber depth), then hydrodissection stops when the nucleus is observed to elevate in the capsular bag, distend and enlarge the CCC, and separate the overlying anterior cortex in a petaloid pattern. At this point, the cannula is withdrawn from the capsule and is used to tamponade the nucleus back into the capsule, causing the posteriorly loculated BSS to be expressed peripherally and anteriorly in the cortical-capsular cleavage plane, hopefully severing equatorial and anterior attachments. The nucleus is not rotated inside the capsule at this point, as the above maneuvers are usually successful in loosening the nucleus enough to allow rotation easily during emulsification. Hydrodelineation is not routinely performed by intention, as the endonuclear fragments produced during chopping separate easily from the epinucleus.

If the lens is a 1+ nuclear sclerotic cataract or a soft posterior subcapsular cataract or the zonule is significantly weak or torn, attempt is made to hydroexpress the nucleus out of the capsular bag. In these cases, the BSS injection does not stop with the completion of the posterior fluid wave, but continues until a pole of the nucleus is expressed through the CCC. The cannula is then used to dial the nucleus out of the bag into the "supranuclear" space. However, no attempt is made to invert the nucleus or "flip" the nucleus, as is performed routinely by Dr. David Brown[11] and recently described by Dr. William Maloney.[12] I have found this flipping maneuver to be somewhat risky for capsular, zonular, and endothelial integrity in the cases of 4+ nuclear sclerosis and in cases where the implant to be used dictates an A-CCC of 5.5 mm or less.

LENS SURGERY

At present, all adult cataract cases are scheduled for ultrasonic phacoemulsification. For eyes with normal corneas and up to 3+ nuclear sclerosis, regular Healon is used for endothelial protection. It has been observed in our practice that corneas

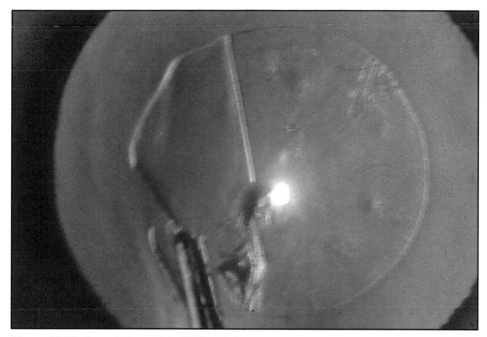

Figure 13-13. Second stage of A-CCC with forceps.

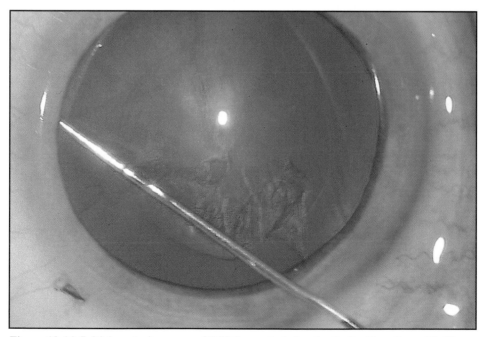

Figure 13-14. Initial posterior wave of BSS for central-cleaving hydrodissection with 30-gauge cannula.

Table 13-1 "1-2-3-4 Vacuum" Settings	
Nucleus	**Vacuum (mmHg)**
1+	100
2+	200
3+	300
4+	400

with guttata occur in approximately 10% of cataract patients and lose twice as many endothelial cells during ultrasonic phacoemulsification than normal healthy corneas. Therefore, in cases of guttata or 4+ nuclear sclerosis, Viscoat, rather than Healon, is injected prior to A-CCC and phacoemulsification.

In Situ Phacoemulsification Technique

Current preferred technique for routine cases involves a Nagahara chopping method[13] using a Haefliger cleaver (Figure 13-15) for nuclei up to 3+. For 4+ nuclei, a Koch stop and chop method is employed, making a wide central groove before bisecting the nucleus; a Koch chopper is then used to bisect, trisect, or quadrisect each heminucleus. A Surgical Design Ocusystem IIe[art] machine (Figure 13-16) is used with a mini-Cobra tip (Figure 13-17) with a spiral cooling sleeve (Figure 13-18) through a 2.5-mm incision. The infusion bottle is stored refrigerated, and is balanced salt solution plain, with gentamicin 8 mg, vancomycin 20 mg, and 0.5 cc of nonpreserved epinephrine.

For initial removal of cortex and epinucleus that are exposed by the A-CCC, the bottle is raised to maximum height, the power is set at 30%, the aspiration at 8 cc/min, and the vacuum at 25 mmHg. The nucleus is then impaled by the 30 degree tip in the central portion closest to the incision (Figure 13-19). For 3+ and 4+ nuclei, bevel-down gives quicker and firmer access to the nucleus. The cleaver is used in the left hand, then placed as distally as the A-CCC will allow into the nucleus to its full extent (Figure 13-20) and is drawn toward the left side of the impaled phaco tip (Figure 13-21). Upon reaching the tip, the two instruments are then separated 180 degrees apart from each other, the cleaver to the surgeon's left and the phaco tip to the right, achieving bisection of the nucleus without pre-grooving (Figure 13-22). The two heminuclei are then rotated 90 degrees (Figure 13-23) and the distal heminucleus is impaled and cleaved into two halves—or now, quadrants of the whole nucleus (Figure 13-24). The aspiration is now changed to 24 cc/min and the vacuum varied according to the density of the nucleus (Table 13-1). Simply, for safety and efficiency, the vacuum is set at 100 mmHg for 1+ nuclei, 200 mmHg for 2+ nuclei, 300 mmHg for 3+ nuclei, and 400 mmHg for 4+ nuclei. The power remains at 30% for all cases except 4+ nuclei, where 40% may be used. Each quadrant may be subdivided to further improve efficiency of emulsification.

Chopping has not only reduced total clock time for emulsification to an average of 2.5 minutes but has also shown a 27% reduction in ultrasound time when compared to the previously used pre-grooving four-quadrant technique.

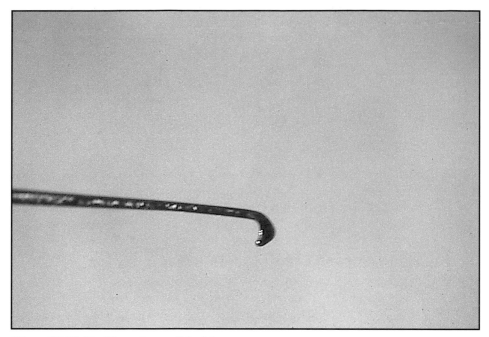

Figure 13-15. Haefliger cleaver (Moria).

Figure 13-16. Surgical Design Ocusystem IIe^{art} ultrasonic phacoemulsification and Ocutine vitrectomy machines with two-bottle set-up for fluid surge prevention.

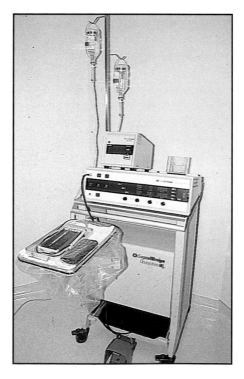

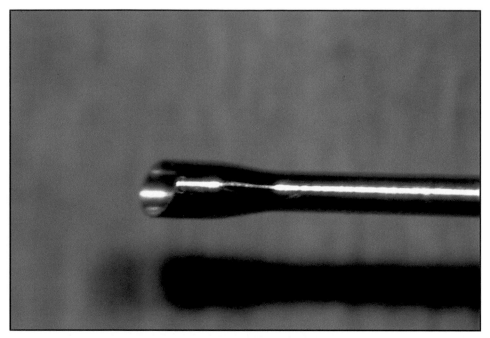

Figure 13-17. Surgical Design Mini-Cobra phacoemulsification tip.

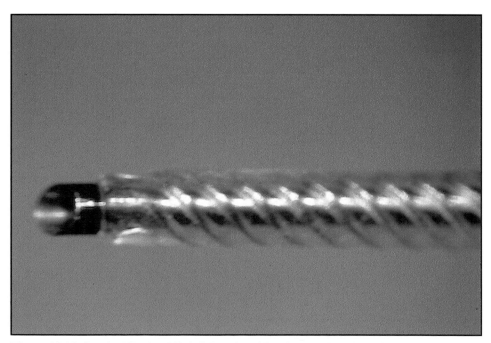

Figure 13-18. Surgical Design Mini-Cobra tip with spiral cooling sleeve for wound burn protection.

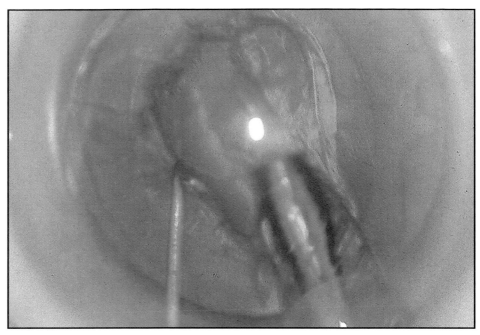

Figure 13-19. Beginning phacoemulsification by impaling the nucleus in preparation for ungrooved bisection with the Haefliger cleaver.

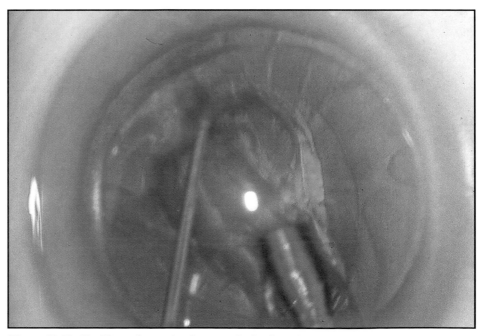

Figure 13-20. Haefliger cleaver in place, ready for first chop or slice.

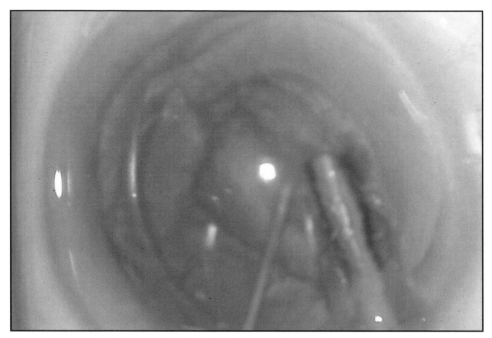

Figure 13-21. First slice completed to side of phaco tip, ready for separation.

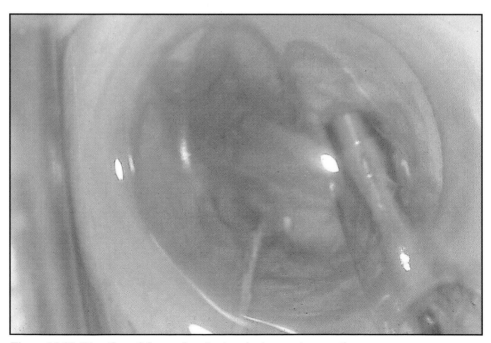

Figure 13-22. Bisection of the nucleus by two-instrument separation.

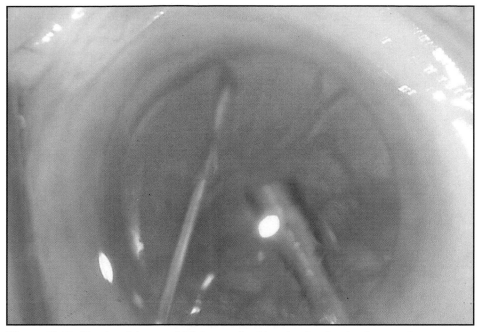

Figure 13-23. Heminuclei rotated 90 degrees for bisection by cleaving into quadrants.

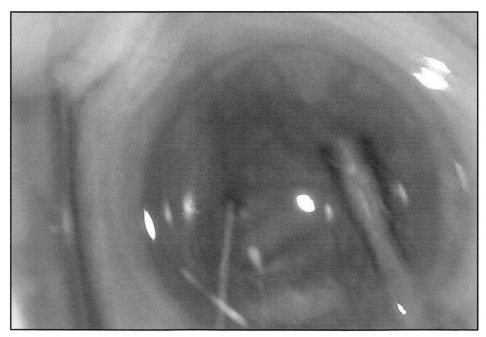

Figure 13-24. First heminucleus cleaved in half to form nuclear quadrants.

Anterior Chamber Phaco Technique

Following successful hydroexpression of a soft nucleus out of the capsular bag, emulsification is performed from outside-in and from back-to-front, using a "cartwheeling" or "carouseling" technique. Attempt is made to circumferentially reduce nuclear size while keeping the nucleus in one piece. The phaco tip is placed bevel-up under the nucleus and the nucleus is gently elevated with a Barraquer iris spatula in the left hand. In this way, all emulsification energy is kept away from the corneal endothelium, as the nucleus is between the phaco tip and the cornea. The irrigation pressure keeps the capsule back and attempt is made to keep the phaco tip continuously occluded until emulsification is complete. Pulsed phaco is often advantageous during this technique. Ultrasound times are extremely low, usually under 1 minute, and total case times are extremely fast, often under 6 minutes.

IMPLANTATION

Following emulsification of the nucleus, viscoelastic is injected in preparation for IOL implantation. If cortex remains, attempt is made to perform cortical-cleaving viscodissection. The anterior chamber, posterior chamber, and capsule must be filled with viscoelastic first. The tip of the cannula is then held against the distended posterior capsule and viscoelastic is injected (Figure 13-25). This will often create a cleavage plane between the cortex and the posterior capsule, and continued injection of viscoelastic (Figure 13-26) can dissect and deposit the posterior cortex into the capsular equator (Figure 13-27).

IOL implantation is then performed (Figure 13-28). For adult eyes without posterior segment pathology, a plate haptic foldable silicone lens with a 5.5-mm optic (Staar AA4207) (Figure 13-29) is injected through the unenlarged 2.5-mm incision with a 60 degree beveled cartridge. If the eye is long or if the patient is known to have large scotopic pupils, a 6.0-mm optic IOL (Staar AA4203) (Figure 13-30) will be used. If posterior segment pathology is present or potential, or a pediatric patient is to be implanted, the collagen copolymer IOL (Staar CC4203) (Figures 13-31 and 13-32) or an acrylic lens (Alcon Acrysof MA60BM) is used. If corneal astigmatism is present, a toric IOL (Staar AA4203T) (see Figure 13-9) is preferred.

Remaining cortex and viscoelastic are removed after IOL implantation using automated irrigation/aspiration through the phaco incision (Figure 13-33) with a 0.2-mm aspiration port. Viscoelastic is removed first from the anterior chamber, posterior chamber, and capsule. The cortex is then removed lateral to the IOL optic, as the cortex that is in the axis of the haptics is compressed in the equator of the bag. Residual cortical remnants are vacuumed from the posterior capsule using free-flow aspiration: the peristaltic pump is turned off and the pinch rollers opened so that the outflow through the port of the I/A tip is determined only by the rate of inflow or bottle height. This system may be a unique feature of the Surgical Design machine, originally conceived by Jack Singer. It makes it virtually impossible to tear the capsule during vacuuming.

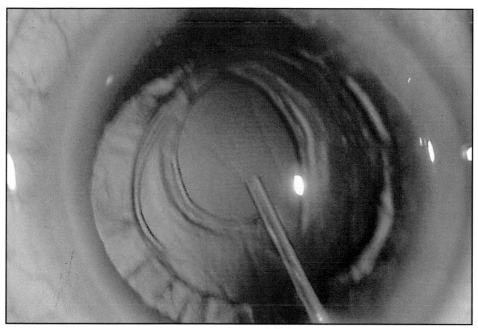

Figure 13-25. Beginning cortical-cleaving viscodissection.

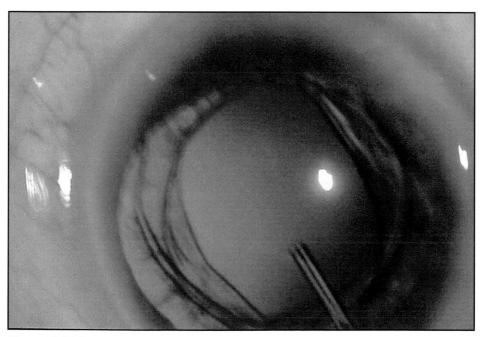

Figure 13-26. Further cortical cleaving by viscodissection.

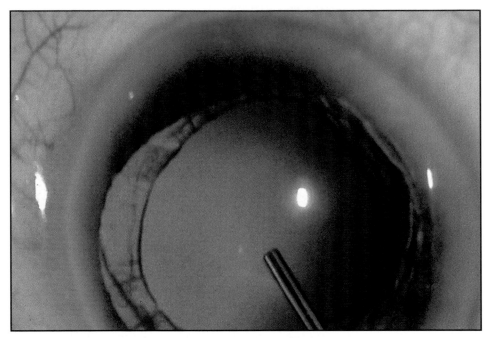

Figure 13-27. Completion of cortical cleaving by viscodissection.

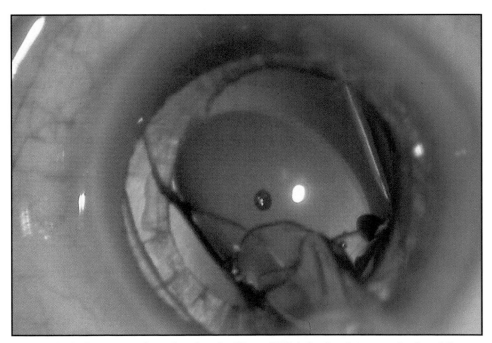

Figure 13-28. Staar one-piece plate haptic silicone IOL injection into capsular bag following cortical cleaving viscodissection and prior to cortical aspiration.

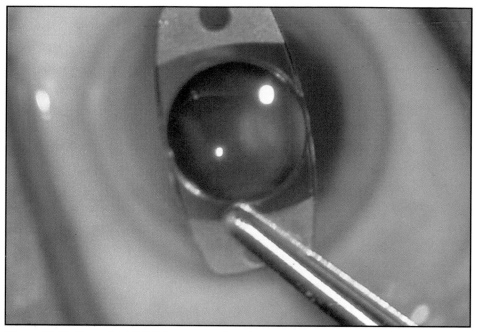

Figure 13-29. Staar AA4207 5.5-mm optic IOL for injection through unenlarged 2.5-mm phaco incision with a 60 degree beveled cartridge.

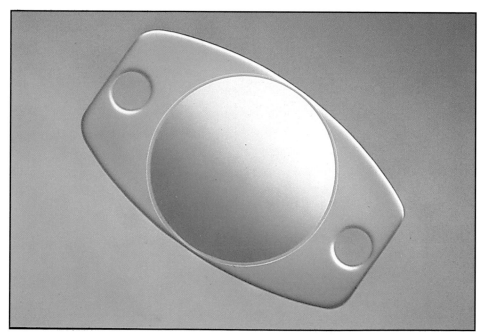

Figure 13-30. Staar AA4203 6.0-mm optic IOL.

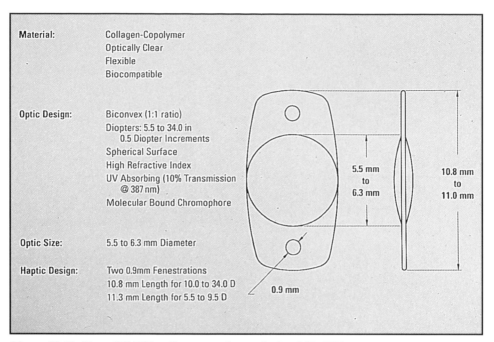

Material:
Collagen-Copolymer
Optically Clear
Flexible
Biocompatible

Optic Design:
Biconvex (1:1 ratio)
Diopters: 5.5 to 34.0 in
    0.5 Diopter Increments
Spherical Surface
High Refractive Index
UV Absorbing (10% Transmission
    @ 387 nm)
Molecular Bound Chromophore

Optic Size:
5.5 to 6.3 mm Diameter

Haptic Design:
Two 0.9mm Fenestrations
10.8 mm Length for 10.0 to 34.0 D
11.3 mm Length for 5.5 to 9.5 D

0.9 mm

5.5 mm
to
6.3 mm

10.8 mm
to
11.0 mm

Figure 13-31. Staar CC4203 collagen copolymer hydrophilic IOL.

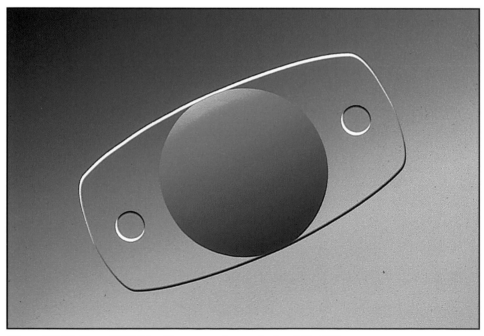

Figure 13-32. Staar CC4203 collagen copolymer hydrophilic IOL.

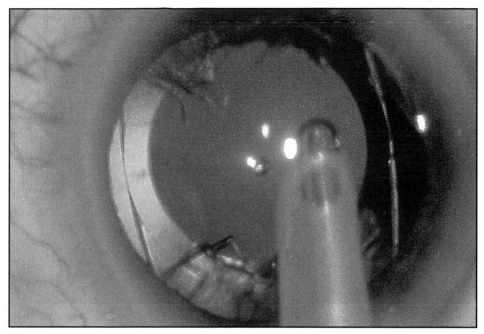

Figure 13-33. Post implantation cortical aspiration with full protection of the posterior capsule by the IOL optic.

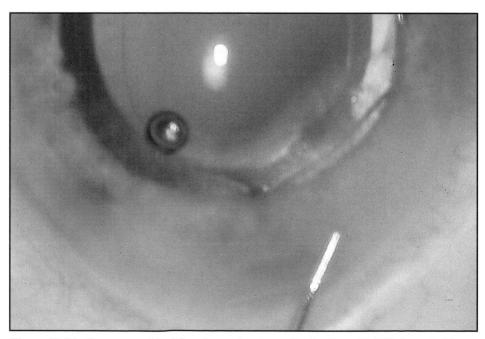

Figure 13-34. Clear corneal incision closure by stromal hydration with BSS through 30-gauge cannula.

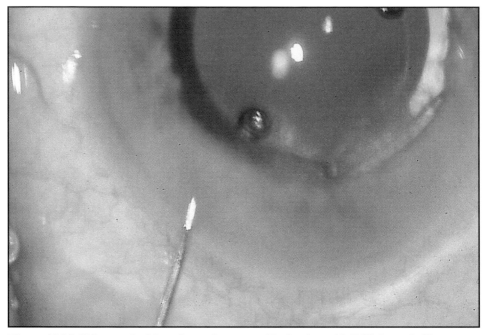

Figure 13-35. Side-port incision closure by stromal hydration with BSS through 30-gauge cannula.

CLOSURE

The initial 2.5-mm temporal clear corneal incision is assumed to have stretched, following phaco and foldable manipulation, to approximately 2.7 mm. Sutureless self-sealing closure is obtained by hydration of the stroma with BSS. The same syringe and 30-gauge cannula are used that were used earlier in the procedure for hydrodissection. The two apices of the incision are injected until the two areas of hydration, as designated by blanching of the stromal lamellae, are in apposition (Figure 13-34). The anterior chamber is then hyperinflated with BSS through the side-port incision, and this incision is hydrated also (Figure 13-35). This usually results in elevation of the IOP, as estimated by tactile tension.

The pressure is then incrementally lowered by introduction of the cannula through the side-port without injection of fluid until the pressure is lowered to about 20 mmHg.

The speculum is then removed by careful elevation of each eyelid separately and slowly, and the eye is observed for a moment through the microscope to be sure anterior chamber depth is maintained. The eye is left unpatched and unshielded. Topical and injectable medications are not administered. The patient is instructed to place no medication in the operated eye until after the first postoperative day examination the morning after surgery and is permitted to resume non-strenuous activity the same day as the operation. The pupil is not constricted, so the vision usually remains unclear for 6 to 8 hours. Most patients report, if they had morning surgery, that they are able to watch the 6 o'clock news on television without wearing their old eyeglasses.

POSTOPERATIVE ROUTINE

The usual simple, uncomplicated routine medication regimen involves resumption of Tobradex ophthalmic drops on the first postop day, following examination. The patient used the Tobradex drops qid for 2 days before surgery and will now use the same drops, from the same bottle, on a tapering schedule for 4 weeks postoperatively: qid for the first week, tid for the second week, bid for the third week, and qd for the fourth week.

If the case was complicated by an open posterior capsule or vitrectomy, Voltaren drops are added tid to the Tobradex, and the schedule of administration is changed. The tapering schedule of the Tobradex is replaced by continuous qid administration for the entire 4-week period. We advise these patients to instill the Tobradex before the three daily meals and at bedtime, and to instill the Voltaren after the three daily meals. This provides these patients with an easy-to-remember schedule. The purpose of the Voltaren is to attempt to preclude the occurrence of cystoid macular edema. The Voltaren is, therefore, also added to the Tobradex, both pre- and postoperatively, in patients with retinal pathology, uveitis, or diabetes mellitus.

REFERENCES

1. Ernest PH, Lavery K, Kiessling LA. Relative strength of scleral corneal and clear corneal incisions constructed in cadaver eyes. *J Cataract Refract Surg*. 1994;20:626-629.
2. Grabow HB. *Clear-Corneal Cataract Surgery & Topical Anesthesia*. Thorofare, NJ: SLACK Incorporated; 1993:50-55.
3. Grabow HB. *Clear-Corneal Cataract Surgery & Topical Anesthesia*. Thorofare, NJ: SLACK Incorporated; 1993:55-58.
4. Williamson C. Presentation at STAAR Surgical course. Plate-haptic implantation techniques. Pre-ASCRS Annual Symposium, April 17, 1998.
5. Dodick J. Laser lens lysis. *Cataract & Refractive Surgery EuroTimes*. 1997;Nov-Dec:2,6.
6. Sanders DR, Grabow HB, Shepherd J. The toric IOL. In: Gills JP, Martin RG, Sanders DR, eds. *Sutureless Cataract Surgery—Evolution Toward Minimally Invasive Technique*. Thorofare, NJ: SLACK Incorporated; 1992:193-197.
7. Gimbel H, Neuhann T. Development, advantages, and methods of the continuous circular capsulorhexis technique. *J Cataract Refract Surg*. 1990;16:31-37.
8. Kratz R. Catarex impeller cataract extraction, Film Festival Winner, ASCRS Symposium, San Diego, 1998. [Video.]
9. Fugo RJ, et al. Focused electromagnetic field cataract surgery (FEFCS). *Ann Ophthalmol*. 1997;29(1):11-18.
10. Fine IH. Cortical cleaving hydrodissection. *J Cataract Refract Surg*. 1992;18:508-512.
11. Brown DC. The nuclear flip techniques. *VJO*. 1994;X:5. [Video.]
12. Maloney WF. Supracapsular and quick-chop phacoemulsification. *VJO*. 1998;XIV:2. [Video.]
13. Nagahara KB. Phaco chop. *VJO*. 1993;IX:3. [Video.]

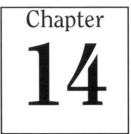

Chapter 14

Clear Corneal Micro Incision Surgery for Cataract and Refractive Implants

Charles H. Williamson, MD, FACS

EVOLUTION AND BASIC PRINCIPLES

My contribution to the surgical technique for clear corneal incision surgery was founded on some basic principles developed early in 1992. Although many authors have described cataract surgery performed through the clear corneal approach, we must credit Dr. I. Howard Fine as the first to suggest using this technique as a routine method of cataract surgery, which he proposed early in 1992. Dr. Fine's technique for single-plane corneal incision was my starting point. I subsequently developed my technique of a stepped clear corneal trapezoidal tunnel performed temporally under topical lidocaine in early 1992, and began teaching this technique in our very first courses that year (Figure 14-1). Although topical anesthesia has been used for more than 100 years, it was Dr. Richard Fichman who championed the idea of using topical tetracaine for conjunctival and scleral tunnel incisions early in 1992. I developed a technique of using topical lidocaine with clear corneal surgery under routine circumstances. Since the beginning I felt that topical lidocaine should be the anesthetic of choice because it allowed the fastest regeneration of the corneal epithelium, as shown by Marr et al[1] in 1957. I believed the regeneration of corneal epithelium was an important point since the stability and strength of the clear corneal wound was questioned early on in the development of this technique.

Dr. Fine's straight beveled clear corneal incision was like a paracentesis (Figure 14-2). I developed the stepped multi-planed trapezoidal incision, not to improve or reduce the incidence of wound leak (I personally had no problems with wound sealability), but rather to provide a thicker edge and roof of the corneal tunnel to prevent

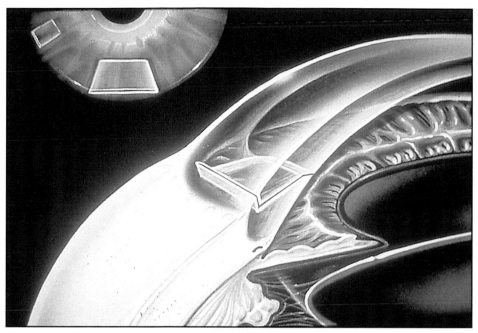

Figure 14-1. Stepped clear corneal trapezoidal incision.

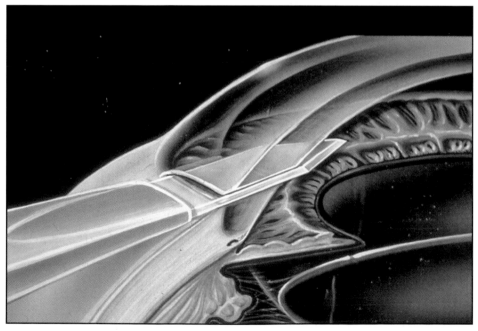

Figure 14-2. Straight beveled incision.

tearing of the wound during instrumentation of the anterior chamber and to make creation of the corneal tunnel easier. The trapezoidal tunnel incision has a small internal wound and larger external wound. It has been the mainstay of my incision technique from the beginning. I felt the development of the trapezoidal corneal tunnel would reduce wound stretch from instrumentation. Kondrot[2] has shown that the strength of wounds decrease significantly after instrumentation (Figure 14-3). This suggests that the wound was stretched. Ruckman[3] and others have confirmed recently that the initial wound the surgeon begins with is larger when measured with metal corneal gauges after phacoemulsification and implantation of the IOL (Figure 14-4). I prefer that all micro incisions be carried out with the smallest wound possible, allowing for the particular lens implant, the injector system, and size of the phacoemulsification tip. A trapezoidal corneal tunnel improves the ergonomics of surgery. The internal wound should be as small as possible as this controls the fluid flow in and out of the eye. The internal tunnel wound must seal well in order to make the eye immediately watertight. The external opening of the tunnel is less critical and can be somewhat larger to allow for ease of instrumentation and prevent corneal stretching which is a major cause of decreased wound strength. The larger external wound diameter allows greater room for maneuverability, better oar locking of the phacoemulsification needle during lens removal (Figure 14-5), and more closely approximates the trapezoid shape of the tapered MicroStaar Injector cartridges used for injecting the Staar AA4203 VF elastic lens (Figure 14-6).

The architecture of the corneal wound in my current surgical technique includes a corneal groove and a multi-planed trapezoidal-shaped 1.9-/2.5-mm micro incision tunnel (Figure 14-7). Dr. David Langerman has described a hinged technique in which the groove is approximately 600 microns in depth to provide a corneal hinge on the interior corneal lip as a method to improve incision sealing (Figure 14-8). All incisions 2.5 mm or less, however, are extremely strong and the hinge is not needed to seal the small wound. All three current corneal incisions, the straight beveled, stepped incision, and the stepped-hinge incision (Figure 14-9), may be used with equal success as long as the incisions are 2.5 mm or less in width. The multi-plane micro incision construction earns its popularity from ease of construction of the corneal tunnel, as well as its resistance to edge tearing or damage from instrumentation.

The first diamond knife system for clear corneal surgery was developed with Ron Dykes of Diamatrix in 1992 in order to fashion the corneal groove, side stab wound, and corneal tunnel using the diamond step-knife (Figure 14-10) and a trapezoid diamond keratome (Figure 14-11). This system allowed the surgeon to reproduce clear corneal wounds of exactly the same dimensions and architecture each time.

A method of arranging the OR and the patient in order to sit laterally to perform the temporal approach we routinely use was developed early on. Clear corneal incisions should be located temporally in order to reduce the amount of induced corneal astigmatism to a minimum. The temporal location is farthest from the visual axis because there is less conjunctival overhang and a slight nasal displacement of the optical axis (Figure 14-12). The temporal corneal tunnel causes a localized flattening postoperatively over the area of the tunnel that may extend only segmentally into

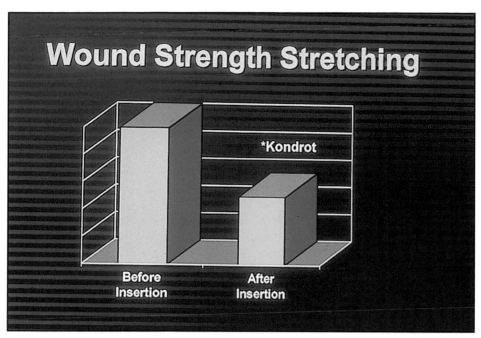

Figure 14-3. Wound strength before and after IOL insertion.

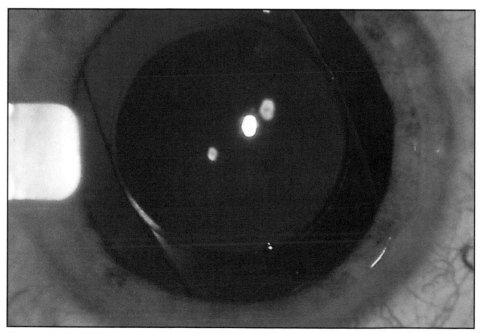

Figure 14-4. Measuring wound with metal corneal gauge.

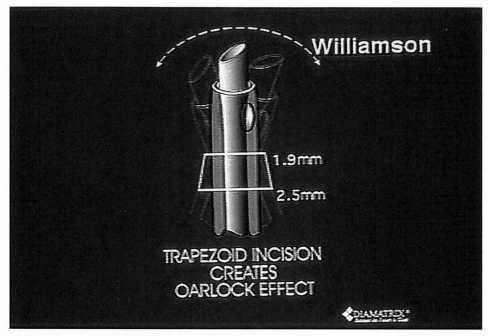

Figure 14-5. Trapezoidal wound better for phaco.

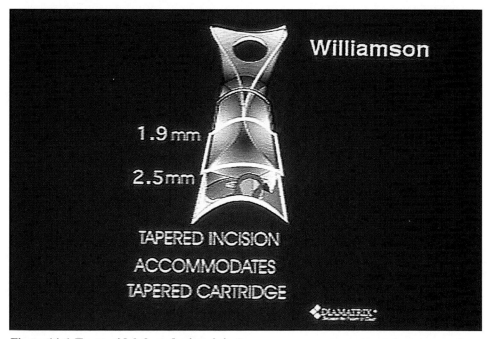

Figure 14-6. Trapezoidal shaped micro injector.

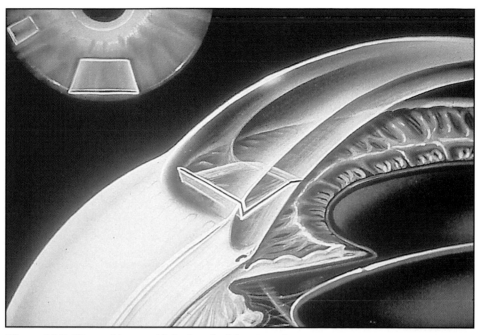

Figure 14-7. Stepped trapezoidal micro incision tunnel.

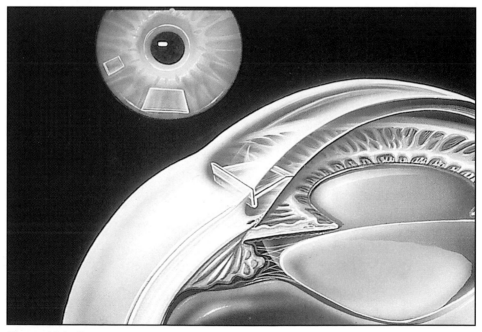

Figure 14-8. Corneal hinge incision.

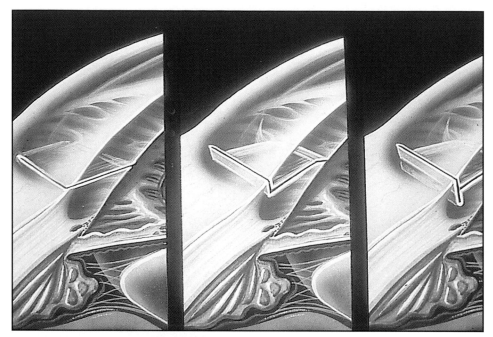

Figure 14-9. Current corneal incision.

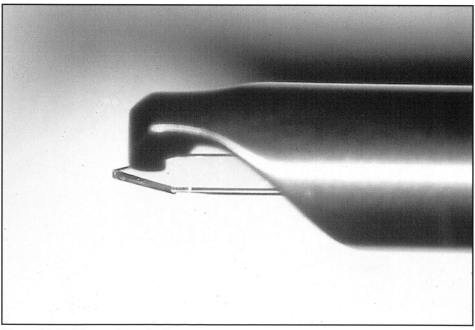

Figure 14-10. Diamond step knife.

Figure 14-11. Williamson trap blade.

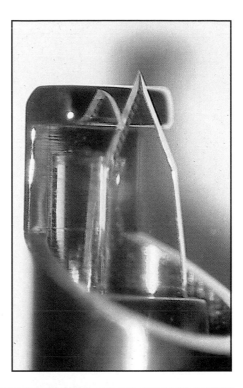

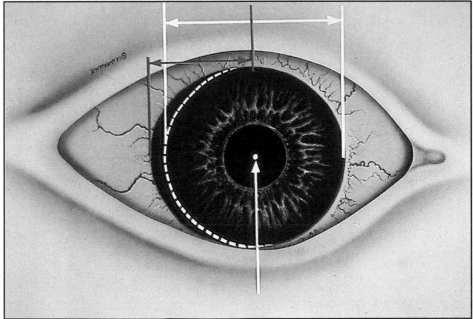

Figure 14-12. Nasal displacement of visual axis (Utrata).

the optical zone in incisions that are 3.0 mm or less (Figure 14-13). For larger incisions, or incisions that are placed superiorly, the degree of flattening and astigmatism induction can not only be more severe but can extend all the way into the visual axis and effect early visual recovery (Figure 14-14). These changes can best be noticed on corneal topography, as they are segmental and therefore can be missed using routine keratometry. In a study I performed using temporal 3.0-mm clear corneal surgery, I found an average of 0.5 D of induced with-the-rule astigmatism. This compared favorably and is slightly less than scleral tunnel incisions of a similar size (Figure 14-15). To produce consistently low or non-existent induced astigmatism, all clear corneal incisions should be performed temporally unless the surgical plan calls for purposeful reduction of astigmatism. In order to reduce pre-existing astigmatism, the surgery may be performed on the axis of the steepest corneal curvature and even combined with astigmatic keratotomy incisions as is discussed elsewhere in this text. The more superior the wound, however, the greater the endothelial cell loss as the phaco tip is positioned closer to the endothelium.

My subsequent contributions were reducing the size of the incisions from small incisions to micro incisions. I coined the term "micro incision surgery" for corneal wounds 2.5 mm or less to make an important distinction in clear corneal incisions. The size of the corneal incision can have a significant effect in clear corneal surgery. In Figure 14-14, a 6.0-mm incision combined with superior location induced a significant amount of irregular astigmatism into the visual axis early in the postoperative period that is readily evident with corneal topography. The larger the incision, the more superior or nasal the incision is placed, the greater the induction of astigmatism. Reducing the incision size of cataract surgery had historically been aimed at reducing iatrogenically induced astigmatism, as well as to allow for greater ease of sutureless closing and the subsequent benefit of rapid visual rehabilitation. I knew that the benefits of incision size in regard to induction of astigmatism and rapid visual rehabilitation disappeared at or about 3.0 mm. My desire to reduce wound size to below 3.0 mm was driven by anecdotal reports of wound leakage and subsequent endophthalmitis in the literature. Reports of wound leak, shallow anterior chambers, and endophthalmitis were discovered to be related to large corneal wounds (greater than 4.0 mm in size) and short corneal tunnels (1.0 mm or less), usually in a superior location. It is my belief that any clear corneal tunnel greater than 4.0 mm in width or less than 1.0 mm in length should be sutured for the sake of safety. The suture may be removed at the slit lamp in the postoperative period. Size matters most when related directly to wound strength and secondarily to wound stability. Ernest[4] performed cadaver studies which showed considerable increase in the strength of a corneal wound as the width of the incision shrank to approximate the tunnel length. His data (in cadaver eye studies) demonstrate that a wound 2.5 mm in width with a 2.0-mm corneal tunnel length is more than twice as strong as a corresponding wound 3.5 mm in width (Figure 14-16). Although these data take into account only non-functioning corneas and dismiss the effect of the endothelial pump mechanism for sealing wounds, the data still provide valuable insight into basic structural studies and tell us that as the tunnel width approximates the size of tunnel length (2.0 mm), the stronger the wound. All my efforts were directed at producing the strongest, most

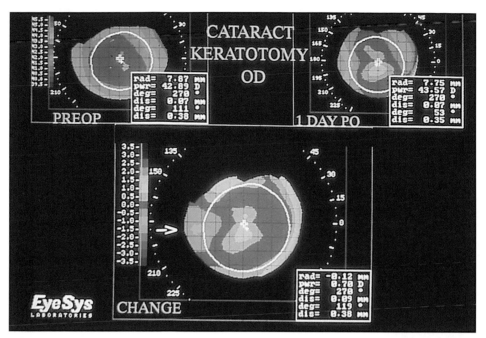

Figure 14-13. Temporal corneal flattening.

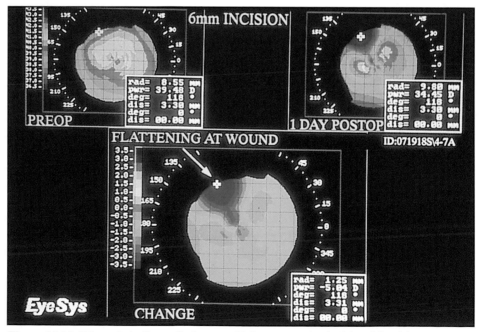

Figure 14-14. Edema into the optical zone with large superior incision (Martin).

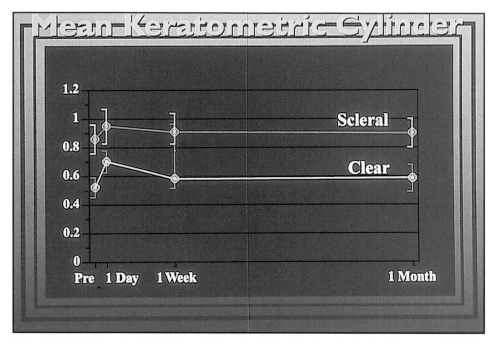

Figure 14-15. Induced astigmatism: clear corneal vs scleral.

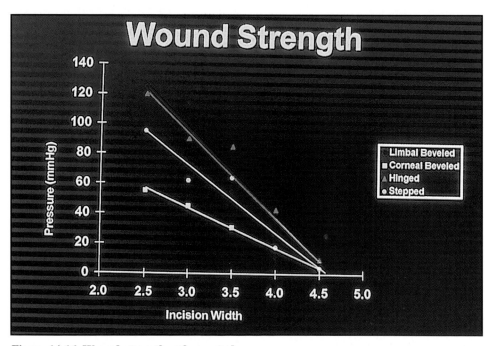

Figure 14-16. Wound strength cadaver study.

stable corneal wound possible, which I felt needed to be multi planed and ideally 2.0 mm or less in width at the internal entrance into the anterior chamber. A micro incision is any wound 2.5 mm or less in width which is produced primarily for the purpose of increasing wound strength, and not primarily for reducing astigmatism or enhancing the speed of visual rehabilitation (Figure 14-17). The development and adaptation in the OR of these principles of wound construction has been fundamental to my surgical technique as it exists today.

THE 1.9-MM UNIVERSAL CLEAR CORNEAL WOUND

My current technique involves reducing the wound size to a 1.9-mm trapezoidal internal incision in order to have the maximum wound strength possible for the creation of a universal system for injecting both pseudophakic implants for cataract as well as refractive phakic implants for myopia or hyperopia into the posterior chamber. After 2 sets of drops of 4% nonpreserved lidocaine are given 5 minutes apart, the eye is prepped and the eyelashes are plastered back under an occlusive plastic drape; a heavy Barraquer wire speculum is inserted (Figure 14-18). The surgeon positions him- or herself temporally on the side of the operative eye (Figure 14-19). Using the Williamson Micro-Trap diamond step knife developed through Diamatrix (Woodlands, Texas) a 2.0-mm long, 300-micron corneal groove is performed temporally at the clear corneal limbus (Figure 14-20). This incision may be curvilinear and follow the curvature of the limbal architecture. The Williamson Micro-Trap diamond step knife is then extended and a 1.0-mm side stab is performed at the clear corneal limbus in a space easily accessible to the non-dominant hand of the surgeon (Figure 14-21).

Viscoelastic is injected into the anterior chamber before creation of the corneal tunnel to prevent anterior chamber collapse during tunnel creation and mute any sudden drops in IOP upon entering the eye. Exchanging aqueous for viscoelastic allows the surgeon to tamponade and flatten the anterior capsule, permitting greater ease of capsulorrhexis. Overfill of the anterior chamber is especially helpful for capsulorrhexis in the thin capsules associated with white mature cataracts and dense black cataracts. The eye is fixated with 0.12 corneal forceps, one prong of the forceps inside the paracentesis and one outside to stabilize the eye during creation of the corneal tunnel. A 1.9-/2.5-mm Williamson Micro-Trap blade is then used to perform the trapezoidal corneal tunnel. The 1.9-/2.5-mm trap blade from Diamatrix has dimensions of 1.9 mm between the first shoulders of the blade, 1.75 mm from the tip of the blade to a line intersecting the shoulders, and a 2.5-mm width at the second shoulders, site of the external wound (Figure 14-22). The blade has a larger bevel superiorly than inferiorly making the entrance into the anterior chamber smoother. This design provides ideal landmarks for consistent reproducible trapezoidal corneal tunnel wounds. The tip of the trap blade is positioned in the corneal groove parallel to the iris plane. Slight downward pressure allows access to the depth of the groove. The blade is then advanced forward into clear cornea, exerting slight downward pressure. The knife traverses from the tip of the blade until the shoulders are just inside the wound creating a trapezoidal corneal tunnel that is approximately 2.0-mm long, 1.9-mm wide internally, and 2.5-mm wide externally (Figure 14-

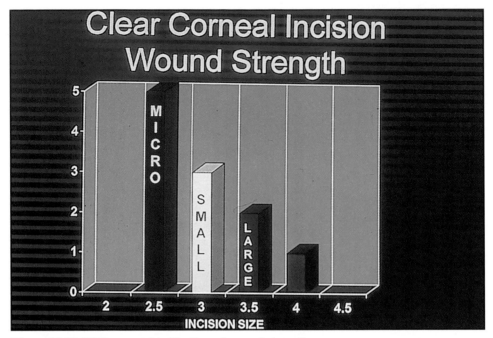

Figure 14-17. Williamson classification of wound strength.

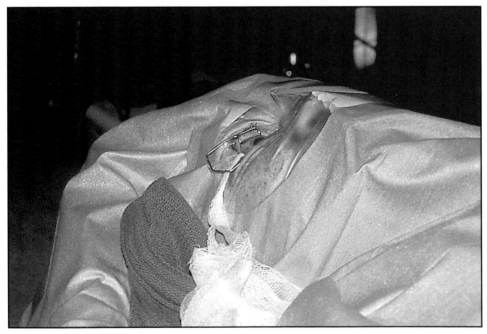

Figure 14-18. Draped patient.

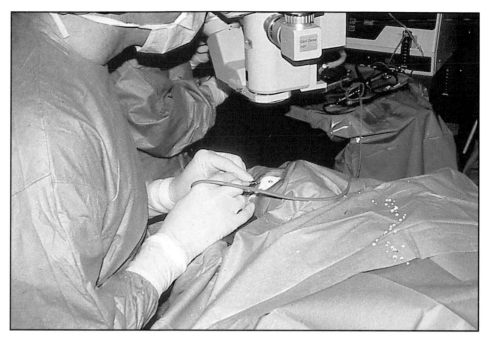

Figure 14-19. Surgeon position.

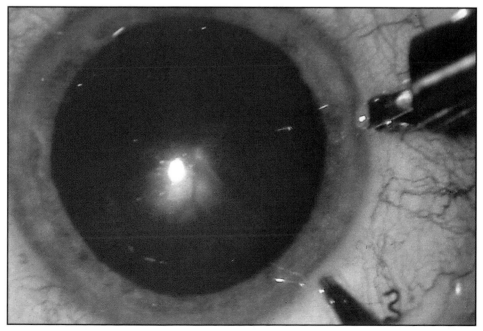

Figure 14-20. Corneal groove.

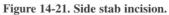

Figure 14-21. Side stab incision.

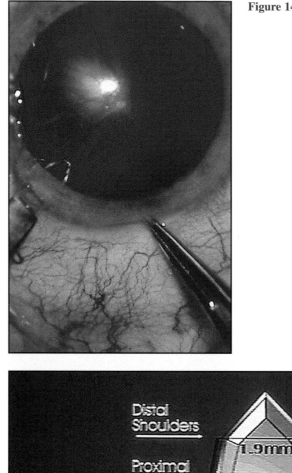

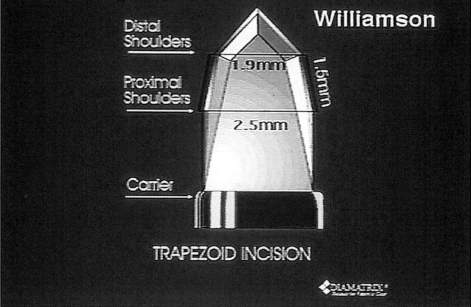

Figure 14-22. 1.9 mm/2.5 mm diamond trapezoid keratome.

23). I should point out that even with a 300-micron groove, the plane of the tunnel never quite reaches the bottom of the incision creating a sort of step-hinge architecture.

A 5-mm capsulorrhexis is performed using a capsulorrhexis forceps. In my technique, a small capsular flap is produced at the mid-point of a line between the center of the capsule and the external corneal wound using a bent needle. The capsular edge is grasped with capsulorrhexis forceps and a continuous circular tear capsulorrhexis is performed (Figure 14-24), moving counterclockwise and smoothly blending the end of the capsulorrhexis with the beginning. If the capsulorrhexis has a notch or extends peripherally into the zonules, it will provide a weak point for the anterior capsule to split during phacoemulsification or lens implantation. A single-wave hydrodissection is performed using BSS on a 30-gauge cannula (Figure 14-25). It is important to use single-wave hydrodissection rather than hydrodelineation in order to eliminate splitting the epinucleus from the harder nuclear material so that phacoemulsification will be easier and more efficient. Avoiding hydrodelineation also increases the ease of cortical cleanup during irrigation/aspiration.

I routinely use a divide and conquer phacoemulsification technique. The lens is divided into four or more pieces, with each piece being emulsified in the deep capsular bag using the bimanual technique. It is most important to use a microtip handpiece especially designed for micro incision surgery. This microtip should be specifically designed to adequately fit through the incision width selected. An incision that is too tight for the phaco tip could unduly stretch the incision, produce increased difficulty in phacoemulsification, tight corneal wounds, inhibit the inflow of fluidics into the eye, and cause potential heating of the cornea with possible wound burn (Figure 14-26).

Machines with which I have had experience in micro incision surgery (sub 2.5 mm) include the Storz Millennium Phaco, the Staar Phaco XL, and the Ocusystem Phaco XL (Figures 14-27 through 14-29). The phaco tip of the Ocusystem Phaco XL can go through a 2.5-mm corneal wound. It has an expanded tip design that increases the efficiency of the emulsification and a corkscrew sleeve that allows fluid flow even through a tight corneal wound. Machine vacuums up to 500 mmHg are available in order to increase the efficiency of the phacoemulsification. The Staar Phaco XL has a similar Super Fineline Phaco Tip allowing phacoemulsification through micro incision wounds. I have found the Storz Millennium using the MicroFlow grooved phaco needle (Figure 14-30) to be an excellent instrument of choice for micro incisions as small as 1.9 mm. The MicroFlow needle developed by Dr. Barrett of Australia allows fluid flow along the sides of the needle, even during total collapse of the sleeve around the phaco needle (Figure 14-31). This even allows phacoemulsification through a 1.9-mm wound and produces a true complete seal preventing fluid egress which stabilizes the anterior chamber even at high vacuum levels of 500 mmHg. The Millennium machine has dual linear emulsification and aspiration for great versatility during phaco.

My technique of divide and conquer involves the initial creation of a vertical groove in the nucleus approximately 4.0 mm in length and 2.0 to 3.0 mm in depth within the confines of the capsulorrhexis (Figure 14-32). It is important not to phaco

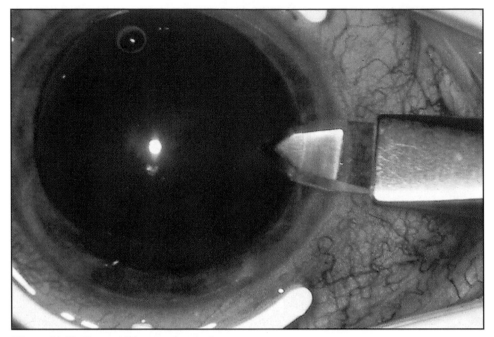

Figure 14-23. Trapezoid corneal tunnel.

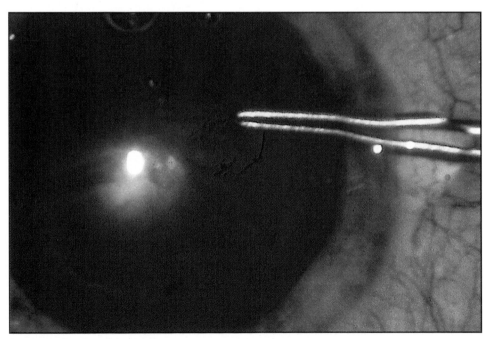

Figure 14-24. Capsulorrhexis.

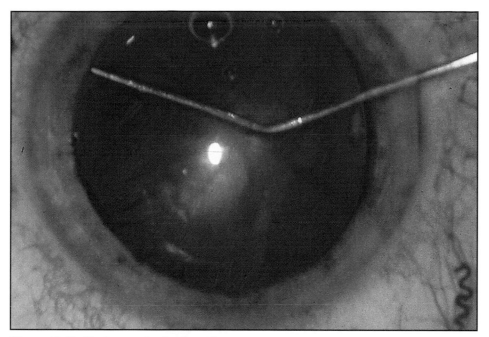

Figure 14-25. Single-wave hydrodissection.

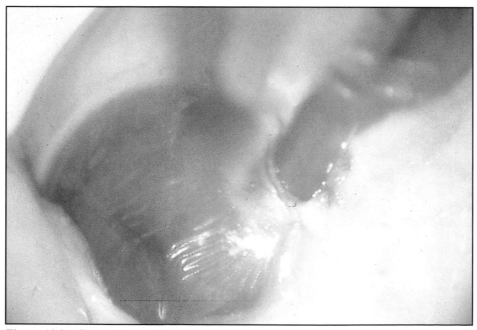

Figure 14-26. Corneal burn (Storz).

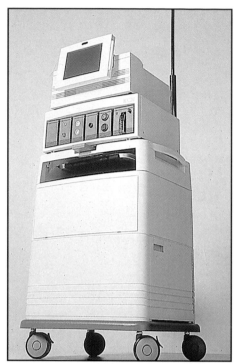

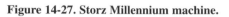

Figure 14-27. Storz Millennium machine.

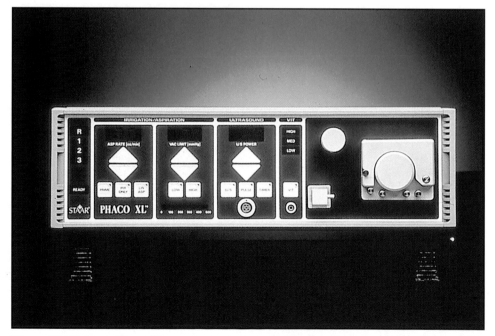

Figure 14-28. Staar Phaco XL.

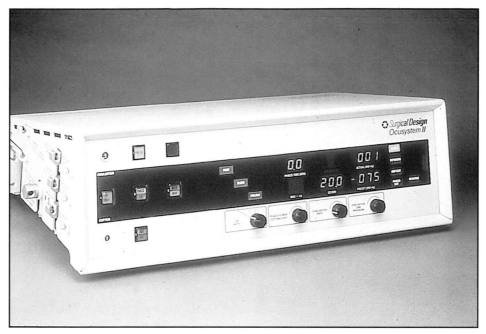

Figure 14-29. Ocusystem Phaco XL.

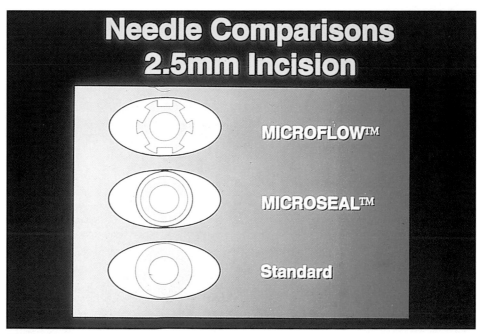

Figure 14-30. Phaco needle design (Storz).

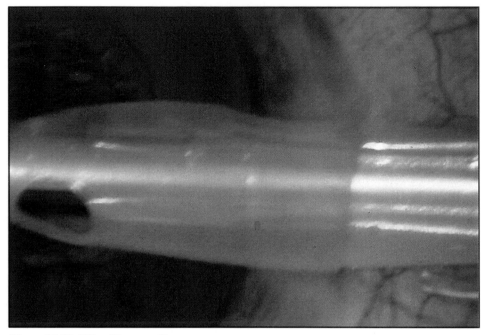

Figure 14-31. MicroFlow needle.

beyond the edge of the capsulorrhexis to prevent accidental breakthrough of the softer parts of the nucleus and potential damage to the posterior capsule. Using a Beckert nuclear spatula through the side stab and the phaco tip, the nucleus is cracked at the floor of the vertical groove starting inferiorly and extending the crack superiorly to completely divide the nucleus into two heminuclear components (Figure 14-33). The heminuclear components are then rotated so that the groove is parallel to the original wound. A small notch is performed at the mid-point of the heminucleus along the full depth of the initial nuclear groove. The phaco tip and Beckert spatula are then used to divide the heminucleus into two quadrants. The spatula is used to move one quadrant to the side while the opening of the phaco tip is applied to the superior edge of the nuclear quadrant allowing suction to tumble the quadrant forward into the deep part of the capsular bag so that the soft posterior side of the nuclear quadrant is exposed for emulsification. The quadrant is quickly emulsified. With dual linear emulsification and aspiration, I may balance high suction with low power emulsification to remove the nuclear quadrant. Aspiration levels of up to 500 mmHg are possible if needed. Once the initial quadrant is removed, the second quadrant is then removed in a similar fashion. The inferior heminucleus is spun in the capsular bag across from the corneal wound positioning it for emulsification. A spatula is used to hold the heminucleus in place and a small notch is once again created in the mid-point of the heminucleus. The nucleus is then divided using the bimanual technique described above and each quadrant is removed. For harder nuclei, more than one groove can be performed in the heminucleus, splitting the nucleus up into four, six, or even eight pieces if necessary. Once the nucleus is com-

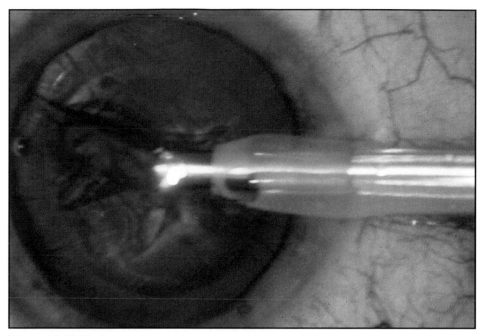

Figure 14-32. Nuclear groove.

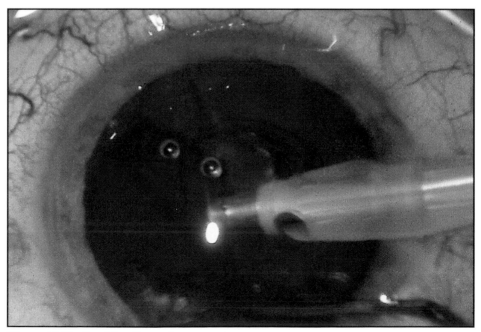

Figure 14-33. Cracking the nucleus.

pletely removed, irrigation/aspiration is performed using a venturi-style pump with a stripping technique at the edge of the capsulorrhexis to efficiently remove all the remaining cortex. I routinely polish the posterior capsule with a Kratz scratcher or use low level aspiration using the I/A tip. Viscoelastic is then placed under the anterior capsular rim to open the capsular bag and deepen the chamber.

IMPLANTATION TECHNIQUE FOR IOL AND ICL

My IOL of choice since the beginning has been the plate haptic lens developed by Staar Surgical. The current models, the AA4203 VF (Figure 14-34) and AA4207 VF lenses, are respectively the 6.0- and 5.5-mm version plate haptic silicone lenses with ultraviolet absorption added and large fixation holes. A recently completed FDA study for the Staar Collamer lens introduces a new collagen-copolymer material for the IOL and ICL, or implantable contact lens. The VF fixation holes allow fibrosis between the anterior and posterior capsule through the large opening (Figure 14-35). The plate lens with VF holes can remain totally stable, even with a large posterior laser capsulotomy performed 3 months after surgery. The plate lens does not rotate in the capsular bag and is the carrier for the Staar toric IOL (Figure 14-36) which is under FDA study protocol for correction of pre-existing astigmatism with cataract surgery. Since clear corneal incision surgery leaves any pre-existing astigmatism undisturbed, it is the procedure of choice for the toric IOL. Early reports have found the toric IOL aligned on the steep corneal axis effectively reduces pre-existing corneal astigmatism improving visual outcome. The Staar AQ2003 V and AQ2010 V three-piece lenses (Figure 14-37) with polyamide haptics are also available in a 12.5-mm length and can be used either as the primary lens of choice or in cases of significant anterior or posterior capsular tear where the plate lens would not be indicated.

The most important part of the IOL implantation is the MicroStaar Injector system. The current MicroStaar Injector cartridge allows for injection of the Staar plate haptic IOL through an internal incision size as small as 1.9 mm (Figure 14-38). The micro cartridge is desirable in all wound sizes 2.5 mm and below to prevent corneal stretching secondary to the injector cartridge tip. Most folding forceps require incision sizes of 3.0 mm or larger. Once the plate haptic IOL is placed into the bag, the viscoelastic is removed from both in front of and behind the lens. The corneal wound is then sealed with hydration of BSS through a 30-gauge cannula (Figure 14-39). The side stab incision is also sealed with hydration. This provides immediate wound seal and virtually guarantees against the possibility of wound leak. In the past 6 years of clear corneal surgery and IOL implantation using the Staar lens, I have not had a single case of shallow chamber, wound leak, or endophthalmitis. The advent of the 1.9-mm corneal wound and corresponding MicroStaar Injector system has allowed the creation of a universal trapezoidal incision with unparalleled wound strength and safety, for delivery of the cataract pseudophakic IOL (Figure 14-40) as well as a posterior chamber refractive phakic Staar ICL (Figure 14-41) through the same injector cartridge and through the same wound size for correction of cataract, cataract with astigmatism, myopia, or hyperopia. This 1.9-mm trapezoidal micro

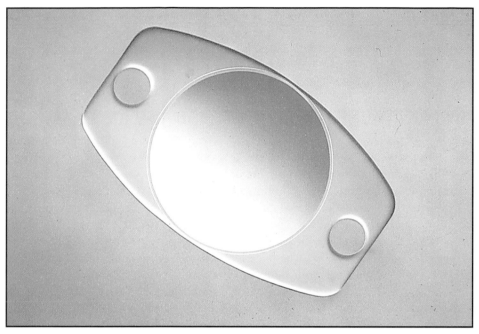

Figure 14-34. AA4203 VF plate lens.

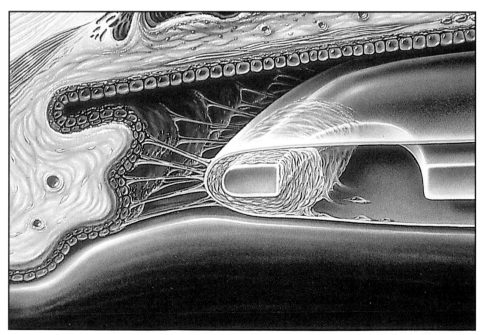

Figure 14-35. VF hole capsular fixation.

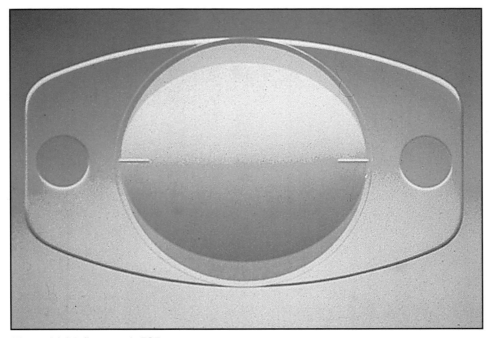

Figure 14-36. Staar toric IOL.

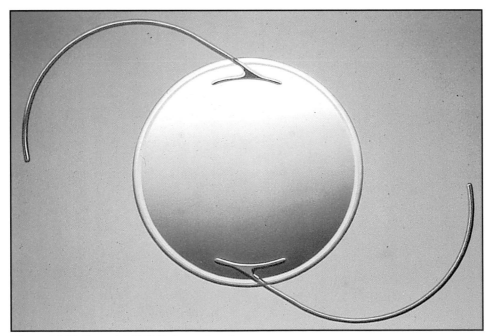

Figure 14-37. Staar AQ2010 V three-piece lens.

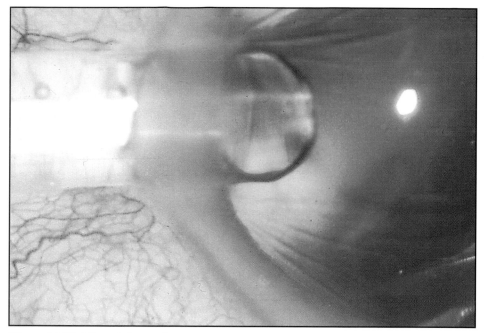

Figure 14-38. Micro injector tip.

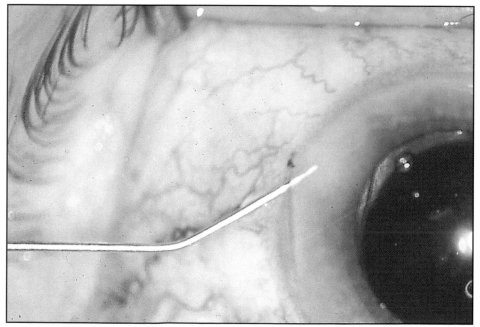

Figure 14-39. Sealing the wound.

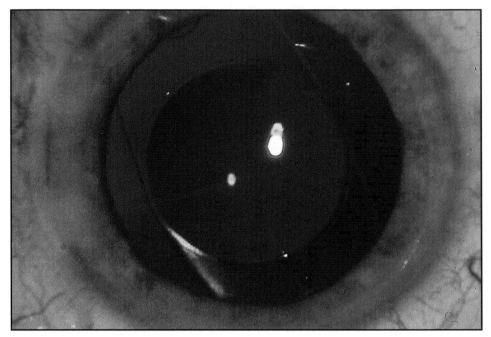

Figure 14-40. Staar plate IOL.

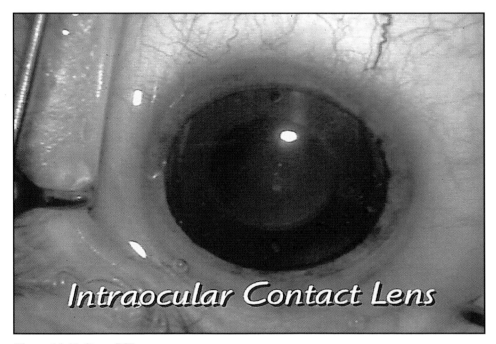

Figure 14-41. Staar ICL.

incision design and MicroStaar injection system is clearly the benchmark for clear corneal incision surgery for cataract and refractive implants.

The hyperopic and myopic Staar ICL is loaded in the MicroStaar Injector cartridge, taking careful note of the orientation of the lens identified by a marker on its right leading haptic. The lens is injected slowly into the anterior chamber of the phakic eye with a widely dilated pupil, taking care to avoid touch of the endothelium or the anterior capsule. The surgeon needs to keep proper anterior-posterior orientation of the ICL as it is vaulted to avoid touch with the anterior lens capsule. Once in the eye, the flexible ICL is easily positioned behind the iris. The pupil is constricted with Miochol, the viscoelastic is removed, and the corneal wound is sealed with hydration in the same manner as the IOL. The patient's vision is immediately stable. The refractive implant procedure provides the most dramatic visual result in ophthalmic surgery and is a welcome addition to our clear corneal surgery techniques.

REFERENCES

1. Marr WG, Wood R, Senterfit L, Sigelman S. Effect of topical anesthesia on regeneration of corneal epithelium. *Am J Ophthalmol.* 1957;43:606-610.
2. Kondrot EC. Rupturing pressure in cadaver eyes with three types of cataract incisions. *J Cataract Refract Surg.* 1991;17:745-748.
3. Ruckman. True incision size and surgically induced refraction change in temporal clear corneal surgery. Presentation at the American Society of Cataract and Refractive Surgery meeting, April 1997.
4. Ernest PH, Fenzel R, Lavery KT, Sensoli A. Relative stability of clear corneal incisions in a cadaver eye model. *J Cataract Refract Surg.* 1995;21:39-42.

Current Personal Phaco Procedure

Richard J. Mackool, MD

CLEAR CORNEAL INCISION
Instrumentation

I prefer the keratome-only technique, without the use of grooves or other means of dissection. Either a metallic or a diamond blade is acceptable.

Technique

Globe fixation is maintained by counterpressure with the left index finger on the nasal portion of the globe (Figure 15-1). A three-plane incision with two graduated transitions is created by altering the angle of the keratome during entry (Figure 15-2). The first stage of the incision requires the keratome to enter the cornea for a distance of 0.3 to 0.5 mm at an angle of 30 degrees. (I prefer to begin the incision at the conjunctival insertion in order to keep the temporal clear corneal incision as peripheral as possible. In order to prevent ballooning of the conjunctiva due to accumulation of incision fluid beneath Tenon's capsule, phacoemulsification and I/A instrumentation which completely seal the incision and prevent leakage during nucleus and cortex removal must be used.) The keratome is then placed nearly flat upon the sclera and advanced for a distance of 2.0 mm. The tip of the keratome is then depressed by elevating the handle, and the third plane is created by advancing the tip slightly into the anterior chamber. At this point, the keratome is redirected so as to be parallel to the iris, and blade entry into the chamber is completed. This results in the creation of a clear corneal incision with the following advantages:

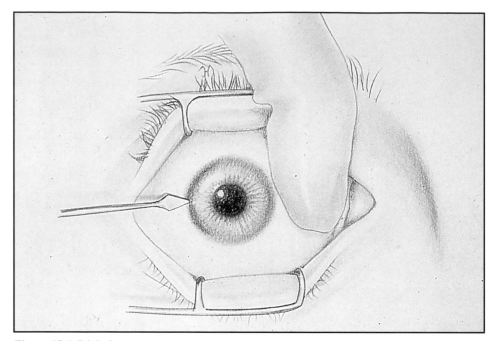

Figure 15-1. Digital counterpressure during keratome use.

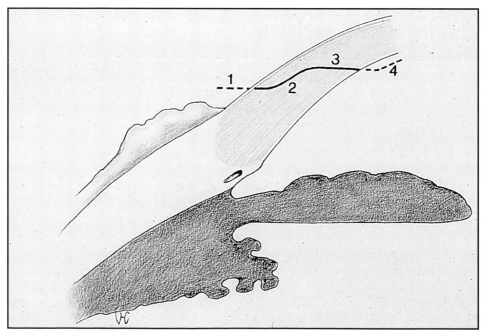

Figure 15-2. Three-plane incision created by single pass of keratome.

- The anterior lip of the incision is reasonably thick, and if necessary may be grasped (Figure 15-3) for insertion of the phaco and/or I/A tip or the IOL. This is due to the fact that the keratome initially entered the cornea at a 30 degree angle rather than a shallower approach which would have created a thinner, more tenuous anterior corneal lip.
- The multi-plane incision, which is 2 mm in length, provides extremely reliable self-sealing.
- The internal opening of the incision is as peripheral as possible, thus permitting the phaco tip to approach the nucleus at a relatively flat angle with subsequent reduction of corneal distortion during phaco and I/A.

This technique may also be employed for superior or oblique corneal incisions. Particularly with superior incisions, a "transconjunctival" approach may be utilized. The keratome is passed through the conjunctiva (which usually inserts 1 to 2 mm more anteriorly than it does temporally), and the incision is created as described above. The transconjunctival technique may be used in any meridian to create a more peripheral incision, and may be preferable for patients with corneal endothelial dystrophy.

Modified "Funnel" Incision

In order to reduce resistance to handpiece motion, the internal aspect of the corneal incision can be enlarged by the creation of an "inverted funnel" incision (Figure 15-4). This is done by withdrawing the shoulders of the keratome into the intrastromal region of the incision after anterior chamber entry has been achieved; the internal incision is then enlarged on one or both sides by redirection and advancement of the keratome. Surgeons who perform one-handed phacoemulsification maneuvers may find this to be an extremely helpful means of reducing globe motion during handpiece movement, and especially during nucleus sculpting. Because the outer aspect of the incision is not enlarged, incision leakage is not increased.

CAPSULORRHEXIS
Instrumentation

The use of any combination of cystotome and forceps is acceptable for performing this critical portion of the procedure. A mature cataract or shallow chamber can make capsulorrhexis much more difficult. An automated capsulorrhexis device under development by Alcon and under the auspices of Dr. Don Serafano promises to provide a valuable addition to our capsulorrhexis armamentarium.

Technique

It is safer to begin the capsulorrhexis centrally. Should the tear begin to extend toward the periphery, this provides a wider margin for error. I prefer a diameter of 3.5 to 5.0 mm, and have been unable to identify any advantage to larger openings. Attempts to create a large diameter tear may increase the risk of peripheral extension.

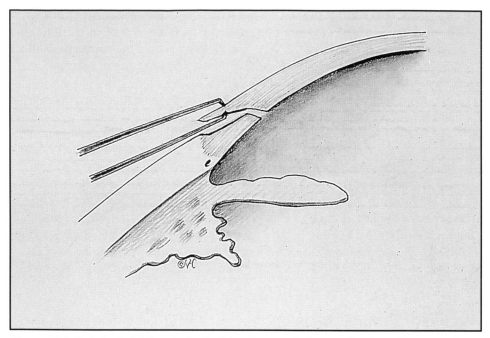

Figure 15-3. Relatively thick anterior incision lip permits forceps fixation without tearing.

Problems

Peripheral Extension

When this occurs, an attempt to salvage the rhexis may be made, unless the tear has extended into the zonule. If it has not, attempted redirection of the tear is most likely to be successful if the anterior chamber is maximally deep. This can be achieved by a combination of viscoelastic injection followed by the insertion of a spatula through a side-port incision. The spatula is used to depress the nucleus, releasing tension on the anterior capsule while redirection of the tear is attempted (Figure 15-5). If the tear extends into the zonule and the capsulorrhexis cannot be salvaged, the capsulotomy can be completed in the opposite direction as shown in Figure 15-6.

When capsulorrhexis extension into the zonule has occurred, nucleus cracking within 90 degrees of the involved meridian by standard divide and conquer (two instrument) techniques is contraindicated; if attempted, extension of the radial anterior capsule tear into the posterior capsule is quite possible, if not likely. A gentle phaco chop technique can be used, however, as less separation of the desired nuclear fragments is required in order to achieve nuclear segmentation with this technique.

Mature Cataract

In this situation, the absence of a red reflex can make it difficult or impossible to observe the advancing margin of the capsule tear. The use of a fiberoptic light, such as those employed during vitreoretinal surgery, can be extremely helpful. The

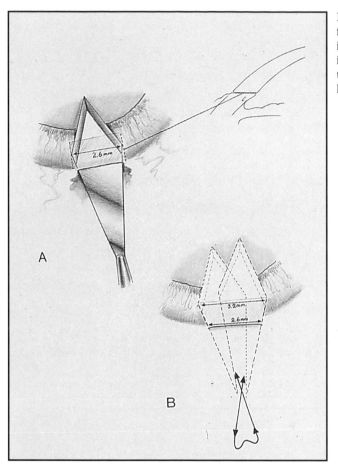

Figure 15-4. The "inverted funnel" incision is wider internally. The external incision remains equal to the diameter of the keratome.

OR and microscope lights are extinguished and the fiberoptic probe is aimed at the eye and redirected as necessary to highlight the margins of the glassy capsular membrane. While somewhat laborious, this technique can literally spell the difference between a successful capsulorrhexis and a peripheral capsular tear extension.

Capsulorrhexis Contracture

This phenomenon generally reaches its maximum by 6 weeks following surgery, and can be readily cured by the creation of radial incisions in the anterior capsule by YAG laser. This laser treatment has no implications for the stability of IOLs with open haptics, but may reduce the stability of some plate haptic IOL designs. Capsulorrhexis contracture is more likely to occur in eyes with lax zonular status (ie, pseudoexfoliation).

Figure 15-5. Nucleus depression during capsulorrhexis redirection.

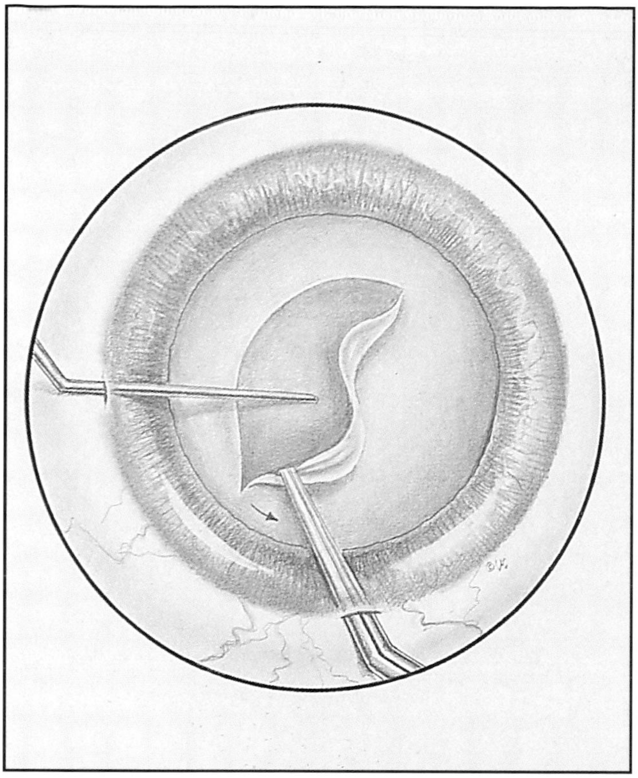

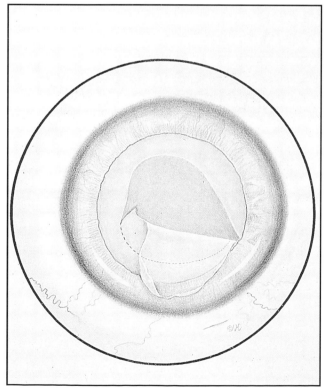

Figure 15-6. If the tear extends into the zonule and the capsulorrhexis cannot be salvaged, the capsulotomy can be completed in the opposite direction as shown.

LENS SURGERY
Instrumentation

My preference is the Alcon Legacy/Mackool System with the 45 degree Kelman Turbosonics MicroTip because of the following.

- The thin wall of this needle and the 45 degree angulation of the beveled port combine to provide superb penetration of even the most dense nucleus. The 45 degree tip, used without ultrasound, is also an extremely efficient instrument for penetrating and then cracking the nucleus during the "soft nucleus phaco chop technique" described below.

- Enhanced cavitational forces greatly improve the ability to sculpt dense nuclei without creating undesirable vector forces which can cause the nucleus to decenter.

- The incision-sealing capacity of this system greatly reduces total fluid flow through the eye, maintains the deepest possible chamber, and improves followability of lens material to the tip. I strongly prefer horizontal orientation (Figure 15-7) of the angulated tip during nearly all of the sculpting process, and for the entirety of the portion of the procedure devoted to nuclear segment removal. The cavitational forces and ultrasonic pressure wave created by the tip are thus maintained in a horizontal direction (not upward toward the corneal endothelium), and these same forces will not have a tendency to push nuclear fragments toward the corneal dome. The tip may be oriented vertically when sculpting the deepest layers of the nucleus, particularly when these layers are firm. Note the recommended orientation of the infusion ports in Figure 15-7.

Technique

I utilize the phaco chop method of nucleus disassembly. The phaco tip is inserted without fixation of the corneal incision; the chopper (Mackool chopper, Duckworth and Kent) is introduced through the side-port incision (which should be 2 clock hours to the left of the surgical incision for a right-handed surgeon), and its presence will stabilize the globe as the phaco tip is inserted. Tip insertion may be accomplished more easily if a gentle to-and-fro rotation of the tip is used as it is advanced.

Moderate or Dense Nuclear Cataracts

My usual method of accomplishing phaco chop for these nuclei employs the following three steps.

1. Creation of a nuclear bowl. A 3-mm wide bowl is sculpted quite deeply so that a reasonably good red reflex is visible through the central nuclear plate. The use of very high magnification is extremely important at this time; the deep layers of the nucleus can be visualized with certainty and shaved with confidence. Rotating the nucleus in order to improve visualization of the various regions at the bottom of the bowl can be extremely helpful. Also, the phaco chopper can be used to gently depress and thus stabilize the nucleus as it is being sculpted.

Figure 15-7. Horizontal orientation of infusion ports with horizontal orientation of angulated Kelman-Mackool MicroTip.

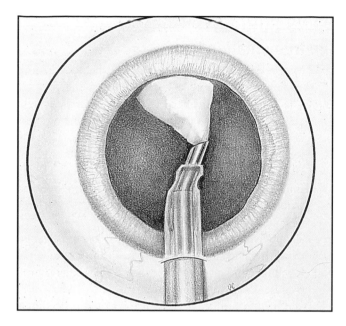

2. Using a relatively high vacuum level (Table 15-1), the posterior half of the nucleus is impaled (Figure 15-8) with the foot pedal briefly in position 3. The tip is embedded approximately 1 mm into the nucleus, and the foot pedal is then rapidly elevated into position 2. The position of the right hand and the right foot are now held constant, maintaining nucleus fixation.
3. The phaco chopper is oriented obliquely (or horizontally, if the chopper is large), then directed beneath the anterior capsule by placing it in cortex before moving it toward the equator of the nucleus. At the equator (or before the equator if the nucleus is not extremely dense), the chopper is turned so that the tip points downward. It is then pulled backward and downward to the phaco tip, and the chopper and tip are then separated (the phaco tip moves to the right and the chopper to the left) so that they are approximately 1 mm apart. If the nucleus has been sculpted deeply and the phaco tip has impaled the posterior half of the nucleus, a successful chop invariably occurs. The nucleus is then rotated and the chop repeated in order to create four or six nuclear segments (the latter is preferred when the anterior chamber is not maximally deep). The fragments are then removed (see Table 15-1 for recommended aspiration flow rate and vacuum levels).

Extremely Dense (Red/Black) Cataracts

Phaco chop is extremely difficult, if not impossible, in these situations. Other surgical options include an excruciatingly slow divide and conquer technique or a much more rapid (and less demanding) iris plane method. Performance of the latter requires either the creation of a relatively large capsulorrhexis or preferably a capsulorrhexis with two relaxing incisions (performed 1 clock hour to the right and to the left of the surgical incision [Figure 15-9]).

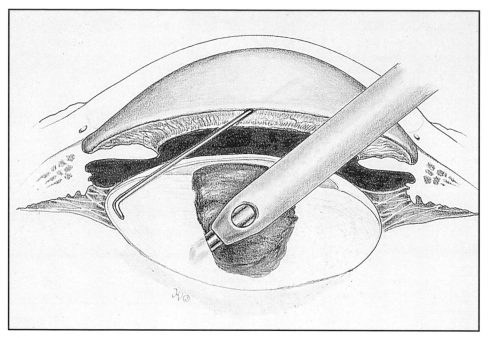

Figure 15-8. Posterior half of nucleus impaled prior to phaco chop.

Table 15-1			
Mackool Phacoemulsification Parameters			
Procedure	**AFR (cc/min)**	**Vac (mmHg)**	**Bottle Height[2] (cm)**
Sculpting[1]	15	20 to 40	60 to 78
Sculpting[3]	15	250	78 to 110
Impaling Nucleus[4]	15	250 to 350	78 to 110
Peripheral Sculpting— One-Handed Technique	15	40 to 150[5]	60 to 110
Nuclear Segment Removal[6]	15 to 35	100 to 350	78 to 110

[1]*Deliberate technique, generally avoiding portal occlusion.*

[2]*Whenever a range for bottle height is present, the higher level is generally preferred.*

[3]*More rapid technique, safely used when sculpting the **central** nucleus, employing portal occlusion. Note: high vacuum level should **not** be used when sculpting in the periphery (ie, near the nucleus equator).*

[4]*Nucleus impaling is commonly performed during phaco chop.*

[5]*One-handed surgeons utilize widely differing vacuum levels. In general, vacuum levels that are two to three times greater than those that the surgeon normally uses with standard handpiece and tip designs may be safely employed.*

[6]*Regardless of settings, a blunt spatula should always be placed behind the last nuclear segment/quadrant as it is removed. This will prevent forward movement of the posterior capsule, which occurs in approximately 1% of phacoemulsification procedures due to infusion misdirection (ie, infusion fluid passing through the zonule and accumulating in the retrocapsular space).*

Figure 15-9.
Capsulorrhexis relaxing
incision is created with
disposable 30-gauge nee-
dle inserted through lim-
bus (not through phaco
incision).

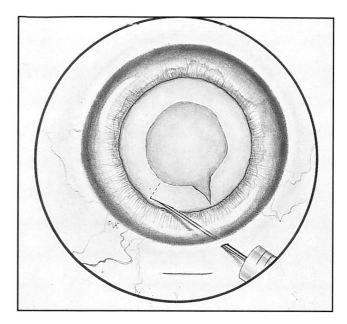

Soft Nucleus

If an attempt is made to fixate a soft nucleus by the use of vacuum forces, a section of nucleus is aspirated and purchase of the nucleus is not obtained. In these eyes, a modification of the standard phaco chop technique can be used to accomplish nuclear segmentation. After sculpting the central bowl as described above, the foot pedal is returned to position 0. The phaco tip is turned horizontally (port sideways) and placed against the vertical sculpted wall opposite the incision; the chopper is then advanced beneath the anterior capsule to the region of the nucleus equator. The chopper and the phaco tip are then moved **toward each other**, thus penetrating the nucleus between them. When the instruments meet, they are separated as described above. In some patients with extremely soft nuclei, this method will not be successful in achieving complete nuclear segmentation. However, significant grooves will be created and the subsequent use of high vacuum will permit the nucleus periphery to be drawn centrally and aspirated. A relatively small nuclear plate will often remain. This can be elevated with the chopper or other instrument and be easily removed.

Retained Nucleus: Prevention

Small pieces of nucleus can be overlooked and remain in the eye following phacoemulsification procedures. To avoid this, remember that there are three situations in which this is more likely to occur:
1.   Eyes with small pupils
2.   Eyes with arcus senilis
3.   Eyes in which the color of the iris and the nucleus are similar

Be sure to inject BSS through the side-port incision at the end of the procedure, as small pieces of nucleus often remain in this region and will be displaced and detected by the injection. Also, washing viscoelastic out from behind the IOL (this is best done with an angulated I/A tip) at the end of the procedure will often reveal the presence of a retained nuclear chip.

Irrigation/Aspiration

Appropriate instrumentation is truly the key to safe, efficient cortex removal. A silicone-sleeved I/A tip can be used to seal the incision (round rigid sleeves cannot deform into the elliptical shape required to accomplish this). An I/A tip that has a 90 degree tip angulation (available from Duckworth and Kent with a 0.25 mm port— this small port reduces the risk of posterior capsule rupture if inadvertent aspiration of the posterior capsule occurs) can be used to remove cortex from any location, and is so much safer than a straight tip design for subincisional cortex removal that one can only wonder how long it will be before the straight I/A tip encounters its extinction. The angulated design facilitates the placement of the aspiration port against the cortex (especially subincisional cortex) and reduces the possibility of inadvertent posterior capsule aspiration. It is also a superior instrument for removing viscoelastic from behind the IOL at the conclusion of the procedure. The sole disadvantage of angulated I/A tips is their inferiority for vacuuming the posterior capsule. When necessary, epithelial cells can be removed from the posterior capsule by gentle rubbing with a Kratz scratcher or similar instrument.

IOL IMPLANTATION

Either a lens injector or forceps can be employed to insert the foldable IOL. The former carries a greater risk of damaging the IOL, and the latter probably increases the risk of corneal incision trauma (tearing) during forceps fixation. If a forceps is used, caution must be employed when grasping the external margin of the incision. The creation of a thick, long corneal lip as previously described permits a 1-mm long portion of the lip to be fixated (see Figure 15-3). Regardless of the injector or forceps design used, all implantations that I have made utilizing equipment available in the United States as of January 1998 result in an incision that is at least 3.0 mm in width. I therefore prefer an incision of at least 2.8 mm for IOL insertion. Insertion through smaller incisions is possible, but may increase the risk of IOL damage or tearing of the incision.

INCISION CLOSURE

When properly created, the clear corneal incision will seal by itself. This can be hastened by stromal hydration, a technique that I have used to seal various corneal incisions since 1976. (I initially used stromal hydration to seal side-port incisions in children, which tend to self-seal poorly. This avoided the problems encountered with corneal sutures in the young, ie, postoperative foreign body sensation from large absorbable sutures, or the need to eventually re-anesthetize the child for removal of non-absorbable material.) Stromal hydration is best accomplished by the placement

of the port of a 27-gauge cannula (more narrow cannulas are too weak for the task) tightly against the lateral wall of the deeper layers of the incision. A forcible injection of fluid via the syringe to which the cannula is attached is then made into the stroma, causing immediate stromal opacification. This same technique can be used to seal the side-port incision. Remember to be patient. All properly created incisions will seal but it may take 1 to 2 minutes for the swollen stroma to oppose properly after incision deformation by IOL insertion. It is always advisable to inject fluid through the side-port incision at the conclusion of the procedure. Nuclear fragments may be hidden in this region, and the injection will usually float them into the central chamber; injecting fluid through the side-port incision will also restore IOP and establish sealing of the clear corneal incision.

Clear Corneal Implant Surgical Techniques

Kenneth J. Hoffer, MD

INTRODUCTION

The present-day success of lens implant (IOL) surgery has benefited from many advances in the surgical techniques for cataract removal. Extracapsular extraction and phacoemulsification were the most significant, but the small clear corneal incision has also been a major advance. The rapid recovery and healing of the eye is the major reason I prefer topical clear corneal, small incision cataract surgery. In my last 475 eyes, best corrected acuity on the first postoperative day was 20/20 in 27%, 20/25 or better in 50%, and 20/40 or better in 70%.

PATIENT SELECTION

Almost every patient is a candidate for this procedure except those patients who have involuntary eye or body movements not easily controlled by mild sedation or patients with severe claustrophobia. I have had to resort to general anesthesia only three times in the past 5 years for such reasons. Even patients initially afraid of proceeding or those with complete language barrier have not been a problem. Some truly one-eyed patients may best be done with general anesthesia (injection anesthesia being an unnecessary risk for such cases).

PREOPERATIVE CONSIDERATIONS

Precise immersion A-scan and personalized theoretic formula selection for IOL power calculation is absolutely essential to maximize the postoperative refraction

prediction accuracy. I strongly recommend a system[1] of using the three modern theoretic formulas:

1. The Hoffer Q formula for eyes shorter than 24.5 mm
2. The Holladay 1 formula for eyes 24.5 to 26.0 mm
3. The SRK/T formula for eyes longer than 26.0 mm

The newer Holladay 2 formula may be helpful in eyes shorter than 19.0 mm but no study has yet demonstrated this because of the rarity of these eyes. I recommend against the use of regression formulas which I have shown[1] to be the major modern cause for ametropic errors. Routine preoperative endothelial cell counts are also performed to discover at-risk corneas. We do routine HIV screening because of the increased susceptibility for endophthalmitis in immunocompromised patients.

Patients are always seen by me personally within 48 hours of surgery (usually 24 hours) to check for any contraindication to surgery and to reconfirm the patient's postoperative refractive wishes. At that time I personally select the exact IOL power for all IOLs that could potentially be needed and answer any questions the patient may have.

OPERATING ENVIRONMENT

I operate in a two-OR ambulatory surgical facility, which is part of my office. The operating table is the gurney the patient relaxes in before and after the surgery, eliminating the need to transfer patients once they are in the surgical facility. Masking tape is used to tape the patient's head to the table as a gentle reminder not to make inappropriate head movements. An anesthesiologist is always present during the procedure.

Operative sheets (pink for right eyes, yellow for left), which are prepared in advance, are hung on the wall (8½ x 11 inches) for the OR staff and are attached just above the oculars of the microscope (3 x 4 inches) for the surgeon. The sheet contains information on the name the patient prefers to be called, allergies, the various IOL powers for each lens style (usually five), the endothelial cell count, the size and axis of cylinder, as well as any warnings or special situations I wish to be reminded of. I can easily glance up from the oculars and reference these data.

We have soft music playing in the background and we talk incessantly. I learned, over many years of being a dental patient, that when there is silence during a major procedure, I grow concerned. As soon as I hear the dentist and his staff discussing mundane issues, I relax because I get the sense everything must be going fine. Therefore, even if there is capsule rupture or nucleus in the vitreous, I keep up a continual conversation about events of the day. In such situations, at the end of the procedure, I always describe to the patient exactly what has happened and what future risks are inherent. I record this discussion in the patient record. This discussion is repeated more thoroughly with the family during the first postoperative visit and again recorded.

Using a silicone plate haptic lens, we always have a duplicate power and style lens on hand in case the lens becomes damaged. We also have a three-piece silicone lens for backup in case the capsulorrhexis is not adequate or there is an opening in

the posterior capsule. All one-piece PMMA lenses are also available if they should be needed, as well as three appropriately powered Kelman Multiflex II anterior chamber lenses. The latter are in 0.5-mm steps in length with the middle size being the pre-measured corneal diameter plus 1 mm. Automated vitrectomy instrumentation is always available and ready for use. We always have a PMMA capsular ring available for cases where there is significant zonular dehiscence.

TECHNIQUE STEPS
1. Topical Anesthesia
2. No Instrument-Touch Technique
3. Oblique Clear Corneal 2.5-mm Incision
4. Dual Viscoelastic Use
5. Circular Capsulorrhexis
6. Hydrodissection
7. One-Handed Quartering Technique
8. Total Cortex Removal
9. Total Capsular Polishing
10. Silicone IOL Injection
11. Sutureless Weck-cel Pressure Closure
12. No Injections
13. No Patch

Topical Anesthesia
Cataract surgery under topical anesthesia was first reported by Redmond and Dallas[2] in England in 1990 and introduced in the United States by Redmond at my Academy cataract course in 1991. Since then, it has gained great popularity. After extensive pupillary dilation, the patient is given topical anesthetic drops starting in the preop area until just before the procedure begins. I have never used ocular decompression routines of any kind. After povidone-iodine prep, a simple 3M drape is taped over the eye, incised between the lids, and the flaps folded under the lids to cover the lashes. The adjusting-lock titanium wire lid speculum (Impex #XYZ-909T, Staten Island, NY) is placed between the lids and the lock adjusted until the patient's ability to reflexively or voluntarily blink is eliminated. There is a certain point of tension whereby patients cease all attempts at trying to blink. A corneal cap fashioned from various materials (latex glove, sponge) is used to shield the retina and keep the cornea from drying out. At various points in the procedure, while waiting for instrumentation, I shield the retina with my index finger.

Although I became very comfortable using topical anesthesia long before Gills introduced the concept of intraocular Xylocaine, I held back trying it until endothelial studies were reported. Without it, patients never experienced pain except to notice a pressure sensation during IOL insertion. I utilized intraocular Xylocaine in a series of cases to see if it would lessen this sensation and it did not. I therefore do not believe it is necessary using my technique. If one starts topical cataract surgery routinely using intraocular Xylocaine, it will be very difficult to discontinue its use

for fear patients will experience pain without it. I have performed pars plana incision, nucleus retrieval, vitrectomy, complete capsular bag removal, iris surgery, and synechia repair under topical without intraocular Xylocaine in cases that have lasted up to an hour without patient discomfort.

No Instrument-Touch Technique

To eliminate any chance of subconjunctival hemorrhage, I have eliminated contacting the eye with any metal instruments except for the keratome and later the phaco tip. For counterpressure while making the incision, I use my gloved index finger 180 degrees from the incision site. It is important not to overwet the conjunctiva just before doing this. I have not appreciated the benefit of fixation rings after having tried several types. Great care is taken so as not to need any instrument to grasp the conjunctiva or cornea throughout the procedure. The phaco tip, I/A tip, and lens injector are inserted without ever grasping the edge of the incision. No injections are made at the conclusion of the procedure.

Oblique Clear Corneal 2.5-mm Incision

A 2.5-mm slit metal keratome blade (Alcon Surgical, Ft. Worth, Texas) is used to make a simple stab incision into clear cornea just above the vascular arcade. The design of the keratome is important. Most keratome tips come to a point at an angle of from 45 to 90 degrees that makes entry through corneal tissue more difficult. I discovered, in 1993, that the Alcon slit blade with a tip angle less than 45 degrees allowed for a smoother, more controlled entry and always created a flat self-sealing incision. The newer Beaver keratomes are quite similar.

The radial length of the incision is approximately 1 mm. Once in the eye, the keratome is rotated to the left and to the right to create a rhomboid shape with the inner incision slightly larger than the external. Care is taken not to damage the anterior capsule with the tip of the keratome. My attempts at using various diamond blades, multi-plane incisions, and a pre-incision perpendicular cut (Langerman) have not been superior to the technique described. A side-port incision is made at the 2 o'clock position using a 1.0-mm diamond blade without counterpressure or grasping the eye.

I find the 10:30 (1:30 for left-handed surgeons) oblique position of the incision the most comfortable for both left and right eyes. It allows me to sit in the usual superior position with easy access to both phaco and microscope foot pedals. The position and approach is therefore the same for either eye. During each step of the procedure, my right hand is in the most normal position as if performing tasks such as writing or using a fork. The back end of the phaco handpiece (with all its tubing) is not pressing into my chest or abdomen, but rather aimed away from my body. Since the whole experience is more natural and comfortable, it immediately reduced my operating time. Theoretically, the patient's nose might cause an impediment when doing left eyes, but so far, this has never occurred.

The oblique incision has all the advantages of a temporal incision and adds the ease of hand position as well as the safety factor of postoperative lid coverage of the

incision. There are exceptions to the oblique position, such as cases with large corneal cylinder or filtering blebs. Over the years, I have learned that I can perform the entire procedure with an incision placed on the right side of the eye, anywhere from 12 to 7 o'clock, while sitting in the usual superior position. Since my astigmatism study of 280 eyes has shown an average flattening of 0.67 D in the axis of the incision at 1 year, I will often move the incision superiorly for with-the-rule cylinder and temporally for against-the-rule. The study also showed slightly more flattening in left eyes (0.73 D vs 0.61 D). My 1980 study[3] of the biometry of 7500 cataract eyes showed that 40% of them have a cylinder of less than 0.50 D, while 50% are between 0.50 D and 2.00 D. Overall mean cylinder was 1.00 (±1.00) D. The remaining 10%, with greater than 2.00 D (3% >3.50 D), might benefit from astigmatic keratotomy at the time of cataract surgery. After performing a series of such cases, I noted both a much longer delay in uncorrected vision recovery and an increase in cystoid macular edema. This led me to defer any astigmatic keratotomy surgery until the eye was completely healed.

Dual Viscoelastic Use

I have used Healon routinely since 1979 when I introduced it in the West. Though recognizing the endothelial protective effect of Viscoat, I encountered greater difficulty performing capsulorrhexis while using it. I performed a small study comparing the ease of capsulorrhexis using all available viscoelastics and discovered Viscoat was the worst and Provisc the best. This stimulated me to switch to DuoVisc, which allows me to first inject Viscoat to cover the endothelium and then use the Provisc cannula to layer a coating of it over the anterior capsule and push the Viscoat to the cornea. The latter is easily aspirated during phacoemulsification while the Viscoat stays attached to the endothelium throughout the procedure. My mean endothelial cell loss rate of 6% (±9) in the last 483 eyes seems to confirm the advantage of this concept.

Circular Capsulorrhexis

The complete circular capsulorrhexis we use today was first described and taught by Dr. Calvin Fercho of Fargo, North Dakota. In my opinion, the capsulorrhexis is the most difficult part of the operation and I have taken several steps to ensure I get the perfect, round, sufficiently large opening I need. I began using a forceps but quickly switched to a prepared bent needle. I begin the tear just in from the pupil at the 5 o'clock position. I proceed to make a series of connecting can-opener cuts until I reach the center of the pupil. I call these relaxing incisions because they cause the fulcrum of the tear to be more central. This allows me to create as large a capsulorrhexis as I want (usually 5 to 6 mm). The capsule piece is removed with Kraff capsule forceps. If the pupil is too small, I perform the Fry pupil stretch technique using an Aker pusher distally and a Bonn hook proximally. After trying various pupil stretching devices and hooks, I feel this simple technique is faster, easier, less traumatic, and more effective.

If the capsulorrhexis tear should stray to where it appears it cannot be recovered, I switch to a 1970s Kelman cystotome and perform connecting can-opener cuts in

the remaining area. The nicks made by the needle can tear backwards but the nicks made by the Kelman cystotome leave a smooth curved area that cannot be torn backward. The instrument creates a strong, serrated margin that leaves an intact complete capsulorrhexis (with a scalloped edge) allowing use of the plate haptic lens.

Hydrodissection

Complete hydrodissection is more important the softer the nucleus is. As taught to me by Dr. I. Howard Fine, I gently lift the edge of the anterior capsule with the BSS cannula until clear capsule is lifted from the cortex. I then irrigate with enough force to see the cleavage plane created behind the lens nucleus. It is important not to irrigate so heavily that an iris prolapse occurs. If it does, it is more safely corrected by gentle posterior pressure with a Wheeler iris spatula on the prolapsed iris covering the posterior lip of the incision. This releases the fluid and flattens the chamber until the iris reposits itself. Attempting to push the iris back into the eye against the pressure of the viscoelastic with an instrument usually leads to iris trauma and loss of large areas of the posterior pigment layer and this may lead to synechia.

One-Handed Quartering Technique

When I first began phacoemulsification in 1972, I used the original Kelman anterior chamber technique with one hand through a 3.5-mm incision. In the early 1980s, I switched to a two-handed technique in the posterior chamber. Since using the Shepherd quartering technique, I noted that the use of two hands to crack the nuclear pieces led to a higher incidence of capsulorrhexis edge split. Determined to accomplish the quartering with one hand I developed a technique to accomplish it. I sculpt the central trough across the nucleus deep enough until I almost reach the posterior capsule. This is done with about 30% power and very low aspiration. I have continued to prefer using the original 15 degree phaco tip. I then rotate the nucleus 90 degrees and cut the perpendicular trough to the same depth. The aspiration is then increased to 100 mmHg and the phaco tip is aimed at the posterior central edge of one of the pie quarters, gently pressed into it with mild ultrasound energy until strongly embedded. The tip is then tipped upward until the quarter cracks away from the remaining nucleus and is then emulsified. The more peripheral, softer nucleocortex is then aspirated with mild intermittent ultrasound energy (as needed) after it is brought centrally. These steps are repeated three more times until the entire nucleus is removed. In 2% of cases, a nucleus is so hard that this will not work, and I resort to a two-handed technique using the Haelfiger nucleus cracker/manipulator (MicroTech, Doylestown, Pa).

Care must be taken if a posterior nuclear plate remains. I lay the mouth of the 15 degree phaco tip posteriorly on the plate and apply strong aspiration until I can lift and twist it into the anterior chamber. In the past 10 years, I have not ruptured the posterior capsule during the removal of the nucleus.

If the zonules should weaken or the capsule tear, I continue slow, gentle emulsification using two hands until it is removed. It may be necessary to create a stab pars plana incision and use the Wheeler iris spatula behind the lens to keep it from

falling back. If the lens should fall back, I leave it, finish the case including IOL insertion, and immediately refer the patient to have nucleus removal by an experienced retinologist within 24 hours. The four cases where I have had this occur in the past 25 years have all resulted in 20/20 vision postoperatively without developing uveitis or glaucoma.

Dr. Richard Mackool encouraged me to switch to a 2.5-mm microseal incision in the early 1990s, and I have used it with standard phaco equipment (CooperVision 9000) and more recently with the Storz microseal handpiece. I have never experienced a case of corneal burn with any incision size, handpiece, or ultrasound time.

Total Cortex Removal

I have always felt it was necessary to remove all of the cortex unless there are extenuating circumstances, such as a moving patient or heavy pseudoexfoliation. Since 1975, I have used the angled I/A tip that was originally made for me by Luminex and Cavitron and is now available from many manufacturers. This allows easier access to cortex near the incision. I find that it is safer to refrain from aspirating cortex that is layered on the posterior capsule. Instead, I always hunt for the piece that is attached to it and lies under the anterior capsule. In cases of pseudoexfoliation, I take care not to pull cortex radially toward the center, but rather to pull it circumferentially to lessen the risk of undue stress on the zonules.

Since cortex removal has the highest incidence of capsular tear, it is extremely important to observe the tip at all times and never let it gobble large amounts of cortex in a rapid, high velocity manner. That is when inadvertent, unexpected splits occur. Also be on the watch for large streaks radiating from the I/A tip which indicate that the aspiration has caught the posterior capsule. Go off aspiration and flush back on the aspiration tubing until the capsule is released.

If cortex must be removed when there is vitreous in the anterior chamber, the vitreous will plug the aspiration tip. Remove the I/A tip, perform an anterior and sub-iris vitrectomy until it is clear, and then finish the cortex removal with the I/A tip. This may need to be repeated several times.

Total Capsular Polishing

I have always felt it was very important to polish the posterior capsule with the Kratz irrigating scratcher to remove any residual epithelial cells or fibrotic plaques. New scratchers should be checked for any sharp barbs, which might open the posterior capsule. It is important that visualization be adequate to polish the capsule vigorously enough without disrupting it. After the posterior capsule is polished, I fill the capsular bag and then the anterior chamber with Provisc. Recently I have begun using the Shepherd-Rentsch ring polishers to carefully remove all the epithelial debris remaining on the underside of the remaining anterior capsule. This is best performed in a viscoelastic-filled anterior chamber. I leave the epithelial debris for final aspiration. I leave epithelial debris until final viscoelastic evacuation. After polishing the anterior capsule, I inject a bolus of Viscoat just inside the incision to protect the endothelium from the injector and silicone lens, as well as keep the iris from pro-

lapsing during the pressure of IOL insertion. Provisc is injected on the center posterior capsule to elevate the epithelial debris so it will wind up behind the IOL. The
Provisc is much easier and quicker to aspirate from the capsular bag than Viscoat,
making this viscoelastic placement scheme much quicker to remove.

Silicone IOL Injection

I measured the width of the incision, in a series of 35 2.5-mm incision eyes,
using the Steinert-Deacon incision gauges (Capitol Instruments, Seattle, Wash) and
discovered most were 2.7 mm just after phaco and 3.1 mm after injector IOL insertion. I continue to use the 2.5-mm keratome because it allows for a microseal incision and less fluid irrigation during phaco. I also fear that if I used a larger initial
incision, the final incision would be even larger than 3.1 mm.

If an anterior chamber lens is necessary, I enlarge the incision to 5.0 mm which
allows the 5.5-mm optic of the Alcon Multiflex II lens a slightly tight squeeze. If a
PMMA lens is needed, I enlarge the incision to 0.5 mm less than the diameter of the
optic. The incision is extended by using the initial metal keratome to slice to the left
and then to the right while measuring with a millimeter caliper.

My primary lens of choice is a silicone plate haptic lens (Staar or Chiron). I have
always found the injector system superior to using folding forceps. The incision
does not have to be enlarged to encompass the forceps nor grasped with an instrument to guide the forceps in. I also like the fact that with the injector the IOL never
comes in contact with the exterior of the eye (contamination). I found the Staar
injector easiest to use but the most recent Chiron injector is fairly comparable. The
60 degree bevel injector tip, first inspired by Daniel Welsh, allows much easier entry
through small incisions. I also prefer the rotating injector to the plunger type because
it allows better control of the injection.

My scrub technician or I load the lens into the injector and the tip is placed at
the incision while gradually angulating, twisting, and pressing it through. I tell the
patient that he or she may experience a sense of pressure just before I exert force to
get it through the incision. Carty has demonstrated that it is not necessary to push
the cartridge through the incision, but merely place it at the incision and inject the
lens through the incision. I have tried this but have found that occasionally the lens
will escape and exit the cartridge externally because I do not use any instrument
counterpressure to hold the eye.

The leading edge of the lens is aimed posteriorly into the distal capsular bag
while the injector handle is twisted. When the majority of the optic has exited the
tip, I twist the plunger handle in the reverse direction and this allows the lens to
escape the plunger grasp and gently exit the tip. A curved Lewicky hook, through
the side-port incision, is used to press the anterior surface of the proximal optic edge
posteriorly to force the proximal plate into the bag. The hook then rotates the lens
into desired position. A straight I/A tip is used to remove all the viscoelastic, remnant epithelial debris from the capsule scrubbing, and any new found pieces of cortex which may have been loosened by the IOL rotation.

Following the suggestion of Gills, in the 1980s, I discontinued performing a peripheral iridectomy for routine extracapsular (phaco) surgery and have yet to see a case of pupillary block glaucoma. It is important, however, to assure a patent iridectomy if an anterior chamber lens is implanted.

Sutureless Weck-cel Pressure Closure

Because the phaco tip, the I/A tip, and IOL injector have forcibly molded the original flat incision into a rounded, fish-mouth form, seldom will the incision automatically seal. This is the reason many surgeons inject the incision edges with BSS to create enough edema and swelling to seal it. Before that concept was described by Fine, I discovered that if I spent a little time pressing the incision flat again with the back end of a dry Weck-cel sponge, I could get the incision to self-seal 90% of the time without injecting with BSS. A significant force must be applied for this to work successfully. When it did not work, I used to place a single suture, but now I simply inject the incision. I have yet to have a flat chamber after a clear corneal incision and because of this, I have become very cavalier about checking for wound leak before removing the lid speculum. Two cases of shallow chamber have reformed spontaneously within 48 hours without treatment or patching.

No Injections

I do not believe there is any scientific evidence that using subconjunctival antibiotic or steroid injections during cataract surgery influences the rate of endophthalmitis. Eyes are white, quieter, and more comfortable without them. We use a steroid/antibiotic drop qid for the first week and discontinue it when it runs out.

No Patch

In 1980, I operated on a truly one-eyed patient and was called to his bedside 2 hours after his surgery because with his patch on he thought he had gone totally blind. I calmed him down, removed his patch, and proved to him he was not. When I inspected his eye, to my surprise, it looked just like eyes do when I remove the patch on the next day. From this experience I began removing patches earlier and earlier until after 6 months I eliminated patching the eye at all. The advantages were:
- Immediate use of the eye
- Normal lid function and tear flow
- The ability to begin the eye drops right away

Eighteen years later I have yet to encounter a disadvantage and have never patched an eye for anterior segment surgery except in cases where there is compromise in the integrity of the corneal epithelium at the end of surgery. Patching is a totally unnecessary exercise in routine modern cataract surgery including sutured extracap.

POSTOPERATIVE REGIME

All patients are examined 24 (usually) to 48 hours after surgery. A manifest refraction is performed using the K readings to find the cylinder and axis. The patient is usually gratified to learn his or her uncorrected and corrected acuity levels. Later extensive refractions are usually unnecessary; simply begin with the last refraction. A pinhole (or no) visual acuity check will not reveal a large ametropic error and this prevents the ability to correct it within the first 2 to 3 days. Today this problem is more easily corrected by using a piggyback lens placed in the bag over top of the other IOL. If the refractive error at the corneal plane is myopic, the power of the corrective lens should be the refractive error multiplied by one. If it is hyperopic, it should be multiplied by 1.5. The chance of a patient instituting legal action with 20/40 or better uncorrected acuity after such an occurrence is extremely negligible.

Slit lamp exam is performed and the fundus checked if the vision is not as expected and this is not explained by corneal edema or preoperative pathology. Applanation pressure is measured and only pressures over 30 mmHg are treated unless the eye has field defects due to glaucoma. The patient is examined again 1 week later when a lens prescription for the operative eye is given. The patient is warned that if he or she experiences any drop in vision, redness, pain, or retinal detachment symptoms, he or she is to come to the office immediately. The patient's return visit is at 3 months after surgery, when the postoperative endothelial cell count is taken and new lenses prescribed if necessary. Finally, they are seen at 6 months later and then annually.

COMPLICATIONS

The benefit of this technique is the extremely low incidence of complications. The major surgical complication specific to this described procedure is silicone lens damage during IOL insertion. This has happened four times, and the first three lenses were left in the capsular bag even with large areas of one plate damaged or missing. In each case, the undamaged plate haptic was left in the inferior position and each eye healed with a well-centered lens. In the last case, the lens was removed and replaced with another lens. The trauma of this additional manipulation led to 4 weeks of inflammation and corneal edema which finally all cleared. I would prefer to leave the lens unless the possibility of fixation is small. Freely mobile fragments must be removed.

My studies of YAG laser posterior capsulotomy with the plate haptic lens show a 12% overall rate at 3 years (475 eyes) and now a rate of 19% at 5 years (625 eyes). The early study showed those out more than 3 years had a 12% rate and now those out more than 3 years have a 39% rate. The mean time to YAG was 1.5 ± 0.5 years. Silicone lenses are more difficult to laser without causing pitting. A ridge on the back of the lens would be very helpful. Ridge silicone lenses have been manufactured and placed successfully in animal eyes but are not available commercially. In the meantime, it is important to carefully focus the laser and begin a circular attack starting in the center and working out to the periphery in a whirl technique, as

described by Shepherd. I have not seen silicone YAG pits decrease visual acuity, but they may have an effect on contrast sensitivity. I have yet to experience a plate haptic lens breaking through the posterior capsule after a YAG capsulotomy. This may be due to the limited size of the opening and/or the fact that I delay all capsulotomies until 1 year after cataract surgery.

CONCLUSION

Many surgeons have contributed to the development of this technique and on behalf of my patients, I thank each and every one of them. I am sure the future will lead to even more successful techniques but today it is pretty hard to beat.

REFERENCES

1.   Hoffer KJ. The Hoffer Q formula: a comparison of theoretic and regression formulas. *J Cataract Refract Surg*. 1993;19:700-712. [Errata 1994;20:677.]
2.   Redmond RM, Dallas NL. Extracapsular cataract extraction under local anesthesia without retrobulbar injection. *Br J Ophthalmol*. 1990;74(4):203-204.
3.   Hoffer KJ. Biometry of 7,500 cataractous eyes. *Am J Ophthalmol*. 1980;90:360-368.

Complications of Clear Corneal and Posterior Limbal Lens Surgery

Thomas Kohnen, MD

The clear corneal tunnel incision is increasingly used as the port of access to the anterior segment by surgeons around the globe. The incision has become very popular because the construction is easy, the incision is convenient for the patient, and the incision is relatively astigmatic neutral.[1-3] However, only the knowledge of proper incision construction, anticipation of critical situations during the operation with this type of incision, and management of complications will allow a successful outcome after corneal tunnel incision cataract surgery. In this chapter, I discuss the elements in the prevention, recognition, and management of the intra- and postoperative complications using clear corneal and posterior limbal incisions.

QUALITY OF THE CUT

Proper construction and quality of the clear corneal[4] or posterior limbal[5] incisions are more critical than with scleral valve incisions because already small mistakes can create problems for this type of incision. The entry is further central to the corneal apex and careful construction is mandatory to achieve a perfect result with the corneal tunnel incisions.

Three items should be considered when starting a corneal tunnel incision:
1. Type of instrument
2. Incision size
3. Incision construction

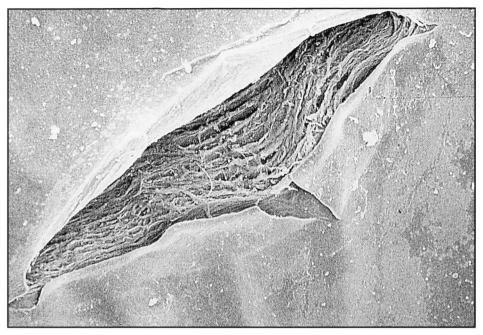

Figure 17-1a. SEM photographs of clear corneal incisions. A 3.0-mm corneal tunnel incision in a cadaver eye cornea following plate haptic IOL (Staar AA4203) insertion with a cartridge/injector system. The limbus is in the upper left-hand side of the photograph. Descemet's membrane appears to be torn at the inferior border of the incision. Stromal collagen has herniated into the anterior chamber, mainly along the upper border of the incision. Both lateral margins show evidence of tearing and disruption of Descemet's membrane. (SEM original magnification: 45x.)

Type of Instrument

Steel blades and diamond knives can be used for the incision. Although steel blades are generally acceptable, I prefer to use diamond knives to construct a clear corneal cut. Advanced designs like the Fine diamond knife (3-D diamond blade) are preferable, because the sloping bevels of the anterior and posterior surfaces of the blade are specially designed to compensate for incising a spherical globe at an angle. With this knife, both internal and external incisions are linear and better wound construction is possible. Radner and colleagues recently showed that the IOL implantation through 3.0-mm clear corneal incisions made with steel keratomes produced corneal trauma that was considerably more severe than implantation through 3.0-mm diamond incisions.[6] They also demonstrated that cutting corneal tissue with diamond tips caused less tissue damage than expanding the incisions with blunt caliper tips.[7] Postoperative wound healing might be better with clean edges of the incision, therefore, my preferred instrument is a diamond knife.

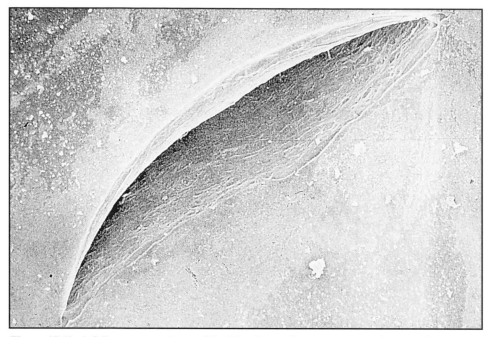

Figure 17-1b. A 3.5-mm corneal tunnel incision in a cadaver eye cornea (same as in Figure 17-1a) following plate haptic IOL (Staar AA4203) insertion with a cartridge/injector system. The limbus is again in the upper left-hand side of the photograph. The incision shows bulging of stromal tissue in the upper part of the incision. The cut edge of Descemet's membrane is smooth and continuous and the lateral borders show little if any evidence of tearing. (SEM original magnification: 45x.)

Incision Size

The incision size plays an important role for postoperative wound stability. The length of the incision is usually between 1.5 and 2 mm; shorter tunnels have the risk to leak, incisions longer than 2 mm can cause vision disturbance during the procedure. The width of the incision is the second parameter in sizing the incision. The enlargement of clear corneal incision used with foldable IOL implantation has been shown in several studies.[8-11] Our studies showed that too small incisions can cause damage to the cornea[10,11] (Figures 17-1a and 17-1b). The laboratory measurements and SEM evaluation indicated that the distortion seen during insertion of foldable IOLs through tight incisions is accompanied by wound enlargement and damage to corneal structures. We concluded, therefore, that the cornea's capacity for true elastic deformation is limited and that the cornea is injured by excessive stretching. Two studies recently showed that the IOL implantation through 3.0-mm clear corneal incisions produced corneal trauma that was considerably more severe than implantation through 3.2-mm wide incisions.[6,11] Thus, an adequate enlargement tailored to each IOL is advisable for clear corneal incisions.

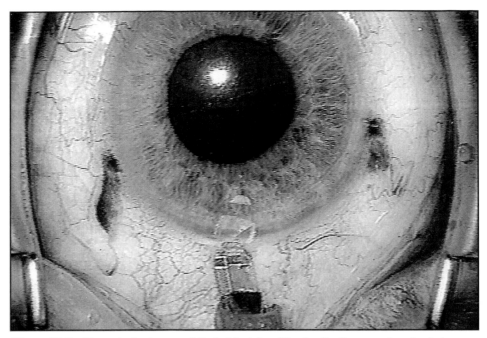

Figure 17-2a. Pre-cut of a temporal limbal incision. The depth of a pre-cut varies between 0.3 and 0.7 mm depending on the surgeon. It can prevent tunnel perforation and enhances wound stability. Intraoperative view of the pre-cut (0.5 mm) using a preset diamond knife.

Tunnel Construction

For improved ocular integrity and corneal stability, the hinged clear corneal incision was introduced.[12] In a cadaver eye study, the better stability of hinged clear corneal incisions compared to beveled clear corneal incisions has been shown.[13] A pre-cut allows a more defined preparation of the incision, and because of these reasons my preferred way currently is a pre-cut of 500 microns followed by a diamond cut (Figures 17-2a through 17-2c). The preparation of the tunnel without a pre-cut can cause improper wound construction (Figures 17-3a and 17-3b).

Detachment of Descemet's membrane is potentially a major complication after cataract surgery resulting in persistent corneal edema and decreased visual acuity. To prevent Descemet's detachment, the surgeon should carefully observe the inner lip (cut edge of Descemet's membrane) at each phase of the clear corneal incision. During enlargement of the wound, a diamond blade that cuts sideways (or a very sharp metal blade) is recommended in order to avoid blunt stripping of Descemet's membrane.

WOUND STABILITY

The most stable place for constructing a cataract wound is the temporal location. To test wound stability of tunnel incisions placed at different locations—scleral and limbal, superior and temporal—Anders et al compared 7-mm wounds using ophthalmodynamometry after 1 and 7 days.[14] They found that temporal scleral incisions

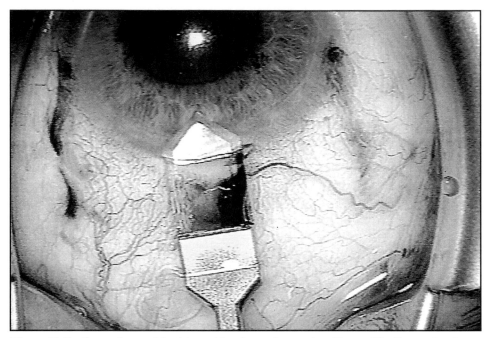

Figure 17-2b. Corneal tunnel incision with a four-edge cutting diamond knife starting in the pre-cut groove.

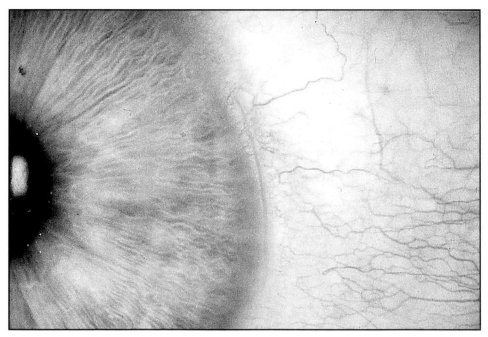

Figure 17-2c. Five days following a 0.5 mm pre-cut at the vascular arcade to construct a corneal tunnel incision.

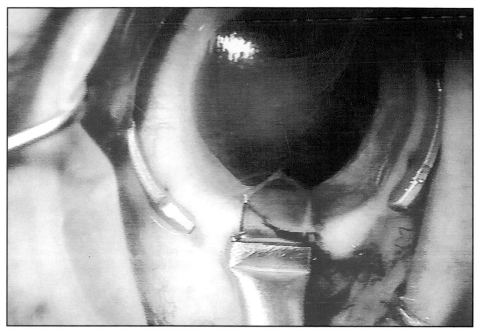

Figure 17-3a. Tunnel perforation. The incision was constructed without a pre-cut and during the clear corneal incision the roof was torn.

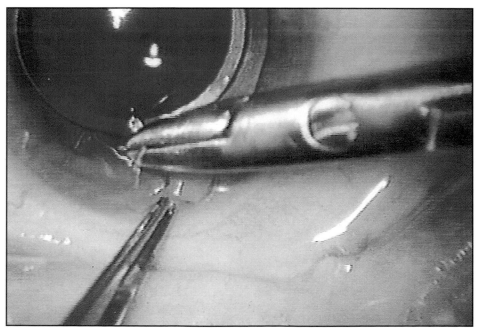

Figure 17-3b. In this case the roof of the clear corneal incision was perforated to both sides and the incision was closed with one radial suture.

yield a maximum wound stability, a result which has also been found in topographical analysis of superior and temporal scleral pocket incisions.[15] Scleral compared to limbal placement of the 7-mm incision resulted in a greater wound strength in both superior and temporal wounds. This has also been demonstrated for smaller incisions in cadaver eye studies,[13] but may only be a theoretical disadvantage for corneal tunnel incisions smaller than 3.5 mm, considering the thousands of sutureless corneal tunnel operations that have been performed. The incisions currently used for small incision phacoemulsification and foldable IOL implantation can be as small as 3.2 mm for almost all cases[11,16] and can be considered to be almost astigmatic neutral, as shown in several studies. These incisions demonstrate a high postoperative wound stability. With the correctly performed construction and size of corneal/limbal tunnel incisions, the wound stability has been excellent in my last 500 cases, in which no postoperative suturing had to be performed or wound leakage occurred.

CLEAR CORNEAL INCISION AFTER PENETRATING KERATOPLASTY OR INCISIONAL REFRACTIVE PROCEDURES

Cataract surgery in eyes following previous penetrating keratoplasty or refractive surgery should be regarded as a difficult procedure. The integrity of a human eye following these procedures is reduced; more reduced after incisional surgery than after other keratorefractive procedures like surface ablation, photorefarctive keratectomy or lamellar surgery like automated lamellar keratotomy or LASIK.[17]

The primary concern for cataract extraction in eyes with previous radial keratotomy or penetrating keratoplasty would be intra- or postoperative wound dehiscence.[18] A compromised intraoperative view due to scarring in the cornea and corneal decompensation following the intraocular intervention should be considered. Preoperatively, these points should be advised to the patient and preoperative evaluation of the eye should include endothelial cell count and careful slit lamp examination of the cornea which would reveal any corneal wound gaps of radial incisions. Manipulation of the eye needs to be as atraumatic as possible. I would use small incision cataract surgery using a self-sealing incision with foldable IOL implantation through an appropriately sized wound.[10,19]

Clear corneal or limbal incisions should only be used if the radial cuts do not extend to the limbus; if they do, the tunnel entry should be further behind the limbus using a corneoscleral tunnel approach. In no case should the groove of the tunnel incision intersect the radial incisions. Of course, this would be more difficult in a 12- or 16-cut radial keratotomy cornea. Postoperative astigmatic changes in an eye with previous incisional corneal surgery are not as predictable as with virgin eyes, therefore, I would not perform any type of astigmatism correction before or at the time of cataract extraction. The incision would be placed temporally, a location that gives the best access to the eye, provides the best postoperative wound stability, induces the least astigmatism, and has the greatest distance from the central corneal dome.[19]

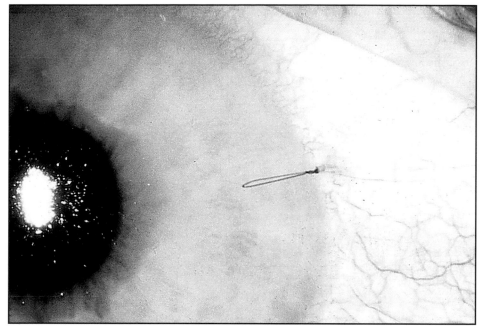

Figure 17-4a. Radial suture of a limbal incision. The suture is placed to prevent postoperative wound leakage or iris prolapse in clear corneal or limbal incisions larger than 4 mm regularly. Suture after 5-mm incision to implant a 5-mm optic PMMA IOL.

If at any time of the procedure wound dehiscence of a radial incision should occur, immediate closing with interrupted 10-0 nylon sutures would be performed. The longer the period since the previous radial keratotomy procedure, the more stable would be the cornea.[20,21]

TUNNEL PERFORATION

Tearing of the roof of the corneal tunnel (Figures 17-4a and 17-4b) predisposes to excessive intraoperative leakage, compromising anterior chamber stability, and to postoperative wound leakage. If the tear occurs at either edge of the roof, then surgery can usually be completed using this incision, proceeding slowly and observing the wound carefully as instruments are introduced or manipulated in the eye. It is usually preferable to suture the incision at the conclusion of surgery, even if the wound is watertight, in order to restore a more normal architecture and prevent external wound gape.

If, however, the roof is perforated in the center of the flap and this is noted prior to entering the anterior chamber, one should consider making a new incision. If the cut is extremely small (eg, <0.5 mm), one can sometimes proceed as noted above with lateral roof tears. Prior to IOL insertion, the opposite margin of the wound is enlarged, and, to prevent further tearing, the incision should be made larger than normal for IOL insertion. Suture closure (radial direction) is usually advisable to restore normal wound architecture (Figures 17-5a and 17-5b).

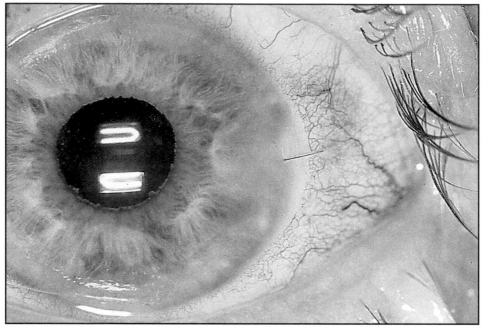

Figure 17-4b. Suture in a case with severe IOP at the end of surgery. The fluorescein test did not reveal any leakage.

IRIS PROLAPSE

With tunnel incisions, the incidence of iris prolapse has been reduced tremendously. If the clear corneal incision is constructed correctly, an iris prolapse is almost impossible. If it occurs, two reasons have to be considered.

Iris prolapse is usually caused by entering the anterior chamber too posteriorly (eg, near the iris root). If this is noted early in the case and interferes with easy introduction of instruments into the eye, it is often advisable to suture the lateral part of the incision and try to finish the case; if not possible, the whole incision should be sutured and a new incision could be created at another location.

A second and more ominous cause of iris prolapse is an acute increase of IOP accompanied by choroidal effusion or hemorrhage. In this instance, the surgeon should attempt to identify the cause and to lower the IOP. Sometimes digital massage on the eye, pressing directly on the incision, can successfully lower the pressure. It is useful to examine the fundus to ascertain if there is a choroidal effusion or hemorrhage. With choroidal effusion, aspiration of vitreous can be helpful, as can be the administration of IV mannitol. If there is a choroidal hemorrhage or the increased IOP from an effusion is resistant to treatment, surgery is usually best terminated. The wound is carefully sutured, and intraocular miotics and a peripheral iridectomy may be performed to assist in repositioning the iris. For effusions, surgery can be deferred until later in the day or until the next day when the fluid dynamics of the eye have returned to a more normal condition. If a limited choroidal hemorrhage has occurred, it is best to wait 2 to 3 weeks prior to further surgery.

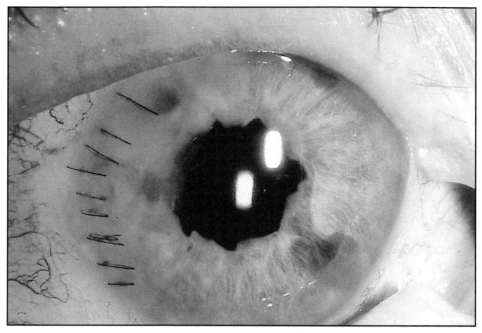

Figure 17-5a. Corneal burn following phacoemulsification. In this patient with an apparent filtering bleb, phacoemulsification was performed through a temporal clear corneal incision. Posterior capsular rupture was suspected, and the surgeon injected a highly retentive viscoelastic agent beneath and in front of the nucleus to minimize the risk of posterior dislocation of the nucleus. Phacoemulsification was instituted with low flow and vacuum settings, and a severe corneal burn was immediately produced due to obstruction of the phacoemulsification tip by the viscoelastic material. The incision was sutured with several interrupted sutures. Many of these pulled through the injured tissue, and additional suturing was required several days later. Postoperatively, the patient has 5 D of surgically induced astigmatism that has persisted for more than 5 years.

Postoperative iris prolapse can occur in unsutured clear corneal incisions that are not self-sealing anymore,[22] therefore, I recommend suturing all incisions larger than 4 mm with one radial suture to prevent this type of complication[2] (see Figures 17-4a and 17-4b).

WOUND DEHISCENCE AND LEAKAGE
Dehiscence

With clear corneal tunnel incisions, preferably hinged, wound dehiscence is relatively uncommon. Creation of an internal corneal valve typically prevents the major complications of wound leakage, inadvertent filtering bleb, and epithelial downgrowth for both scleral and clear corneal incisions. The wound healing process varies according to the site of the posterior entry.

For corneal incisions, closure of the external wound is by apposition or, in areas of wound gape, by an epithelial plaque. A gradual process of remodeling then occurs, consisting of fibrocytic metaplasia of keratocytes with deposition of new

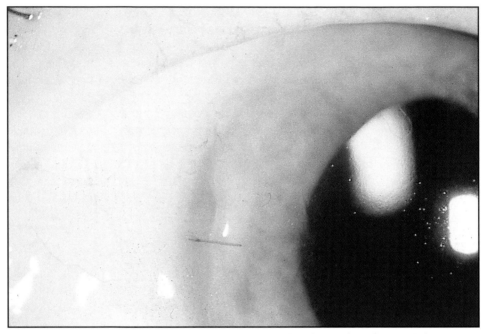

Figure 17-5b. Corneal burn during the procedure resulted in melting of corneal tissue, which had to be resutured at the end of the case.

collagen again parallel to the incision, followed over a period of years by remodeling similar to that seen with scleral incisions.[23] In the absence of vascular tissue, this process occurs much more slowly than in scleral or limbal tissue.[24] Therefore, my technique of corneal incision has changed over the past 6 years from a real clear corneal incision to an entry of the incision in the vascular arcade. During the first minutes of the procedure, a slight bleeding of the limbal vessels can be seen (see Figures 17-2a and 17-2b); this will enhance postoperative wound healing.[24] Postoperative abnormalities in wound structure are produced by defects in the tunnel architecture or to defective wound healing due to systemic disorders, pre-existing tissue abnormalities (eg, excessively thin or weak tissue), and/or incarceration of material such as lens, vitreous, or iris in the wound, inhibiting the normal wound healing process.

Leakage

Intraoperative wound leakage can cause anterior chamber fluctuations, sometimes even an anterior chamber collapse during the procedure. Intraoperative difficulties during the whole case could be created and postoperatively corneal problems might occur. Therefore, meticulous preparation of the clear corneal or limbal incision with the appropriate size for the used phaco tip diameter is essential to prevent intraoperative leakage.

A wound leak that occurs in the immediate postoperative period is usually due to inadequate suture closure for a specific wound configuration. This entity is rare

with tunnel constructions. Corneal incisions as small as 3.5 mm in width seal remarkably well, even though intraoperative pinpoint posterior lip pressure in these eyes can often induce a wound leak. Some surgeons perform hydration of the corneal stroma to minimize the wound leak that can be elicited with posterior lip pressure; however, this hydration clears within a few minutes to hours, and it is uncertain if in fact this has any actual clinical value.

Medical management of corneal wound leaks may include decreasing or stopping corticosteroid therapy; administration of prophylactic topical antibiotics; pressure patching; insertion of a collagen shield, bandage lens, or disposable contact lens; and administration of aqueous inhibitors. Suturing of a leaking wound is usually necessary if the leak persists after 5 to 7 days or there is a flat anterior chamber, iris prolapse, extensive external tissue gape, or excessive against-the-wound astigmatism.

THERMAL BURNS

Thermal burns will occur much quicker in corneal/limbal incisions than in scleral tunnel cases. Part of the energy produced by the phacoemulsification tip is dissipated as heat. This heat is conducted into the eye along the titanium tip and is cooled by the ongoing flow of the I/A fluid. If for any reason the cooling is blocked, a corneal burn can occur within 1 to 3 seconds. The most common cause is inadequate flow through the phaco tip obstructed by a retentive viscoelastic agent due to use of low flow and vacuum settings. The critical warning sign is the appearance of milky fluid that is produced around the phaco tip as emulsification is begun.

To avoid corneal burns, the surgeon should always test phacoemulsification and I/A functions before entering the eye. The surgeon can aspirate some of the viscoelastic material overlying the nucleus prior to beginning emulsification to ensure that aspiration is adequate. To prevent constriction of the irrigating sleeve, one should select an incision size appropriate for each particular phacoemulsification tip. New sleeves that are not compressible avoid the occurrence of corneal burns during surgery. If a burn has occurred, meticulous suturing of the wound with multiple radial sutures (see Figures 17-5a and 17-5b) is required. A bandage contact lens may assist with wound closure. Severe postoperative astigmatism can result.

RUPTURED POSTERIOR CAPSULE
AND CONVERSION TO EXTRACAPSULAR PROCEDURES

Although posterior capsule rupture is the most common serious intraoperative complication of cataract surgery, proper management can result in minimal morbidity to the patient. After residual lens and/or cortical material removal and anterior vitrectomy,[25] the surgeon can choose based on the status of the capsular remnants the implantation of a posterior chamber IOL in the bag, in the ciliary sulcus, or as sutured posterior chamber IOL. The fourth option would be an anterior chamber IOL. If a foldable IOL is used, the incision should be slightly larger than the regular incision size for the chosen IOL; this is done to manage safe and atraumatic IOL implantation. If, however, a rigid IOL (posterior or anterior chamber IOL) is

implanted, the incision has to be enlarged to 5.5 to 6 mm. In order to maintain as much of the self-sealing properties of a clear corneal/limbal incision as possible, it should be enlarged by maintaining the length of the tunnel. A side-cutting diamond knife or a sharp steel blade is used to open the tunnel construction almost limbus parallel. Following IOL implantation the incision should be sutured with two to three radial sutures to prevent iris prolapse, postoperative wound leakage, or further complications (Figure 17-6). The sutures can be removed after 2 to 4 weeks.

If a conversion to extracapsular procedures is necessary, the surgeon should proceed as described above with the appropriate enlargement to deliver the nucleus out of the anterior chamber. The incision should be closed also with several radial sutures which can be removed after 4 to 8 weeks.

ANTERIOR SEGMENT HEMORRHAGE

The incidence of anterior segment hemorrhage (intraocular bleeding, postoperative hyphema, endocapsular hematoma) is reduced with clear corneal incisions.

- Intraocular blood decreases the surgeon's view during the procedure, stimulates postoperative inflammation and synechia formation, and accelerates capsular opacification. To minimize the risk of bleeding, one can consider discontinuing anti-coagulant therapy prior to surgery if this does not pose a significant medical risk to the patient. The sites of anterior segment hemorrhage are either the wound or the iris. Steps to minimize or eliminate bleeding from the wound include careful cautery of bleeding vessels in the vicinity of the incision, creation of an adequate internal corneal valve to minimize the likelihood of scleral blood entering into the anterior chamber, and performing a clear corneal incision.
- Postoperative hyphema is caused by a bleeding vessel from the wound or iris. Bleeding from the wound can be avoided by the usage of clear corneal incisions. Late hyphema or microhyphema is most often caused by chafing of the IOL against the iris or ciliary body.[26] A rare cause of postoperative bleeding is hemorrhage from vascularization of the internal margin of the incision (Swan's syndrome[27]); this can be diagnosed by noting neovascularization of the wound by gonioscopy and can be treated by argon laser photocoagulation.
- Endocapsular hematoma is a postoperative entrapment of blood between the posterior surface of the IOL and the posterior capsule.[28] It is a variant of hyphema with the exception that the blood can become entrapped within the capsular bag for months or even permanently.

ENDOTHELIAL CELL LOSS, CORNEAL EDEMA, AND BULLOUS KERATOPATHY

Possible disadvantags of phacoemulsification through a corneal tunnel incision include thermal damage from the phacoemulsification tip, greater mechanical stress on the cornea, and the proximity to the corneal endothelial cell layer. However, the endothelial cell loss following phacoemulsification through a temporal clear corneal tunnel compared favorably with endothelial cell loss rates after other cataract extraction procedures.[29]

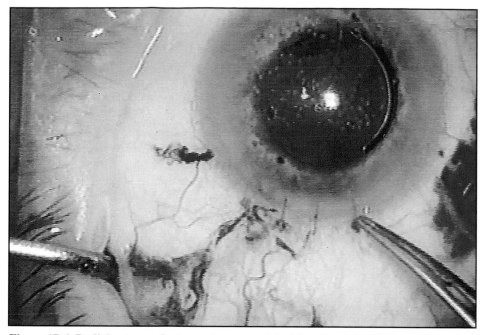

Figure 17-6. Radial sutures of a large clear corneal incision. Several radial sutures were placed in this patient who had a capsular rupture, extracapsular cataract extraction, required anterior vitrectomy and implantation of a PMMA IOL for sulcus implantation with 6-mm incision. The sutures are placed to ensure wound closer.

Factors that predispose to corneal edema following cataract surgery include prior endothelial disease or cell loss, intraoperative mechanical endothelial trauma, excessive postoperative inflammation, and prolonged postoperative elevation of IOP. Preoperatively, patients should be carefully examined to determine if there is any evidence of Fuchs' dystrophy or other conditions that produce a low endothelial cell count. Although most patients with Fuchs' dystrophy have guttata that are readily visible with slit lamp examination, in rare instances, patients can have low endothelial cell counts in the absence of guttata. It is often advisable to obtain an endothelial cell count in the fellow eye.

There are several measures that can be taken intra- and postoperatively to minimize the risk of corneal injury. For some surgeons, extracapsular cataract extraction may be safer than phacoemulsification. Techniques to remove the nucleus in the posterior chamber seem to minimize endothelial cell loss,[30] and there is evidence that highly retentive viscoelastic agents are more protective when surgical removal of the nucleus occurs near the endothelium. Postoperatively, inflammation should be aggressively treated with topical corticosteroids, and IOP should be controlled below 20 mmHg. Mechanical factors, such as Descemet's detachment or retained nuclear fragments in the angle touching the endothelium, should be addressed. For symptomatic relief, hypertonic saline ointment is sometimes helpful as a temporizing measure. Sequential corneal pachymetry is an excellent means of documenting the progress of postoperative corneal edema. Postoperative corneal edema may take as long as 3 months to clear, so it is usually advisable to wait at least this long prior to recommending penetrating keratoplasty.

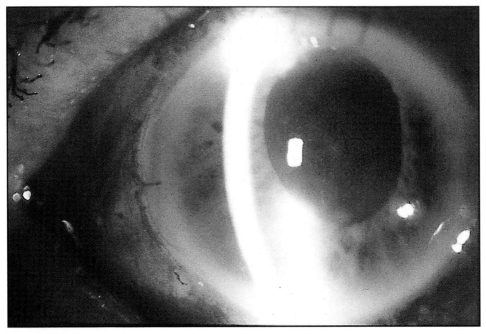

Figure 17-7. Postoperative endophthalmitis. This patient developed an acute postoperative endophthalmitis after clear corneal cataract surgery and PMMA posterior chamber IOL implantation. During cataract surgery a capsular break occurred, and an anterior vitrectomy was performed. The patient was successfully treated with vitrectomy and injection of intravitreal antibiotics combined with postoperative topical antibiotic therapy. Final visual acuity was 20/50.

ENDOPHTHALMITIS

In the beginning of the clear corneal incision era, several postoperative endophthalmitis cases were reported. However, most of these cases had an incorrect wound construction with postoperative wound leaks or dehiscence (Figure 17-7). Now, as most surgeons are aware of the potential complications and treat the wound under the above described conditions, the rate has not been found to be higher than with scleral tunnel incisions.

REFERENCES

1. Long DA, Monica ML. A prospective evaluation of corneal curvature changes with 3.0- to 3.5-mm corneal tunnel phacoemulsification. *Ophthalmology.* 1996;103:226-232.
2. Kohnen T, Dick B, Jacobi KW. Comparison of induced astigmatism after temporal clear corneal tunnel incisions of different sizes. *J Cataract Refract Surg.* 1995;21:417-424.
3. Masket S, Tennen DG. Astigmatic stabilization of 3.0 mm temporal clear corneal cataract incisions. *J Cataract Refract Surg.* 1996;22:1451-1455.
4. Fine IH. Self-sealing corneal tunnel incision for small-incision cataract surgery. *Ocular Surgery News.* 1992;10(9):38-39.

5. Ernest PH, Neuhann T. Posterior limbal incision. *J Cataract Refract Surg*. 1996;22:78-84.
6. Radner W, Menapace R, Zehetmayer M, Mallinger R. Ultrastructure of clear cornea incisions. Part I: effect of keratomes and incision width on the corneal trauma after IOL-implantation. *J Cataract Refract Surg*. 1998;24:487-492.
7. Radner W, Amon M, Mallinger R. Diamond-tip versus blunt-tip caliper enlargement of clear corneal incisions. *J Cataract Refract Surg*. 1997;23:272-276.
8. Steinert RF, Deacon J. Enlargement of incision width during phacoemulsification and folded intraocular lens implant surgery. *Ophthalmology*. 1996;103:220-225.
9. Mackool RJ, Russell RS. Effect of foldable intraocular lens insertion on incision width. *J Cataract Refract Surg*. 1996;22:571-574.
10. Kohnen T, Lambert JR, Koch DD. Incision sizes for foldable intraocular lenses. *Ophthalmology*. 1997;104:1277-1286.
11. Kohnen T, Koch DD. Experimental and clinical evaluation of incision size and shape following forceps and injector implantation of a three-piece high-refractive-index silicone intraocular lens. *Graefes Arch Clin Exp Ophthalmol*. In press.
12. Langerman DW. Architectural design of self-sealing corneal tunnel, single-hinge incision. *J Cataract Refract Surg*. 1994;20:84-88.
13. Ernest PH, Fenzel R, Lavery KT, Sensoli A. Relative stability of clear corneal incisions in a cadaver eye model. *J Cataract Refract Surg*. 1995;21:39-42.
14. Anders N, Pham DT, Antoni HJ, Wollensak J. Postoperative astigmatism and relative strength of scleral tunnel incisions: a prospective clinical trial. *J Cataract Refract Surg*. 1997;23:332-336.
15. Kohnen T, Mann PM, Husain SE, Abarca A, Koch DD. Corneal topographic changes and induced astigmatism resulting from superior and temporal scleral pocket incisions. *Ophthalmic Surg Lasers*. 1996;27:263-269.
16. Olson R, Cameron R, Hovis T, et al. Clinical evaluation of the Unfolder. *J Cataract Refract Surg*. 1997;23:1384-1389.
17. Peacock L, Slade S, Martiz J, Chuang A, Yee R. Ocular integrity after refractive procedures. *Ophthalmology*. 1997;104(7):1079-1083.
18. Budak K, Friedman NJ, Koch DD. Dehiscence of a radial keratotomy incision during clear corneal cataract surgery. *J Cataract Refract Surg*. 1998;24:278-280.
19. Kohnen T. After RK, many patients are maturing and developing cataracts. What incision method would you choose after 8-incision RK? Do you modify your approach for 12 or 16 incisions? Does the length of time after RK surgery matter? In: Masket S, ed. Consultation section. *J Cataract Refract Surg*. 1998;24:150-151.
20. Deg JK, Zavala EY, Binder PS. Delayed corneal wound healing following radial keratotomy. *Ophthalmology*. 1985;92:734-740.
21. Binder PS, Nayak SK, Deg JK, Zavala EY, Sugar J. An ultrastructural and histochemical study of long-term wound healing after radial keratotomy. *Am J Ophthalmol*. 1987;103:432-440.
22. Menapace R. Delayed iris prolapse with unsutured 5.1 mm clear corneal incisions. *J Cataract Refract Surg*. 1995;21:353-357.
23. Koch DD, Smith SH, Whiteside SB. Limbal and scleral wound healing. In: Beuerman RW, Crosson CE, Kaufman HE, eds. *Healing Processes in the Cornea*. Houston, Texas: Gulf; 1989;165-182.
24. Ernest PH, Tippermann R, Eagle R, et al. Is there a difference in incision healing based on location? *J Cataract Refract Surg*. 1998;24:482-486.
25. Kohnen T, Friedman NJ, Koch DD. The lens. Complications of cataract surgery. In: Yanoff M, Duker J, eds. *Ophthalmology*. London, England: Mosby. In press.

26. Johnson SH, Kratz RP, Olson PF. Iris transillumination and microhyphema syndrome. *Am Intra-Ocular Implant Soc J*. 1984;10:425-428.

27. Swan KC. Hyphema due to wound vascularization after cataract extraction. *Arch Ophthalmol*. 1973;89:87-90.

28. Hagan III JC, Menapace R, Radax U. Clinical syndrome of endocapsular hematoma: presentation of a collected series and review of the literature. *J Cataract Refract Surg*. 1996;22:379-384.

29. Dick HB, Kohnen T, Jacobi FK, Jacobi KW. Long-term endothelial cell loss following phacoemulsification through a temporal clear corneal incision. *J Cataract Refract Surg*. 1996;22:63-71.

30. Koch DD, Liu JF, Glasser DB, Merin LM, Haft E. A comparison of corneal endothelial changes after use of Healon or Viscoat during phacoemulsification. *Am J Ophthalmol*. 1993;115:188-201.

Clear Lensectomy

Robert H. Osher, MD

The idea of removing a clear crystalline lens for the sole purpose of correcting a refractive error was radical. When Verzella advocated this surgical alternative for high myopia in the mid-1980s, surgeons were either intrigued or downright hostile.[1] There was no middle group. The proponents said that severe myopia was a major visual disability that could be managed by a standard surgical approach. The opponents quoted studies where the incidence of retinal detachment following cataract surgery in myopes was unacceptably high, and which could not be justified.[2-4] While the debate was heating up for the high myopes, a 43-year-old chemist was referred to me with a history of contact lens intolerance. He was terribly unhappy wearing "coke bottle" spectacles to correct his 11 D of hyperopia.

His symptoms were identical to those of aphakic patients with contact lens intolerance in whom a secondary implant provided a wonderful solution to their high hyperopia. If we could justify the risks to allow selected aphakes to become deliriously happy, why not apply the same rationale to the phakic high hyperope. After all, the incidence of serious complications such as retinal detachment associated with clear lens extraction in the high myope was not comparable, and small incision surgery using phacoemulsification had elevated the safety and success of lens extraction to unprecedented levels.

Armed with these convictions, I initially operated upon a small series of high hyperopes whose refractive error was between +7.5 D and +11 D. The axial length measured 20.0 mm or less and the selected IOL power was between +31 D and +37 D. These patients were fully informed and their uncomplicated lensectomies

were followed by implantation of single-piece PMMA lenses placed within the capsular bag. Each patient was highly satisfied with his surgical outcome...even though I was not. Regardless of the IOL formula selected, the intended refractive error was missed by as much as 4 D of residual hyperopia. One patient experienced a reduction in visual acuity due to a swollen optic disc without an afferent pupil or visual field defect that resolved after 5 months. Even with this complication, the surgery provided a valid alternative to an unacceptable refractive problem that resulted in improved functional vision. The indications for surgical intervention were sound and each patient was happy so I had no regrets despite harsh criticism from a handful of colleagues.

In 1987, I presented a paper summarizing the preliminary results of hyperopic lensectomy at the annual meeting of the American Society of Cataract and Refractive Surgery (ASCRS). I updated this series with longer follow-up data 2 years later at the ASCRS meeting and published a representative case in "Controversies in Cataract Surgery" on the *Audiovisual Journal of Cataract & Refractive Surgery* in 1989.[5] I became more comfortable in the OR performing phacoemulsification upon the small eye with a shallow anterior chamber that often had a tendency toward positive pressure. I also became more aware of the importance of selecting the IOL power when the axial length was 21 mm or less. In addition to consulting some of the leading experts who have published their formulas for IOL selection in short eyes (Drs. Kenneth J. Hoffer,[6] Jack Holladay[7]), we developed a database correlating axial length and an additive "fudge factor" necessary to achieve emmetropia from which the IOL could be selected empirically.

Other ophthalmic surgeons also experienced favorable results following clear lens extraction in hyperopic eyes. Lyle and Jin reported six hyperopic eyes with a range from +4.25 D to +7.87 D who underwent routine phacoemulsification.[8] The mean axial length was 20.86 mm and the mean IOL power was 29.50 D. No intra- or postoperative complications were encountered and all six eyes achieved a postoperative uncorrected Snellen visual acuity of 20/40 or better. The mean postoperative spherical equivalent was -0.42 D and all eyes were within 1 D of emmetropia.

A subsequent publication by the same authors expanded their series to 20 eyes.[9] Uncorrected visual acuity improved from 20/200 preoperatively to 20/30 postoperatively. Eighty-nine percent of eyes achieved an uncorrected visual acuity of 20/40 or better and all eyes corrected to 20/25 or better. There were no surgical or postoperative complications with a mean follow-up of 23.2 months. The Holladay formula proved the most accurate, resulting in the mean postoperative spherical equivalent of -0.21 ± 0.89 (SD) when the surgeon aimed for -1.00 D sphere.

Dr. Paul Koch reported a similar series at the ASCRS meeting in 1993. He performed a clear lensectomy on 10 eyes of six patients with hyperopia ranging between +1.50 D and +10.50 D with a mean of +4.75 D. The average axial length was 22.3 mm and the mean IOL power was +28.0 D. No intraoperative complications were encountered, but additional surgery was required in four eyes because of residual refractive errors. An IOL exchange was performed in two eyes, radial keratotomy after IOL exchange in one eye, and astigmatic keratotomy for induced astigmatism in one eye. We combined our data in a collaborative presentation to the

European Society of Cataract and Refractive Surgery in Innsbruck, Austria, during September 1994.

Siganos and associates from Greece have presented their experience in a series of 17 eyes at the 1993 annual meeting of the International Society of Refractive Keratoplasty and later discussed their approach on the *Audiovisual Journal of Cataract & Refractive Surgery*.[10] In several related publications[11,12] they published their results in 35 eyes of 21 patients with a hyperopic spherical equivalent of +9.19 ± 0.34 D and a range of +6.75 D to +13.75 D. Refraction was aimed at emmetropia by targeting -1.50 D using the SRKII and SRKT formulae in 17 and 18 eyes, respectively. Follow-up was up to 5 years. The results showed a mean unaided visual acuity in all eyes of 20/25, and 91.4% were within ±1 D of emmetropia. One eye required IOL exchange and myopic photorefractive keratectomy was performed on another eye because of an IOL miscalculation greater than 2 D.

Another series has been published by Isfahani, Salz, and coworkers[13,14] in which 18 hyperopic eyes of 10 patients underwent phacoemulsification with posterior chamber lens implantation using the Hoffer Q formula. The mean spherical equivalent was +6.17 D with a range of +4.25 D to +9.62 D. The mean axial length was 21 mm with a range from 17.64 to 22.65 mm. The mean postoperative spherical equivalent was 0.21 D, and all eyes achieved an uncorrected visual acuity of 20/40 or better. No intra- or postoperative complications were reported, although two patients lost 2 lines of best corrected visual acuity (20/30) without any identifiable reason.

The limiting factor in improving the success of hyperopic lens extraction is the relative inaccuracy of modern IOL calculation formulas for the short eye. In the Siganos series, the surgeon deliberately selected a postoperative refractive error of -1.50 D. In the Isfahani series, the IOL error margin was approximately +0.8 D. While current third-generation formulas (Holladay, SRK-T, and Hoffer Q) are more accurate, Holladay is convinced that newer formulas that use additional anterior segment measurements, such as corneal diameter, anterior chamber depth, and lens thickness, will be required for improved accuracy because the anterior segment is often not proportional to the axial length.[7]

There has also been a problem with the availability of high-powered IOLs in the United States. Gayton introduced the concept of piggybacking IOLs in 1993.[15] He initially used two plano-convex lenses and fit the two plano sides together to make one biconvex lens, placing the posterior-most IOL in the capsular bag and the haptics of the second IOL in the sulcus. He subsequently modified his surgical technique using either two single-piece biconvex PMMA lenses or two acrylic foldable lenses placing both within the capsular bag. Gills expanded the concept by implanting multiple IOLs into an eye. He also corrected the underpowered pseudophake by implanting a secondary IOL anterior to the original implant.[16]

There is one other condition that warrants mention in the discussion of hyperopic lensectomy. The nanophthalmic eye with its small cornea, shallow anterior chamber, and short axial length is not only a difficult eye upon which to operate but also has a higher risk of intra- and postoperative complications.[17,18] Phacoemulsification probably minimizes these risks even though the surgeon should be prepared for a challenging phaco with positive pressure and chamber

collapse. Should the surgeon encounter a uveal infusion, he or she should be familiar with a sclerotomy technique.[19]

CONCLUSION

Perhaps the future of refractive surgery for the high hyperope will bring new and exciting alternatives such as phakic implantation, the subject of other chapters. At the present time, clear lens extraction using small incision cataract surgery remains a valid alternative to contact lens and spectacle intolerance in our severely farsighted patients. As I concluded in 1987 and in subsequent presentations: "We must keep an open mind and a willingness to explore...as we venture along the untrodden path that leads into the frontier of refractive surgery."[20-22]

REFERENCES

1. Verzella F. Refractive surgery of the lens in high myopes. *Refract Corneal Surg.* 1990;6:273-275.
2. Lindstrom RL. Refractive surgery for the high myope: controversy and concern. [Editorial.] *J Refract Surg.* 1987;3:77-78.
3. Lindstrom RL. Ophthalmologic debate: is it reasonable to remove a healthy lens to improve vision? *JAMA.* 1987;257:2005.
4. Goldberg MF. Clear lens extraction for axial myopia: an appraisal. *Ophthalmology.* 1992;99(suppl):108.
5. Osher RH. Controversies in cataract surgery. *Audiovisual Journal of Cataract & Refractive Surgery.* 1989;5(3).
6. Hoffer KJ. The Hoffer Q formula: a comparison of theoretic and regression formulas. *J Cataract Refract Surg.* 1993;19:700-712.
7. Holladay JT, Gills JP, Leidlein J, Cherchio M. Achieving emmetropia in extremely short eyes with two piggyback posterior chamber intraocular lenses. *Ophthalmology.* 1996;103:1118-1123.
8. Lyle WA, Jin GJC. Clear lens extraction for the correction of high refractive error. *J Cataract Refract Surg.* 1994;20:273-276.
9. Lyle WA, Jin GJC. Clear lens extraction to correct hyperopia. *J Cataract Refract Surg.* 1997;23:1051-1056.
10. Siganos DS. Refractive cataract surgery. *Audiovisual Journal of Cataract & Refractive Surgery.* 1995;11(1).
11. Siganos DS, Siganos CS, Pallikaris IG. Clear lens extraction and intraocular lens implantation in normally sighted hyperopia eyes. *J Refract Corneal Surg.* 1994;10:117-121.
12. Siganos DS, Pallikaris IG, Siganos CS. Clear lensectomy and intraocular lens implantation in normally sighted highly hyperopic eyes: three-year follow-up. *Eur J Implant Ref Surg.* 1995;7:128-133.
13. Isfahani AHK, Salz JJ. Clear lens extraction with intraocular lens implantation for the correction of hyperopia. In: Sher N, ed. *Surgery for Hyperopia and Presbyopia.* Baltimore, Md: Williams & Wilkins; 1997.
14. Isfahani AHK, et al. Surgical correction of hyperopia. In: Abbott R, Hwang D, eds. *Refractive Surgery—Ophthalmology Clinics of North America.* Philadelphia, Pa: WB Saunders Co; 1997.
15. Gayton JL, Sanders VN. Implanting two posterior chamber lenses in a case of microphthalmos. *J Cataract Refract Surg.* 1993;19:776-777.
16. Gills JP. Implantation of multiple intraocular lenses to optimize visual results. In: Best Papers of 1995 Symposium on Cataract, IOL, and Refractive Surgery.

J Cataract Refract Surg. 1995;(suppl):42-47.

17. Brockhurst RJ. Cataract surgery in nanophthalmic eyes. *Arch Ophthalmol.* 1990;108:965-967.

18. Nishida A, Uchida S, Onishi T. Cataract surgery for nanophthalmic eye. *Jpn J Clin Ophthalmol.* 1995;49:509-511.

19. Jin JC, Anderson DR. Laser and unsutured sclerotomy in nanophthalmos. *Am J Ophthalmol.* 1990;109:575-580.

20. Osher RH. Discussant. Management of patients with high ametropia who seek refractive surgical correction. *Eur J Implant Ref Surg.* 1994;6:298-299.

21. Osher RH. Clear lens extraction. [Letter.] *J Cataract Refract Surg.* 1994;20:674.

22. Osher RH. Hyperopic lensectomy: an update. Presented at American Academy of Ophthalmology Annual Meeting, San Francisco, 1997.

Implantable Contact Lens

Roberto Zaldivar, MD, Susana Oscherow, MD,
Giselle Ricur, MD

INTRODUCTION

We have all witnessed the tremendous progress in refractive surgery during these past years. Many surgical techniques have come and gone leaving behind invaluable information and teachings.

Basically, refractive surgery can be divided into two main groups: keratorefractive techniques and lenticular refractive procedures. The advantages of the latter are:

- Their precision, predictability, and reversibility
- Immediate onset of desired effect
- Long-term stability
- Little or no adverse effects on corneal stabilization
- Clear optic zone
- Relatively painless postop
- Cost efficiency

Obviously, we are all aware of open eye surgery disadvantages such as risk of intraoperative complications, cystoid macular edema, endophthalmitis, retinal detachment, as well as loss of accommodation in pre-presbyopic patients as in clear lens extraction.[1-3]

The first modern experiences with phakic IOLs were made in the late 1950s and 1960s by Barraquer, Strampelli, and Choyce.[4-12] Many patients (phakic and aphakic) required lens explantation within the first 3 years due to the development of corneal decompensation or the uveitis-glaucoma-hyphema syndrome.[5,13-17] In our opinion, the main causes of the adverse reactions these investigators encountered were:

- Poor lens design technology which made them very rigid, not allowing adequate positioning in the angle
- Large or inadequately sized lenses
- Lack of knowledge and therefore decreased emphasis on achieving and maintaining a safe distance between the implant and corneal endothelium

The state of surgical technology at the time (eg, the absence of high-grade surgical microscopes, delicate sutures such as 10-0 nylon, and viscoelastic substances) also hindered the investigators.

In cataract surgery, initial experiences with anterior chamber lenseswere also poor worldwide.[5,8,9,14] The complications that ensued were difficult to resolve. We feel that contributing factors to this were:

- Anterior chamber lenses were too rigid, or the loops so flexible, that they caused intermittent touching of the corneal endothelium
- Rigidity of the IOLs caused neovascularization of the angle and pain due to lack of lens elasticity

Afterwards, improvement in lens technology, such as the Multiflex lens of Kelman, showed better results.[18,19] Due to the emerging posterior chamber lens industry, further research and development of anterior chamber lenses were practically abandoned. The consequences were:

- Technically poor anterior chamber lenses at the end of the 1960s, such as the first-generation anterior chamber lenses (eg, Choyce's Mark I lens) or the rigid lenses of the 1970s and early 1980s[14,20]
- The use of anterior chamber lenses as secondary implants, or when complications appeared with first-generation posterior chamber lenses

The association of anterior chamber lenses with surgical and post surgical complications made the study of their use as phakic implants difficult.[5,13-15,17,21-23] Their tarnished image may have been avoided with continued improvements in quality and technology.

In the late 1980s, we became interested in treating high ametropias, such as high myopia. Our first experiences were made with clear lens extractions (CLE).[24] The results were acceptable, but problems with CLE included:

- Loss of accommodation in young patients
- Posterior capsule opacity, which made exams of the vitreous and peripheral retina difficult
- High YAG capsulotomy rates, with increased risk of retinal detachments
- Difficulties in lens power calculations[22,25]
- Need for implanting more than one IOL (piggyback technique) in cases of extreme refractive errors[26-28]

Although CLE offers the advantage of relatively deepening the anterior chamber as opposed to the anterior chamber lenses, the difficulties encountered persuaded us to try phakic anterior chamber lenses.[9,29,30]

Renewed interest in these lens began with Baikoff's new angle supported PMMA anterior chamber lens in 1986.[29,31-34] Other anterior chamber lenses developed were the Momose spider glass lens and the Worst iris claw PMMA lens.[35-39]

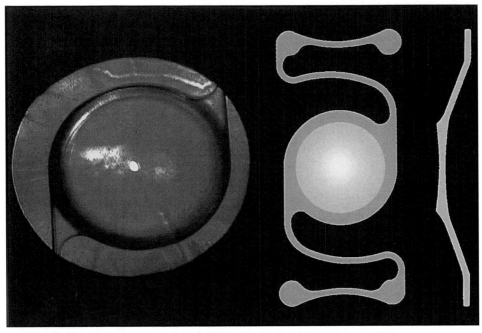

Figure 19-1. Baikoff anterior chamber phakic IOL. Model Domilens ZB5M.
Photograph on the left is a retroilluminated image (retroillumination mode) captured with the Nidek EAS 1000 camera. The sketch on the right shows the IOL. Optic diameter of 5.0 mm (effective optical diameter: 4.0 mm). Lengths vary in size from 12.5 to 13.5 mm.

We began our experience with the first-generation Domilens Model ZB.[11,12,34,40] At first we had excellent optical results. Afterwards, we began to notice that certain patients, especially ones with high diopter models, showed endothelial alterations attributed to the closeness of the anterior chamber lens. Eye rubbing would provoke direct contact of the ZB with the endothelium and cell loss patterns resembled the outline of the implant.

These models were discontinued and replaced with the ZB5, and very shortly afterwards with the Chiron/Domilens Model ZB5M (Figure 19-1). The differences between the ZB5M and its predecessors were:
- Optic diameter of 4.5 mm and decreased optic thickness
- Polished edges
- Ring around the optics to prevent it from getting close to the endothelium
- New IOL shoulder angle of 20 degrees, instead of 25 degrees, which also kept it farther away from the cornea

This new design permitted direct compression of the eye without producing forward intraocular movement of the lenses associated with the other models. The endothelial response was quite acceptable in patients with uneventful surgery. Later, the third-generation Baikoff anterior chamber lens was developed by Bausch & Lomb Surgical/Chiron Vision. Model NuVita MA20 and its initial studies revealed stable results and non-progressive corneal endothelium damage.[34]

After 6 years of experience with anterior chamber lenses and over 2000 implanted, our cell loss rate did not exceed an overall of 10%, with only 3.5% loss intraoperatively. Compared to the physiological loss, there was no significant difference, nor was it progressive. The future of phakic anterior chamber lenses appeared promising.[11,12]

As time went on, complications arose, which diminished their use. The major complaints were:

- Night halos, caused by the 4.5-mm optics, were found in 100% of the patients inquired; only 35% of the patients referred to them spontaneously
- Need of daily pilocarpine to reduce the halos
- 12.6% incidence of irregular pupils

One of the basic problems was that due to its 4.5-mm diameter, the majority of patients complained about night halos, which eventually were overcome with daily instillation of diluted pilocarpine. If the iris root suffered ischemia, pupils would be oval or "cat-like." Pupillary ovalization could occur immediately after surgery caused by iris tuck or 1 to 2 years postoperatively caused by progressive iris root ischemia.

Another difficulty was selecting the appropriate lens length. Indirect measuring of the anterior chamber with white-to-white measurement was not precise. If oversized lenses were placed, pupillary ovalization would occur. On the other hand, if too small, rotation could favor high risk of endothelium cell loss, making explantation necessary.

Pupillary block, either intra- or postoperative, occasionally would occur attributed to the absence of iridotomies. Small wound leaks would often cause shallow anterior chambers and subsequent occlusion of the pupillary space with the anterior chamber lens. The consequent increase in IOP was easily preventable with preoperative iridotomies.

The multitude of difficulties spurred our search for a better treatment of extreme ametropia.

In the late 1980s, Fyodorov started working with silicone posterior chamber lenses to correct high myopia in phakic patients.[41-43] They resembled a mushroom with the optics in the anterior chamber and the loops in the posterior chamber. Although initial results were good, complications appeared, such as corneal touch and anterior capsule opacities, attributed to the lens design. Consequently, a new phakic was developed with both optics and haptics in the posterior chamber. In 1992, a clone was developed in Germany by Fechner.[35,44]

Many posterior chamber models were developed during the early 1990s with newer and more biocompatible material, such as those that included collagen in their composition.[42,45-47]

In 1991, at a Moscow refractive surgery convention (IRTC Microsurgery Complex), I (RZ) had the opportunity to meet Dr. Fyodorov and his team. I was then able to observe surgery and examine many of their patients with collagen posterior chamber lenses. I was truly impressed. The surgical technique was straightforward, however, the lenses had unpolished edges and sometimes were trimmed intraoperatively with scissors. Postoperative results were impressive considering the quality of the lenses used.

ICL EVOLUTION

During the last months of 1993, four investigators (Christian Skorpic in Austria and Vicenzo Assetto, Paolo Pesandro, and Stefano Benedetti in Italy) and myself (RZ) began our experience with ICLs, or implantable contact lenses.[2,45,46,48]

In 1992, with past and current technology in hand, Staar Surgical AG (Nidau, Switzerland) began development of new kind of posterior chamber lens called the Staar Surgical AG Implantable Contact Lens.[49,50]

The ICL is composed of collamer: a porcine collagen/HEMA copolymer with a refractive index of 1.45 at 35°C. The plate haptic design resembles the Fyodorov model. The foldable implant is introduced into the anterior chamber of the eye through a 3.0-mm corneal incision under peribulbar or topical anesthesia. The central concave/convex optic has sizes from 4.5 to 5.5 mm in diameter, depending on the lens power. Lens power ranges from –3.0 D to –20.0 D for myopic lenses, and +3.0 D to +17.0 D for hyperopic lenses. There are five lengths available to accommodate different eye sizes: 10.8 to 13.0 mm. Its positioning in the posterior chamber maintains the normal anatomy of the eye.

Both the lens design and our implantation technique evolved over the following years. In December 1993, we implanted our first three ICLs. A flat insertion technique was used on two patients. The third had the first folded ICL implant through a 3-mm incision. All were placed through a superior incision, rotated temporally and tucked beneath the iris—the rotational insertion technique (Figure 19-2). The lens shape resembled Fyodorov's, with a rectangular shape and smooth ends.

Problems encountered were:
- Difficulty in adequate size selection
- Rotation and decentration
- High incidence of pupillary block

In February 1994, prophylactic YAG iridotomies were performed 1 week prior to surgery. March 1994 saw the implantation of the first hyperopic ICL, and in September of that same year, the second myopic generation ICL was developed with a larger optic and a decreased IOL haptic-optic angle profile (Figures 19-3 and 19-4).

In January 1995, the third-generation ICL had some of my (RZ) suggestions incorporated, such as distal "footplates" to avoid rotation and improve central positioning (Figure 19-5). We also developed the non-rotational insertion technique which included a temporal clear corneal incision in the same location as the implant position (Figure 19-6).

In March 1995, we implanted the first ICL with topical anesthesia. This was somewhat more difficult than in phacoemulsification, due to the photophobia these patients experienced. Dr. Harry Grabow assisted me with this problem, contributing his experience and teachings in this type of anesthesia, and I also referred to Dr. I. Howard Fine's description of the technique and recommendations published in *Clear-Corneal Cataract Surgery & Topical Anesthesia*.[51]

In July 1995, the fourth-, fifth-, and sixth-generations of ICLs began development with profile changes, such as slightly wider plates with increased stability (Figure 19-7).

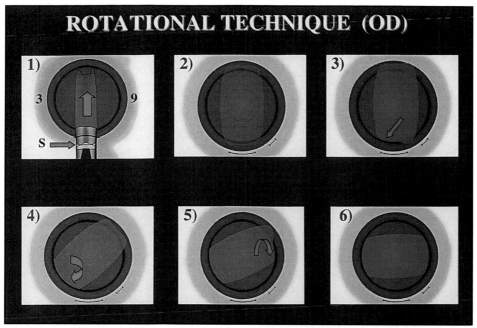

Figure 19-2. Rotational technique. The six-step technique begins with: 1) introduction of the ICL folded in the injector, through a 12 o'clock corneal incision. Peripheral iridotomy at 1 o'clock. Merocel sponge wedge inside injector (S). 2) ICL unfolded anterior to the iris plane. Paracentesis 11 o'clock. 3) through 5) The arrows show the direction of the dial-in maneuver of the ICL. 6) ICL positioned temporally in the posterior chamber.

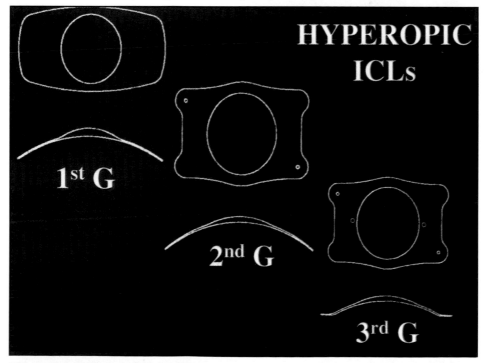

Figure 19-3. Hyperopic ICL models. The three generations of hyperopic ICLs are shown. Courtesy of Staar Surgical AG, Dr. Vladimir Feingold.

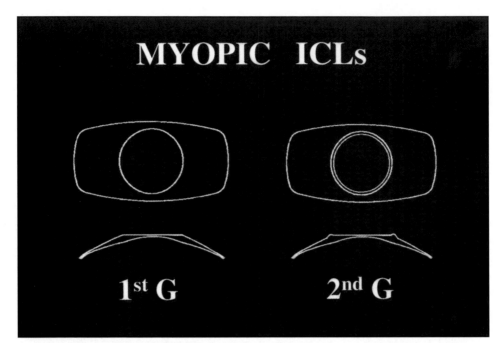

Figure 19-4. Myopic ICL models. First- and second-generation myopic ICLs. Courtesy of Staar Surgical AG, Dr. Vladimir Feingold.

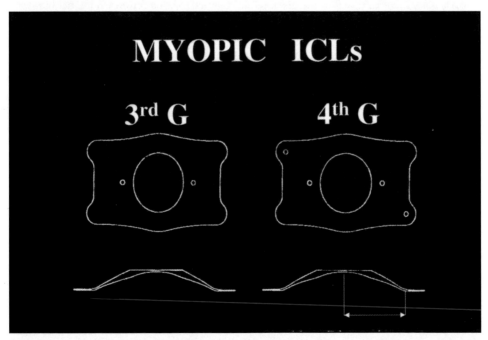

Figure 19-5. Myopic ICL models. Third- and fourth-generation myopic ICLs. Courtesy of Staar Surgical AG, Dr. Vladimir Feingold.

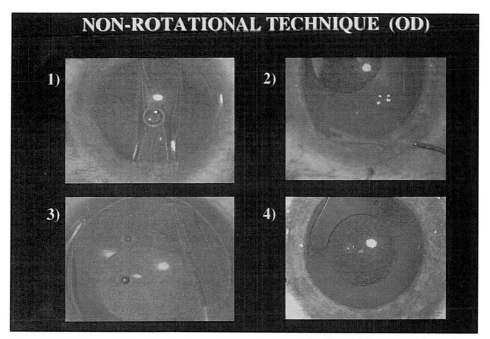

Figure 19-6. Non-rotational technique. 1) Introduction of the ICL through a temporal clear corneal incision. 2) Bechert hook used to place the proximal (left) footplate behind the iris plane. 3) Placement of the distal (right) footplate with a Sinskey hook behind the iris. 4) ICL unfolded and positioned in the posterior chamber.

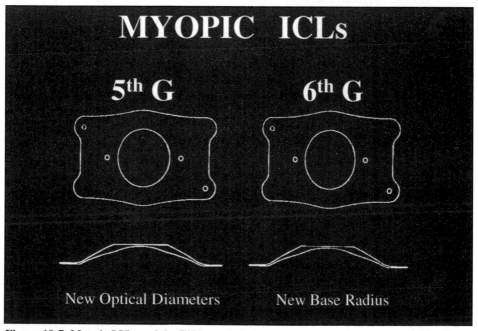

Figure 19-7. Myopic ICL models. Fifth- and sixth-generation myopic ICLs. Courtesy of Staar Surgical AG, Dr. Vladimir Feingold.

In March 1996, intraocular lidocaine, as taught to us by Dr. James Gills, was added to supplement topical anesthesia.

April 1996 saw the advent of Bioptics. I created this procedure to assist in treating extreme myopia.[11,12,40,48,52] The highest lens power available was only –21.0 D, with an average correction range of approximately –19.0 D. Many of our patients exceeded this range. In Bioptics, two optical systems—lens and cornea—are addressed to correct these individuals. Our current technique combines ICL implantation with planned LASIK at 1 month aimed to correct the anticipated post ICL residual refractive errors.

This procedure is indicated in myopic patients with spherical equivalents of -15.0 D or greater, patients with high levels of preoperative astigmatism (>2.0 D), hyperopes over +5.0 D, and patients in whom lens power availability is a problem.

The advantages of combining these procedures are:
- ICL large optical zone
- ICL preciseness
- LASIK large optical zone and its advantages[53-55]
- Higher optical quality (less optical aberrations)
- Less corneal ablation (diminished ablation depths)

Four years of experience have taught us how to select and operate the appropriate patients by determining:
- Adequate anterior chamber depths
- Correct type of iris
- Mandatory iridotomies
- Correct power calculation (Olsen formula modified by a personal constant)
- Accurate white-to-white measurements
- Appropriate ICL lengths based on white-to-white measurements (myopic ICLs should be 0.5 mm greater than measured and hyperopic lens should be the same or 0.5 mm less)
- Correct folding of the ICL in the cartridge and our "Merocel sponge technique" to avoid lens tear during the insertion (Figures 19-8 and 19-9)

We also gained intraoperative management experience with:
- Pupillary block
- IOP elevations
- Shallow or collapsed anterior chambers
- Lens rotation during insertion

Our postoperative experience taught us the need for:
- Postoperative medication refinement
- Better regulation of the implant vaulting (Figure 19-10)
- Bioptics improvements to more accurately deal with the residual refractive errors

PATIENT WORK-UP AND SURGICAL TECHNIQUE

At present, I have performed over 300 ICL and 112 Bioptics procedures in our Institute.

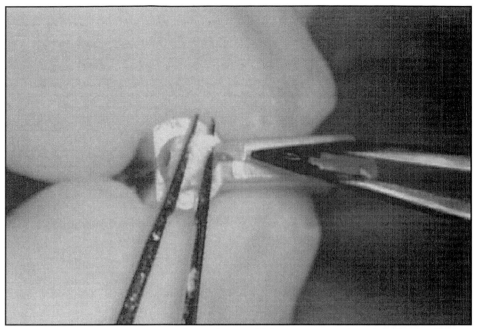

Figure 19-8. Merocel sponge technique. Wedge of Merocel sponge placed behind the folded ICL in the cartridge.

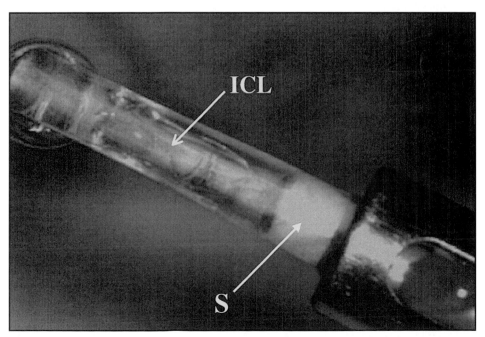

Figure 19-9. ICL in the cartridge. The folded ICL within the injector. Wedge of surgical sponge.

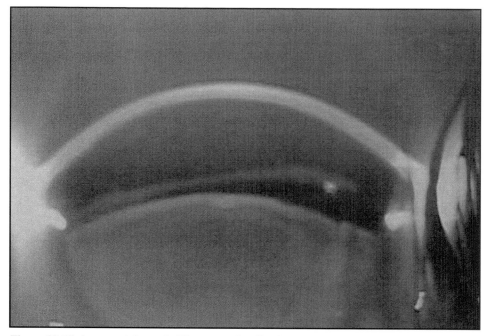

Figure 19-10. Asymmetric vault. The space that lies between the ICL and the anterior surface of the crystalline lens (vault) is asymmetric. The Nidek EAS 1000 (slit-mode) photograph reveals more space on the right side than on the left. On the lateral extremes of the crystalline lens, one can see the light beam that passes through the ICL is projected on the lens surface.

Patient Selection

Patients under 19 years of age with previous intraocular surgery, visually significant lenticular opacities, glaucoma, proliferative diabetic retinopathy, retinal breaks, or systemic diseases are all excluded from ICL implantation or Bioptics procedures.

ICL Procedure

ICL Prep-Up

Hard contact lenses and rigid gas permeable contact lenses should be discontinued for at least 2 weeks before surgery. Preoperative examination includes uncorrected visual acuity, best spectacle corrected visual acuity with both manifest and cycloplegic refraction, keratometry, slit lamp biomicroscopy, applanation tonography, dilated fundoscopic examination, corneal topography with color and tangential maps (EyeSys Corneal Topographer, EyeSys Technologies, Houston, Texas), corneal diameters (white-to-white), pachymetry, non-contact specular microscopy (Konan Noncon Robo-CA), and A-scan ultrasonography. If necessary, gonioscopy and B-scan ultrasonography are also performed.

ICL Power Calculation

The lens power calculations are made based upon Olsen's formulas modified by a personal constant made by taking into account our previous experience accumulated during all these years.

The independent variables in the formula are preoperative spherical equivalent, vertex distance, average keratometry, and actual anterior chamber depth. The final choice of lens power is determined following adjustments based on target postoperative refraction and our personal experience. The length of ICL implanted is determined based on the patient's corneal diameter.

ICL Surgical Technique

In order to decrease the incidence of postoperative pupillary block, in June 1994, we began performing a single superior laser iridotomy at least 4 days preoperatively. In August 1995, two superior iridotomies were positioned 60 degrees apart in order to decrease the risk of iridotomy occlusion by the ICL haptics. At first, only the Nd:YAG laser was used; subsequently in mid 1996, we began using the argon-green laser prior to applying the Nd:YAG spots in order to decrease pigment deposition on the ICL or related IOP increase.[12]

ICLs were implanted with our routine technique, and if required, intraoperative astigmatic keratectomies were also performed. Tropicamide 1%, phenylephrine 2.5%, diclofenac, and gentamicin are applied serially beginning 1 hour preoperatively. Anesthesia is achieved with either peribulbar or topical lidocaine. When good dilation, anesthesia, and akinesia are obtained, patients are taken to the OR, and a lid speculum is placed. A superior paracentesis and a 2.8-mm temporal clear corneal incision is made with the ZAP knife (Zaldivar Anterior Procedure diamond knife, ASICO, USA) (Figure 19-11). In cases where topical anesthesia is used, a supplement of intraocular lidocaine is instilled into the anterior chamber.

We use Staar Collamer ICLs in all cases. Under direct visualization with the operating microscope (Carl Zeiss, Germany), the ICL is positioned in the lens insertion cartridge (Figure 19-12). A 1.0-mm diameter wedge of microsurgical sponge is cut and placed behind the cartridge within the lens injector in order to protect the ICL from the injector arm; we call this the "Merocel sponge technique" (see Figures 19-8 and 19-9).

The injector tip is placed within the wound, previous injection of hydroxypropyl methylcellulose (Ocucoat) into the anterior chamber. The lens is slowly injected anterior to the iris plane. During insertion, the ICL tends to rotate upside down. Current ICL models have a certain angulation and only proper positioning will suffice. To assist in this, the ICL has two dimples on its surface and positioning holes next to the footplates: one hole next to the distal (right) footplate and a second next to the proximal (left) footplate. An upside-down lens would show inversion of the positioning of these holes. Often, it is really difficult to assess positioning in the injector and one way to overcome poor alignment is to rotate the injector while inserting the ICL, maintaining proper lens position throughout the whole procedure.

A Bechert Nucleus Rotator hook is used to place the temporal haptic beneath the iris, with gentle posterior pressure. The nasal haptic is then positioned in a similar

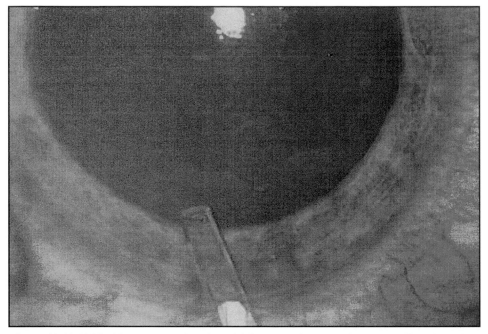

Figure 19-11. ZAP. Clear corneal incision of 2.8 mm performed with the Zaldivar Anterior Procedure diamond knife.

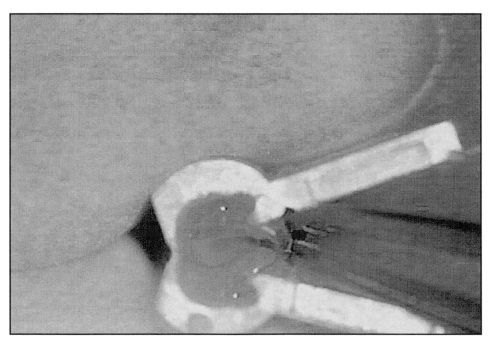

Figure 19-12. Folding of the ICL. The ICL is folded inside the special cartridge.

fashion with a Sinskey hook. When proper lens orientation is verified, acetylcholine is injected into the anterior chamber. Remaining viscoelastic is then removed with gentle irrigation/aspiration with the AMO Prestige Phacoemulsification System (Irvine, Calif) (see Figure 19-6).

Topical tobramycin-dexamethasone and gentamicin, in addition to 500 mg of oral acetazolamide, are given at the conclusion of the surgery. Eyes that received peribulbar anesthesia are patched, as opposed to those who were operated with topical anesthesia. The latter remain uncovered, and patients are given protective eye shields for night use only.

Postoperative medication includes:

- 0.3% dibekacina qd for 1 week
- 1% prednisolone qd for 1 month
- Beta-blocker, ie, 0.5% timolol bid for 1 month

ICL Follow-Up

Routine postoperative examinations are scheduled at 1 day, 1 month, 6 months, and then once a year following surgery. Of all the patients treated, 91.34% had at least 1 month of follow-up.

All follow-up examinations detailed subjective complaints. Uncorrected visual acuity, best corrected visual acuity, automated keratometry, slit lamp biomicroscopy, and applanation tonometry are all performed at each visit. Postoperative specular microscopy, ICL vaulting and positioning, pupil size and light response, patent iridotomies, pigment dispersion, and crystalline lens clarity are documented. Gonioscopy and dilated funduscopy are performed if needed.

Bioptics Procedure

This procedure combines ICL implantation with programmed LASIK 1 month afterwards, aimed at correcting the anticipated post ICL residual refractive error.

Laser Delivery Systems

The lasers used are the Nidek EC-5000 (Nidek Co Ltd, Aichi, Japan) and the Chiron Technolas Keracor 116 (Chiron Vision, Irvine, Calif). Both are argon-fluoride excimer lasers with an output wavelength of 193 nm.

The Nidek EC-5000 utilizes a scanning slit delivery system with a variable fluency (100 to 140 mJ) and a repetition rate of 10 to 50 Hz (we use a rate of 40 Hz). A 5.5-mm treatment zone with a 7.0-mm transition zone was used in most myopic patients treated with this laser.

The Chiron, with the PlanoScan software, uses a scanning spot delivery system (2-mm diameter spot) with a pulse duration of 18 ns and a repetition rate of 50 Hz. Optical zones of 5.2 mm with transitional zones of 8.7 mm are used in myopic patients. In hyperopes, optical zones are 5.7 mm with transitional zones of 9.2 mm. Toric ablations use optical zones of 5.0 x 8.0 mm.

With both lasers, patients are instructed to look at the helium-neon beam to facilitate centration.

LASIK Surgical Technique

One half hour prior to treatment, 1 drop of pilocarpine 1% is instilled into the treatment eye. Ten minutes before treatment, proparacaine HCL 1% drops are instilled followed by copious irrigation with balanced salt solution containing gentamicin and vancomycin to remove debris from the fornices and eyelashes. The fellow eyelid is taped closed. Patients are taken to the OR and positioned in the supine position under the laser.

Proparacaine HCL 1% drops are, once again, instilled into the treatment eye. A rigid eyelid speculum is used. Three radial marks and two diagonals are made with gentian violet on an eight-point radial marker and then gently imprinted on the corneal epithelium.

We use two different microkeratome systems depending on the refractive error treated: the Automated Corneal Shaper (ACS) or the Hansatome System both from Chiron Vision (Irving, Calif). The ring is placed on the eye concentric to the geometric center of the cornea. The suction pump is activated to a pressure of 22 to 24 mmHg in the ACS or to 25.5 mmHg approximately with Hansatome. Intraocular high pressures are verified with the Barraquer tonometer. Several drops of the irrigating solution are applied to the suction ring track prior to placement of the microkeratome head.

The microkeratome head is then placed into the groove of the suction ring and a 160-micron flap is dissected by activating the forward motion on the foot pedal. A slow smooth pass is performed until the microkeratome reaches the permanent stop. Reverse action on the foot pedal permits retraction of the microkeratome head. Suction is released, and the microkeratome head and suction ring are removed together.

The corneal flap is manipulated according to the microkeratome used. It is usually everted using 0.12 Castroviejo forceps, exposing the underlying corneal stroma. Flap size is verified using a modified Holladay-Godwin corneal gauge. The ACS cuts a flap size of 8.25 mm and the Hansatome a 10-mm flap. A Visitec microsurgical eye sponge is used to dry the stromal bed of conjunctival fornix fluid that occasionally moves to the stromal surface via capillary attraction. The everted flap is laid flat with minimal wrinkling across the nasal or superior limbus.

Treatment parameters are inputted into the laser's computer based on the type of refractive error treated and our personal nomograms. Photoablation is then carried out in the stromal bed. During ablation, holding the microsurgical sponge just above the exposed stromal surface at the flap's hinge protects the flap. During and after ablation, the stroma is wiped clean with the same sponge. Several drops of the irrigating solution are placed on the stromal bed and back surface of the flap. The corneal flap is repositioned with the blunt 27-gauge cannula by lifting the everted flap from its epithelial surface, and the interface is then irrigated with irrigating solution on the 27-gauge cannula. Gentle massage over the corneal surface with the Barraquer spatula facilitates fluid egress from the interface. The periphery of the flap is dried using an additional eye sponge and then with a blow of oxygen (fast, but low).

Topical tropicamide 1%, diclofenac 1%, and tobramycin-dexamethasone solu-

Table 19-1
ICL Perioperative Complications

Intraoperative	Postoperative
Pupillary block	ICL-induced IOP spike
Flipped ICLs	Steroid-induced IOP spike
ICL rotation	Pupillary block
ICL decentration	ICL decentration
Broken ICL	Irregular pupils
Pigmentary dispersion	Atonic pupils
	Lens capsule opacities
	Pigmentary dispersion

tion are instilled into the treatment eye. The lid speculum is removed, and the patient is given a protective eye shield for night use only.

Patients are controlled 15 minutes postoperatively and then discharged. Postoperative medication includes tobramycin-dexamethasone qd for 1 week.

Post LASIK Follow-Up

Examinations are scheduled for 1 day, 1 to 6 months, and once a year postoperatively. Routine examination, as described in ICL follow-up, is performed at all visits. Special attention is paid to the flap, and any epithelial, stromal, or interface alterations are documented.

Data Analysis and Results

ICL patients with preoperative myopia and hyperopia are analyzed separately, as well as with the Bioptics patients.

Refractive outcome and postoperative visual acuity can be analyzed as measures of the procedure's efficacy. Baseline refraction (spherical equivalent and cylinder) and visual acuity (uncorrected and best corrected) are compared to the refraction and visual acuity at the patient's last visit. Only patients with at least 1 month of follow-up post ICL are considered.

The stability of both procedures is addressed by examining the refractive result of the patients with 6 months to 4 years of follow-up in ICL patients, and 1 to 2 years in Bioptics patients.

Complications were analyzed as a measure of the safety of the procedures. Table 19-1 lists the complications we have encountered in the past 4 years.

ICL Results

We will analyze here 284 eye processes that received ICL implantation. Eighty-seven patients were female and 55 were male. Of all the cases treated, 245 were myopic eyes and 39 eyes were hyperopic. Mean age at surgery was 37 years. Once again, only patients with at least 1 month of follow-up post ICL were considered for this analysis.

Baseline Refraction. The myopic population showed a mean preoperative spherical equivalent and refractive cylinder of -17.76 D and -3.03 D, respectively.

Hyperopic patients presented a mean preoperative spherical equivalent of +6.56 D and a refractive cylinder of +1.37 D.

Refractive Outcome. At 1 year, the mean postoperative spherical equivalent and refractive cylinder were -0.22 D and -0.19 D for the myopic group and +0.22 D and -0.41 D for the hyperopic group, respectively.

The patients who returned after 2 years of surgery showed the following postoperative refraction:

- Myopic group: mean postoperative spherical equivalent of -0.12 D and a refractive cylinder of -0.88 D
- Hyperopic group: mean postoperative spherical equivalent of -0.02 D and a refractive cylinder of -0.75 D

Of those patients in which the target postoperative refraction was plano, our mean error was ±0.75 D (Figure 19-13). Stability of the spherical equivalent refraction can be observed in Figure 19-14.

Visual Acuity. Preoperative uncorrected visual acuity was 20/200 or worse in all the myopic patients. At 1 year, 66.65% presented uncorrected visual acuity of 20/40 or better (total number of eyes controlled: 81). A gain of 1 or more lines was seen in 59.25% and loss of 1 or more lines of best corrected visual acuity was found in 23.45% of the eyes controlled at 1 year.

All the hyperopic cases presented preoperative uncorrected visual acuity of <20/80. After 1 year of surgery, 14 eyes were controlled and 42.85% of them obtained uncorrected visual acuity of 20/40 or better. Gain in best corrected visual acuity of 1 line or more was seen in 35.61% and loss of 1 or more lines of best corrected visual acuity in 21.42%. Of those who returned for their 2-year control (6 eyes), gain of 1 or more lines was registered in 33.35% and none lost 1 or more lines of best corrected visual acuity.

In Figures 19-15 and 19-16 you can observe uncorrected and best corrected visual acuity both pre- and postoperatively. Figures 19-17 and 19-18 show best corrected visual acuity gain and loss, respectively.

Please note that travel constraint was the main cause of patient loss during follow-up. Over 70% of our patient population lives more than 600 km from the Institute.

Bioptics Results

Since April 1996, 112 eyes have been treated with the Bioptics procedure. To analyze these results, one must take into account both the ICL and the LASIK portions of the Bioptics procedure. The LASIK portion deals with the intended residual post ICL refractive error. The residual myopia is calculated trying to optimize the large optic of the ICLs and the larger and more acceptable optical zones in myopic LASIK.

The laser delivery system chosen in each particular case depended on the refractive error. As you can see in Figure 19-19, 88 myopic eyes were treated with the Nidek EC-5000 laser. The Chiron Keracor 116 PlanoScan was used for 16 myopes and eight hyperopes. Because the Nidek treatment group was statistically more significant, I will refer to the results obtained with this laser. In this series, 62 patients

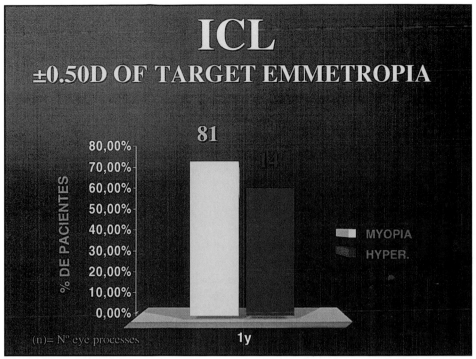

Figure 19-13. Deviation from target emmetropia. The graphic shows the ±0.50 D deviation from target emmetropia at 1 year. On top of each column are the total number of eye processes controlled.

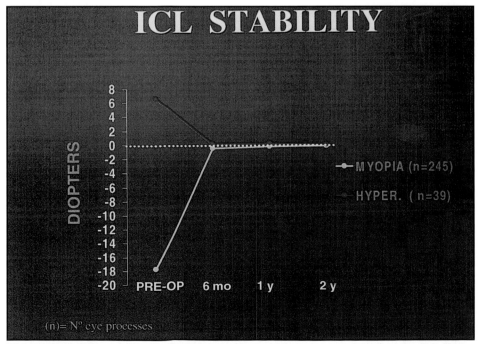

Figure 19-14. ICL stability. Both myopic and hyperopic series are plotted on the time line. The stability of this intraocular procedure is demonstrated in the graphic.

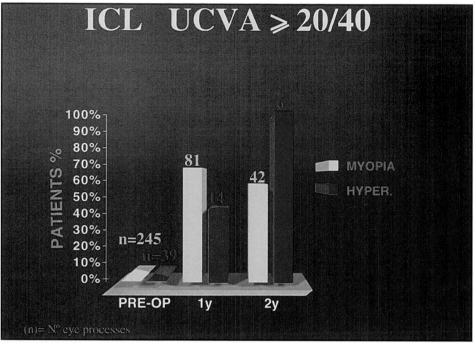

Figure 19-15. Uncorrected visual acuity of 20/40 or better in ICL. Myopic and hyperopic eyes treated with ICL obtained improvement in their uncorrected visual acuity. Shown are the total number of eye processes controlled at each follow-up exam. (Note: travel constraint was the main cause of patient loss during follow-up.)

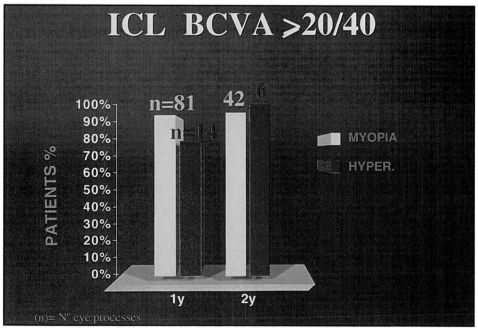

Figure 19-16. Best corrected visual acuity of 20/40 or better in ICL. Gain in best corrected visual acuity of 20/40 or better in myopic and hyperopic eyes treated with ICL. Shown are the total number of eye processes controlled at each follow-up exam. (Note: travel constraint was the main cause of patient loss during follow-up.)

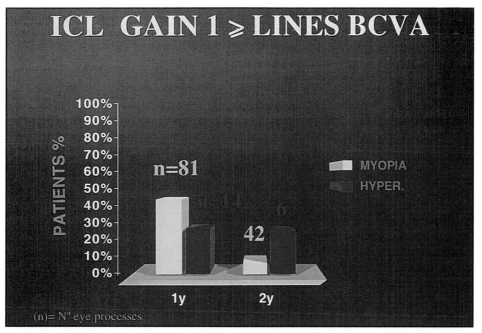

Figure 19-17. ICL gain of 1 or more lines of best corrected visual acuity at 1 and 2 years of follow-up. The first pair of columns show the gain in percentage of best corrected visual acuity of 1 or more lines in both population groups (myopic and hyperopic) at 1 year, and the second pair, at 2 years.

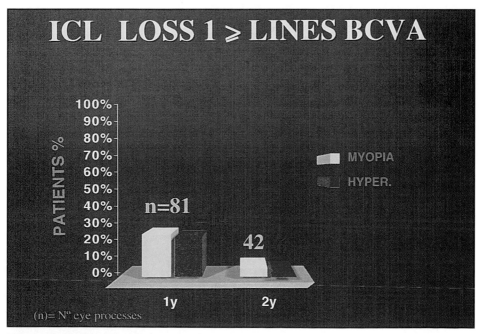

Figure 19-18. ICL loss of best corrected visual acuity of 1 line or more at 1 and 2 years of follow-up. The small percentage of loss in best corrected visual acuity and its tendency towards stability at 2 years. (Note: this loss corresponds to the patients with capsular opacities, retinal complications, and one case of secondary angle closure glaucoma.)

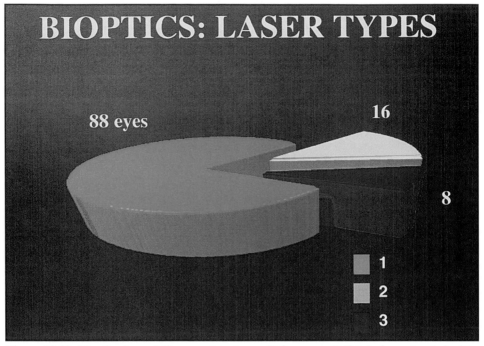

Figure 19-19. Bioptics laser delivery system types. References: 1) Total of eyes treated with the Nidek EC-5000 (green). 2) Total of eyes treated with the Chiron (yellow). 3) Total of eyes treated with the Chiron Technolas Keracor with the hyperopic PlanoScan software (blue).

were female and 26 male. Mean age at surgery was 35.5 years.

Baseline Refraction. The myopic population showed a mean pre ICL spherical equivalent of -21.70 D. The mean pre ICL refractive sphere was -20.80 (max: -35.00 D, min: -12.00 D). The mean pre-ICL refractive cylinder was -1.85 D.

Refractive Outcome. Post ICL refraction at 1 month revealed a mean spherical equivalent of -5.34 D, with a mean refractive sphere and cylinder of -4.50 D and -1.71 D, respectively.

Post LASIK refraction day 1 showed a mean spherical equivalent of +0.14 D with a mean refractive sphere and cylinder of +0.24 D and -0.21 D, respectively.

Only 63 Bioptics eye processes (71.60%) were controlled at 1 month. Mean spherical equivalent was plano, and the mean refractive sphere and cylinder were +0.14 D and -0.28 D, respectively. At 1 year, the mean postoperative spherical equivalent and refractive cylinder were -0.13 D and -0.04 D, respectively, in 13 eyes controlled (14.77%) (Figure 19-20).

Figure 19-21 demonstrates the stability of the Bioptics procedure during the first year analyzed. Mean spherical equivalent, pre- and postoperatively, are plotted on the graph.

Once again, patient loss during follow-up was mainly caused by travel inconveniences.

Visual Acuity. Pre ICL uncorrected visual acuity was 20/200 or worse in all cases, and best corrected visual acuity was only 20/40 or better in 21.6% of the eye

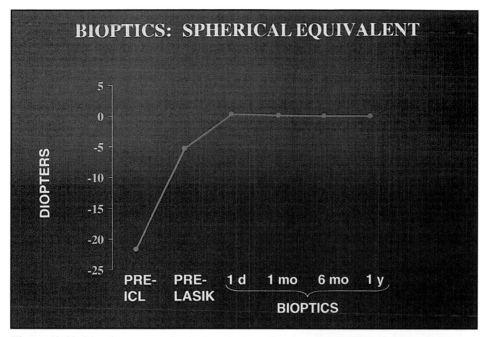

Figure 19-20. Bioptics mean spherical equivalent. One can observe the marked gain in postoperative refraction following the Bioptics procedure. The mean spherical equivalents are plotted along on the time line. Post ICL and post LASIK gains are dramatic, and their stability at 1 year can be evidenced with this graphic.

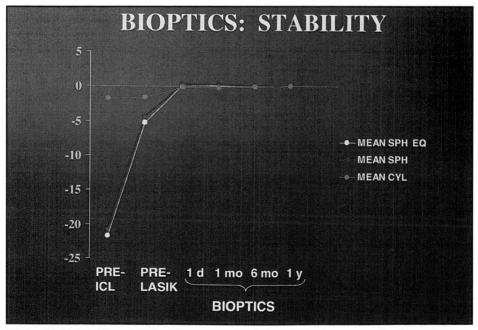

Figure 19-21. Bioptics stability. The mean spherical equivalents, mean refractive sphere, and mean refractive cylinder are plotted along on the time line. Marked gain and stability can be observed. Note the particular improvement of the refractive cylinder after the Bioptics (LASIK portion) procedure.

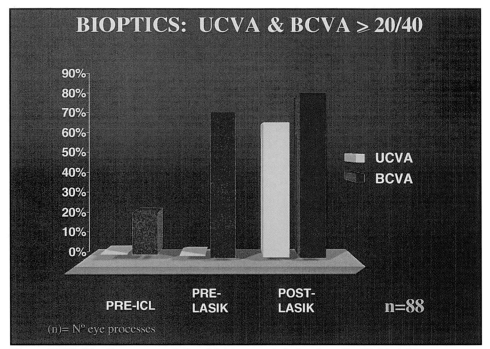

Figure 19-22. Bioptics uncorrected and best corrected visual acuity. Eight-eight eye processes treated with the Nidek EC-5000 can be analyzed pre-ICL, pre-LASIK, and at 1 month post LASIK. Columns show the percentage of gain in uncorrected or best corrected visual acuity. Uncorrected visual acuity does not improve at first, due to the intended residual myopia calculated from the beginning, but shows great improvement after the LASIK portion of the Bioptics procedure. On the other hand, best corrected visual acuity gain is marked from the very beginning, post ICL, and continues to do so after LASIK.

processes. At 1 month, post ICL, best corrected visual acuity was already 20/40 or better in 75% of eyes controlled. One year later, the Bioptics group showed gain in both uncorrected and best corrected visual acuity of 20/40 or better in 69.26% and 84.65% of eye processes controlled, respectively (Figures 19-22 and 19-23).

Complications

Perioperative complications can be divided into two groups: either intra- or postoperative complications. Both ICL and Bioptics share the intraocular procedure related complications, and the latter may also share complications inherent to the LASIK procedure. We have selected the complications we consider the most interesting and presented them as "mini" case reports.

Subjective Complaints

In general terms, the subjective complaints referred by patients with more than 1 month of follow-up were glare, monocular diplopia, and mild ocular pain. Decentration of more than 1 mm and torn ICLs were the main causes of glare and diplopia, and pain was reported in those patients who presented IOP spikes.

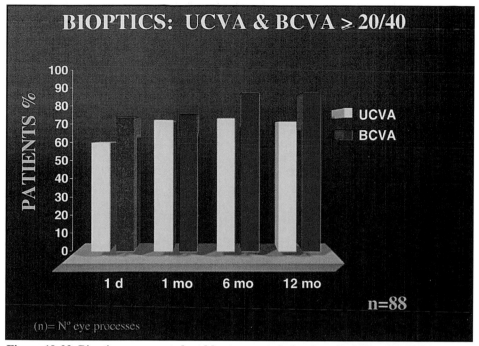

Figure 19-23. Bioptics uncorrected and best corrected visual acuity follow-up. Follow-up examinations scheduled at day 1, 1 month, 6 months, and 1 year are shown with the percentage of gain in both uncorrected and best corrected visual acuity. Eighty-eight eye processes were controlled at day 1, 63 at 1 month, 38 at 6 months, and 13 at 1 year. (Note: travel constraint was the main cause of patient loss during follow-up.)

Mini Case Reports

Intraoperative Pupillary Block. We had a case in which surgery had been uneventful until we injected BSS to reform the anterior chamber. Immediately, the eye began to feel tense and the anterior chamber collapsed. The injection of more further shallowed the anterior chamber! (I could only remember a similar episode while implanting an anterior chamber lens.) This event required an intraoperative iridectomy, which immediately resolved the problem. Of the utmost importance is the ability to recognize these intraoperative signs of ICL-induced pupillary block. If missed, the great amount of fluid injected will make resolution of the block more difficult afterwards. The prophylactic YAG iridotomies can almost eliminate the risk of pupillary block.

Postoperative Pupillary Blocks. After many successful cases, our first pupillary blocks appeared in 1994. ICL surgical technique initially did not include peripheral iridotomies. Patients were left resting for 3 hours after surgery, examined, and pressure elevations were addressed at that time. One of our first cases with pupillary block presented after surgery with pain and IOP of 45 mmHg. Slit lamp examination revealed:

* Mild corneal edema
* Shallow anterior chamber
* Angle closure due to suspected ICL-induced pupillary block

We were suspicious of this complication owing to previous reports of pupillary blocks by Russian authors (personal communication). We managed the complication with immediate YAG laser iridotomies which provoked instant increase in the anterior chamber depth, an open angle, and a decreased IOP.

Another patient had such severe corneal edema that performing laser iridotomy was impossible. A surgical iridectomy was necessary to resolve the problem.

The increase in IOP is usually caused by pupillary blocks, "ICL-related," or post-steroid medication. The last is the most frequent cause we have documented in our series, at 1 month postop follow-up examinations. Most of the patients with steroid-induced IOP spikes did not refer symptoms during their follow-up controls. Only 2% referred glare and mild ocular pain. Withdrawal of the steroid medication and administration of a beta-blocker (timolol 0.5%) returned IOP to normal levels. Very few cases presented ICL-related IOP spikes in which no other cause could be identified.

Lens Tear. In late 1993 and early 1994, the first ICLs implanted were inserted with a metal head injector. Due to lens fragility, passage through the metal tip occasionally caused partial or complete tears of the implants. The damaged ICLs had to be explanted and replaced.

We have had two cases in the past 4 years:

1. A 37-year-old male patient presented, during the injection of the ICL into the anterior chamber, a tear in one of the footplates. Due to the smallness of the defect, surgery was completed in a regular fashion. Subjective complaints during the postop follow-up included halos, image distortion, decrease of uncorrected visual acuity, and monocular diplopia. Slit lamp examination revealed a decentered ICL. ICL was finally explanted and exchanged for a new one, 7 months after the original surgery. Uncorrected visual acuity was recovered and has remained stable.

2. The second case we had was a 25-year-old female, whose implant suffered a tear during its injection. Based on my previous experience, the ICL was immediately exchanged.

Pigmentary Dispersion. An interesting case of pigmentary dispersion occurred in a female diabetic (well controlled) with fair irides and a mid dilated pupil during surgery. A large amount of pigment was liberated just as the lens was placed beneath the iris. Based on my previous experience, this was clearly abnormal. Postoperative day 1 revealed large amounts of pigment in the angle with a consequent IOP increase. Beta-blocker and trabeculoplasty were necessary in order to control the secondary open-angle glaucoma. At 1 month, the IOP remained elevated with continued pigment dispersion. Shortly afterwards, the lens was removed and the pressure and refraction returned to normal levels.

"Crowded" Anterior Chamber. A 27-year-old female patient presented a preoperative uncorrected visual acuity of 20/800 and her best corrected visual acuity was 20/40. Spectacle refraction was +8.00 +2.00 x 110°. Preoperative IOP was 14 mmHg and anterior chamber depth was 2.80 mm. Axial length was 18.90 mm. The ICL surgical technique was performed in a regular fashion, with special attention

paid due to the smallness of the eye.

Twenty-four hour follow-up exam revealed IOP elevation of 45 mmHg, without pupillary block, that was untreatable with the routine anti-glaucomatous medication. Gonioscopy showed total closure of the angle structure. ICL explantation was performed the following day. IOP and visual acuity returned to preoperative levels.

Secondary Angle Closure Glaucoma. A hyperopic patient presented IOP elevation, presumably ICL-related, 1 month after surgery. Despite treatment with repeated laser iridotomies, two trabeculectomies, and final ICL removal with phacoemulsification and posterior chamber lens implantation, the optic nerve showed cupping and neovascularization of the angle occurred. Best corrected visual acuity loss of 3 lines (20/60) of the patient's preop refraction occurred. At 18 months, IOP was under control on topical medications (16 mmHg) and his visual acuity currently remains stable.

Atonic Pupil. We observed two cases of patients who presented with non-responsive dilated pupils postoperatively. In both cases the viscoelastic substance used during surgery was Healon. In our opinion, improper storage or handling led to a breakdown product that may have caused extensive postoperative mydriasis and IOP increase. Halo complaints were attributed to the dilation and the patient's perception of the ICL's edges. The lenses were explanted, phacoemulsification performed, and a 6.5-mm posterior chamber lens was successfully implanted.

Capsular Opacities. We have had only six cases of capsular opacities since we began implanting ICLs 4 years ago. Obviously, the concerns of cataractogenesis are heightened in phakic posterior chamber lens surgery as opposed to anterior chamber lens surgery.

Two (one anterior and another posterior) appeared related to perioperative maneuvers. Another one developed a peripheral anterior subcapsular opacity close to one of the iridectomies. A fourth case of postoperative central anterior subcapsular opacity was related to an inverted ICL.

Two myopic cases had improperly sized, small lenses implanted. Postoperatively, photographs with the Nidek EAS 1000 (Nidek Co Ltd, Aichi, Japan) camera caused us to realize that the white-to-white measurements did not adequately coincide with the actual posterior chamber dimensions. This contributed to improper vaulting (Figure 19-24). Both patients developed anterior subcapsular opacities in the following 6 months. The opacities were circular and mirrored the border of ICL's optic zone.

It is my (RZ) theory that due to the optic shape of myopic ICLs, inadequately sized, the optic's shoulder can come in contact with the crystalline lens. It is my belief that this led to a lack of the circulation between the implant and the lens that may have promoted opacity formation (Figure 19-25). Both patients underwent ICL explantation and clear corneal phacoemulsification from a temporal approach.

On the other hand, in hyperopic ICL implantations, one of our primary concerns was the closeness of the implant to the crystalline lens in these short eyes. Due to the shape difference between the hyperopic and myopic ICL, circulation is not impaired. To date, no hyperopic ICL-induced opacities have been documented (Figures 19-26 through 19-28).

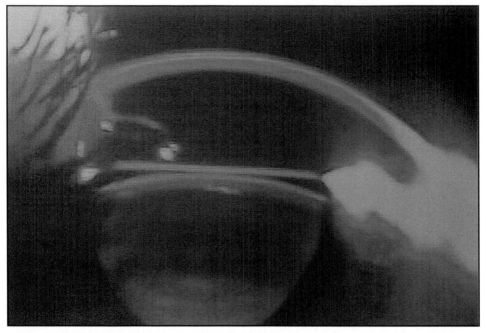

Figure 19-24. Improper vault. Nidek EAS 1000 photograph (slit-mode) reveals inadequate vault in a myopic patient. White-to-white measurements did not reflect real anterior chamber dimensions, and therefore the ICL length was inadequate (undersized) with the consequent improper vaulting.

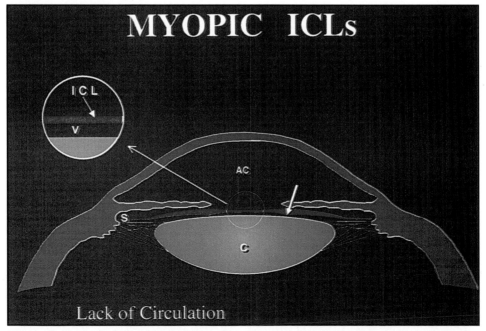

Figure 19-25. Lack of circulation theory. The schematic diagram intends to show the lack of space or vault (V) between the myopic ICL and the crystalline lens (C) (circle). If inadequately sized, the biconcave optic favors contact of the IOL shoulder with the lens (arrow). The lens footplates rest in the sulcus (S). Anterior chamber (AC).

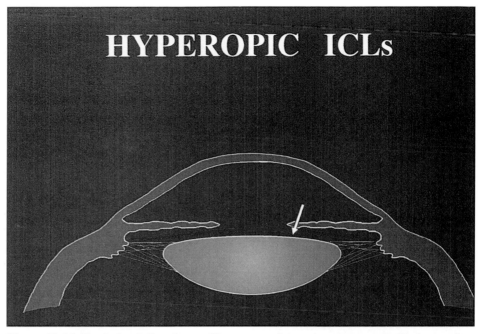

Figure 19-26. Good circulation theory. The arrow points out a proper vault. The convexity of the hyperopic ICL optic favors sufficient space for circulation and decreases the possibility of lens touch.

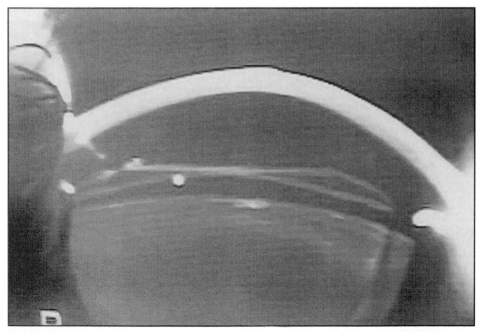

Figure 19-27. Appropriate vault. Nidek EAS 1000 photograph reveals a proper vault in an adequately sized myopic ICL.

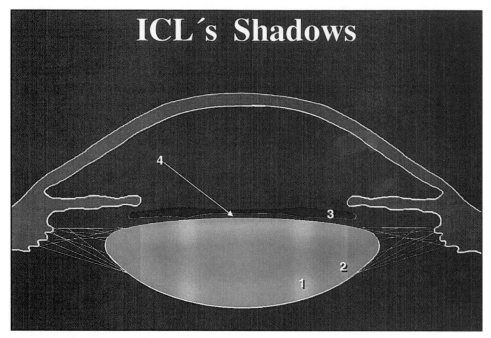

Figure 19-28. ICL's shadow. The schematic diagram represents the outline of the photograph seen in Figure 19-27. As light projects itself through the ICL (3), it will generate, in a dilated patient, the shadow of the ICL's shoulder on the surface of the crystalline lens. This will cause image distortion known as night halos. ICL shoulder (1) and footplates (2) shadows are projected on the lens. Vault (4).

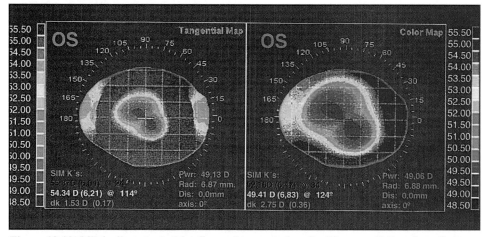

Figure 19-29. ICL/epikeratophakia. Corneal topography of a 36-year-old female patient who was referred for evaluation. She presented an epikeratophakia procedure on her left eye.

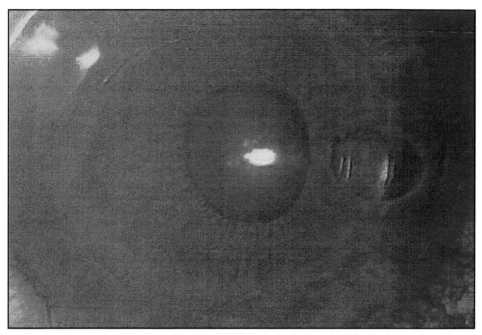

Figure 19-30. ICL/epikeratophakia. Digital photograph shows the border of the ICL through the peripheral surgical iridectomy, positioned at 12 o'clock. Two argon Nd:YAG laser iridotomies can be observed at 10 and 2 o'clock positions. The corneal trace of the epikeratophakia procedure is also clearly seen.

Retinal Complications. So far, only two patients have presented retinal complications, presumably ICL-unrelated.

One patient presented a macular hemorrhage. It occurred 1 month after surgery and apparently was unrelated to the procedure. Best corrected visual acuity decreased from 20/40 to 20/50. Three months later, the hemorrhage cleared up and the patient's refraction returned to its preoperative level.

An extreme myope presented a macula-off rhegmatogenous retinal detachment 3 months postoperatively with a decrease in his best corrected visual acuity (20/800). His preoperative spherical equivalent was –22.25 D and presented an axial length of 32.87 mm. The patient was referred to a retina specialist for adequate treatment, and has not yet returned to our Institute.

Special Case Report: ICL/Epikeratophakia. A 36-year-old female patient with bilateral non-aggressive keratoconus was treated successfully with an epikeratophakia procedure in the left eye. Regression occurred over the years and she was referred to our office for evaluation. Best corrected visual acuity was 20/200 in the left eye. Manifest refraction was -17.00 -5.00 x 125°. Central pachymetry revealed a corneal thickness of 638 microns. Figure 19-29 shows the patient's topography.

I (RZ) proposed an ICL procedure, which was performed and accompanied by relaxing incisions (AK) in the steepest meridians. Postop day 1, the uncorrected visual acuity was 20/40, and at 1 week 20/30. The patient, with a past history of contact lens intolerance, was overwhelmed with her uncorrected visual acuity (Figure 19-30).

Special Tips

One must also mention the following events as special tips in order to avoid them from occurring.

Endothelial Cell Loss

A skilled surgeon and a polished technique are essential in order to avoid initial endothelial cell loss due to surgical trauma. ICL-induced cell loss in our experience, due to intermittent ICL-cornea touch or chronic inflammation, is theoretically of less concern than with the anterior chamber lenses. Our average loss in mean endothelial cell density was 4.38 ± 6.90 cells/mm^2.[11,12]

Inadequately Sized Lenses

Many times while inserting oversized lenses, you can see evidence of anterior displacement of the iris and shallowing of the anterior chamber. Always remember that the latter can be caused usually by either non-patent iridotomies or oversized implants. One should always replace the improperly sized lenses.

Undersized lenses can easily rotate and decenter. Lack of experience may cause this to be overlooked during surgery and only visualized the day after. These cases all require explantation in order to avoid the diplopia provoked by looking through the borders of the ICL.

Flipped Lens

The rotation of the lens during the insertion is something that must be detected and resolved immediately. One must not intend to maneuver the lens inside the anterior chamber. The inverted implant should be removed and replaced before continuing with the surgical procedure.

ICL Exchange. ICLs must be explanted when improperly fit, flipped, dislocated, or torn. The surgical technique applied for ICL exchange is quite simple:

- Slow injection of viscoelastic substance underneath the ICL, taking special care in avoiding all contact of the anterior capsule of the crystalline lens
- Once the implant is floating, Kelman-McPherson forceps should be used to grasp the ICL and explant it through the original incision
- The new ICL is folded and implanted in a regular fashion

DISCUSSION AND CONCLUSIONS
Efficacy and Predictability

Based on our experience treating extreme refractive errors, it is unquestionable that the best optical quality is obtained with IOL procedures.

There is no doubt that when using keratorefractive procedures for treating extreme ametropias, the excessive flattening of the central cornea and the reduction in the optical zone size cause important visual aberrations. This results in decrease of visual quality and a poor refractive outcome.

Cataract surgeons have all evidenced that when operating extreme myopes,

these patients recover their preoperative best corrected visual acuity and usually even gain 1 to 2 lines of best corrected visual acuity. This same refractive outcome is experienced by those operated with phakic posterior chamber lenses.

Since performing ICL implantation or Bioptics, the marked gain in uncorrected visual acuity compared to the patient's preoperative best spectacle corrected visual acuity has always surprised us. This may be attributed to the elimination of spectacle-induced minification experienced preoperatively. Holladay stipulates that minification decreases 1 line for every 10 D corrected. This still does not explain, in some cases, the marked gain of 3 to 4 lines. Most probably, the optical system obtained with these procedures permits a better resolution and improved macular alignment of the image.

Good efficacy and predictability, as seen in Figure 19-13, have been constants in all our cases studied. Seventy-five percent of the patients at 1 year presented a mean spherical equivalent within ±0.50 D of target emmetropia at last visit. Taking in account that other investigators have achieved lower spherical equivalent refraction, I think that more accurate lens power calculation formulas should be developed.[45]

This leads me to conclude that in terms of obtaining a better visual quality and refractive outcome, phakic IOLs offer the best results.

Safety

The perioperative complication rate has decreased over the years due to all the improvements in lens design and surgical techniques.

The phakic IOLs offer clear advantages over the aphakic lens:
- Maintenance of accommodation in pre-presbyopic patients
- Absence of posterior capsule opacification
- Decreased risk of retinal detachment (due to the anterior displacement of the posterior capsule post CLE)
- Decrease of macular edema incidence

On the other hand, the potential risks of phakic lens are:
- Crystalline lens opacification (ICL-induced)
- Pigmentary dispersion
- IOP elevation

After 4 years of ICL experience with different IOL models and surgical approaches, our incidence of ICL-induced cataractogenesis is still very low (2%). This complication is, in my (RZ) opinion, the only real risk that this procedure presents if compared with other procedures. My preliminary conclusion is that adequate designs and size selection, as well as proper vaulting, are essential for preserving crystalline transparency.

We also have a very low incidence of pigmentary dispersion, one case in 300 procedures performed during these past years. This patient obviously presented a pathological type of iris pigment. With this in mind, I can conclude that this procedure has very little or no influence in pigmentary dispersion and related IOP increase.

Regarding the pupillary blocks, these occurred at the beginning when prophylactic iridotomies were not routinely performed. Their incidence has decreased notably since combined argon and Nd:YAG preoperative peripheral iridotomies are performed. Hyperopes are especially sensitive to this possible complication due to their smaller anterior chambers. The combination of both laser types for the iridotomies decreased the pigment dispersion and deposit on the ICL's surface. Also, the current non-rotational technique has diminished surgical trauma pigmentary dispersion and related IOP increase.

Topical steroid medication was the main cause of IOP spikes during the first month of surgery. Adequate pressure control during follow-up examinations is critical for early detection of this possible complication. Withdrawal of the steroids and prescription of beta-blockers usually overcomes this event and IOP usually returns to normal levels without consequences on visual acuity.

Endothelial cell loss, as described before, is infrequent if the surgeon is skilled and surgical trauma is reduced to a minimum. The posterior chamber location of the ICLs should prevent corneal endothelium damage from occurring, provided absence of chronic inflammation.[13]

The retinal detachment and macular hemorrhage cases described previously were apparently unrelated to the ICL procedure. In our series, the incidence of retinal complications is only 0.66% and found only in myopic patients. High and extreme myopes are obviously predisposed to suffer myopic retinopathy and therefore the risk of spontaneous retinal detachment is increased. Detailed dilated funduscopic examination must be routinely performed in these patients. If one bares in mind the poor preoperative visual quality these extreme myopes present, the risk-benefit ratio must be well assessed.

If we compare managing ICL-induced opacities with the management of all the other complications that keratorefractive procedures can present in treating extreme myopia, ICLs still offer an enormous advantage. For example, these other procedures can produce:
- Corneal ectasia
- Severe endothelial cell loss (deep ablations)
- Optical aberrations (due to small optical zones and a flat central cornea)

The above complications are very difficult to resolve, and in many cases require penetrating keratoplasty for their resolution. Keeping in mind that the original treatment procedure was performed to correct a refractive error, indicating a penetrating keratoplasty will imply a posteriori, an even greater refractive defect. We now have an additional and serious problem: uncorrection of the primary refractive error and a new secondary refractive defect. Under the hypothetical case of an ICL-induced opacity, its solution and refractive outcome is easy to achieve: routine phacoemulsification with posterior chamber lens implantation.

Loss of best corrected visual acuity occurred only in the ICL patients that presented capsular opacities, small regressions of the secondary procedures (eg, RK, AK, PRK), retinal complications, and the case of secondary angle closure glaucoma.

In the myopic group, 23.45% loss 1 or more lines at 1 year and 4.75% at 2 years. The total number of eyes decreased in each one of these controls. Eighty-one eyes

(n = 245) were controlled at the 1-year follow-up examination and only 42 another year afterwards.

Of the 14 hyperopic eyes controlled (n = 39) at the 1-year follow-up exam, only three had lost 1 or more lines of best corrected visual acuity. On the other hand, no loss of best corrected visual acuity was registered in the six eyes controlled at 2 years.

The Bioptics group did not experience any vision-threatening complications. Our results, so far, show short- and mid-term safety. Further studies are needed to evaluate possible late complications.

Stability

Phakic IOL surgery has demonstrated its long-term stability not only in the correction of high myopia, but in hyperopia as well. Regression, common in keratorefractive procedures, does not exist with the use of phakic IOLs.

Initially, in cases of extreme ametropias, residual refractive errors were addressed with secondary refractive procedures (eg, RK, AK, PRK), but low-grade undercorrections and regression occurred. This led us to improve power calculation formulae and lens design, and develop increased lens power models. Currently the combination of LASIK 1 month post ICL implantation (Bioptics), along with the above improvements, has turned this procedure into a precise, predictable, efficient, stable, and safe means of treating extreme refractive errors.

CONCLUSION

All our experiences indicate that ICL implantation is the most adequate refractive procedure for the correction of high ametropias, both myopia and hyperopia, with or without astigmatism. Gain in best corrected visual acuity is common, and our results show good refractive outcome, stability, and safety.

Future development of newer surgical techniques, power calculation formulas, and lens designs will permit improvement of results obtained as well as decrease the incidence or eliminate possible complications.

For extreme myopia, Bioptics offers the precision not yet found with any other refractive procedure, and patients visually handicapped can benefit from an excellent visual prognosis. Further studies are needed to evaluate the results of the Bioptics procedure in the correction of extreme hyperopia and mixed astigmatisms.

Note: Thanks to Hugo Micarelli, who collaborated with the photographic and digital art material.

REFERENCES

1.   Barraquer C. Re: Future of procedures. ISRS Online Forum [message posted on-line]. Available at: http://www.isrs.org/interact/boards/members/index.cgi. Accessed January 18, 1998.
2.   Grabow H. Intraocular correction of refractive errors. Presented at Staar ICL Training Seminar, April 25-26, 1996, Mendoza, Argentina.
3.   Werblin TP. Future of procedures. ISRS Online Forum [message posted on-line]. Available at: http://www.isrs.org/interact/boards/members/index.cgi. Accessed January 13, 1998.
4.   Azar D, ed. *Refractive Surgery*. Stanford, Conn: Appleton & Lange; 1997.

5.   Barraquer J. Anterior chamber plastic lenses. Results and conclusions from five years experience. *Trans Ophthalmol Soc UK*. 1959;79:393-424.
6.   Barraquer J. Historia de la cirugía refractiva. In: Barraquer J, ed. *Cirugía Refractiva de la Cornea*. Vol 1. Bogotá, Colombia: Instituto Barraquer de América; 1989.
7.   Bores LD. *Refractive Eye Surgery*. Boston, Mass: Blackwell Scientific Publications; 1993.
8.   Jaffe NS, Galin MA, Hirschman H, Clayman HM. History of pseudophakos. In: *Pseudophakos*. St. Louis, Mo: The CV Mosby Co; 1978:35-52.
9.   Kwitko M, Praeger DL, eds. *Pseudophakia Current Trends and Concepts*. Baltimore, Md: Williams & Wilkins Co; 1980.
10.   Strampelli B. Sopportabilits' di lenti aciliche in camera antriore nella afachia e nei vizi di refrazicne. *Ann Ottalmol Clin Ocul*. 1954;80:75-82.
11.   Zaldivar R, Davidorf JM, Oscherow SA. Intraocular contact lens. In: Buratto L, ed. *LASIK: Principles and Techniques*. Thorofare, NJ: SLACK Incorporated; 1998.
12.   Zaldivar R, Davidorf JM, Oscherow SA. Posterior chamber phakic IOL for myopia of −8 to −19 diopters. *J Refract Surg*. 1998;14:294-305.
13.   Alio JL, de la Hoz F, Ismail MM. Subclinical inflammatory reaction induced by phakic anterior chamber lenses for the correction of high myopia. *Ocular Immunology and Inflammation*. 1993;1:219-223.
14.   Apple DJ, Brems RN, Park RB, et al. Anterior chamber lenses. Part I: complications and pathology and review of designs. *J Cataract Refract Surg*. 1987;13:157-174.
15.   Baikoff G, et al. Damage to the corneal endothelium using anterior chamber intraocular lenses for myopia. *Refract Corneal Surg*. 1990;6(5):383.
16.   Drews RC. Risk benefit analysis of anterior chamber lenses for the correction of myopia in phakic patients. *Eur J Implant Ref Surg*. 1991;3:171-194.
17.   Minouni F, Colin J, Koffi V, Bonnet P. Damage to the corneal endothelium from anterior chamber intraocular lenses in phakic myopic eyes. *Refract Corneal Surg*. 1991;7:277-281.
18.   Baikoff G, Colin J. Intraocular lenses in phakic patients. *Ophthalmol Clin North Am*. 1992;5:789-795.
19.   Helsin KB, Kelman CD. Kelman anterior chamber lens. In: Kwitko M, Praeger DL, eds. *Pseudophakia Current Trends and Concepts*. Baltimore, Md: Williams & Wilkins Co; 1980.
20.   Choyce DP. Choyce Mark VIII anterior chamber implant. In: Jaffe NS, Galin MA, Hirschman H, Clayman HM, eds. *Pseudophakos*. St. Louis, Mo: The CV Mosby Co; 1978:111-125.
21.   Alio JL, Ruiz-Moreno JM, Artola. Retinal detachment as a potential hazard in surgical correction of severe myopia with phakic anterior chamber lenses. *Am J Ophthalmol*. 1993;115:143-148.
22.   Drews RC. Reliability of lens implant power formulas in hyperopes and myopes. *Ophthalmic Surg*. 1988;19:11-15.
23.   Saragoussi JJ, et al. Damage to the corneal endothelium by minus power anterior chamber intraocular lenses. *Refract Corneal Surg*. 1991;7:282-285.
24.   Fukala V. Operative Behandlung der hochstgradigen Myopie durch Aphaquie (Surgical treatment of high degrees of myopia through Afaquia). *Graefs Arch Ophthalmol*. 1980;36:230-244.
25.   Olsen T, Thim K, Corydon L. Accuracy of the newer generation intraocular lens power calculation formulas in long and short eyes. *J Cataract Refract Surg*. 1991;17:187-193.
26.   Holladay JT, et al. Achieving emmetropia in extremely short eyes with two piggyback posterior chamber intraocular lenses. *Ophthalmology*. 1996;103:1118-1123.
27.   Lyle WA, Jin GJ. Clear lens extraction for the correction of high refractive error. *J Cataract Refract Surg*. 1994;20:273-276.
28.   Siganos DS, Siganos CS, Pallikaris IG. Clear lens extraction and intraocular lens implantation in normally sighted hyperopic eyes. *Refract Corneal Surg*. 1994;10:117-121.
29.   Baikoff G, Joly P. Comparison of minus power anterior chamber intraocular lenses and

myopic epikeratoplasty in phakic eyes. *Refract Corneal Surg*. 1990;6:252-260.

30. Risco JM, et al. Dislocation of a phakic intraocular lens. *Am J Ophthalmol*. 1994;118(5):666-667.

31. Baikoff G, et al. Surgical correction of severe myopia using an anterior chamber implant in the phakic eye. Concept-results. *Bull Soc Belge Ophtalmol*. 1989;233:109-125.

32. Baikoff G. Phakic anterior chamber intraocular lenses. *Int Ophthalmol Clin*. 1991;31(1):75-86.

33. Baikoff G, Samaha A. Phakic intraocular lens. In: Azar D, ed. *Refractive Surgery*. Stanford, Conn: Appleton & Lange; 1997.

34. Baikoff G, et al. Angle-fixated anterior chamber phakic intraocular lens for myopia of –7 to –19 diopters. *J Refract Surg*. 1998;14(3):282-293.

35. Fechner PU, Strobel J, Wichmann W. Correction of myopia by implantation of a concave Worst-iris claw lens into phakic eyes. *Refract Corneal Surg*. 1991;7:286-298.

36. Gelender H. Corneal endothelial cell loss, cystoid macular edema, and iris-supported intraocular lenses. *Ophthalmology*. 1984;91:841-846.

37. Jaffe NS, Galin MA, Hirschman H, Clayman HM. *Pseudophakos*. St. Louis, Mo: The CV Mosby Co; 1978.

38. Krumeich JH, Daniel J, Bast R. Closed-system technique for implantation of iris-supported negative-power intraocular lens. *J Refract Surg*. 1996;12:334-340.

39. Perez-Santonja JJ, et al. Surgical correction of high myopia in phakic eyes with Worst-Fechner myopia intraocular lenses. *J Refract Surg*. 1997;13(3):268-281.

40. Zaldivar R. Posterior chamber ICL follow-up: three years of experience and results with ICL and Bioptics. Presented at ACES QS XI Meeting, February 13-16, 1997, Ft. Lauderdale, Fla.

41. Fyodorov SN, et al. Intraocular correction of high-degree myopia. *Vestn Oftalmol*. 1988;104(2):14-16.

42. Fyodorov SN, Zuev VK, Aznabayev BM. Intraocular correction of high myopia with negative posterior chamber lens. *Ophthalmosurgery*. 1991;3:57-58.

43. Fyodorov SN, Zuyev VK, Tumanyan NR, Suheil AJ. Clinical and functional follow-up of minus IOL implantation in high-grade myopia. *Ophthalmosurgery*. 1993;2:12-17.

44. Fechner PU. "Phakic PCL is promising for high myopia." by Schonfeld AR. *Ocular Surgery News*. International ed. 1993;Dec:4-12. Presented at the European Society of Cataract and Refractive Surgeons annual symposium, September 1993, Innsbruck, Austria.

45. Assetto V, Benedetti S, Pesando P. Collamer (TM) intraocular contact lenses for high myopia. Presented at: XII Congress of the European Society of Cataract and Refractive Surgeons, September 18-22, 1994, Lisbon, Portugal.

46. Assetto V, et al. Collamer intraocular contact lens to correct high myopia. *J Cataract Refract Surg*. 1996;22(5):551-556.

47. Erturk H, et al. Phakic posterior chamber intraocular lenses for the correction of high myopia. *J Refract Surg*. 1995;11(5):388-391.

48. Zaldivar R. The intraocular contact lens (ICL). Presented at I Staar ICL Training Seminar, April 25-26, 1996, Mendoza, Argentina.

49. Fechner PU, et al. Posterior chamber myopia lenses in phakic eyes. *J Cataract Refract Surg*. 1996;22(2):178-182.

50. Feingold, V. Feasiblility studies for the implantable contact lens for high myopia. Presented at Staar ICL Training Seminar, April 25-26, 1996, Mendoza, Argentina.

51. Fine IH, Fichman RA, Grabow HB, eds. *Clear-Corneal Cataract Surgery & Topical Anesthesia*. Thorofare, NJ: SLACK Incorporated; 1993.

52. Wilson SE. The correction of myopia with phakic intraocular lenses. *Am J Ophthalmol*. 1993;115(2):249-251.

53. Zaldivar R, et al. Laser in situ keratomileusis for low myopia and astigmatism with scanning spot excimer laser. *J Refract Surg*. 1997;13(7).

54. Zaldivar R, Davidorf JM, Oscherow SA. Laser in situ keratomileusis for myopia from -5.50 to -11.00 diopters with astigmatism. *J Refract Surg*. 1998;14(1).
55. Zaldivar R, et al. Results and complications of laser in situ keratomileusis by experienced surgeons. *J Refract Surg*. 1998;14(2).

BIBLIOGRAPHY

Buratto L, Ferrari M, Genisi C. Myopic keratomileusis with the excimer laser: one year follow-up. *J Refract Corneal Surg*. 1993;9:12-19.

Colin J, Mimouni F, Robinet A, Conrad H, Mader P. The surgical treatment of high myopia: comparison of epikeratoplasty, keratomileusis and minus power AC lenses. *Refract Corneal Surg*. 1990;6:245-251.

Davidorf JM, Zaldivar R, Oscherow SA. Posterior chamber phakic intraocular lens for hyperopia of +4 to +11 diopters. *J Refract Surg*. 1998;14:306-311.

Dvali ML. Intraocular correction of high myopia. *Vestn Oftalmol*. 1986;102(6):29-31.

Fechner PU, et al. Intraocular lens for the correction of myopia of the phakic eye. *Klin Monatsbl Augenheilkd*. 1988;193(1):29-34.

Fechner PU, et al. The correction of myopia by lens implantation into phakic eyes. *Am J Ophthalmol*. 1989;107(6):659-663.

Fechner PU. Intraocular lenses for the correction of myopia in phakic eyes: short-term success and long-term caution. *Refract Corneal Surg*. 1990;6(4):242-244.

Kashani AA. Phakic posterior chamber intraocular lenses for the correction of high myopia. *J Refract Surg*. 1996;12(4):454-456.

Landesz M, Worst JGF, Siertsema JV, van Rij G. Correction of high myopia with the Worst myopia claw intraocular lens. *J Refract Surg*. 1995;11:16-25.

Marinho A, et al. Posterior chamber silicone phakic intraocular lens. *J Refract Surg*. 1997;13(3):219-222.

Neumann AC. "Update on three IOLs for myopia," by Schonfeld AR. *Ocular Surgery News*. 1993;Dec 1. Presented at European Society of Cataract and Refractive Surgeons annual symposium, September 1993, Innsbruck, Austria.

Perez-Santonja JJ, Iradier MT, Sanz-Iglesias L, Serrano JM, Zato MA. Endothelial changes in phakic eyes with anterior chamber intraocular lenses to correct high myopia. *J Cataract Refract Surg*. 1996;22:1017-1022.

Praeger DL. Innovations and creativity in contemporary ophthalmology: preliminary experience with the phakic myopic intraocular lens. *Ann Ophthalmol*. 1988;20(12):456-462.

Praeger DL. Phakic myopic intraocular lens—an alternative to kerato-lenticulorefractive procedures. *Ann Ophthalmol*. 1988;20(7):246.

Praeger DL, et al. Thirty-six month follow-up of a contemporary phakic intraocular lens for the surgical correction of myopia. *Ann Ophthalmol*. 1991;23(1):6-10.

Salz J, ed. *Corneal Laser Surgery*. St. Louis, Mo: CV Mosby Co; 1995.

Waring GO III. Phakic intraocular lenses for the correction of myopia—where do we go from here? *Refract Corneal Surg*. 1991;7(4):275-276.

Waring GO III, ed. *Refractive Keratotomy for Myopia and Astigmatism*. St. Louis, Mo: CV Mosby Co; 1992.

Wichmann W. Correction of high myopia by implantation of minus-power intraocular lenses in phakic eyes. *J Refract Surg*. 1996;12(6):672-673.

Wilson SE. The correction of myopia by lens implantation into phakic eyes. *Am J Ophthalmol*. 1989;108(4):465-466.

Zaldivar R. Three years of experience with anterior chamber implants for the correction of high myopia. Winner of the Storz Award at the Second Video Festival SBIIO '92, Sao Paolo, Brazil.

Zaldivar R. Our experience "Prelimanary results in phakic posterior chamber lens for high myopia." Presented at IV Reunion Anual, Sociedad de Egresados de Oftalmología, February 4-5, 1994, Monterrey, Mexico.

Zaldivar R, et al. The current status of phakic intraocular lenses. *Int Ophthalmol Clin.* 1996;36(4):107-111.

Zaldivar R. ICL demands attention in correction of high myopia. *Eye World International.* 1997;2(3).

Zaldivar R. ICL offers up to four lines of improvement in BCVA. *Ocular Surgery News.* 1997;8(5).

Zaldivar R. Experts discuss history and what's new in phakic IOL's. *Ocular Surgery News.* 1997;8(9).

Zaldivar R, et al. Posterior chamber lens implantation in phakic patients: a report of 220 patients treated with the intraocular contact lens. Submitted for publishing to *J Cataract Refract Surg.*

Phakic Refractive Intraocular Lenses

Paul S. Koch, MD

Using IOLs to correct refractive errors started more than 40 years ago. Strampelli began clinical trials of an anterior chamber phakic implant in 1953.[1] In 1959, Barraquer reported on 239 phakic implants, most of which had to be removed.[2] Though consistent with the technology of the time, those implants used were, by modern standards, primitive. They were rigid, thick, and poorly polished. When placed in the anterior chamber angle, they touched both the cornea and the iris, causing corneal edema, chronic iridocyclitis, or hyphema. These trials were quickly abandoned. Interestingly, many of the Barraquer lenses were preserved by an OR nurse and were available to be examined by Drews in 1982.[3]

The experience of patients receiving these early phakic implants was similar to that of aphakic patients who had implants and corresponded to the technology of IOL manufacture. The exciting history of IOLs for the treatment of aphakia is one of technological advancement, bringing us to our present state in which we have excellent implants that are tolerated nearly perfectly by the eye. Rigid lenses have been replaced by flexible ones, thick by thin ones, and poorly polished ones by lenses that are exquisitely smooth.[4,5] Therefore, it is without surprise that the subject of phakic IOL is revisited.

It is reasonable, then, to reevaluate the use of IOLs to treat refractive errors, to determine if the technology of IOL manufacture is up to the task, and to decide how IOL insertion compares with corneal refractive surgery. We certainly have excellent corneal refractive procedures for myopia up to 10 D, but there is a limit to the practical application of corneal flattening as a means of affecting refractive chance.

Phakic IOLs have the potential to unlock an entire range of refractive correction, which heretofore have been inaccessible to us.

The first modern implant in a phakic eye was performed by Worst in 1980, but it was not for refractive purposes. A patient with intractable diplopia received an opaque iris fixation lens to inhibit vision from one eye. Examined 9 years later, the eye showed no problems. Visual acuity was undisturbed, as recorded around the implant through a dilated pupil. The natural lens showed no opacification.[6]

Dvali reported the use of an anterior chamber phakic implant in 1986.[7] Baikoff presented his anterior chamber lens in 1988 (Sixth Congress of the European Intraocular Implant Lens Council in Copenhagen, August 14-18), and later reported a comparison of his lens to epikeratoplasty.[8,9] About the same time, Fyodorov described his results with a thin lens floating in the posterior chamber between the iris and natural lens.[10,11]

There are certainly many attractions to the use of phakic IOLs. A manufactured plastic lens gives us excellent refractive quality and accuracy. The predictability of a plastic lens' power is guaranteed, while the accuracy of a corneal refractive procedure is anticipated. Compared to lensectomy and lens implantation, accommodation in young patients is preserved. The surgical techniques necessary to implant a phakic IOL are common and performed regularly by most anterior segment surgeons. The procedure is reversible (implant removal) and adjustable (implant exchange). The technique does not require large and expensive laser systems, nor the payment of royalties when performed.

All clinical studies of refractive IOLs have several well-defined goals:

- To determine the postoperative visual acuity, short- and long-term, of eyes receiving these implants while the natural lens remains in place
- To determine which postoperative complications may occur
- To identify the appropriate groups in whom to implant such a lens, and in whom not to implant

Most clinical trials are designed to evaluate the use of phakic implants in eyes with myopia. However, the use of phakic IOLs to treat hyperopia is also under investigation.

OPTICS

The optic shapes of implants designed for myopia and hyperopia are different. The implants designed to correct hyperopia are biconvex, so the anterior surface of the optic follows the contour of the cornea's back surface. Most implants for myopia, on the other hand, have a concave front surface, with edge thickness increasing along with the power of the lens. This means the distance between the edge of the optic and the endothelium narrows as the lens power increases. The Worst myopia claw lens, on the other hand, has evolved from one with a biconcave optic to one having a concave back surface and a convex front surface, so it more closely mimics the surface characteristics of a lens for hyperopia, and avoids some of the edge thickness questions.[12] The ability to correct high refractive errors with a phakic IOL may depend on the maximum thickness lens that can be implanted in a

human eye before the optic/endothelium separation narrows to a critical point—this thickness being determined by the lens power and the anterior chamber depth.

Saragoussi et al have analyzed the qualitative and quantitative anatomic relationships of an anterior chamber phakic IOL to the cornea, angle, iris, and lens in myopic eyes.[13] High-resolution ultrasound was used to measure the actual clearance between the optic and cornea in 13 eyes that had a Baikoff anterior chamber implant with a power ranging from -9.00 D to -15.00 D. The mean distance from central cornea to optic was 2.05 ± 0.18 mm (range: 1.80 to 2.47 mm). The mean distance from peripheral cornea to implant was 1.56 ± 0.17 mm (range: 1.33 to 1.95 mm). The mean distance from the natural lens to the implant was 0.58 ± 0.12 mm (range: 0.48 to 0.81 mm). Theoretical calculations derived using the Worst myopia indicate that with a 3.2-mm anterior chamber depth, the optic has clearance from the cornea estimated to be 2.05 mm with a 10 D implant, and 1.86 mm with a 20 D.[14]

CALCULATION

The distance from the cornea is also important in calculating the power of the lens to be used. van der Heijde has calculated the implant power needed to correct a refractive error. The factors important in the calculation are the patient's refraction, the corneal curvature, and the anterior chamber depth. The anterior chamber depth in this case is defined as the distance from corneal back surface to the implant front surface, and varies in a single eye depending on the style and location of the phakic IOL to be implanted. For a given eye, the calculated anterior chamber depth will be shorter when an anterior chamber IOL is used, and longer when a posterior chamber IOL is used. The anterior chamber depth is calculated by performing a standard A-scan to determine the natural, pre-surgical anterior chamber depth, and then subtracting the anticipated distance of the anterior surface of the implant from the anterior surface of the natural lens. Matrix nomograms tabulating the calculations to determine the lens power have been published.[15]

Among van der Heijde's observations is that the power of a lens needed to correct aphakia increases as it moves from the spectacle plane toward the retina. There is a significant increase in required lens power once it reaches the anterior chamber. The power of a lens to correct myopia, on the other hand, peaks at the corneal plane, and decreases when moving either toward the retina or away from it. The power of a minus lens at vertex distance 12 mm anterior to the cornea is roughly equal to the power of a lens 4 mm behind the cornea. Therefore, the power of a lens to correct myopia is roughly the same whether it is placed in a spectacle or in the anterior chamber.

ACCURACY

The most challenging step in determining the appropriate power implant to use is the patient's refraction. As the refractive error increases, the accuracy of the refraction decreases. The endpoint becomes vague when eyes have posterior staphylomata, myopic degeneration, and macular changes. As a result, the accuracy of phakic IOL implantation is less in the more myopic eyes, and better in the less myopic eyes.

Marinho reported 71% of eyes receiving the Adatomed silicone posterior chamber IOL had a final refraction of -1.00 D to +1.00 D.[16] The preoperative range was -7.00 D to -28.00 D. Fechner, also using the Adatomed lens, reported 53 eyes with a final refraction of +0.07 ± 1.05 D.[17] In another report, Fechner, this time using the Worst-Fechner lens found the final correction to be within 10% in 47 of 62 eyes (76%), and within 20% of desired correction in all eyes.[18] Perez-Santonja reported on 32 eyes with the Worst-Fechner lens. Seventy-six percent were within 1 D of target.[19] Landesz observed 55.5% of his eyes within 1 D and 25% were greater than 2 D.[12] He attributed this to inaccuracies with the preoperative refraction.

RETINAL IMAGE SIZE

The relationship between lens location and retinal image size is an important one. Compared to lenses placed at the corneal plane, plus lenses for hyperopia provide more magnification as they move away from the retina. Minus lenses for myopia cause minification as they are moved away from the retina and relative magnification as they are moved closer. Image sizes in myopia increase as a patient goes from spectacles to contact lenses and increases further when a patient goes from contact lenses to phakic IOLs. van der Heijde has calculated image size changes when correcting 18 D of myopia.[15] Compared to a contact lens, a spectacle with a 12-mm vertex distance would give 20% minification. A phakic IOL with a 4-mm anterior chamber depth would give 8% magnification.

IMPROVED BEST CORRECTED VISUAL ACUITY

One advantage of phakic IOLs for myopia is the almost universal finding that many of these eyes have an improvement in best corrected visual acuity. This is because of the placement of the optic closer to the retina. van der Heijde has calculated a myopia lens would actually cause a magnification, compared to a contact lens, of 8% at 18 D.[15]

The magnification provided by a phakic implant compared to a contact lens is noticed by the patient in terms of improved best corrected visual acuity. Marinho et al found 63% of eyes had improved best corrected visual acuity of 2 lines or more with a silicone posterior chamber phakic IOL.[16] With the Worst myopia lens approximately 40% of eyes either stayed the same or improved by 1 line, another 40% improved by 2 to 4 lines, and an additional 11% improved by more than 4 lines of best corrected visual acuity. Three to 8% of eyes lost 1 or more lines of vision by the end of 3 years, which may reflect the natural course of extreme myopia.[14] Perez-Santonja reported mean improvement of best corrected visual acuity of 1.6 lines in a report of 32 eyes, preoperative refractions ranging from -9.50 to -27.00, that received the Worst myopia lens.[19] Six of 10 patients had improved best corrected visual acuity in the Staar Implantable Contact Lens (ICL) study, and in the Baikoff anterior lens study, 57.7% of patients were correctable to 20/40 prior to surgery compared with 90% following surgery (company data). Virtually the same findings were obtained in the Worst claw lens study, 56.7% correctable to 20/40 prior to surgery, and 87.4% after surgery.[14]

CELL LOSS

The presence of an iris fixation or an angle fixated IOL naturally causes concerns about endothelial cell loss. The original Fechner-Worst lens was modified in response to cell loss. The biconcave optic was replaced with a concave/convex optic in order to avoid the thick edges of a biconcave lens. Another problem with the Worst myopia lens is the difficulty implanting this lens in some cases. This can cause immediate cell loss from surgical trauma, which may not be progressive.

Perez-Santonja reported on cell loss with the Worst-Fechner lens and with the Baikoff lens.[19] With the Worst lens they observed 7.2% loss at 3 months, 10.6% at 6 months, 13.0% at 12 months, and 17.6% at 24 months. The corresponding numbers for a Baikoff angle fixated lens were 7.5%, 10.9%, 12.3%, and 12.3%, respectively. Menezo prospectively measured the cell counts of 90 eyes in 70 patients who received the Worst myopia lens.[20] Central and mid-peripheral measurements were taken, and both counts and morphology were studied. The loss of cells was 3.3% at 6 months, 5.5% at 1 year, and 7.63% at 2 years. Landesz reported cell loss with the claw lens at 5.6% at 6 months and 8.9% at 1 year.[12]

Werblin reported endothelial cell loss following cataract surgery as being 8.8% at 1 year, increasing to 11.5% at 3 years, then plateauing.[21] These numbers are comparable with those reported for the Worst myopia lens and the Baikoff angle fixated lens, but it is not known yet whether the cell counts plateau in these eyes as they do in aphakic eyes.

Fechner discussed cell loss with the Worst lens and contemplated whether a posterior chamber lens would be better.[22] In another report he and coauthors discussed cell loss with the Worst lens and felt that it may be more of a problem than with the lens in aphakic eyes because the myopia lens sits closer to the cornea.[17] If a patient has myopia, with low scleral rigidity, and rubs the eye, there can be temporary implant-endothelial contact. Therefore, they recommend that patients receiving these lenses be advised not to rub their eyes. Landesz reported a case of corneal edema and echoed the opinion that patients should be counseled not to rub their eyes.[12]

CLINICAL INVESTIGATIONS

There are three types of phakic implants undergoing clinical trials: posterior chamber, iris fixated, and anterior chamber. Each has specific advantages and disadvantages.

Posterior Chamber Implants

Fyodorov, who proposed a thin, buoyant lens that would float between the iris and the natural lens, originally described the posterior chamber implant.[10,11] It was hoped this lens would neither irritate the iris, liberate pigment, damage the cornea, or cause a cataract. However, Wiechens has reported one case of bilateral cataract after phakic posterior chamber top hat-style silicone IOL implanted in Russia.[23] When the implants were removed there were membranes on the posterior surface of the implants. Presence of the implant prevented accurate preoperative axial length

measurement prior to cataract surgery. Eventually, the cataract was removed and then the patient had intraoperative retinoscopy to determine the appropriate aphakic lens power.

This report notwithstanding, modern posterior chamber phakic IOLs have the advantage of being extremely flexible and thus can be folded and injected through a very small incision. The small incision required minimizes, if not eliminates, induction of astigmatism as a significant factor in eventual visual recovery. On the other hand, the insertion technique is difficult, requiring gentle placement of the lens through a dilated pupil. Even with meticulous surgical technique there remains concerns about inducing cataracts. Fechner has reported an 18% rate of new lens opacities within 2 years following implantation of a silicone posterior chamber implant.[24] Also, fixation is a challenge because the lens floats in the posterior chamber. This raises the possibility of pigment dispersion, chronic low-grade iritis, cataract formation, and chronic glaucoma. He recommended that, to avoid marked decentration, the best length of the implant should equal the horizontal diameter of the cornea (white-to-white).

Another question about posterior chamber phakic implants revolves around the movement of the natural lens during accommodation. As the lens thickens, the anterior surface moves forward as much as 0.6 mm, sometimes moving through the pupil anterior to the iris.[15] Phakic implant designs have to allow for this movement and to provide for sufficient clearance so this is not a problem. Iris fixation and anterior chamber phakic IOL can easily be vaulted to ensure clearance, but it is likely that there is intermittent touch between the natural lens and the posterior chamber phakic implant during accommodation. Whether this will eventually affect the clarity of the natural lens is unknown, but there is suspicion that this was a factor in the termination of the Adatomed silicone lens trials.

Among the first posterior chamber implants to undergo clinical investigation were a Collagel implant from Staar and a silicone implant from Adatomed/Chiron. There are others being developed, including a prototype foldable PMMA implant, but the two lenses mentioned are the furthest along in their trials.

Adatomed Silicone Implant

A silicone posterior chamber implant from Adatomed/Chiron has been in clinical trials. Marinho reported its use in 38 eyes with myopia range from -7.00 D to -28.00 D.[16] There were no problems with the lens, only occasional problems caused by the surgical technique. There were no cataracts as of 24 months postop, nor any vision-threatening complications. Seventy-one percent were within 1 D of target refraction. Sixty-five percent of eyes had improved best corrected visual acuity by at least 2 lines.

Fechner reported his results with 69 Adatomed implants.[24] Eight eyes developed central subcapsular opacities after 1 to 2 years. These were assumed to be implant induced.

At this time we do not know whether there is an actual causal relationship between implant and natural lens opacity, or what the nature of the relationship would be. There could have been a material incompatibility, or it could have been a matter of the natural lens pressing against the implant during accommodation. Nevertheless, the clinical investigation of the Adatomed lens was terminated in 1997.

Staar ICL

The phakic implant from Staar is different in that it is made of a proprietary material consisting of collagen and hydrogel (Figure 20-1). The lens is extremely soft and is injected into the anterior chamber through a small incision. Once in the eye it unfolds slowly and can be gently directed under the iris. The surgeon must be careful not to touch the natural lens out of concern for causing a cataract to form.

The implant is designed to float in the posterior chamber between the iris and the natural lens. Initial results of clinical trials show that this is the case. In order to prevent pupillary block, it is recommended that eyes receiving these implants have two iridectomies or iridotomies, 90 degrees apart.

The US clinical trials of the Staar implant for myopia began in February 1997. Ten patients were enrolled who had refractions ranging from -7.25 to -9.375 D with a mean of -7.75 D.

Nine of the 10 patients ended up within 0.5 D of emmetropia and all were within 0.75 D. Seven patients had 20/20 uncorrected vision, and two others were 20/25. The 10th patient saw 20/60 without correction due to pre-existing astigmatism. With correction, all patients were 20/20 or better within 1 week. Six patients had improved best corrected visual acuity by at least 1 line.

The US clinical trials of the Staar implant for hyperopia also began in February 1997. These 10 patients had refractions ranging from +2.50 D to +10.875 D with a mean of +6.63 D.

Eight of the 10 patients were within 0.5 D of emmetropia, and all were within 1.125 D. Prior to surgery five patients had uncorrected vision of count fingers, and eight were 20/70 or worse. At final visit, all patients saw 20/40 or better without correction with eight seeing 20/25 or better and six seeing 20/20 or better. Two patients had improvement of best corrected visual acuity by 3 lines.

Iris Fixated Implants

The iris fixation implant has been with us for the longest period of time. This implant is based on a design by Worst that dates to 1978.[25] Worst had previously designed a pupil fixation lens (Worst medallion lens) (Figure 20-2) which had two holes in the peripheral optic through which fixation sutures were placed. When the synthetic sutures he used failed because they dissolved, he decided to try stainless steel sutures. He could not, however, easily use the holes with the wire so he replaced the holes with notches (Figure 20-3). Later, he noticed several patients had iris incarceration in the notches, and this provided lens stability. He incorporated little claws in some of his later IOLs, precursors of the later design (Figure 20-4).

In 1978 he introduced the Worst claw lens, which had small notches on either side into which to incarcerate a small amount of mid-peripheral iris for fixation. The Worst lens for aphakia proved popular in Europe and across the Middle East and Asia with several hundred thousand being implanted.

The first placement of an iris fixation lens in a phakic eye came in 1980, when an opaque implant was implanted to occlude the pupil in a patient with diplopia[6] (Figure 20-5). Nine years later, examination showed no problems. Visual acuity was

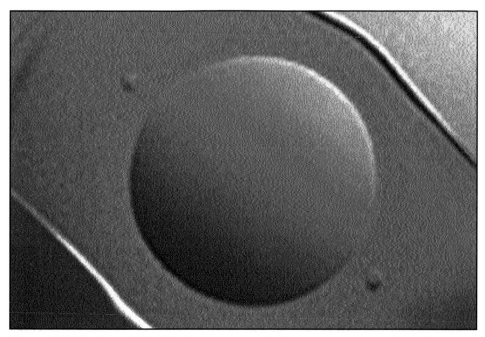

Figure 20-1. The Staar ICL. This lens is made of Collagel, a proprietary collagen/hydrogel material. It is designed to float between the natural lens and the posterior iris.

Figure 20-2. The Worst medallion lens. The two small holes in the optic were designed for a soft, flexible suture.

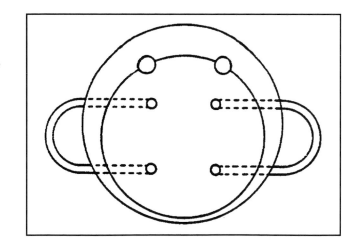

undisturbed, as recorded around the implant through a dilated pupil, and the natural lens showed no opacification.

The iris fixated lens should not be confused with the old pupil fixated lenses. The pupil is a very mobile structure and the problem found with pupil fixated implants are not those found with iris fixated lenses. The other end of the iris, the iris root, is secured to the scleral spur and is completely non-mobile. Between the

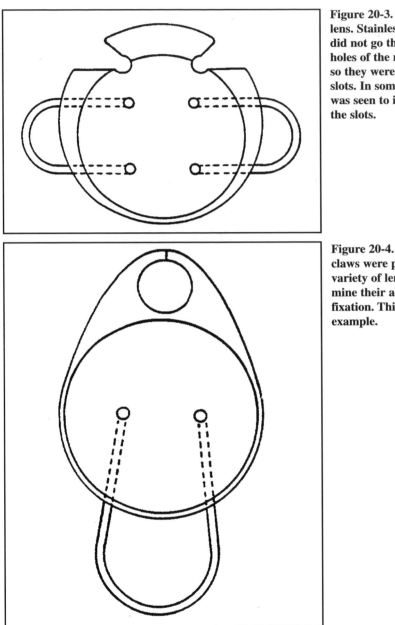

Figure 20-3. The Worst slot lens. Stainless steel suture did not go through the holes of the medallion lens, so they were replaced with slots. In some cases iris was seen to incarcerate in the slots.

Figure 20-4. The original claws were placed on a variety of lenses to determine their adequacy for fixation. This is just one example.

iris root and the pupil is the mid-peripheral iris, which is relatively non-mobile. It barely moved even during dilation, because when the pupil dilates the pupil is pulled to the periphery. The iris proximal to the iris root barely moves.

That makes the anterior mid-peripheral iris a place where a lens can be fixated comfortably. Unlike anterior chamber implants, there are no concerns about the lens being wedged against the cornea, and there are no concerns about localized synechi-

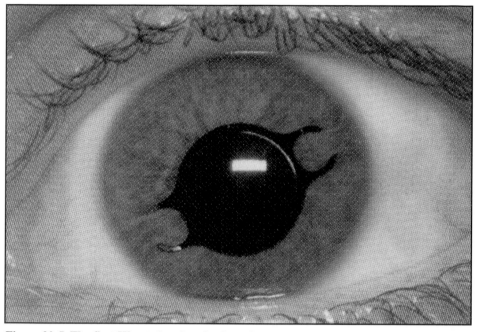

Figure 20-5. The first Worst claw lens implanted was an opaque lens, designed to eliminate double vision in a patient with intractable diplopia.

ae occluding the angle. There are no sizing issues, and one size implant length suits all eyes.

Concerns about securing an implant on the mid-peripheral iris are more akin to concerns about the placement of sphincterotomy sutures or of a McCannel suture.[17] These are routinely placed without concerns about localized inflammation.

Nevertheless, there is always a concern about the effects of iris fixation of an IOL on the iris, because of its greater size and mass. Fechner studied 109 eyes with the Worst lens after at least 1-year follow-up. Iris angiography showed no vascular leaks. The flare cell meter showed results of the same magnitude as that seen following cataract surgery with in-the-bag lens implantation at least 6 months postoperatively: protein below 20 counts, cells 4.5 ± per 0.075 mm². Examination for signs of chronic inflammation (Tyndall phenomenon, cells in the anterior chamber) was negative. The long-term findings in eyes with Worst claw lenses generally do not demonstrate synechiae, iris atrophy, or flourescein leakage at the enclavation sites.[17]

Perez-Santonja, on the other hand, found evidence of chronic inflammation in 15 eyes that received the Worst-Fechner lens.[19,26,27] The authors noted no postoperative complications, including cystoid macular edema. All clinical signs of inflammation disappeared between 3 and 5 weeks following surgery. The eyes were evaluated using fluorometry. The fluorescein concentration in the anterior vitreous was significantly higher than preoperatively as late as 14 months following surgery. There was also a mild decrease in lens transmittance. In another study they compared the laser flare measurements of 30 eyes with Worst-Fechner lenses with 30

eyes having Baikoff implants. Compared with 13 phakic eyes, the surgical eyes had more flare as late as 24 months following surgery.[27] These studies did not include a comparison group of eyes receiving lens implants for aphakia, but noted previous studies indicating a return to baseline by 6 to 12 months in the cataract surgery population.[28-31]

The intraocular environment has been impressively hospitable to IOLs for aphakic correction, and it is difficult to imagine that with the sole difference being an encapsulated natural lens the phakic eye should react any differently. Still, any findings related to chronic inflammation cannot be dismissed in the phakic eye. While sub-clinical inflammation in an aphakic eye cannot cause a cataract to form, we do not know whether it can in a phakic eye.

In 1986, Fechner modified the Worst aphakia implant to treat myopia. The original Worst-Fechner lens had a biconcave optic with little vaulting on its footplates. Clinical results were underwhelming. The biconcave optic, even without much vaulting came too close to the cornea and progressive cell loss was documented. Also, the lens sat too close to the pupil, impeding aqueous flow and leading to increased IOPs. In 1990, the Fechner-Worst lens was redesigned. The new lens, called the Worst myopia lens had not only adjusted vaulting, but also a convex/concave optic. This lens worked better and remains the design used today[12] (Figures 20-6 and 20-7).

Aside from its unconventional appearance, the main difficulty with this lens is placement. The implantation is noticeably more difficult than with angle fixated implants. The 5 mm-wide lens is placed through a 6-mm incision and positioned directly over the constricted pupil. The implant is grasped with forceps while a bent needle is used to establish fixation. The enclavation needle pushes against the peripheral iris and then pulls upward, capturing a fold of iris on its tip. The fold is lifted into the claw while at the same time the lens is slightly depressed against it. When the fold of iris is engaged, enclavation is complete. The process is repeated on the other side, watching to be sure the optic stays centered. If the enclavation is insufficient, the iris can be removed and the steps repeated. Likewise, enclavation can be repeated if the lens is not centered. It can even be repeated at a later date, if necessary (Figures 20-8 through 20-10).

Angle Fixated Implants

Angle fixated lenses have many potential advantages. They, like other phakic IOLs, are associated with accuracy, predictability, and reversibility. There is a very long history of using lenses of this design in treating aphakia. The haptic design and the fixation methods are well established.

Angle fixated phakic implants are by far the easiest to implant. The technique is virtually exactly the same as implanting angle fixated lenses for aphakia. The pupil is constricted prior to surgery. An incision is made slightly larger than the optic. A Sheets' Glide can be placed to protect the pupil, if desired. The implant is placed in the anterior chamber and secured in the angle.

Anterior chamber lenses for aphakia have historically been associated with

Figure 20-6. The Worst myopia lens. An evolution from the lens used for aphakia, this lens has improved vaulting and a convex/concave optic.

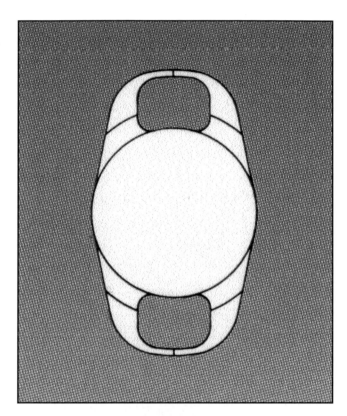

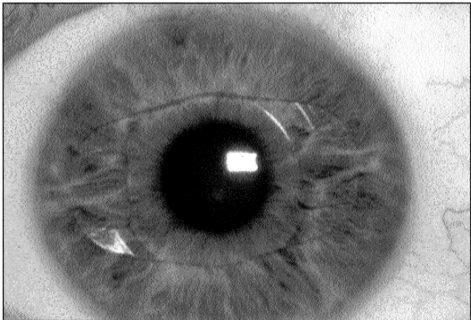

Figure 20-7. The Worst myopia lens in situ. A small bridge of iris holds the lens. The effect on iris tissue is similar to the effect exerted when an iris suture is left in place.

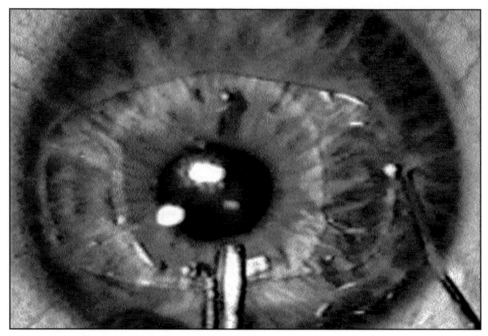

Figure 20-8. When securing the Worst myopia lens, forceps are used to hold the optic in position while enclavation is performed.

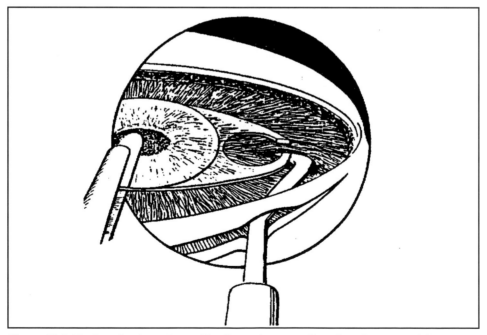

Figure 20-9. Enclavation is performed by first using a needle to bunch up some iris. Push inferiorly a little with the tip of the needle to gather some iris on its tip.

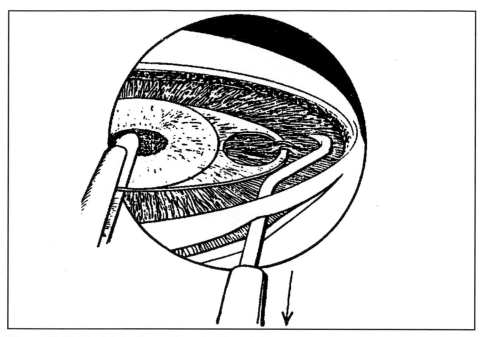

Figure 20-10. The iris is slipped into the claw of the lens, where it is secured and held gently. The lens will not move, but if it needs to be positioned, the iris can be easily slipped out.

problems including uveitis, glaucoma, hyphema, cell loss, and glare. Modern designs have essentially eliminated these problems in aphakia, and so we should not anticipate significant problems when these lenses are used in phakia, with perhaps only a few exceptions.

Glare is a function of the relationship between optic size and pupil size. Young, phakic patients tend to have larger and more easily dilatable pupils, so glare should be expected in some patients, regardless of lens design.

Pupil distortion can be a problem with anterior chamber implants, caused by incorrect sizing or inappropriate stiffness of the lens. Pressure in the angle leads to localized ischemia, manifested by iris change and pupil elongation. This problem is avoided by selecting a lens of appropriate size and flexibility. How to ensure this remains a topic of clinical investigations and manufacturer research and development.

Another design characteristic concerns how the lens sits in the angle. Critical to acceptance as a phakic implant will be assurance that the footplates neither rub the corneal endothelium, nor chafe against the iris.

Baikoff Anterior Chamber Lens

The Baikoff-Kelman lens remains a popular lens worldwide, being investigated in a number of locations. Originally associated with stiffness and glare, the lens has been modified with a larger optic and more flexible haptics, resolving, it is hoped, some of the early difficulties.[8,9]

The original Baikoff lens, the ZB, was associated with a high incidence of

endothelial cell loss, believed to be caused by contact between lens optic and endothelium. The lens was redesigned as the ZB5M, a second-generation lens, which was evaluated in a multicenter 5-year prospective study in France. This lens is a single-piece, biconcave anterior chamber lens with a 5-mm optic, having an effective diameter of 4 mm. It was available from -7.00 D to -20.00 D. In the study, however, the range of lenses used was -7.00 D to -15.00 D with an average of -11.08 ± 2.1 D (Figure 20-11).

Spherical equivalent refraction averaged approximately -1.00 D over the 3 years of follow-up and no eyes were overcorrected by more than 1 D. After 3 years, 88.2% of patients were still within 2 D of intended correction and 58.8% were within 1 D of intended correction.

The prospective study demonstrated a marked improvement in both near and distance uncorrected visual acuity, increasing from 20/400 to 20/40 at distance and 20/100 to 20/30 at near. Ninety percent of treated eyes had vision of 20/40 or better at each postoperative visit, contrasted to only 57.7% prior to surgery. A few eyes had an apparent decline in distance visual acuity, attributable to natural progression of myopia in some eyes and/or disproportionate representation of patients having poor outcome implanted during the early phase of the protocol. There was no evidence that the decreased visual acuity was lens related.[32]

At 3 years, the mean endothelial cell loss was 4.6%. There was an immediate drop of 3.4%, reflecting the effects of surgery. After that, there was an additional decline of 0.69% per year. This is slightly higher than the 0.33% to 0.53% per year estimate occurring in normal eyes in patients of comparable age, but it is still well below the 1.5% per year reduction postulated as producing corneal decompensation in a 95-year-old patient implanted with a phakic IOL at 25 years of age, who experienced a 12% cell loss at the time of implantation.[33-36]

There were quite a few visual complications; 27.8% of eyes presented with halos, glare, and similar phenomena at some time over the course of the study (about 15% at any visit) and pupillary ovalization was observed in 22.6% of eyes, the incidence increasing with years following surgery.

Predictability was measured by the actual error in refractive correction (achieved minus intended), which was <-0.4 D over the first 2 years of follow-up, increasing slightly to -0.6 D at the 3-year visit. Also, 58.8% to 76.9% of eyes were within 1 D of intended correction and 88.2% to 98.7% were within 2 D of intended correction.

The third-generation lens, the NuVita MA20, is an evolution of the ZB5M model designed to address the problem of halos and glare (Figure 20-12). The effective optical diameter is increased from 4.0 to 4.5 mm, without changing the overall optical diameter, and the posterior edge of the optic is subjected to a patented process termed Peripheral Detail Technology to reduce the incidence of reflected or refracted glare to zero. Ovalization of the pupil was addressed by changing the vaulting of the haptics from a step vault to a curved angulation, and by redesigning the haptic footplates to better conform to iridocorneal angle geometry.

Peripheral Detail Technology is a treatment designed to reduce edge glare. The light intensity at the retinal plane caused by the angle of incidence of an illuminating beam and the IOL is demonstrated in Figures 20-13 and 20-14. Initially, there is

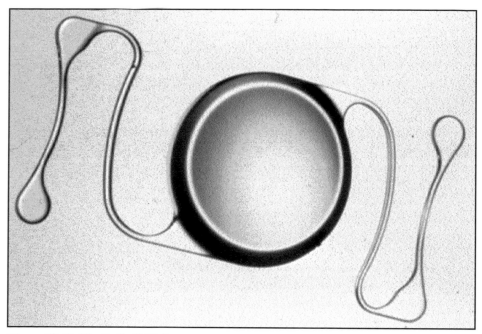

Figure 20-11. The Baikoff ZB lens used in a multicenter 5-year prospective study in France.

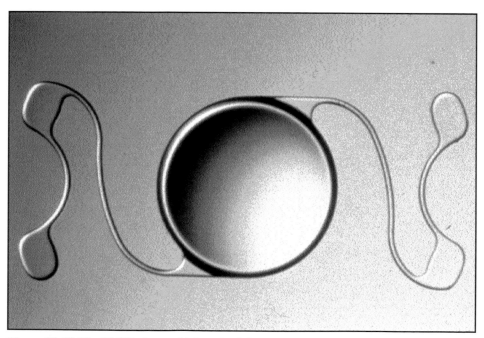

Figure 20-12. The NuVita lens, which evolved from the ZB lens. This model has an enlarged effective optical diameter, while keeping the actual diameter at 5 mm. Step vaulting gave way to curved angulation, and the footplates were modified to better conform to the angle.

a definite peak of light intensity, demonstrating edge glare. This is resolved after the edge treatment.

ThinOptx Thin Lens

The edge thickness of an anterior lens seems to be a concern in all of these lens designs, causing problems ranging from glare to lenticular endothelial touch. A wonderful advance would be the elimination of the edge completely. This is a project undertaken by ThinOptX, which is developing a PMMA lens of previously undreamed thinness. For example, a standard 20 D lens has a central thickness of approximately 1000 microns. The center thickness of the Thin Lens with the same power, is approximately 50 microns.

Conceivably, a posterior chamber phakic implant could be made that would fit comfortably between the natural lens and the iris. While there is certainly not enough space to place a typical posterior chamber phakic implant of usual thickness, there may be adequate space to place a lens that is only 50 microns thick.

In the anterior chamber, the thickness of a standard meniscus lens could be decreased from about 750 microns to approximately 50 microns. This would improve the distance from lens to cornea by an additional 700 microns, and could possibly allay concerns about lens-corneal touch (Figures 20-15 and 20-16).

Removing the bulk and retaining the surfaces creates the Thin Lens. For example, consider a lens in which the front surface carries the power and the back surface is plano. Light is bent at the front surface toward the central axis in proportion to the radius of curvature and the index of refraction of the lens and its surrounding media. If the posterior surface is plano, the light is bent slightly toward the central axis, so all the parallel light rays entering the back of the lens come to focus at one point. The bulk of the optic is removed by carving out several small steps of plano backed surfaces, leaving the implant with a curved front surface and a plano back surface (Figures 20-17 and 20-18).

Customary lenses generate several optical imperfections, from spherical aberrations, from the thickness of the lens, and from peripheral aberrations due to the edges of the lens. It is conceivable that making the lens extremely thin will eliminate these aberrations and improve its optical quality. If this is the case, lens diameter will be a less critical factor because there will be less concern about edge glare. Smaller optic sizes may be possible.

ThinOptX hopes to begin US clinical trials in late 1998 or early 1999.

Galin Lens

Another angle fixated implant is the Galin lens, which is somewhat similar. It is carried on a standard Kelman-style carrier and has a heparin-coated 6-mm optic. The haptics are extremely flexible so there is only gentle pressure in the chamber angle. This is expected to minimize localized point ischemia and pupil ovalization. The slightly larger optic is designed to reduce the incidence of glare, especially in dim light conditions. International clinical trials have begun, with FDA-sanctioned US trials anticipated to begin in 1998 (Figure 20-19).

Assuming the historical problems with angle fixated implants are resolved, the

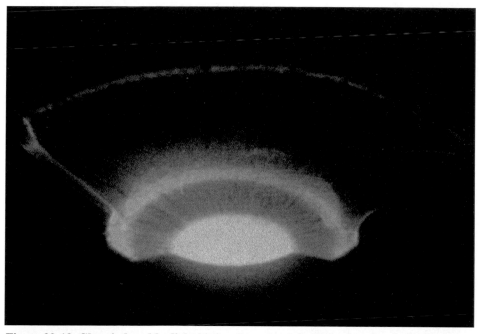

Figure 20-13. Glare induced by light hitting the untreated, thick edge of a phakic lens for myopia.

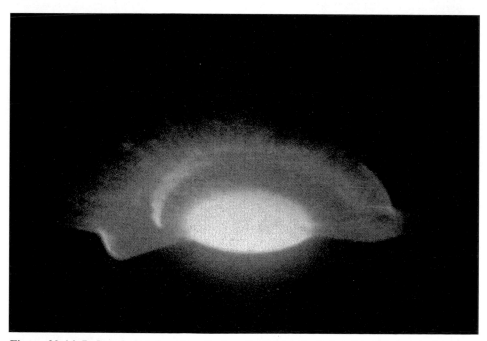

Figure 20-14. Induced glare is reduced when the thick edge is treated with a proprietary method, Peripheral Detail Technology. This is designed to reduce edge glare.

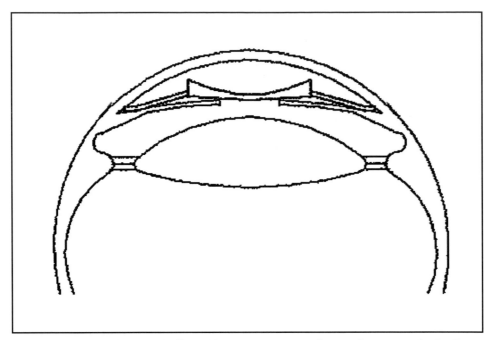

Figure 20-15. A meniscus angle fixated lens can come very close to the cornea. As the diameter increases, the thick edges come closer to the peripheral cornea.

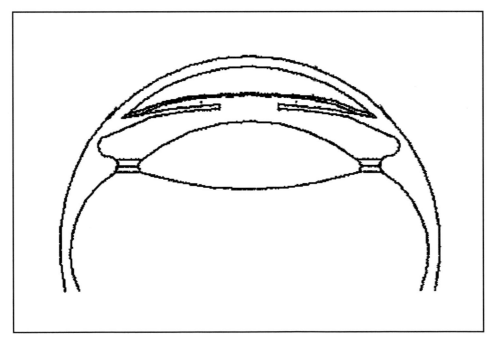

Figure 20-16. The Thin Lens would eliminate the thick edges, permitting an implant of a very high power to sit in the anterior chamber without coming close to the cornea.

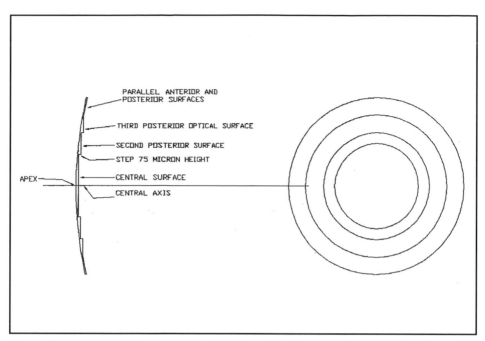

Figure 20-17. The Thin Lens is designed with a series of steps, each concentric ring designed to work as a complete lens system. Each point on the lens focuses light to the exact same focal point.

Figure 20-18. The Thin Lens maintains a curved front surface and a plano back surface. The steps allow the back of the lens to be removed in the manufacturing process.

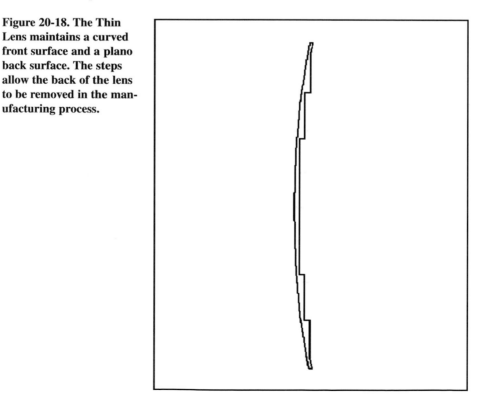

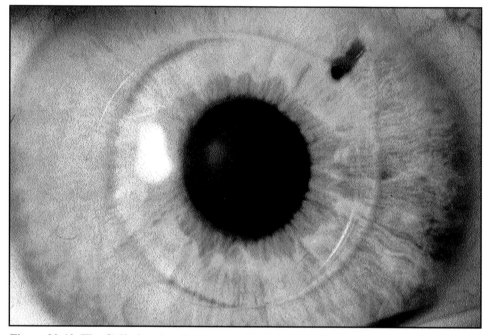

Figure 20-19. The Galin lens is a 6-mm angle fixated IOL.

only factor which might lead to phakic lens failure is the unique position of the iris relative to these lenses. Angle-fixated lenses are typically placed in aphakic eyes in which the iris has collapsed posteriorly due to removal of the natural lens. In phakic eyes the iris remains convex, and possibly even moves slightly anterior during accommodation. The footplates and the vault must be designed to avoid chronic iris chafe, which could lead to chronic inflammation, cataract formation, and so forth.

These lenses were initially placed through superior scleral or corneal incisions, but with a 5.0- or 6.0-mm optic there is the potential for surgically induced astigmatism. Alternatively, a temporal corneal incision can be used. Once secured with two or three sutures, this incision will be very stable. One disadvantage of a temporal incision is the relative difficulty of making a peripheral iridotomy. One way is to introduce small scissors through the incision and directed toward 12 o'clock. The lower blade can tent some iris and lift it up, away from the natural lens. The tented iris can be snipped, making a small, but wholly adequate, iridectomy. Alternatively, a laser iridotomy can be made a week or so prior to lens implantation.

SUMMARY

Clinical research is ongoing regarding the safety and efficacy of phakic IOLs. The eye has shown itself to be a marvelous host of IOLs for eyes with aphakia, so hopefully it will be for phakic eyes, also. Two major differences between these eyes make these investigations necessary. First, the presence of the natural lens changes the anatomy of the anterior segment. The iris is convex, and the natural lens moves forward during accommodation. The pupil is in just close proximity to both the nat-

ural lens and the implant that interference with aqueous flow is a concern. Early designs were associated with elevated IOPs. Even with the newer implants, a peripheral iridectomy or iridotomy is a necessity. Second, the presence of a clear natural lens mandates that we keep it that way. Whether these lenses cause, or are associated with, sub-clinical inflammation of such an extent that the natural lens may be compromised is a topic requiring investigation. There is also a concern about intermittent natural lens-plastic lens touch during accommodation. Preliminary reports are very encouraging in both regards, regardless of the lens style used.

Each of the three styles has its advantages and disadvantages. Compared to corneal refractive surgery they have several important features. Plastic lenses can be manufactured to high degrees of precision and accuracy, and the procedure can be adjustable or reversible. The techniques used for implantation are common to all anterior segment surgeons. Expensive equipment and royalty payments are unnecessary. Best corrected visual acuity, at least in myopia, improves in the majority of eyes.

REFERENCES

1. Strampelli B. Supportabilita di lenti acriliche in camera anteriore nella afachia e nei vizi di refrazione. *Annali di Ottalomologia e o Clinica Oculistica*. 1954;80:75-82.
2. Barraquer J. Anterior chamber plastic lenses: results and conclusions from five years' experience. *Trans Ophthalmol Soc UK*. 1959;79:393-424.
3. Drews C. The Barraquer experience with IOLs. *Ophthalmology*. 1982;89:386-393.
4. Apple DJ, Brems RN, Park RB, et al. Anterior chamber lenses. Part I: complications and pathology and a review of design. *J Cataract Refract Surg*. 1987;13:157-174.
5. Apple DJ, Hansen SO, Richards SC, et al. Anterior chamber lenses. Part II: a laboratory study. *J Cataract Refract Surg*. 1987;13:175-189.
6. Worst JGF, Van der Veen G, Los LI. Refractive surgery for high myopia. *Documenta Ophthalmologica*. 1990;75:335-341.
7. Dvali MD. Intraocular correction of high myopia. *Vestnik Ophthalmologij*. 1986;102:29-31.
8. Baikoff G, Joly P. Comparison of minus power anterior chamber IOLs and myopic epikeratoplasty in phakic eyes. *Refract Corneal Surg*. 1990;6:252-260.
9. Baikoff G. Phakic anterior chamber IOL. *Intl Ophthalmol Clin*. 1991;31:76-78.
10. Fyodorov SN, Zuev VK, Tumanyan ER, Larionoy YeV. Analysis of long-term clinical and functional results of intraocular correction of high myopia. *Ophthalmosurg*. 1990;2:3-6.
11. Fyodorov SN, Zuev VK, Aznabayev BM. Intraocular correction of high myopia with negative posterior chamber lens. *Ophthalmosurg*. 1991;3:57-58.
12. Landesz M, Worst JGF, Siertsema JV, Van Rij G. Negative implant, a retrospective study. *Documenta Ophthalmologica*. 1993;83:261-270.
13. Saragoussi JJ, Puech M, Assouline M, Berges O, Renard G, Pouliquen YJ. Ultrasound biomicroscopy of Baikoff anterior chamber phakic IOLs. *J Refract Surg*. 1997;13:135-141.
14. Surgical correction of high myopia in the phakic eye with the 206W Worst Myopia Claw Lens, Interim Results, Ophtec, Groningen, Holland, March 1997.
15. van der Heijde GL. Some optical aspects of implantation of an IOL in a myopic eye. *Eur J Implant Ref Surg*. 1989;1:245-248.
16. Marinho A, Neves MC, Pinto MC, Vaz F. Posterior chamber silicone phakic IOL. *J Refract Surg*. 1997;13:219-222.
17. Fechner PU, Strobel J, Wichmann W. Correction of myopia by implantation of a concave Worst-iris claw lens into phakic eyes. *Refract Corneal Surg*. 1991;7:286-298.
18. Fechner PU, van der Heijde GL, Worst JGF. The correction of myopia by lens implantation

into phakic eyes. *Am J Ophthalmol.* 1989;107:659-663.

19. Perez-Santonja JJ, Bueno JL, Zato MA. Surgical correction of high myopia in phakic eyes with Worst-Fechner myopia IOLs. *J Refract Surg.* 1997;13:268-281.

20. Menezo JL, Cisneros AL, Cervera M, Harto M. Iris claw phakic lens—intermediate and long-term corneal endothelial changes. *Eur J Implant Ref Surg.* 1994;6:195-199.

21. Werblin TF. Long-term endothelial cell loss following phacoemulsification: model for evaluating endothelial cell damage after intraocular surgery. *J Cataract Refract Surg.* 1993;9:29-35.

22. Fechner PU, Wichmann W. Correction of myopia by implantation of minus optic (Worst Iris Claw) lenses into the anterior chamber of phakic eyes. *Eur J Implant Ref Surg.* 1993;5:55-59.

23. Wiechens B, Winter M, Haigis W, Happe W, Behrendt S, Rochels R. Bilateral cataract after phakic posterior chamber top hat-style silicone IOL. *J Refract Surg.* 1997;13:392-397.

24. Fechner PU, Haigis W, Wichmann W. Posterior chamber myopia lenses in phakic eyes. *J Cataract Refract Surg.* 1996;22:178-182.

25. Worst JGF. Evolution of iris fixation and the application of the iris claw principle. Ophtec, Groningen, Holland.

26. Perez-Santonja JJ, Hernandez JL, Benitez del Castillo JM, Rodriguez-Bermejo C, Zato, M. Fluorophotometry in myopic phakic eyes with anterior chamber IOLs to correct severe myopia. *Am J Ophthalmol.* 1994;118:316-321.

27. Perez-Santonja JJ, Iradier MT, Benitez del Castillo JM, Serrano JM, Zato MA. Chronic subclinical inflammation in phakic eyes with IOLs to correct myopia. *J Cataract Refract Surg.* 1996;22:183-187.

28. Miyake K, Asakura M, Kobayashi H. Effect of IOL fixation on the blood-aqueous barrier. *Am J Ophthalmol.* 1984;98:451.

29. Sanders DR, Kraff MC, Lieberman HL, Peyman GA, Tarabishy S. Breakdown and reestablishment of blood-aqueous barrier with implant surgery. *Arch Ophthalmol.* 1982;100:588.

30. Kaiya T. Observation of blood-aqueous barrier function after posterior chamber IOL implantation. *J Cataract Refract Surg.* 1990;16:320.

31. Landesz M, Worst JGF, Siertsema G, Van Rij G. Correction of high myopia with the Worst myopia claw IOL. *J Refract Surg.* 1995;11:16-25.

32. NuVita phakic lens. Product monograph. Chiron Vision Corp.

33. Bourne WM, Kaufman HE. Specular microscopy of human corneal endothelium in vivo. *Am J Ophthalmol.* 1976;81:319-323.

34. Wilson RS, Roper-Hall, MJ. Effect of age on the endothelial cell count in the normal eye. *Br J Ophthalmol.* 1982;66:513-515.

35. Yee RW, Matsuda M, Schultz RO, Edelhauser HF. Changes in the normal corneal endothelial cellular pattern as a function of age. *Curr Eye Res.* 1985;4:671-678.

36. Werblin TP. Long-term endothelial cell loss following phacoemulsification: model for evaluating endothelial damage after intraocular surgery. *Refract Corneal Surg.* 1993;9:29-35.

Phakic Intraocular Lenses

George O. Waring III, MD, FACS, FRCOphth

DEFINITION

IOLs of special design can be placed in an eye with a normal crystalline lens to correct refractive errors.

TERMINOLOGY AND CLASSIFICATION

The term intraocular lens, or IOL, indicates the implantation of a synthetic lens with refractive power inside the eye to decrease ametropia. Phakic IOL designates the placement of an IOL in an eye with a normal crystalline lens. The term refractive IOL designates any IOL, whether placed in a phakic or in an aphakic eye, since all IOLs have refractive power.

Each lens style has its own designation, often an eponym (eg, Baikoff or Worst lens), a description of the appearance of the lens (eg, lobster claw lens), the general configuration of the lens (eg, multiflex or plate), the composition of the lens (eg, silicone or hydrogel), the location of the lens (eg, anterior chamber or posterior chamber), or trade names (eg, NuVita).

Inaccurate jargon or marketing terms used to designate a plate lens placed in the posterior chamber (such as "intraocular contact lens"—an IOL is not a contact lens), will probably emerge as the field develops, but should be avoided, except as they help in colloquial communication to patients.

HISTORY AND DEVELOPMENT

The development of phakic IOLs has occurred during two periods of time.

1953 to Approximately 1963

During this nascent period of IOL development for cataract surgery and aphakia, some surgeons thought the new technology could be used to correct refractive errors. Approximately two dozen styles of anterior chamber IOLs were designed—including Strampelli, Dannheim, Joaquin Barraquer—and were implanted in hundreds of patients. Strampelli of Italy began to implant his rigid anterior chamber lens in 1953, but after a period of quiescence in the eye, approximately two thirds of the eyes developed corneal edema within 5 years. This was due to late endothelial damage, starting in the periphery because of compression by the haptic support of the lens. Strampelli tried several modifications, and the best known was an anterior chamber implant with external fixation and tiny threads that were buried in the sclera under a conjunctival flap. The lens was roughly rectangular, 5 x 13 mm. It had three tips, resting in the chamber angle with the optic in front of the haptic support, vaulting anteriorly. The absence of microsurgical techniques and viscoelastics, the cruder design and poorer quality of manufacture of the lenses, and the poor understanding of the corneal endothelium led to complications such as corneal edema, chronic uveitis, and intractable glaucoma. Barraquer also failed to achieve good long-term results with various anterior chamber lenses. In 1959, he reported on 411 cases: 342 Strampelli, 60 Dannheim, and nine of his own design. This series contained 239 phakic eyes for the correction of myopia. The complication rate with these phakic cases was higher and as time went on, the incidence of endothelial damage and corneal edema increased. Barraquer removed an increasing number of lenses from 1956 to 1970, removing approximately half of the lenses implanted.

The number of anterior chamber lenses implanted in Europe between 1953 and 1963 is unknown. The technique of phakic IOLs fell into disrepute.[1,2]

1986 to Present

Improvements in IOL design, manufacture, and surgical techniques led to a resurgence in interest, with the emergence of new lens styles implanted in informal clinical trials.

Four ophthalmic surgeons were prominent in the revival of interest in phakic IOLs:

1. Fechner of Germany, who in 1986 suggested new designs for phakic IOLs
2. Worst of the Netherlands, whose iris claw lens had been used for the correction of aphakia and was modified to correct myopia
3. Baikoff of France, who modified the four-point fixation multiflex anterior chamber lens to correct myopia
4. Fyodorov of Russia, who introduced a plate-style IOL for insertion in the posterior chamber with fixation in the ciliary sulcus

All of these lens styles have undergone subsequent modifications in design (Table 21-1).

Table 21-1
Stages in the Development of Current Styles of Phakic IOLs

Style	Eponym	Manufacturer	First Stage	Second Stage	Third Stage
Anterior chamber, angle fixated, quadriflex	Baikoff	Domilens, France; Chiron, USA	ZB 4.5 mm biconcave optic; high optic shoulder, step vault; endothelial damage	ZB5M 4 mm biconcave effective optic; lower optic shoulder, step vault; fluorine-treated; minimal endothelial damage; iris retraction-oval pupil	MA20 4.5 mm effective meniscus optic; no optic shoulder; curved angulation; anti-glare edge treatment; larger curved footplate fluorine-treated
Iris fixated, claw enclavation of stroma	Worst	Ophtec, The Netherlands	Worst/Fechner, 4.5 mm biconcave optic; higher shoulder		206W Worst claw convex—concave optic; 5 and 6 mm optic; lower shoulder
Posterior chamber, ciliary sulcus fixated, plate	Fyodorov	Eye Microsurgical Institute, Russia; Staar, Switzerland	Silicone; collar button into pupil; cataracts	Flat, plate (abandoned in Russia); multiple Staar designs	IC2020 hydrogel and 0.01% collagen copolymer; flat plate, thin haptic; foldable 5.0 mm effective meniscus optic

BASIC PRINCIPLES

Phakic IOLs work like aphakic IOLs, focusing images on the retina to correct ametropia. IOLs that correct myopia have minus power whereas those for aphakia have plus power. Implanting an IOL has the advantage of leaving corneal curvature normal, whereas corneal refractive surgery creates an abnormal corneal shape with the induction of optical aberrations.

Phakic IOLs preserve accommodation, in contrast to clear lens extraction. Phakic IOLs must fit within the space available in the anatomically normal anterior ocular segment, in contrast to an aphakic IOL which can fit in the space vacated by the removed cataract; this increases the challenge for phakic IOL design, to obviate damage to the corneal endothelium, anterior chamber angle, iris, and crystalline lens (Table 21-2).

To highlight contrasting and complementary aspects of corneal refractive surgery and phakic IOLs, Table 21-3 provides a qualitative tabular comparison. The content of Table 21-3 is oversimplified and represents my own opinions, but it serves as a point of departure to monitor the competitive struggle over the next 5 to 10 years between refractive corneal surgery and IOL surgery. Of course, in the reality of clinical practice, the two techniques are complementary and supplemental, as Zaldivar and Davidorf demonstrate in their forthcoming article reporting the correction of

Table 21-2	
Some Ideal Qualities of Phakic IOLs	
Ideal Quality	**Clinical Effect**
Superior (?aspheric) optics	Excellent quality vision
7-mm diameter functional optic	No edge effect
No glare design	No glare, halos
Foldable	Small, self-sealing incision
Bicompatible design, material, and manufacture	No endothelial, iris, or lens damage
Free flow of aqueous	No pupillary block
Easy to implant	Fewer intraoperative complications
Easy to exchange	Adjustable
Spherocylindrical	Correct astigmatism
Negative and positive powers	Correct myopia and hyperopia
Multifocal	Correct presbyopia without reduced quality of vision
Affordable	Fair profits

Reprinted with permission from Waring GO III. Comparison of refractive corneal surgery and phakic IOLs. J Refract Surg. 1998;14:279.

high myopia with combined LASIK and phakic IOLs,[3] as most cataract surgeons know who combine transverse keratotomy for astigmatism with aphakic IOL implantation.

REFRACTIVE ERROR TREATED

Current styles have minus power designed to treat myopia. Plus power phakic IOLs are being designed, but because space between the crystalline lens and the cornea is less than the space between the posterior capsule and the cornea in an aphakic eye, the overall volume of the lens must be smaller.

Currently, phakic IOLs have the most utility in treating high myopia of more than -12.00 D, because there is no other surgical technique to treat such high refractive errors without inducing marked optical aberrations. As modern technology proves increasingly safe and effective, IOLs will be used to treat smaller and smaller refractive errors.

Theoretically, a cylindrical lens could be made to treat astigmatism, but such a lens does not now exist. No phakic IOLs are available for presbyopia, although monovision is an option for patients with bilateral implantation.

DEVICES AND INSTRUMENTS

The most important device is the IOL (see Tables 21-1 and 21-4).

There are currently three sites of fixation: anterior chamber angle (Figures 21-1a through 21-1c), iris surface (Figures 21-2a through 21-2c), and ciliary sulcus (Figure 21-3). Centration on the pupil, diameter of the optic, and edge design all must be optimal to minimize optical aberrations. The lens should be exchangeable.

The distance between the lens and the endothelium must be 2.5 mm or greater to avoid endothelial damage. The lens must not damage tissue at the point of fixa-

Table 21-3
Qualitative Comparison of Corneal Refractive Surgery and Phakic IOLs

Topic	Corneal Surgery	Phakic IOL
Refractive Disorder Treated		
Myopia	-1 D to -15 D	-1 D to -25 D
Astigmatism	0.50 D to 5 D	Requires cylindrical IOL
Hyperopia	+1 D to +5 D	+1 D to +10 D
Presbyopia	No	Multifocal IOL
Surgical Setting		
	Topical anesthesia	Topical anesthesia
	Office	OR
Surgical Complexity		
	Less familiar to surgeon	More familiar to surgeon
	Highly complex	Medium complex
	Microkeratome	Manual instruments
	Excimer laser	Phakic IOL
Accuracy of Refractive Outcome		
Present ±0.50	66%	45%
Future ±0.25	Possible with individualized LASIK	Possible with improved formulas
Freedom from Full-Time Distance Optical Correction		
	90%	Not published
Individualized Custom Surgery		
	Theoretically possible	No
Stability of Refraction		
Excellent	LASIK, intracorneal ring	Phakic IOL
Good	RK, PRK	
Fair	TKP	
Corneal Contours Postoperatively		
	Abnormal	Normal
Quality of Vision		
	Good	Good to excellent
Adjustability		
	Yes: myopia, hyperopia, cylindrical LASIK	Yes: IOL exchange but no astigmatism adjustment
Reversibility		
	No: RK, PRK, LASIK, TKP	Yes
	Yes: Intracorneal ring	
Vision-Threatening Complications		
	Irregular astigmatism	Endothelial damage
	Corneal scar	Cataract
	Keratitis	Endophthalmitis
Cost		
Of location	Lower—clean room	Higher—sterile OR
Of equipment	LASIK, PRK: very high	Low
	RK, ring: low	
Of device and disposables	Medium	Medium
Patient Satisfaction		
	High	Very high
Published Results		
	Extensive	Few

The opinions in this table apply generally; there are exceptions. Reprinted with permission from Waring GO III. Comparison of refractive corneal surgery and phakic IOLs. J Refract Surg. *1998;14:278.*

Table 21-4
Comparison of Three Phakic IOLs, 1998

Style	Model/ Manufacturer	Material	Optic Diam.	Haptic	Powers	Sizing	IOL Power Calculation Formula
Anterior chamber, multiflex	NuVita MA20 Bausch & Lomb Surgical, Claremont, Calif	PMMA fluorine-coated	5 mm	12.0 to 13.5 mm, 4-point fixation in anterior chamber	-7 D to -20 D	Horizontal, white-to-white +1 mm	van der Heijde in clinical nomogram by manufacturer
Iris claw	Worst 206W Ophtec, Groningen, The Netherlands	PMMA	5 mm	8.5 mm, 2-point fixation of iris stroma	-3 D to -20 D +3 D to +12 D	One size (8.5 x 5.0 mm)	van der Heijde by manufacturer
Posterior chamber plate	Implantable "Collamer" contact lens IC2020 Staar, Widav, Switzerland	HEMA bovine collagen (0.03%) copolymer	4.5 to 5.5 mm	11.5 to 13.0 mm, 4-point fixation in ciliary sulcus	-3 D to -20 D +3 D to +17 D	Horizontal, white-to white +0.50 mm	Manufacturer or Holladay 2

HEMA=hydroxyethylmethacrylate (35% water).

tion, so an angle fixated lens must not cause trabecular damage, peripheral anterior synechiae, or iris tuck or retraction; a lens attached to the anterior surface of the iris must not cause iris atrophy; and a lens placed in the posterior chamber must not cause a cataract, iris chafing, or pigment dispersion.

The sizing of the lens must be appropriate for each eye. A lens style in which one size fits all eyes is probably optimal, such as the Worst iris claw lens. Angle fixated and ciliary sulcus fixated lenses have the danger of being too large with ocular pain or too small with lens decentration or rotation, because it is not practical to measure accurately the diameter of the anterior or posterior chamber using current clinical methods. A lens with a flexible haptic that fits in the anterior or posterior chamber might decrease problems with sizing.

The optic ideally should have a 6-mm or greater functional diameter and be able to be centered on the pupil to diminish edge glare which is often seen by the patient as halos or ghost images when the pupil is dilated.

The design of phakic IOLs will undergo many changes in the next decade. Lenses that can be inserted through a small internal corneal valve sutureless incision will allow the minimal surgical trauma and maximal rate of recovery of vision that is now enjoyed with modern cataract surgery. Lens materials are in rapid evolution, including classic PMMA, silicones, hydrogels, copolymers, and thin diffractive wafers.

Hand instruments used for lens implantation are similar to those used in cataract surgery. Some lenses may require special instruments, such as the Krumeich spreader used for the Worst iris claw lens and the injectors used for foldable lenses.

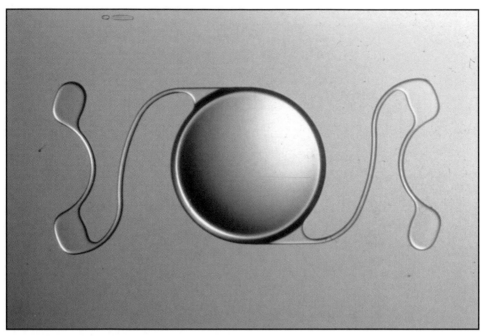

Figure 21-1a. Baikoff MA 20 (NuVita) anterior chamber phakic IOL. Reprinted with permission from Leibowitz, Waring GO III. *Corneal Disorders, Clinical Diagnoses, and Management.* **2nd ed. Philadelphia, Pa: WB Saunders; 1998:1083.**

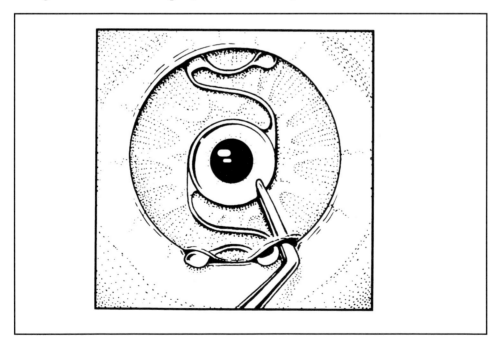

Figure 21-1b. Insertion of IOL into anterior chamber. Reprinted with permission from Leibowitz, Waring GO III. *Corneal Disorders, Clinical Diagnoses, and Management.* **2nd ed. Philadelphia, Pa: WB Saunders; 1998:1083.**

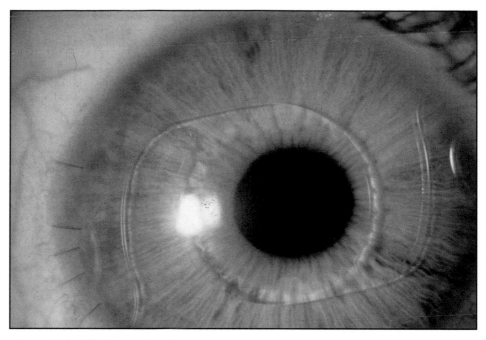

**Figure 21-1c. IOL in place in the anterior chamber. Wound closed by sutures (arrow).
Reprinted with permission from Leibowitz, Waring GO III.** *Corneal Disorders, Clinical
Diagnoses, and Management.* **2nd ed. Philadelphia, Pa: WB Saunders; 1998:1083.**

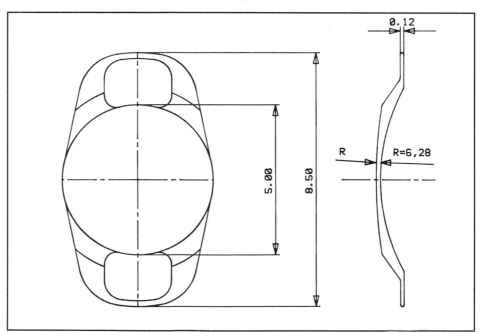

**Figure 21-2a. Worst iris claw phakic IOL. Configuration and measurements of IOL.
Reprinted with permission from Leibowitz, Waring GO III.** *Corneal Disorders, Clinical
Diagnoses, and Management.* **2nd ed. Philadelphia, Pa: WB Saunders; 1998:1084.**

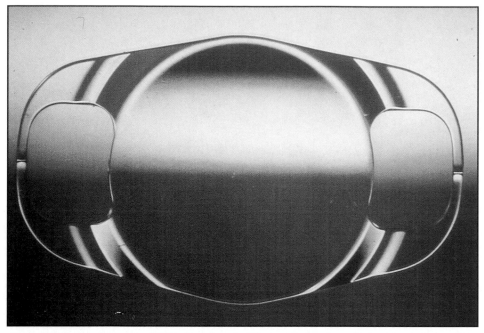

Figure 21-2b. Photograph of IOL. Reprinted with permission from Leibowitz, Waring GO III. *Corneal Disorders, Clinical Diagnoses, and Management.* **2nd ed. Philadelphia, Pa: WB Saunders; 1998:1084.**

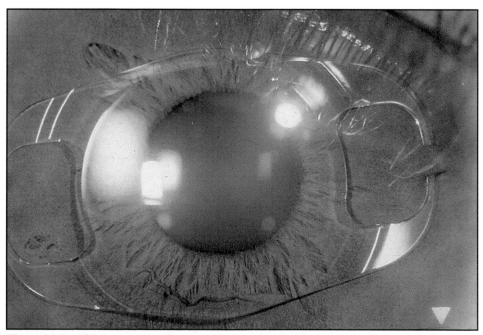

Figure 21-2c. IOL in anterior chamber. Iris is enclavated between the claws of the IOL (arrows). Reprinted with permission from Leibowitz, Waring GO III. *Corneal Disorders, Clinical Diagnoses, and Management.* **2nd ed. Philadelphia, Pa: WB Saunders; 1998:1084.**

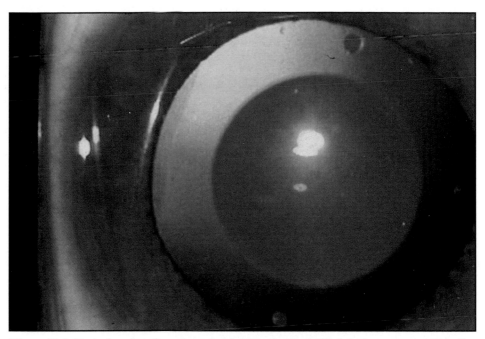

Figure 21-3. Posterior chamber plate phakic IOL. Optic of IOL is between arrows. P indicates the edge of the pupil. Arrowhead points to positioning hole. Reprinted with permission from Leibowitz, Waring GO III. *Corneal Disorders, Clinical Diagnoses, and Management.* **2nd ed. Philadelphia, Pa: WB Saunders; 1998:1084.**

In comparision to lamellar refractive corneal surgery, which requires technically complex and expensive lasers and microkeratomes that cost hundreds of thousands of dollars, and in comparison to refractive keratotomy which requires tens of thousands of dollars of investment, phakic IOLs require minimal upfront investment for the surgeon or eyecare facility.

PREOPERATIVE PLANNING

Calculation of IOL power should be more accurate for phakic IOLs than that required for IOLs in cataract surgery, because refractive surgical patients want to have 20/20 or better uncorrected visual acuity and be free of wearing spectacles or contact lenses, whereas cataract patients are more willing to wear glasses after surgery. Calculation of phakic IOL power also should be more accurate because the final location of the lens in the eye has less variability than that during cataract surgery.

Calculation of the lens haptic diameter for angle and sulcus fixated lenses currently depends on a white-to-white limbal measurement. This measurement is not accurate because the amount of scleral overriding on the anterior surface of the cornea is quite variable, because the point selected for the white-to-white measurment varies from one surgeon to another, and because the calipers used for such measurements are not very accurate. There is a need to develop imaging methods,

such as anterior ocular segment ultrasound, that can accurately measure the diameter of the anterior chamber from scleral spur to scleral spur and of the ciliary sulcus. For the iris claw lens, the 8.5-mm diameter fits all eyes, and it is useful to use a laser to mark the iris at exactly the 3 and 9 o'clock positions 8.5 mm apart and equidistant from the pupil, which helps the surgeon quickly identify the proper location for the lens during surgery.

Theoretical and empirical formulas for power and size calculation are being derived for each lens style. These methods range from a simple nomogram based on spectacle refraction to formulas based on ocular biometry. Standard IOL power calculation formulas used for aphakic IOLs are inaccurate for the high minus power phakic IOLs.

SURGICAL STEPS AND SEQUENCES
Pupil Size

For anterior chamber and iris surface fixated lenses, the pupil is constricted preoperatively with topical pilocarpine. For posterior chamber lenses, the pupil is dilated widely preoperatively with mydriatics.

Anesthesia

Ideally, phakic IOLs could be implanted using topical anesthesia with supplemental intracameral nonpreserved 1% Xylocaine, as is done for cataract surgery. However, ocular movements during surgery, especially in younger, anxious patients, may have more disastrous consequences—particularly if one is placing a posterior chamber phakic IOL. Development of these techniques is in progress.

Peribulbar anesthesia decreases intraoperative eye movements, but in highly myopic eyes, posterior staphylomas and enlarged globe diameter present dangers for any intraorbital needle. Retrobulbar anesthesia should be avoided or used with great caution. Episcleral anesthesia with a blunt cannula provides a compromise between topical and intraorbital techniques.

Ocular compression is applied for 5 minutes.

Anterior Chamber Angle Fixated Lenses
Internal Corneal Valve Incision

After fixating the globe with forceps or a fixation ring, a 5.5-mm incision is made parallel to the limbus through the corneal limbal vascular arcade to a depth of approximately 200 to 300 microns, using a calibrated diamond knife or a knife of the surgeon's choice. Dissection is carried into the cornea approximately 1.5 mm with a diamond blade or rounded steel blade. The anterior chamber is entered with a 5-mm wide keratome at the central edge of the dissection by depressing the tip of the keratome to depress the posterior cornea and pushing the keratome into the anterior chamber. The anterior chamber is filled with viscoelastic, without getting any behind the iris. The keratome can then be used to enlarge the wound to 5.5 mm by pushing the sharp edge of the keratome against the shoulders of the wound to enlarge it.

Limbal Incision

A 5.5-mm, 250-micron deep limbus parallel incision is made, followed by entry into the anterior chamber with a diamond or disposable knife. The anterior chamber is filled with viscoelastic, and the slightly beveled two-plane incision is enlarged with a knife or scissors.

The lens is grasped with an IOL forceps at the edge of the optic. The lens is slid in parallel to the iris, placing first the curved end of the haptic, then the free end, taking care not to catch the haptic on the edge of the pupil and not to touch the corneal endothelium. The haptic is inserted into the anterior chamber angle without deforming the pupil.

There are two ways to insert the trailing haptic:

1. Place a collar button or similar IOL manipulator in the concave recess of the haptic, and push the lens straight in. Once each shoulder of the haptic is in the anterior chamber, move the IOL manipulator slightly posteriorly and retract it toward the wound so the two shoulders seat themselves into the angle beneath the wound without distortion of the pupil.
2. Grasp each end of the haptic with a Kelman/McPherson-style smooth forceps, retract the posterior edge of the incision with a hook, and push the shoulder centrally and slightly posteriorly, seating it in the angle. This is done first with the corneal end of the haptic and then second with the free end. If the pupil is oval, the iris is probably tucked. Using an IOL hook in the concave crotch of the haptic, displace the haptic centrally to release the iris tuck and position the haptic into the angle on the scleral spur.

An intraoperative goniolens can be used to verify the position of the footplates, which should sit on the scleral spur at the base of the iris insertion without displacing the iris.

If an internal corneal valve is used, close the wound with one to four interrupted 10-0 nylon sutures. Once the wound is secure, a Simcoe-style cannula is used to remove the viscoelastic. This is extremely important because excess viscoelastic in the eye can cause a severe rise in IOP resulting in ischemia of the iris sphincter and permanent mydriasis with disastrous consequences in terms of glare and visual function.

Iris Claw Lens

A superior incision 5.5- to 6.0-mm wide of the surgeon's choice is made and the anterior chamber filled with viscoelastic. The lens is inserted into the anterior chamber onto the iris surface and the wound is sutured (Figures 21-4a and 21-4b). There are two techniques of enclavating the iris:

1. Use a Krumeich spreader to spread the claws, press them down on a previously tented iris, and obtain a large bite of anterior stroma.[4]
2. Use the Worst two-handed method of holding the lens optic with one instrument and use a bent needle to push the iris up into the claws.[5] The wound is sutured and viscoelastic removed. A peripheral iridectomy is optimal.

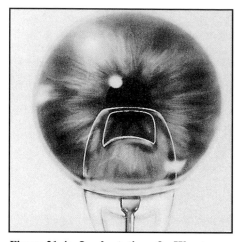

Figure 21-4a. Implantation of a Worst claw lens using the closed-system approach. After making a 4.5- to 5.0-mm corneoscleral incision, the lens is inserted into the anterior chamber while the endothelium is protected by viscoelastic. Reprinted with permission from Krumeich et al. Negative-power intraocular lens. *J Refract Surg*. 1996;12:337.

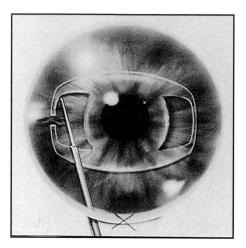

Figure 21-4b. The anterior chamber is closed with a shoelace suture, using the keratoscope to control suture tension. After insertion of the Krumeich-Koch spreader, an iris fold is created and the haptic positioned over these folds. Reprinted with permission from Krumeich et al. Negative-power intraocular lens. *J Refract Surg*. 1996;12:337.

Posterior Chamber Plate Lenses

A peripheral iridotomy (YAG or surgical) is necessary before IOL insertion to prevent intra- and postoperative pupillary block. In general, these lenses are folded, so a 3- to 4-mm wide incision with an internal corneal valve can be used.

Viscoelastic is injected to deepen the anterior chamber. In some techniques, it is injected between the iris and the crystalline lens, to elevate the iris and make room for insertion of the lens. The lens is inserted through a shooter/injector. The surgeon manipulates the inferior haptic beneath the inferior iris by pressing down gently and inserts the superior haptic beneath the superior iris. This is ideally done without pressing on the crystalline lens, but in reality the IOL is briefly pushed across the surface of the lens; this does not cause a cataract within the first year after surgery if done properly. Viscoelastic is then aspirated through a separate stab incision. The wound is self-sealing or a suture is placed.

IOL Exchange and Removal

If IOL power calculations are accurate, repeated surgery should be unnecessary. However, if lens power is unacceptable or if the lens is malpositioned, it is possible to either reopen the previous wound or to create a new surgical wound, fill the anterior chamber with viscoelastic, release the lens from its points of fixation, slide it out of the eye, and replace it with a lens of appropriate power or size. Every intraocular

Table 21-5
Endothelial Cell Density After Implantation of a
Baikoff ZB5M Phakic Anterior Chamber IOL

Postoperative Exam	Central Cornea, Mean ± SD (Range)
Baseline	2935 ± 307 (2160 to 4150)
6 months	2841 ± 330 (2200 to 3950), -3.3 ± 6.7 (-20.0 to +21.3), 6 eyes (6.3%)
12 months	2761 ± 315 (2060 to 3950), -4.5 ± 7.4 (-28.5 to +19.4), 6 eyes (6.9%)
18 months	2757 ± 283 (2200 to 3800), -3.8 ± 7.3 (-16.4 to +25.9), 2 eyes (3.1%)
24 months	2744 ± 368 (2000 to 3978), -5.6 ± 8.8 (-23.1 to +32.4), 6 eyes (10.5%)
36 months	2763 ± 259 (2340 to 3628), -5.5 ± 10.2 (-24.8 to +16.7), 4 eyes (14.8%)

Mean ± standard deviation and ranges given for both absolute counts (expressed as cells/mm²) and percent change from baseline, along with the number and percentage of eyes with greater than 15% cell loss. Adapted from Baikoff G, Arne JL, Bokobza Y, et al. Angle-fixated anterior chamber phakic intraocular lens for myopia of -7 to -19 diopters. J Refract Surg. 1998;14:282-293.

intervention increases the chance of endothelial and crystalline lens damage and of endophthalmitis, but one of the enormous advantages of phakic IOLs is the ease with which they can be removed or replaced, making them an adjustable, reversible form of refractive surgery.

POSTOPERATIVE COURSE AND WOUND HEALING

Early postoperatively, there is minimal inflammation (assuming uncomplicated surgery), and recovery of vision is rapid. Postoperatively, topical antibiotics and topical corticosteroids are administered for approximately 1 week. Mydriatics are unnecessary. Topical nonsteroidal anti-inflammatory agents may decrease postoperative discomfort. Topical or oral anti-glaucoma medication may be used to decrease IOP.

Refraction is extraordinarily stable, because the position and power of the IOL do not change over time.

Astigmatism can change if a wound 5- to 6-mm long is used and sutured, as occurs in extracapsular cataract surgery, but as foldable phakic IOLs become available, surgeons will use smaller (2.5- to 3.0-mm) wounds that do not need sutures and that do not affect astigmatism.

PUBLISHED RESULTS
Baikoff Multiflex Anterior Chamber Phakic IOL

The early designs of the Baikoff-style IOL, particularly the ZB (Domilens, Lyon, France) had a high vault and thick edges to the minus power optic, which produced progressive endothelial cell damage in the paracentral cornea.[6,7] The redesigned lens with a lower vault and thinner optic (model ZB5M) has been studied in a prospective multicenter trial lasting 3 years.[8] One-hundred twenty patients (133 eyes) with a mean

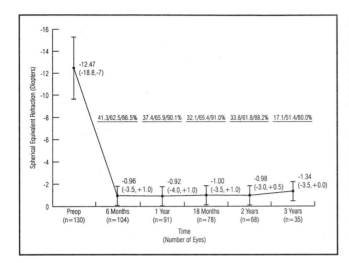

Figure 21-5. Mean (range) spherical equivalent manifest refraction over 3 years after implantation of the Baikoff ZB5M phakic IOL. Proportion of eyes within ±0.50, ±1.00, and ±2.00 D of emmetropia are underlined. Reprinted with permission from Baikoff G, Arne JL, Bokobza Y, et al. Angle-fixated anterior chamber phakic intraocular lens for myopia of -7 to -19 diopters. *J Refract Surg.* **1998;14:285.**

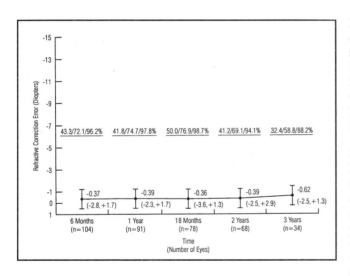

Figure 21-6. Refractive correction error is presented as the difference between achieved and intended refractive outcome. Means (ranges) are provided, and the proportion of eyes within ±0.50, ±1.00, and ±2.00 D of emmetropia are underlined. Reprinted with permission from Baikoff G, Arne JL, Bokobza Y, et al. Angle-fixated anterior chamber phakic intraocular lens for myopia of -7 to -19 diopters. *J Refract Surg.* **1998;14:286.**

spherical equivalent refractive error of -12.50 D (range: -7.00 D to -18.80 D), a preoperative cell density of 2500 cells/mm^2 or greater, and an anterior chamber depth of 3 mm or more were studied. The Chiron/Domilens ZB5M 5-mm optic diameter, 12.5- to 13.5-mm haptic length lens was used, with IOL power calculations derived from van der Heijde.[9] The mean error in refractive correction, as measured by the mea difference between achieved and intended correction was substantially less than 1.00 D over the entire study. At 3 years follow-up, 88.2% (117 eyes) were still within ±2.00 D of intended correction, 58.8% (78 eyes) were within ±1.00 D, 32.4% (43 eyes) were within ±0.50 D, and the maximum overcorrection was +1.30 D (Figures 21-5 and 21-6).

The reduction in mean endothelial cell density centrally and peripherally averaged 3.3% at 6 months and declined by approximately 1% to 2% over the remaining 2.5 years of follow-up—consistent with normal aging. Approximately 15% of eyes lost 15% or more central endothelial cell density at 3 years, but only three eyes had a cell density below 2000 cells/mm^2 (Table 21-5).

Approximately 27% of patients described halos and glare, which was attributed to the 5-mm diameter optic that was not always centered over the pupil, because it centered on the anatomical cornea as determined by the anterior chamber angle anatomy.

The most common serious complication was progressive retraction of the iris that produced an oval pupil in approximately 6% of eyes at 1 month, rising to 28% at 3 years. The direction of the iris retraction was along the meridian of the haptic orientation. The retraction progressed in some eyes in spite of removal of the IOL was not associated with a rise in IOP, and was sometimes associated with a gray membrane on the surface of the iris, suggesting that endothelial cell migration onto the iris surface with retraction may have occurred (similar to the iridocorneal endothelial syndrome). The cause was not mechanical tucking of the iris (Figure 21-7).

Other complications occurring in less than five eyes each included transient corneal edema, iridocyclitis, and pupillary block (all of which resolved spontaneously or with medical treatment), implant rotation or displacement treated by implant or IOL exchange, and implant removal because of halos or a flat anterior chamber.[10]

A new design of the Baikoff lens, representing a third major design revision (MA20, NuVita) (see Table 21-4) features a larger diameter optic (5.5 mm with 5.0-mm active optical zone), a large footplate that decreases contact with the iris, lower shoulder height of the optic to increase distance from the corneal endothelium, increased flexibility to make sizing easier, and a peripheral treatment of the optic to decrease glare.

Iris-Supported Negative Power IOL (Worst Iris Claw)

Krumeich reported 35 eyes in a prospective study with a preoperative spherical equivalent refraction of -6.00 D to -21.25 D (mean: -12.50 + 5.25 D).[4] The lens was inserted using the Krumeich spreader through a superior corneoscleral incision.

At 6 months, with 27 eyes being followed, approximately 90% of eyes were within 1.00 D of emmetropia and the correlation coefficient between expected and achieved refraction was 0.98. At 6 months, with 30 eyes followed, 70% were within 0.50 D, 83% within 1.00 D, and 100% within 2.00 D of emmetropia. The refraction remained stable during 1 year of follow-up. The endothelial cell counts centrally showed a 1% decrease over baseline at 12 months.

Landesz found similar results in a series of 35 eyes with a preoperative refraction ranging from -6.00 D to -28.00 D, with 20 eyes followed for 12 months[5] (Figure 21-8). The two-handed technique of implantation was used, pushing the iris into the claws with a curved needle. The mean postoperative refraction was -0.93 D (SD: 2.90 D). Nineteen of the 35 eyes (54%) had a refraction within +0.50 D and 26 (74%) within +1.00 D. The refraction was stable for 1 year. Objective measurements showed no increase in glare. Endothelial cell counts showed a mean cell loss of 5% at 6 months, and of 9% at 12 months (range: +0.77 to -23.5%). Statistically, there was not a significant cell loss in the entire population, although two eyes showed cell loss of over 20% at 12 months, without corneal edema. A subjective satisfaction

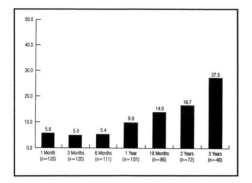

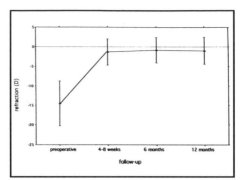

Figure 21-7. Percentage of eyes with iris retraction and pupillary ovalization over 3 years after implantation of the Baikoff ZB5M phakic IOL. Reprinted with permission from Baikoff G, Arne JL, Bokobza Y, et al. Angle-fixated anterior chamber phakic intraocular lens for myopia of -7 to -19 diopters. *J Refract Surg*. 1998;14:289.

Figure 21-8. Mean (error bars, 1 SD) refractive outcome in 20 eyes with a Worst claw IOL followed for 1 year. Reprinted with permission from Landesz M, Worst JGF, Siertsema JV, van Rij G. Correction of high myopia with the Worst myopia claw intraocular lens. *J Refract Surg*. 1995;11:20.

questionnaire was completed, with a mean overall satisfaction rating of 7.5 (range: 1 [very poor] to 10 [excellent]) and a mean subjective disturbance by glare or distortion of 1.0 to 2.7. One eye lost 2 or more lines of spectacle corrected visual acuity, but 20 eyes gained 2 or more lines, presumably because of changes in magnification.

In 1997, Menezo and colleagues[12] reported 97 eyes of 62 patients with baseline myopia greater than -7.00 D who underwent Worst-Fechner IOL implantation. Mean follow-up time was 48.9 months (range: 36 to 72 months). Three years after surgery, 58 eyes (61%) had an uncorrected visual acuity of 20/40 or better, and 77 eyes (82%) gained 2 or more lines of spectacle corrected visual acuity from baseline; 75 eyes (79%) were within ±1.00 D of emmetropia and 46 eyes (48%) were within ±0.50 D of emmetropia. The mean endothelial cell loss was 17.9% at 5 years after surgery, while the percentage of hexagonality and the coefficient of cell variation tended toward preoperative levels. No vision-threatening complications were reported.[12-14]

From these reports, complications with the iris claw lens appear rare. One eye had persistent postoperative inflammation that gradually cleared. However, subtle estimates of the postoperative status of the iris claw lens raises some questions. Perez-Santonja[11] studied 32 eyes and found similar refractive and stability outcomes, but noticed an increase in endothelial cell loss: 7.2% at 3 months, 10.6% at 6 months, 13% at 12 months, and 17.6% at 24 months. Using a flare cell meter, the values were significantly higher for eyes implanted with the iris claw lens than in those of control eyes. A decentation greater than 0.5 mm was present in 43 eyes and halos in 56%.

Posterior Chamber Phakic IOL

Zaldivar and colleagues[13] examined the efficacy, predictability, stability, and safety of posterior chamber phakic IOL implantation in patients with extreme myopia and presented their results of 124 eyes that received a posterior chamber hydrogel collagen plate phakic IOL (Staar ICL) for the correction of myopia. Emmetropia was the target postoperative spherical equivalent refraction, and mean follow-up was 11 months (range: 1 to 36 months). The mean preoperative spherical equivalent refraction was -13.38 D ± 2.23 D (range: -8.50 D to -18.63 D). Mean postoperative spherical equivalent refraction at last examination was -0.78 D ± 0.87 D (range: +1.63 D to -3.50 D); 86 eyes (69%) were within ±1.00 D and 55 eyes (44%) were within ±0.50 D of emmetropia. The refraction remained stable with a statistically insignificant change (p>0.05 at each interval) during follow-up. A gain of 2 or more lines of spectacle corrected visual acuity was seen in 45 eyes (36%) at last examination. One eye (0.8%) lost 2 or more lines of spectacle corrected visual acuity from a retinal detachment.

For the correction of hyperopia, Davidorf and colleagues[14] examined the efficacy, predictability, stability, and safety in 24 eyes that received a posterior chamber hydrogel-collagen plate phakic IOL (Staar ICL), the goal being emmetropia. Mean follow-up was 8.4 months (range: 1 to 18 months). The mean preoperative spherical equivalent refraction was +6.51 D ± 2.08 D (range: +3.75 D to +10.50 D). Mean postoperative spherical equivalent refraction at last examination was -0.39 D ± 1.29 D (range: +1.25 D to -3.88 D); 19 eyes (79%) were within ±1.00 D and 14 eyes (58%) were within ±0.50 D of emmetropia. Postoperative uncorrected visual acuity at last examination was 20/40 or better in 15 eyes (63%). A gain of 2 or more lines of spectacle corrected visual acuity was seen in two eyes (8%) at last examination. One eye (4%) lost 2 or more lines of spectacle corrected visual acuity due to progressive neovascular glaucoma initiated by early postoperative pupillary block. Large, patent iridotomies are important in hyperopic eyes to lower the risk of postoperative pupillary block. Improved phakic IOL power calculation formulas will refine predictability of refractive outcome.

Changes in Spectacle Corrected Visual Acuity

A consistent theme in reports of phakic IOL implantation is increase in spectacle corrected visual acuity, with substantial numbers of patients showing 2 lines or more improvement. Clinicians should avoid the term best corrected visual acuity and use either the term spectacle corrected visual acuity or contact lens corrected visual acuity. The majority of patients who receive phakic IOLs wear contact lenses preoperatively, and therefore the proper baseline comparison for improvements in visual acuity would be contact lens corrected visual acuity. This is not reported in the literature, but rather best spectacle corrected visual acuity (usually called best corrected visual acuity) is reported. While surgeons can be proud of the improvement over spectacles achieved postoperatively, the improvement is somewhat exaggerated, because the comparison for improvement should be contact lens corrected preoperative visual acuity.

COMPLICATIONS
Residual Refractive Error

Residual myopia or hyperopia can be treated by IOL exchange, using IOL power calculations that adjust for the ametropia. Residual myopia can be treated by refractive keratotomy[15] and residual myopia or hyperopia can be treated by excimer laser PRK or LASIK. Indeed, for power corrections over approximately -20.00 D, Zaldivar has suggested an intentional division of the correction between the IOL (approximately two thirds of the correction) and LASIK (approximately one third of the correction).[16] Residual astigmatism can be corrected with arcuate transverse keratotomy or excimer laser ablation.

Endothelial Damage

Contact between the IOL and the endothelium intraoperatively can cause acute cell loss, and persistent contact postoperatively causes progressive cell loss, which could result in corneal edema. Modern phakic IOL designs have not caused corneal edema. Surgical techniques are being improved to decrease intraoperative damage and lenses are being constantly redesigned to create a lower profile to decrease the chance of endothelial damage. Viscocoelastic filling the anterior chamber during surgery helps protect the endothelium by giving the surgeon plenty of room in which to work. Long-term specular microscopy of the endothelium will be required to document that the rate of endothelial cell loss does not exceed that of normal aging. (Endothelial damage for specific lens styles is previously reported.)

Decentration

A decentered lens, with the edge of the optic overlying the pupil, creates optical aberrations, glare, and ghost images. One advantage of the Worst iris claw lens is that it can be centered over the entrance pupil, whereas the anterior chamber angle fixated and posterior chamber plate lenses center on the anatomic ring of the limbus—which usually places the pupil slightly nasal from the center of the optic. Decentration greater than 0.5 mm can occur from 40% to 50% of eyes.[17-19] Decentration can be reduced by proper sizing, proper placement and fixation, modification in edge design that decreases optical aberrations, and increased optic diameter from the current 4.5 to 5.0 mm to 6.0 mm or greater (assuming a low profile of the larger optic).

Iris Tuck and Pupillary Distortion

Angle fixated lenses can cause a reaction focally where the footplates contact the peripheral iris, resulting in progressive iris retraction and distortion of the pupil. A poorly placed angle fixated IOL can tuck the iris and distort the pupil acutely. The iris claw lens can produce pupillary distortion if the iris is stretched between the claws. These complications can be avoided by accurate placement of the IOL haptics and by design of haptics that do not irritate the peripheral iris or corneal endothelium.

Cataract

Damage to the crystalline lens during insertion of the IOL can produce focal cataract. Gentle contact with a hydrogel posterior chamber lens seems unlikely to produce a cataract in the short-term. This matter requires great judgment and skill on the part of the surgeon. Whether posterior chamber lenses chronically alter the metabolic status of the crystalline lens and produce a nonmechanical cataract over time remains to be determined. Current designs of posterior chamber plate phakic IOLs contain a significant vault, with 200 to 300 microns between the anterior lens capsule and the IOL. However, beneath the iris, it is probable that the IOL contacts the surface of the crystalline lens, and this may increase during accommodation when the iris root moves backward and the crystalline lens moves forward. There is lifelong contact between the posterior surface of the iris and the crystalline lens without the formation of focal cataracts (even in the pigment dispersion syndrome in which the crystalline lens and zonules are displaced forward and rub actively enough on the posterior iris to scrape off the pigment). If a cataract occurs, it is possible to remove the phakic IOL, remove the cataract, and implant a plus power aphakic IOL.

Iridocyclitis

A mild postoperative iridocyclitis may occur as in any intraoperative procedure, but this may be severe if there has been marked manipulation of the iris. Concerning long-term follow-up, the flare-cell meter has shown increased flare and cell after the implantation of the Baikoff and the Worst lenses, but this appears to be of sub-clinical severity, and it is unknown whether the cells represent leukocytes or pigment cells. There are no reports of chronic low-grade iridocyclitis producing clinical damage over 2 to 3 years after surgery, but a long-term effect over decades is unknown.[11,20] Fluorophotometry has shown a slight increase in crystalline lens density over 2 years after implantation of a Worst iris claw lens, but it is unknown whether this has clinical significance.[11]

Dislocation and Inadequate Sizing

An angle fixated or posterior chamber phakic IOL may rotate if the size is too small. An anterior chamber IOL footplate may disclocate into a peripheral iridectomy, damaging the zonules and causing pigment dispersion; such lenses should be removed, with or without a replacement lens of proper size. An iris claw lens requires a large firm bite of iris stroma; a small superficial bite can result in dislocation of the lens,[21,22] with possible secondary endothelial damage if the lens contacts the back of the cornea.

Too large an anterior chamber lens may cause pain and tenderness in the eye from pressure in the angle. Too large a posterior chamber lens may cause anterior buckling of the lens with rubbing on the iris. Some surgeons intentionally oversize a posterior chamber plate lens to induce a greater vault in an attempt to avoid contact with the crystalline lens.

Pigment Dispersion

Iris pigment epithelium dispersion can occur acutely during surgery or chronically from contact with the IOL. This occurs more markedly in patients with diabetes. In general, this is of little clinical consequence, and pigment that settles on the IOL gradually disappears, presumably removed by aqueous convection currents or macrophages. If extreme and persistent, however, the pigment could theoretically clog the trabecular meshwork and produce elevated IOP, as occurs with pigment dispersion syndrome in myopes. Myopes with pre-existing pigment dispersion should be considered at greater risk for implantation of a phakic IOL.

Elevated IOP

Acute elevations of IOP can occur postoperatively from leaving too much viscoelastic in the eye. Very high pressure spikes can cause necrosis or ischemia of the sphincter of the pupil, producing a permanently dilated and fixed pupil, with severe consequences of glare and visual distortion. Therefore, viscoelastic must be aspirated thoroughly at the end of the procedure. There is no evidence that a properly designed and placed phakic IOL increases the risk of long-term glaucoma.

Wound Problems and Endophthalmitis

All limbal wounds are subject to similar types of complications: wound leak, cystic blebs, and scarring or gaping with induction of astigmatism, and the like. As wounds become smaller with the protection of an internal corneal valve, these complications become less common, as demonstrated by modern cataract surgery. All intraocular surgery is subject to potential endophthalmitis. The risk for this can be reduced by antibiotic prophylaxis and good surgical technique.

Retinal Detachment and Cystoid Macular Edema

Since the lens-iris diaphragm remains in place, it is unlikely that a retinal detachment or cystoid macular edema will occur after implantation of a phakic IOL. However, once an eye is opened, the pressure and structural dynamics can change, and there may be a small risk of these complications—one that has not yet been statistically demonstrated.

FUTURE TRENDS AND UNFINISHED BUSINESS

Phakic IOLs are in active evolution and represent the new frontier of refractive surgery in the latter 1990s. Improvements in design will be varied, rapid, and creative, just as they were for aphakic IOLs in the 1970s and 1980s. The fact that a well-trained cataract surgeon can implant a phakic IOL without much extra training and that a large capital outlay is not required will make the technology more attractive to surgeons. The exchangeability and removability of the implant will make them attractive to patients, although the requirement for intraocular surgery will create foreboding (see Table 21-3).

REFERENCES

1. Leonard P, Rommel J. *Lens Implantation: 30 Years of Progress*. The Hague: W. Junk; 1982:7-14.
2. *Bull Soc Belge Ophthalmol*. 1982;194:177.
3. Zaldivar R, Davidorf J, Oscherow S. Combined posterior chamber phakic intraocular lens implantation and laser in situ keratomileusis: the bioptics procedure for extreme myopia. *J Refract Surg*. In press.
4. Krumeich JH, Daniel J, Gast R. Closed-system technique for implantation of iris-supported negative-power intraocular lens. *J Refract Surg*. 1996;12:334-340.
5. Landesz M, Worst JGF, Siertsema JV, van Rij G. Correction of high myopia with the Worst claw intraocular lens. *J Refract Surg*. 1995;11:16-25.
6. Mimouni F, Colin J, Koffi V, Bonnet P. Damage to the corneal endothelium from anterior chamber intraocular lenses in phakic eyes. *Refract Corneal Surg*. 1991;7:277-281.
7. Saragoussi JJ, Cotinat J, Renard G, et al. Damage to the corneal endothelium by minus power anterior chamber intraocular lenses. *Refract Corneal Surg*. 1991;7:282-285.
8. Baikoff G, Arne JL, Bokobza Y, et al. Angle-fixated anterior chamber phakic intraocular lens for myopia of -7 to -19 diopters. *J Refract Surg*. 1998;14:282-293.
9. van der Heijde GI. Some optical aspects of implantation of an IOL in a myopic eye. *Eur J Implant Ref Surg*. 1989;1:245-248.
10. Saragoussi JJ, Puech M, Assouline M, Berges O, Renard G, Pouliquen YM. Ultrasound biomicroscopy of Baikoff anterior chamber phakic intraocular lenses. *J Refract Surg*. 1997;13:135-141.
11. Perez-Santonja JJ, Bueno J, Zato MA. Surgical correction of high myopia in phakic eyes with Worst-Fechner myopia intraocular lenses. *J Refract Surg*. 1997;13:268-284.
12. Menezo JL, Avino JA, Cisneros A, Rodriguez-Salvador V, Martinez-Costa R. Iris claw phakic intraocular lens for high myopia. *J Refract Surg*. 1997;13:545-555.
13. Zaldivar R, Davidorf J, Oscherow S. Posterior chamber phakic intraocular lens for myopia of -8 to -19 D. *J Refract Surg*. 1998;14:294-305.
14. Davidorf J, Zaldivar R, Oscherow S. Posterior chamber phakic intraocular lens for hyperopia of +4 to +11 diopters. *J Refract Surg*. 1998;14:306-311.
15. Choyce DP. Residual myopia after radial keratotomy successfully treated Baikoff ZB5M IOLs. [Letter.] *Refract Corneal Surg*. 1993;9:475.
16. Zaldivar R, Davidorf J. Bioptic technique of correcting high myopia with combined phakic intraocular lens and laser in situ keratomileusis. *J Refract Surg*. In press.
17. Harto MA, Menezo JL, Pérez L, Cisneros A. Corrección de la alta miopía con lentes intraoculares (Worst-Fechner) en ojos fáquicos. *Arch Soc Esp Oftalmol*. 1992;62:267-274.
18. Perez-Torregrosa VT, Menezo JL, Harto MA, Maldonado MJ, Cisneros A. Digital system measurement of decentration of Worst-Fechner iris claw myopia intraocular lens. *J Refract Surg*. 1995;11:26-30.
19. Perez-Santonja JJ, Bueno JL, Meza J, García-Sandoval B, Serrano JM, Zato MA. Ischemic optic neuropathy after intraocular lens implantation to correct high myopia in a phakic patient. *J Cataract Refract Surg*. 1993;19:651-654.
20. Perez-Santonja JJ, Iradier M. Chronic subclinical inflammation in phakic eyes with intraocular lenses to correct myopia. *J Cataract Refract Surg*. 1996;22:183-187.
21. Risco JM, Cameron JA. Dislocation of a phakic intraocular lens. *Am J Ophthalmol*. 1994;118:666-667.
22. Ibrahim O, Waring GO. Successful exchange of dislocated phakic intraocular lens. *J Refract Surg*. 1995;11:282-283.

Index

A-CCC, 197
  technique, 193–195
Adatomed silicone implant
  phakic IOLs, 330
adjunctive astigmatic reduction
  techniques
  clear corneal surgery transition,
    56–57
anesthesia
  intraocular
    clear corneal cataract surgery,
      59–68
  phakic IOLs, 359
  regional, 66
  topical
    clear corneal implant surgical
      techniques, 253–254
    clear corneal surgery transition,
      54–56
    corneal surgery, 43–57
angle fixated implants
  phakic IOLs, 335–345
anterior chamber angle fixated
  lenses
  phakic IOLs, 359
anterior chamber phaco technique,
  203
astigmatic keratotomy, 187
astigmatism
  against-the-rule
    high degree, 192
    mild, 187, 192
    moderate, 192
  clear corneal incisions, 21–42
  oblique-axis, 192
  post cataract surgery, 35–42
  reduction techniques
    clear corneal surgery transition,
      56–57
  with-the-rule, 192
astigmatism management
  sub 3.0-mm phaco, 187–192
atonic pupil
  ICLs and bioptic complications,
    312

Baikoff
  phakic IOLs, 351t
Baikoff anterior chamber lens,
  338–341
Baikoff lens ZB, 338–339
Baikoff MA 20
Baikoff multiflex anterior chamber
  phakic IOL, 362–364
Baikoff-Kelman lens, 338
biocompatbility, 151
bioptics procedure

complications, 309–316
  ICLs, 300
  results, 303–309
blades
  clear corneal cataract technique,
    95–97
  clear corneal incision, 132
  clear corneal micro incision
    surgery, 217- 218
  Davison's clear corneal temporal
    incisions, 164–165
  Feaster, 190
  Masket's clear corneal incision,
    127
  sub 3.0-mm phaco, 190
  technologies, 14–19
  Williamson trap, 218
blunt tip cannula, 19
Brown-Grabow forceps, 194
bullous keratopathy
  clear corneal or posterior limbal
    incision complications,
    275–276

capsular opacities
  ICLs and bioptic complications,
    312
capsular polishing
  clear corneal implant surgical
    techniques, 257–258
capsulorrhexis, 135
  incision, 138
  Mackool phaco procedure,
    241–244
  principles, 136
  procedural categories, 135–136
  sub 3.0-mm phaco, 193–195
capsulorrhexis contracture
  Mackool phaco procedure, 243
cartridge injector systems, 44
cataract access
  illustrations, 24–26
cataract extraction
  clear corneal incisions, 29
cataract pseudophakic IOL, 233
cataract removal, 139–149
  hydrodissection, 139–140
  phaco quick chop, 140–144
cataract surgery
  astigmatism adjustment, 35–42
  corneal incisions, 21–23
  corneal surgery, 2
cataracts
  clear corneal micro incision sur-
    gery, 211–238
  Mackool phaco procedure
    dense nuclear, 245–246

  extremely dense (red/black),
    246
  phakic IOL complications, 367
CCC, 193
cell loss
  phakic IOLs, 329
Chan wrist rest, 49
Choo-Choo chop and flip phacoemulsification technique, 71–82
chopping
  vs. pre-grooving four-quadrant
    technique, 197
circular capsulorrhexis
  clear corneal implant surgical
    techniques, 255–256
clear cornea
  clear corneal surgery transition,
    51–54
clear corneal cataract extraction
  ideal patient, 51
clear corneal cataract incisions
  surgeons' survey, 4
clear corneal cataract surgery
  intraocular anesthesia, 59–68
clear corneal cataract technique
  Hunkeler's personal, 95–97
clear corneal implant surgical techniques, 251–261
  complications, 260–261
  operating environment, 252–253
  patient selection, 251
  postoperative regime, 260
  preoperative consideration,
    251–252
  technique steps, 253–259
clear corneal incisions
  approach
    three categories, 131
  astigmatism, 21–42
  cataract extraction, 29
  complications, 263–277
  controversies regarding, 7–18
  corneal shape control rules,
    29–32
  definitions, 23–29
  effects, 32–34
  equipment, 131–133
  individuality, 29
  IOL implantation and cataract
    extraction
    principles, 23
    requirements, 23
  keratometry, 34
  location, 134–135
  Mackool phaco procedure,
    239–241
  Masket's method, 121–130

self-sealing, 8
sutures, 35
technique, 134
three-plane, 38
clear corneal lens surgery, 1–4
clear corneal micro incision surgery
  basic principles, 211–222
  cataract and refractive implants,
    211–238
  implantation technique, 233–238
  universal clear corneal wound,
    1.9-mm, 222–233
clear corneal surgery
  cataract surgery, 2
  temporal
    topical anesthesia transition,
      43–57
  vs. phakic IOLs, 353t
clear corneal temporal incisions
  cataract surgery, 157
clear lensectomy, 281–284
closure, 179
  incision, 153–154
  Mackool phaco procedure,
    249–250
  sub 3.0-mm phaco, 209
conjunctiva, 12
continuous circular capsulorrhexis,
  193
corneal edema
  clear corneal or posterior limbal
    incision complications,
    275–276
corneal incisions, 24
  cataract surgery, 21–23
  deep groove, 85–93
corneal shape control rules, 29–32
corneal shelf, 2
corneal tunnel incisions
  classifications, 8–10
  history, 85–87
cortex removal
  clear corneal implant surgical
    techniques, 257
crowded anterior chamber
  ICLs and bioptic complications,
    311–312
cyclodialysis spatula, 175, 177
cystoid macular edema
  phakic IOL complications,
    368–369

Davison's clear corneal temporal
  incisions, 157–184
decentration
  phakic IOL complications,
    366–367
deep groove corneal incision, 85–93
Descemet's membrane, 13, 17
diamond step knife, 217
dual viscoelastic use
  clear corneal implant surgical
    techniques, 255

elevated IOP
  phakic IOL complications, 368
emmetropia, 29
endophthalmitis
  clear corneal or posterior limbal
    incision complications, 277
  phakic IOL complications, 368
endothelial cell density, 362t
endothelial cell loss
  clear corneal or posterior limbal
    incision complications,
    275–276
  ICLs and bioptic complications,
    317
endothelial damage
  phakic IOL complications, 366
epikeratophakia
  ICLs and bioptic complications,
    316
equipment. See also instruments
  clear corneal incision, 131–133

Feaster blade, 190
Fechner-Worst lens, 335
fibrovascular response, 12
Fine cortical-cleaving hydrodissection, 195
Fine phacoemulsification parameters, 72t, 73t
Fine universal III forceps, 47
Fine-Thornton ring, 13, 71–72
Fine/Nagahara chopper, 73
foldable IOLs, 95
foldables
  clear corneal surgery transition,
    44–46
  instruments, 44
Fyodorov
  phakic IOLs, 351t

Galin lens, 341–345
grooved biplanar clear corneal
  incision, 187

Haefliger cleaver, 197
hinge incision, 85
  components, 86, 87
  physiology, 87
  procedure, 87–89
  surgical procedure, 89–93
Hoffer Q formula, 252
Holladay 1 formula, 252
Hunkeler's clear corneal cataract
  technique, 95–97
hydrodissection
  cataract removal, 139–140
  clear corneal implant surgical
    techniques, 256
  sub 3.0-mm phaco, 195
hyperope, high
  refractive surgery, 281–284

ICLs, 287–320
  bioptics procedure, 300

complications, 309–316
data analysis and results, 302
history, 287–295
implant vaulting, 295
Merocel sponge technique, 295
patient work-up and surgical
  technique, 295–300
safety, 318–320
stability, 320
implant vaulting, 295
implantable contact lens, 287–320
implantation
  sub 3.0-mm phaco, 203–208
incisions
  capsulorrhexis, 138
  clear corneal
    astigmatism, 21–42
    cataract extraction, 29
    complications, 263–277
    controversies regarding, 7–18
    corneal shape control rules,
      29–32
    definitions, 23–29
    effects, 32–34
    equipment, 131–133
    individuality, 29
    IOL implantation and cataract
      extraction principles, 23
    keratometry, 34
    location, 134–135
    Mackool phaco procedure,
      239–241
    self-sealing, 8
    sutures, 35
    technique, 134
  clear corneal approach
    three categories, 131
  clear corneal micro cataract
    surgery, 211–238
  clear corneal or posterior limbal
    complications, 263–277
  clear corneal or posterior limbal
    incision complications
    construction, 266
    quality, 263–265
    size, 265
  clear corneal temporal
    cataract surgery, 157
  closure, 153–154
  corneal
    cataract surgery, 21–23
  corneal tunnel
    classifications, 8–10
    history, 85–87
  enlargement, 178
  hinge, 85–93
  internal corneal valve
    phakic IOLs, 359
  inverted funnel, 243
  limbal
    phakic IOLs, 360
  limbal relaxing, 96–97
  Mackool phaco procedure,
    239–241

Masket's method, 121–130
modified funnel
    Mackool phaco procedure, 241
oblique clear 2.5-mm
    clear corneal implant surgical
        techniques, 254–255
on-axis, 187
paracentesis, 162
posterior limbal
    complications, 263–277
scleral, 24
side stab, 225
size, 32
size and insertion ease, 152–153
step, 86-87
sub 3.0-mm phaco, 185–192
surgeons' survey
    clear corneal cataract, 4
types, 23–29
induced astigmatism, 36
instruments. *See also* equipment
    clear corneal or posterior limbal
        incision complications,
        263–265
    foldables, 44
    Mackool phaco procedure, 239
        capsulorrhexis, 241
        lens surgery, 245
        phakic IOLs, 352–358
internal corneal valve incision
    phakic IOLs, 359
intraocular anesthesia
    clear corneal cataract surgery,
        59–68
intraocular lidocaine
    clinical studies, 60–65
    side effects, 65–66
intraoperative pupillary blocks
    ICLs and bioptic complications,
        310
inverted funnel incision, 243
IOL exchange and removal
    361-362
IOL implantation, 178–179
    corneal incisions, 23
iridocyclitis
    phakic IOL complications, 367
iris claw lens
    phakic IOLs, 360
iris fixated implants
    phakic IOLs, 331–335
iris prolapse
    clear corneal or posterior limbal
        incision complications,
        271–272
iris supported negative power IOL,
    364–365
iris tuck
    phakic IOL complications, 367

keratometry
    clear corneal incisions, 34
keratorefractive techniques, 287
keratotomy, 39
knuckle, 11

Koch chop, 197
Kratz iris plane method, 99, 100

laser delivery systems
    ICLs, 300
laser thermal keratotomy, 39
LASIK surgical technique
    ICLs, 301–302
Lehner II inserter and loader, 48
lens implantation, 150
lens insertion technology, 44
lens surgery
    sub 3.0-mm phaco, 195–203
lens tear
    ICLs and bioptic complications,
        311
lensectomy
    clear, 281–284
lenses
    ICLs and bioptic complications
        flipped, 317
        inadequately sized, 317
lenticular refractive procedures, 287
lidocaine, intraocular
    clinical studies, 60–65
    side effects, 65–66
light source
    non-coaxial, 137–138
limbal incision
    phakic IOLs, 360
limbal relaxing incisions, 96–97
Lindstrom's tilt and tumble
    phacoemulsification, 99–119
LTK, 39

Mackool phaco procedure, 239–250
    capsulorrhexis, 241–244
        instrumentation, 241
        problems, 242–244
        technique, 241
    clear corneal incision, 239–241
        instrumentation, 239
        technique, 239–241
    closure, 249–250
    IOL implantation, 249
    lens surgery, 245–249
        instrumentation, 245
        irrigation/aspiration, 249
        retained nucleus prevention,
            248–249
        technique, 245–248
    modified funnel incision, 241
Mackool/Kelman MicroTip, 72
manufacturers
    phakic IOLs, 351t
Masket's clear corneal incision,
    121–130
    surgical method, 126
mature cataract
    capsulorrhexis problems
        Mackool phaco procedure,
            242–243
Merocel sponge technique, 295
mini-Cobra tip, 197
modified funnel incision

Mackool phaco procedure, 241
modified Langerman, 107f
myopia
    phakic IOLs

Nagahara chopping method, 197
Nichamin II inserter and loader, 47
non-coaxial light source, 137–138

Ocusystem Phaco XL, 226
on-axis incisions, 187
optics
    phakic IOLs, 326–327

paracentesis incision, 162
patient selection
    clear corneal implant surgical
        techniques, 251
peripheral extension
    capsulorrhexis problems
        Mackool phaco procedure, 242
peripheral iridotomy, 361
phaco chop, traditional
    vs. phaco quick chop, 143
phaco needle design, 230
phaco procedure
    Mackool, 239–250
phaco quick chop, 145, 147–148
    cataract removal, 140–144
    vs. traditional phaco chop, 143
phaco technique
    anterior chamber, 203
phacoemulsification, 166
    non-occluded phase, 166–171
    occluded phase, 171–177
    tilt and tumble
        Lindstrom's, 99–119
phacoemulsification technique
    in situ, 197
phakic implantation, 284
phakic IOLs, 325–346, 349–369
    accuracy, 327–328
    calculations, 327
    cell loss, 329
    complications, 366–369
    corrected visual acuity, 328, 366
    definition, 349
    devices and instruments, 352–358
    future trends, 369
    history and development, 350
    ideal qualities, 352t
    IOL comparison, 354t
    optics, 326–327
    preoperative planning, 358–359
    principles, 351–352
    published results, 362–365
    qualitative comparison, 353t
    refractive error treated, 352
    retinal image size, 328
    style development, 351t
    surgical steps and sequences,
        359–362
    terminology and classification,
        349
    types, 329–345

angle fixated implants, 335–345
iris fixated implants, 331–335
posterior chamber implants,
    329–331
vs. corneal surgery, 353t
phakic refractive intraocular lenses,
    325–346, 349–369
pigment dispersion
    phakic IOL complications, 368
pigmentary dispersion
    ICLs and bioptic complications,
    311
pinpoint pressure
    validity, 10
post cataract surgery astigmatism
    adjustment, 35–42
posterior chamber implants
    phakic IOLs, 329–331
posterior chamber plate lenses
    phakic IOLs, 361
posterior corneal lip, 2
posterior limbal incisions
    complications, 263–277
postoperative pupillary blocks
    ICLs and bioptic complications,
    310–311
preoperative procedures
    clear corneal cataract surgery, 67
pterygium, 125
pupil size
    phakic IOLs, 359
pupillary distortion
    phakic IOL complications, 367

quartering technique
    clear corneal implant surgical
    techniques, 256–257

refractive implants
    clear corneal micro incision
    surgery, 211–238
refractive surgery
    high hyperope, 281–284
residual refractive error
    phakic IOL complications, 366
retinal complications
    ICLs and bioptic complications,
    316
retinal detachment
    phakic IOL complications,
    368–369
retinal image size
    phakic IOLs, 328

safety
    ICLs, 318–320
sclera-less corneal tunnel approach,
    85
scleral incision, 24
secondary angle closure glaucoma
    ICLs and bioptic complications,
    312
Seidel test, 130
self-sealing clear corneal incisions, 8
side stab incisions, 225
silicone IOL injection

clear corneal implant surgical
    techniques, 258–259
silicone posterior chamber implant
    phakic IOLs, 330
single-plane incision, 23
Six Steps to Sphericity, 187–192
size
    phakic IOL complications, 368
soft nucleus
    lens surgery technique
        Mackool phaco procedure, 248
spherical eyes, 187
spiral cooling sleeve, 197
SRK/T formula, 252
Staar AA4203 VF, 233
Staar AA4203T, 191
Staar AQ2003 V, 233
Staar AQ2010 V, 233
Staar ICL, 233
    phakic IOLs, 331
Staar Phaco XL, 226
Staar Surgical AA4207VF, 79, 82
Staar toric IOL, 233
step incision, 86–87
Storz Millennium Phaco, 226
stromal hydration, 19, 85, 183
    Masket's clear corneal incision,
    128
Sturm's conoid, 29
sub 3.0-mm phaco, 185–210
    capsulorrhexis, 193–195
    closure, 209
    hydrodissection, 195
    implantation, 203–208
    incision, 185–192
    lens surgery, 195–203
    postoperative routine, 210
superior scleral tunnel cataract
    extraction
    temporal clear corneal surgery
        topical anesthesia transition,
        43–57
Surgical Design Ocusystem IIe
    machine, 197
surgical practice
    clear corneal cataract surgery
        new patterns, 67–68
surgical procedures
    clear corneal cataract surgery, 67
sutureless Weck-cel pressure closure
    clear corneal implant surgical
    techniques, 259
sutures
    clear corneal incisions, 35

temporal clear corneal surgery
    superior scleral tunnel cataract
    extraction
    topical anesthesia transition,
    43–57
temporal surgery
    clear corneal surgery transition,
    46–51
thermal burns
    clear corneal or posterior limbal
    incision complications, 274

ThinOptic thin lens, 341
three-plane incision, 23
tilt and tumble, 99–119
    indications, 102
    key steps, 118–119
    operative procedure, 104–116
    postoperative care, 117
    preoperative preparation,
    102–104
    topical anesthesia
        clear corneal implant surgical
        techniques, 253–254
        clear corneal surgery transition,
        54–56
topical anesthesia transition
    temporal clear corneal surgery
        superior scleral tunnel cataract
        extraction, 43–57
topographical analysis
    clear corneal incisions, 7–8
toric IOLs, 187, 192
traditional phaco chop
    vs. phaco quick chop, 143
trapezoid keratome, 225
trapezoidal corneal tunnel, 85
tunnel perforation
    clear corneal or posterior limbal
    incision complications, 270
two-plane incision, 23, 86, 87

ungrooved uniplanar clear corneal
    incision, 187
universal clear corneal wound
    clear corneal micro incision sur
    gery, 222–233

vision quality, 150

Williamson trap blade, 218
Worst
    phakic IOLs, 351t
Worst claw lens
    phakic IOLs, 331
Worst iris claw, 364–365
Worst iris claw phakic IOL, 356
Worst medallion lens
    phakic IOLs, 331
Worst myopia lens, 335
Worst slot lens
    phakic IOLs, 333
wound closure, 179
wound dehiscence and leakage
    clear corneal or posterior limbal
    incision complications,
    272–274
wound healing
    phakic IOLs, 362
wound stability
    clear corneal or posterior limbal
    incision complications,
    266–269
wound strength
    Williamson classification, 223
wounds
    phakic IOL complications, 368
wrist rest, 49

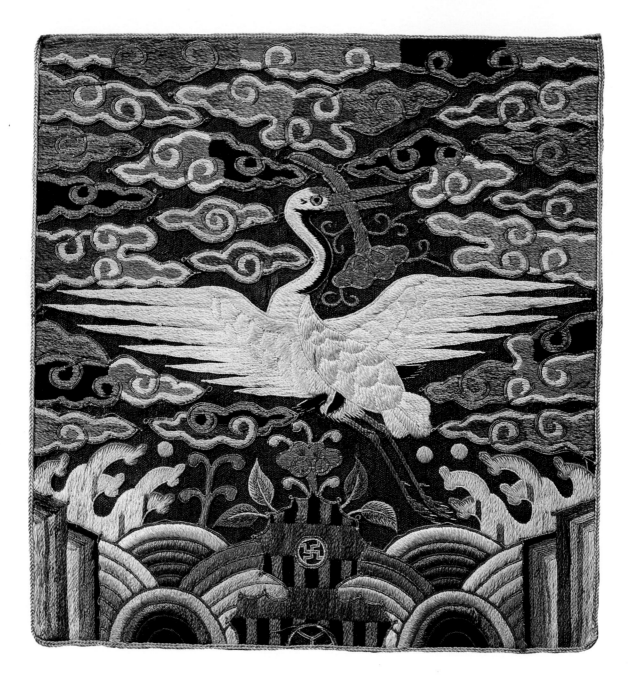

98. Two Pairs of Mandarin Squares *(Hyungbae)*
(detail)

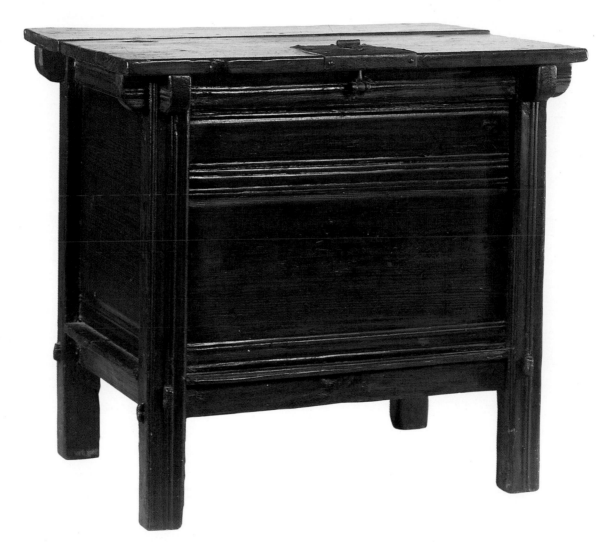

83. Rice Chest *(Ssal tuiju)*

Pine; iron fittings
H. 22″, W. 23⅝″
Yi Dynasty, 19th century
Lent by Dr. John Lyden   TL1986.40.3 a&b

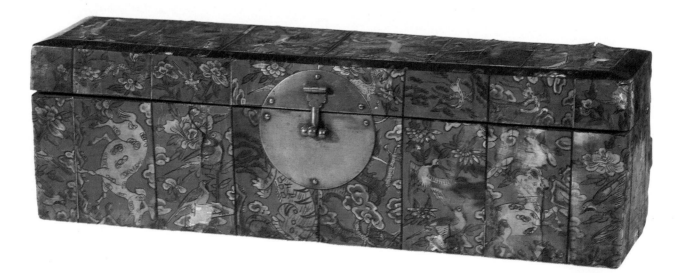

87. Ox-horn *(Hwagak)* **Document Box** *(Soryu Ham)*

Back-painted ox horn, on wood; brass fittings
H. 5⅛", L. 16⅝"
Yi Dynasty, 19th century
Lent by Dr. John Lyden   TL1986.40.2

81. Chest *(Chang)*
Red lacquer inlaid with mother-of-pearl, on wood;
brass fittings
H. 32⅝", W. 30⅜"
Yi Dynasty, late 18th–early 19th century
Lent by Mr. & Mrs. David Drabkin   TL1984.83 a&b

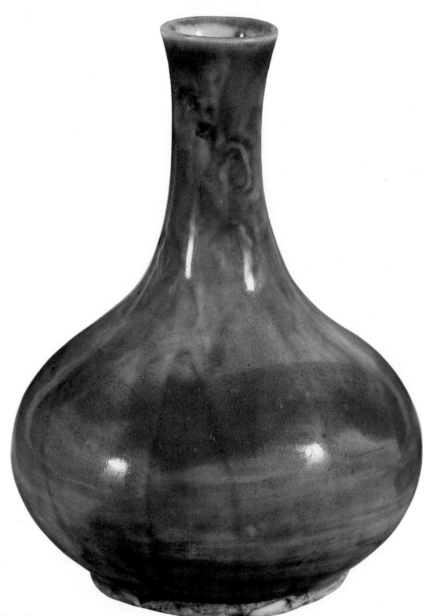

71. Porcelain Wine Bottle

White porcelain brushed with
cobalt under a clear glaze
H. 6″, W. 4¼″
Yi Dynasty, 18th century
Lent by Dr. John Lyden   TL1986.56.1